Understanding YOUR Health

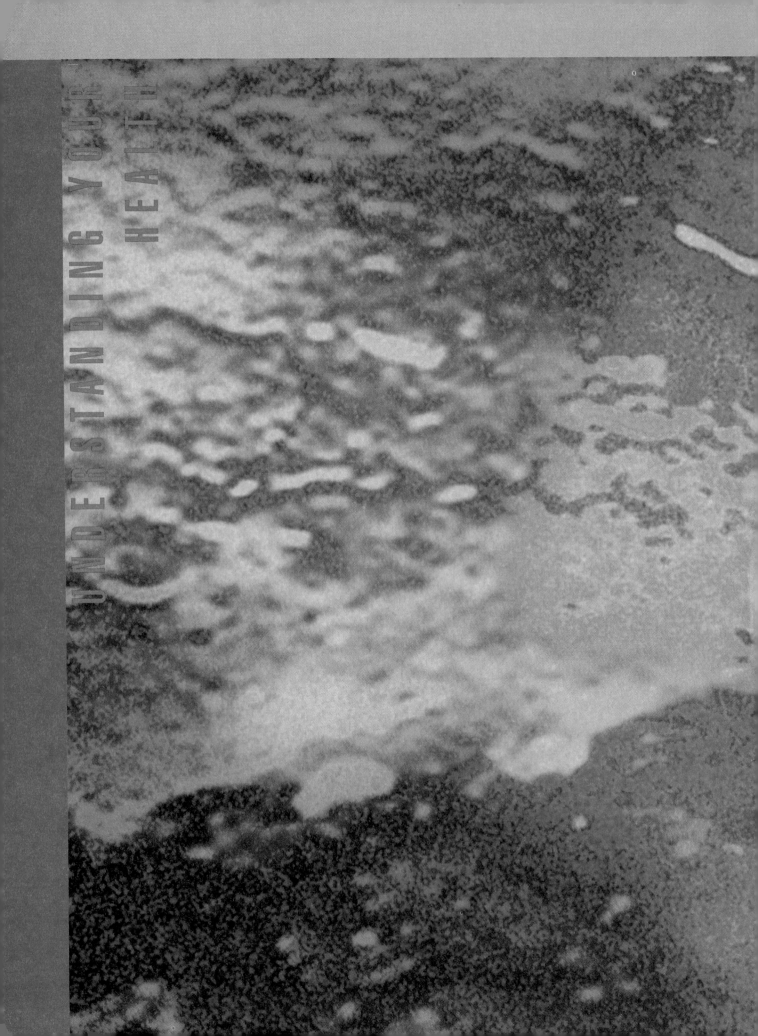

UNDERSTANDING YOUR HEALTH

Understanding YOUR Health

Wayne A. Payne, Ed.D. ▼ **Dale B. Hahn, Ph.D.**

BALL STATE UNIVERSITY, MUNCIE, INDIANA

FOURTH EDITION

Illustrated

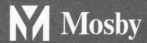 Mosby

St. Louis   Baltimore   Boston   Carlsbad   Chicago   Naples   New York   Philadelphia   Portland
London   Madrid   Mexico City   Singapore   Sydney   Tokyo   Toronto   Wiesbaden

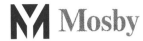

Dedicated to Publishing Excellence

Publisher: James M. Smith
Acquisitions Editor: Vicki Malinee
Sr. Developmental Editor: Michelle Turenne
Project Manager: Linda McKinley
Senior Production Editor: Gail Brower
Designer: Elizabeth Fett
Illustrator: Donald O'Connor Graphic Studios
Cover Design: AKA Design Incorporated

Credits for all materials used by permission appear after the index.

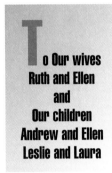

To Our wives
Ruth and Ellen
and
Our children
Andrew and Ellen
Leslie and Laura

Fourth Edition

Copyright © 1995 by Mosby-Year Book, Inc.

Previous editions copyrighted 1986, 1989, 1992

Printed in the United States of America

Composition by Graphic World, Inc.
Color separation by Color Dot Graphics, Inc.
Printing/binding by Von Hoffman Press, Inc.

Mosby-Year Book, Inc.
11830 Westline Industrial Drive
St. Louis, Missouri 63146

International Standard Book Number 0-8151-6716-4

95 96 97 98 99 / 9 8 7 6 5 4 3 2 1

Instructor Preface

As a personal health instructor, you already understand how important health issues are for today's college students. For the media-oriented students of the mid 1990s, however, the messages about health can be confusing. Complementing the personal health course in its potential to expand student knowledge, *Understanding Your Health* helps students clearly see how important health is to their daily lives. This is accomplished with a direct and practical approach to health behavior—an approach that is pedagogically sound and visually stimulating.

Three highly successful editions of this book have paved the way for this comprehensive and exciting fourth edition of *Understanding Your Health*. Students who use this text will be able to examine their lifestyles and attitudes pertaining to health issues and decide how they can modify their behavior to improve their overall health status and perhaps prevent or delay undesirable health conditions.

Approach

Understanding Your Health continues its unique framing of health content around two independent but related focuses: the multiple dimensions of health and the developmental tasks of college students. Only when using this text will students be able to consistently consider health information from the physical, emotional, social, intellectual, and spiritual dimensions. *Understanding Your Health* also clearly and consistently reminds students that their health allows them to achieve personally satisfying lives by helping them master the important developmental tasks that confront them:

▼ Forming an initial adult identity
▼ Assuming responsibility
▼ Establishing independence
▼ Developing social skills
▼ Developing intimacy

Authorship

Understanding Your Health accomplishes this task with a carefully composed, well-documented manuscript written by two health educators who teach the personal health course to nearly 1000 students each year. We understand the teaching issues you face in the classroom on a daily basis and have written this text with your concerns in mind.

We have also been able to maintain the highest level of content integration and consistency of writing style. Reviewers clearly indicate that *Understanding Your Health* is written in a manner that conveys accuracy, clarity, and sensitivity.

Audience

This text is written for both traditional-age college students and nontraditional-age students. We have not ignored the increasing number of nontraditional students who have decided to pursue a college education. Frequently, points within the discussion concern the lives of these nontraditional students. For example, with so many nontraditional students in college in the 1990s, it became increasingly important to add a developmental task specifically for these students. Therefore, the fourth edition of *Understanding Your Health* introduces the developmental task of "developing intimacy" in Chapter 1 and applies it at the completion of each unit. This inclusion helps make the content consistently meaningful for students beyond the traditional college-age years.

New Features In This Edition

The fourth edition of *Understanding Your Health* incorporates several new features that will appeal to your students.

New chapter on violence and safety

Unlike any other time in our nation's history, personal safety issues represent a monumental health issue for today's citizens. To meet the needs of students in this area, *Understanding Your Health* contains a new chapter on violence and safety. Topical coverage consists of intentional injuries (such as homicide, domestic violence, gang violence, bias and hate crimes, rape and assault), campus safety, and unintentional injuries (including residential safety, recreational safety, and automobile safety). New Chapter 19, "Violence and Safety: Coping in Today's Society," enables your students to think more critically about protecting their safety and helps them apply this information through numerous tips and suggestions.

Learning from all cultures

Recognizing the importance of learning information from a multicultural perspective, students are encouraged to view their health within a broader context with the addition of new boxes in every chapter titled "Learning from All Cultures." The information in these boxes allows students to examine health-related topics from the perspectives of others from different racial or ethnic backgrounds and to recognize that the world is filled with many fascinating people whose

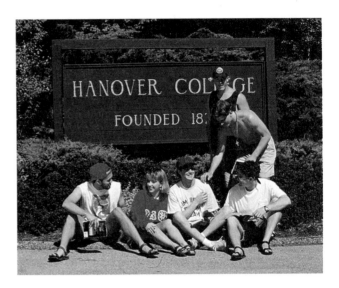

views and approaches to life and health may be different from those with whom they are already familiar.

Real life, real choices

The fourth edition introduces a unique and practical new feature at the beginning of every chapter: applications using real-life situations that engage students in applying the chapter content. Students may recognize family, friends, or even themselves in these scenarios. After reading the content, *Your Turn* questions at the end of the chapter relate back to these situations and ask students what choices they would make and why. This feature provides another "hands on" method that positively affects students' attitudes and behaviors toward health.

Healthy people 2000 objectives

Healthy People 2000 is the government document that outlines 300 health objectives for the nation to achieve by the year 2000. Each chapter in this new edition begins with approximately five objectives that relate to that chapter's content. Awareness of these objectives will enable students to become part of the national push to achieve better health.

Design

We know how important it is to visually "grab" the student's attention. With its dynamic and exciting design, your students will enjoy looking through this text as well as reading it. The fourth edition now includes a double-column format and provides boxed definitions and helpful pronunciation guides for selected terms.

In addition, the artwork is drawn with a three-dimensional appearance that both enhances the learning process and provides a visually appealing presentation.

Photographs have been selected to convey current health issues and to show a wide diversity of people.

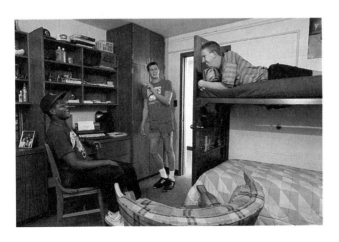

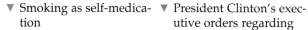

Current issues and topics

In addition to updating information that appeared in the third edition of *Understanding Your Health* (for example, HIV infection and AIDS, cancer, heart disease, drug information, and contraceptives), we have added more than 50 new topics. Some of these topics include:

Chapter 1
▼ The concept of health empowerment
▼ Developing intimacy for midlife adults

Chapter 2
▼ Shyness
▼ Expanded discussion of spiritual development

Chapter 3
▼ Time management and tips for reducing test anxiety
▼ Cultural conflict as a basis for stress
▼ The concept of "hardiness"

Chapter 4
▼ Steroid "stacking"
▼ Static vs. ballistic stretching
▼ Power nap

Chapter 5
▼ Vitamin supplementation and antioxidants
▼ Food technology

Chapter 6
▼ Obesity related health conditions
▼ Life-time control of weight and body composition
▼ FTC restraint against weight loss claims

Chapter 7
▼ Updated data about college students' drug use
▼ Addictive behaviors
▼ Smart drinks and raves
▼ Cocaine-related hospital episodes

Chapter 8
▼ Zero tolerance laws
▼ Binge drinking
▼ Ice beer
▼ New definition of alcoholism
▼ 12-step and secular recovery programs

Chapter 9
▼ Transdermal nicotine patches
▼ Joe Camel

▼ Smoking as self-medication
▼ Chippers

Chapter 10
▼ Women and heart disease
▼ Alcohol and heart disease
▼ Physical inactivity as a risk factor
▼ Excimer laser use on clogged arteries

Chapter 11
▼ PSA test
▼ Breast implants

Chapter 12
▼ HIV in the health care setting
▼ Hantavirus pulmonary syndrome
▼ Pneumonia, mumps, tuberculosis

Chapter 14
▼ Homosexuals in the military

Chapter 15
▼ Depo-Provera injectable progesterone
▼ Updated information on the female condom

▼ President Clinton's executive orders regarding abortion
▼ Updated contraceptive effectiveness chart

Chapter 16
▼ Updated section on pregnancy tests
▼ HIV and breastfeeding caution
▼ Revised success rates for IVF-ET and GIFT

Chapter 17
▼ Animal and human research in drug development

Chapter 18
▼ Off-road vehicle engine pollution
▼ Electromagnetic radiation concerns
▼ Wetlands destruction
▼ Selecting sunglasses

Chapter 20
▼ Hip replacement
▼ The elderly driver

Chapter 21
▼ New generic living will
▼ Updated funeral costs

Successful Features

Along with our new features, *Understanding Your Health* presents a number of existing unique features that enhance student learning:

Two central themes

As mentioned earlier, two central themes (the multiple dimensions of health and the developmental tasks of college students) are woven throughout this text. Each unit of *Understanding Your Health* starts with a one-page discussion of how the five dimensions of health are related to the information in the unit. Each unit ends with a one-page description of how the unit's information may help students achieve their developmental tasks.

Health action guides

These unique boxes provide health behavior strategies or guidelines that students can use to improve their own health habits. These guidelines enliven the text material in every chapter to make the content especially applicable to students.

Flexibility of chapter organization

The fourth edition of *Understanding Your Health* has 21 chapters organized into 7 units. The first chapter stands

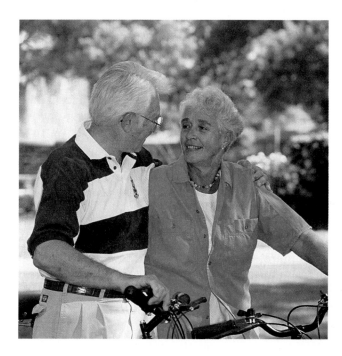

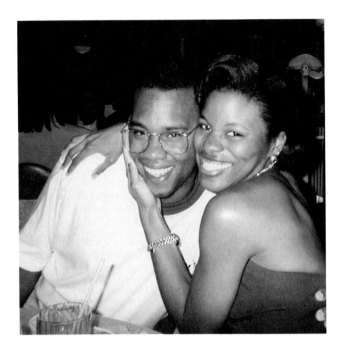

alone as an introductory chapter that explains the focus of the book. This arrangement of the chapters and units follows the recommendations of both the users of earlier editions of *Understanding Your Health* and the reviewers for this edition. Of course, individual professors can choose to arrange the chapters in any order that suits the needs of their own courses.

Health reference guide

This guide lists the most commonly used resources that may have an impact on health. Perforated and laminated, this guide provides information students can keep for later use, such as national hotline phone numbers.

Pedagogical aids

In addition to the new pedagogical features previously discussed, the fourth edition of *Understanding Your Health* incorporates a variety of proven learning aids that enhance student understanding. Each box or feature is easily identified by a particular design element or symbol.

Star boxes. In each chapter special material in "star" boxes encourages the student to delve into a particular topic or to closely examine an important health issue.

Personal assessment inventories. Each chapter contains at least one personal assessment inventory, starting with a comprehensive inventory ("A Personal Profile: Evaluating Your Health") in Chapter 1. These inventories serve three important functions: they capture the attention of the student, they serve as a basis for introspection and behavior change, and they provide suggestions to carry the applications further.

Definition boxes. Key terms important to the student's understanding and application of the material are in boldface type and are defined in corresponding boxes. Pronunciation guides are provided where appropriate.

Other significant terms in the text are in italics for added emphasis. Both approaches facilitate student vocabulary comprehension.

Chapter summaries. To help the student pull the chapter material together, each chapter concludes with a bulleted summary of the key ideas and their significance or application. The student can then return to any part of the chapter for repeated study or clarification as needed.

Review questions. To help the student check for overall understanding, questions are provided after each chapter for review and analysis of the material presented.

Think about this. . . This feature poses questions that encourage students to apply what they have learned in the chapter to determine appropriate solutions.

Your turn. Follow-up questions that correspond with the *Real Life Real Choices* scenarios at the beginning of each chapter ask students to expore how they would resolve the identified problem based on their understanding of the chapter content. These questions also promote classroom discussion.

Documentation. We believe that it is critical both for instructors and for students to be convinced that the material presented in the textbook is scientifically accurate, fully documented, and as up-to-date as possible. *Understanding Your Health* provides this kind of solid documentation by fully referencing the information at the end of each chapter.

Suggested readings. Because some students desire further reading in a particular area of interest or research, *Understanding Your Health* provides an annotated reading list at the end of each chapter. This list is made up of current books that can be readily obtained in bookstores or public libraries.

Appendixes. *Understanding Your Health* includes five appendixes that are valuable resources for the student:

- ▼ **Commonly used over-the-counter products.** Popular categories of over-the-counter drugs are discussed in detail, with recommendations for the consumer of these products.
- ▼ **First aid.** This Appendix outlines first aid procedures to follow for injury situations.
- ▼ **A look at Canadian health.** Statistical information pertinent to the health of Canadians is presented. These statistics include information about a variety of health-related topics.
- ▼ **Mental disorders.** Categories of mental disorders and therapeutic approaches are outlined.
- ▼ **Body systems.** The anatomical systems of the human body have also been prepared with a three-dimensional appearance to highlight more difficult concepts.

Comprehensive glossary. At the end of the text, all terms defined in the boxes, as well as pertinent italicized terms, are merged into a comprehensive glossary. This glossary improves the overall usefulness of the text.

Ancillaries

An extensive ancillary package is available to adopters to enhance the teaching-learning process. We have made a conscious effort to produce supplements that are extraordinary in utility and quality. This package has been carefully planned and developed to assist instructors in deriving the greatest benefit from the text. To that end you will find several unique features within them and a quality that enhances the use of this book. Each of these ancillaries has been thoroughly reviewed by personal health instructors, and we have subsequently refined them to ensure clarity, accuracy, and a strong correlation to the text. We encourage instructors to examine them carefully. Beyond the following brief descriptions, additional information on these helpful packages may be obtained from Mosby.

Instructor's manual and test bank

Prepared by Nancy Geha, Ed.D., the Instructor's Manual features chapter overviews, learning objectives, suggested lecture outlines with recommended notes and activities for teaching each chapter, personal assessments, issues in the news, individual activities, community activities, suggestions for guest lectures, activities for nontraditional students and special populations, current media resources including software, and 65 full-page transparency masters of helpful illustrations and charts. The Test Bank contains multiple choice, true/false, matching, and essay test questions. The manual is perforated and three-hole punched for convenience of use. The Instructor's Manual is also available for use on IBM and Macintosh computers.

Student study guide

For the fourth edition, the Student Study Guide was prepared by James F. McKenzie, Ph.D., M.P.H., and Bonita L. McKenzie, M.Ed., both of Ball State University. With an emphasis on test preparation, the comprehensive manual includes content and vocabulary reviews, self-quizzes, and flashcards to provide students with more self-testing questions. Your students will be better prepared for examinations after working through self-tests and exercises that reinforce content knowledge.

Computerized test bank

This software provides a unique combination of user-friendly aids that enables the instructor to select, edit, delete, or add questions, as well as construct and print tests and answer keys. The Computerized Test Bank package is available to qualified adopters of the text for the IBM and Macintosh microcomputers.

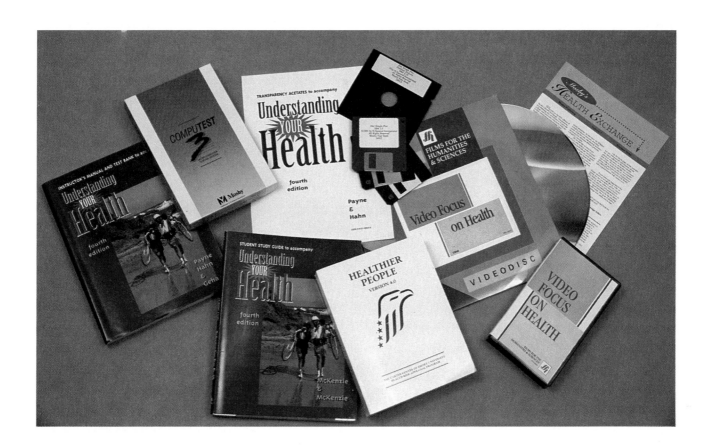

Overhead transparency acetates

Important illustrations and graphics are available as acetate transparencies. Attractively designed in full-color, these useful tools facilitate learning and classroom discussion. They were chosen specifically to help explain difficult concepts. This package is available to qualified adopters of the text.

Mosby's Health Exchange

This new newsletter provides instructors with the latest information concerning "hot" health topics to supplement their Mosby health, fitness, sexuality, drugs, and wellness books. Published twice a year, the newsletter covers numerous health and wellness areas. In addition to being a useful resource for instructors, each edition will include a pullout center section with information designed for student use.

Personal assessment software

For an additional charge, your students can also receive the 26 Personal Assessments from the text on an IBM 3.5 or 5.25 disk; free to adopters.

Videodisc

Approximately 60 minutes in total, this visual presentation enhances classroom discussion with numerous film clips on health issues facing students today. The videodisc is also available in videotape (VHS) format to qualified adopters.

Mosby Diet Simple

This program calculates nutritive analyses of single foods or combinations of foods that may be classified

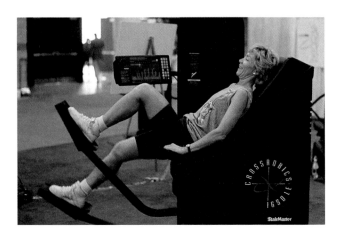

as recipes, meals, menus, or complete diets. Analyses include weight and percent of RDAs according to age and sex for 32 nutrients. The Client Activity Profile portion of the program allows one to calculate energy expenditures, excesses, and deficits. (Available to qualified adopters.)

Healthier People version 4.0 software

This software is a state-of-the-art health risk appraisal program that provides Participant Reports highlighting health risks affecting life expectancy and pinpoints risks an individual can control. (Available to qualified adopters.)

Acknowledgments

REVIEWERS

Our goal throughout this project has been to provide the most accurate, up-to-date, and useful personal health text available. We have constantly called on the expert assistance of many noted colleagues in health research and instruction. Their contributions are present in every chapter of this text. We would like to express our sincere appreciation for their valuable insight and critical and comparative readings.

For the fourth edition

Rosemary C. Clark
*City College of San
  Francisco*

Marianne Frauenknecht
*Western Michigan
  University*

Nancy Geha
*Eastern Kentucky
  University*

Jeffrey S. Hallam
Ohio State University

Dawn Larsen
Mankato State University

Loretta M. Liptak
*Youngstown State
  University*

Bruce M. Ragon
Indiana University

J. Lynn Wolfe
*Georgia Southern
  University*

For the third edition

Charles A. Bish
Slippery Rock University

G. Robert Bowers
*Tallahassee Community
  College*

Donald L. Calitri
*Eastern Kentucky
  University*

Shae L. Donham
*Northeastern Oklahoma
  State University*

P. Tish K. Doyle
University of Calgary

Judy C. Drolet
*Southern Illinois
  University—Carbondale*

Dalen Duitsman
Iowa State University

Mary A. Glascoff
East Carolina University

Sonja S. Glassmeyer
*California Polytechnic State
  University—San Luis
  Obispo*

Health Education Faculty
Cerritos College

Norm Hoffman
Bakersfield College

C. Jessie Jones
University of New Orleans

Jean M. Kirsch
Mankato State University

Duane Knudson
Baylor University

Doris McLittle-Marino
University of Akron

Juli Lawrence Miller
Ohio University

Victor Schramske
*Normandale Community
  College*

Janet M. Sermon
Florida A&M University

Myra Sternlieb
DeAnza College

Mark G. Wilson
University of Georgia

Focus group participants

Danny Ballard
Texas A&M University

Robert C. Barnes
East Carolina University

Jacki Benedik
University of Southwestern Louisiana

Kathie C. Garbe
Youngstown State University

Virginia Peters
University of Central Oklahoma

Les Ramsdell
Eastern Kentucky University

James Robinson III
University of Northern Colorado

Linda Schiller-Moening
North Hennepin Community College

For the second edition

Dan Adame
Emory University

Judith Boone Alexander
Evergreen Valley College

Judy B. Baker
East Carolina University

Robert C. Barnes
East Carolina University

Loren Bensley
Central Michigan University

Ernst Bleichart
Vanier College

Shirley F. B. Carter
Springfield College

Vivien C. Carver
Youngstown State University

Cynthia Chubb
University of Oregon

Janine Cox
University of Kansas

Dick Dalton
Lincoln University

Sharron K. Deny
East Los Angeles College

Emogene Fox
University of Central Arkansas

George Gerrodette
San Diego Mesa College

Ray Johnson
Central Michigan University

James W. Lochner
Weber State College

Linda S. Myers
Slippery Rock University

Virginia Peters
University of Central Oklahoma

James Robinson III
University of Northern Colorado

Merwin S. Roeder
Kearney State College

James H. Rothenberger
University of Minnesota

Ronald E. Sevier
El Camino Community College

Reza Shahrokh
Montclair State College

Albert Simon
University of Southwestern Louisiana

Dennis W. Smith
University of North Carolina—Greensboro

Loretta R. Taylor
Southwestern College

For the first edition

Stephen E. Bohnenblust
Mankato State University

Neil Richard Boyd, Jr.
University of Southern Mississippi

William B. Cissell
East Tennessee State University

Victor A. Corroll
University of Manitoba

Donna Kasari Ellison
*University of Oregon
Umpqua Community College*

Neil E. Gallagher
Towson State University

Susan C. Girratano
California State University—Northridge

Raymond Goldberg
State University of New York College at Cortland

Marsha Hoagland
Modesto Junior College

Carol Ann Holcomb
Kansas State University

Sharon S. Jones
Orange Coast College

Daniel Klein
Northern Illinois University

Susan Cross Lipnickey
Miami University of Ohio

Gerald W. Matheson
University of Wisconsin—La Crosse

Hollis N. Matson
San Francisco State University

David E. Mills
University of Waterloo

Peggy Pederson
Montana State University

Valerie Pinhas
Nassau Community College

Jacy Showers
Formerly of Ohio State University

Parris Watts
University of Missouri—Columbia

Wayne E. Wylie
Texas A&M University

SPECIAL ACKNOWLEDGMENTS

Understanding Your Health could not have been written and published without the assistance of numerous people. Among these are our department colleagues at Ball State University who continue to keep us abreast of new information in areas related to personal health. A special thanks goes to Dr. James F. Comes and his staff at the Ball State Health Science Library.

We wish to acknowledge Richard W. Harris, Director of Disabled Student Development at Ball State University, for his preparation of the discussion of students with disabilities and Elisabeth Boone for her role in developing the *Real Life Real Choices* situations and the accompanying *Your Turn* questions. We appreciate their research and writing contributions to the text.

We also wish to acknowledge the contributions of Bonnie McKenzie. Bonnie played a key role in the development of the new multicultural information boxes. We appreciate her research and writing efforts in this important area.

A note of thanks must also be given to Hanover College, Hanover, Indiana, and to Gary Rice for selected photographs used in this edition of the text.

A variety of dedicated people at Mosby deserve thanks. Among them are Publisher, Jim Smith, for his vision that this book will continue to be a major success; our Acquisitions Editor, Vicki Malinee, whose direction and guidance have been welcomed; and Senior Developmental Editor, Michelle Turenne, whose constant enthusiasm and prodding we have grown to appreciate.

Many people in the production end of this project also deserve recognition. Their expertise and dedication have made *Understanding Your Health* well organized and visually appealing for today's college students. Linda McKinley's leadership as the Project Manager was superb.

Special kudos go out to Gail Brower and Elizabeth Fett. As Senior Production Editor, Gail made certain every manuscript detail was clear and every deadline was met. As our Senior Designer, Elizabeth created an exciting and inviting appearance for this book.

Finally, we would like to thank our families for the continued support and love they have given us. More than anyone else, these people know the energy and dedication it takes to write and revise textbooks. To them we offer our sincere admiration and loving appreciation. Thanks a lot !

Wayne A. Payne
Dale B. Hahn

Student Preface

*W*e're not all the same . . . Because we all have different health needs, *Understanding Your Health* addresses today's relevant health issues to help you make informed decisions that will positively affect your attitudes and behaviors toward your own health. Our goal is to help you improve your overall health, and even to delay and avoid possible adverse conditions, through an exciting and lively presentation.

Features

We have included the following helpful features in *Understanding Your Health*:

▼ **Current Topics.** We address those health issues likely to have the greatest impact on the health of today's college students: from managing test anxiety to your cholesterol intake; from using drugs to passive smoking; and from the latest information on AIDS, contraception, and abortion to suggestions for personal and home safety.

▼ **Personal Assessments.** *Understanding Your Health* includes Personal Assessments that conclude with recommendations to help you apply the chapter content to your own lifestyle.

▼ **Full-color Presentation.** The use of full-color throughout *Understanding Your Health* provides a presentation that is both instructional and visually exciting.

Pedagogy

Understanding Your Health includes tools called *pedagogy* to help you learn. The next pages graphically illustrate how to use these study aids to your advantage.

Ancillaries

▼ **Student Study Guide.** A Student Study Guide is available that includes self-quizzes and flashcards to help you prepare for classroom examinations.

▼ **Mosby Diet Simple.** Your instructor may request that you purchase this software to help you determine your daily nutritional habits.

▼ **Personal Assessment Software.** The 26 Personal Assessment activities from the text are also available on software to help you evaluate your own health behaviors, and determine where improvement is needed.

▼ **Diet Analysis Quick Reference.** This pocket-size quick reference is a handy nutrition evaluation tool which is available free with every *new* purchase of this text.

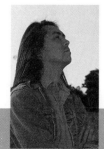
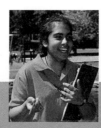
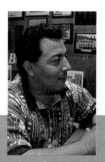

CHAPTER 19

Violence and Safety
Coping in Today's Society

As recently as 15 years ago, the suspicious disappearance of a school-age child or the death of a bystander during a drive-by shooting was virtually unheard of. In the mid-1990s, violent crimes are committed so frequently in the U.S. that they rarely make front page headlines. However, in June of 1994, the brutal deaths of Nicole Brown Simpson (former wife of football Hall of Famer O.J. Simpson) and her friend put one form of violence—domestic violence—back on the front page. Domestic violence directed at women and children seems to be increasing, and many persons fear being a random victim of a homicide, robbery, or carjacking. Law enforcement officials contend that gang activities and hard core drug involvement are major factors that have increased violent behavior in our society.

VIOLENCE AND SAFETY

The following objectives will be covered in this chapter:

▼ Reduce homicides to no more than 7.2 per 100,000 people. (Age-adjusted baseline: 8.5 per 100,000 in 1987; p. 278.)

▼ Reduce physical abuse directed at women by male partners to no more than 1,000 couples (Baseline: 30 per 1000 in 1985; p. 233.)

▼ Reduce assault injuries among people age 12 and older to no more than 10 per 1000 people. (Baseline: 11.1 per 1000 in 1986; p. 233.)

▼ Reverse to less than 25.2 per 1000 children the rising incidence of maltreatment of children younger than age 18. (Baseline: 25.2 per 1000 in 1986; p. 232.)

HEALTHY PEOPLE 2000 OBJECTIVES

Chapter openers feature overviews and objectives.

A new chapter on *Violence and Safety* provides a complete discussion of this crucial topic.

414

UNIT SIX • Consumerism and Environment

Health ACTION Guide

Preventing a Carjacking

In the past 5 years a new form of violence has reached the streets of America. This crime is popularly called carjacking. Unlike auto theft, in which a car thief attempts to steal an unattended parked car, carjacking involves a thief's attempt to steal a car with a driver still behind the wheel.

Most carjacking attempts begin when a car is stopped at an intersection, usually at a traffic light. A carjacker will approach the driver and force him or her to give up the car. Resisting an armed carjacker can be extremely dangerous. Law enforcement officials offer the following tips to prevent carjacking:

▼ Drive only on well-lit and well-traveled streets, if possible.

▼ Always keep your doors locked when driving your car.

▼ Observe traffic for any vehicles that you think that may be following you. If you to locate a police officer or a busy, populated area to seek help.

▼ If someone approaches your car and you cannot safely drive away, roll the window down only slightly and leave the car running and in gear. If the situation turns bad, use your wits and quickly flee the scene, either in the car or on foot. *Remember: your life is worth more than your car.*

▼ If another car taps the rear of your car (a common carjacking maneuver to get you to exit your car) and you feel uncomfortable about getting out of your car, tell the other driver that you are driving to the police station to complete the accident report.

Bias and Hate Crime

One sad aspect of any society is how some segments of the majority treat certain people in the minority. Nowhere is this more violently pronounced than in bias and hate crimes. These crimes are directed at persons or groups of persons solely because of a racial, ethnic, religious, or other difference attributed to the victims. Victims are often verbally and physically attacked, their homes are spray painted with various slurs, and many are forced to move from one neighborhood or community to another.

Typically, the offenders in bias or hate crimes are fringe elements of the larger society who believe that the presence of someone with a racial, ethnic, or religious difference is inherently bad for the community, state, or country. Examples of groups commonly known to commit bias and hate crimes in the U.S. are white supremists, skinheads, and the Ku Klux Klan. Increasingly, state and federal laws have been enacted to make bias and hate crimes serious offenses.

With a small but growing presence of neo-Nazi groups in Europe and clear evidence of so-called ethnic cleansing taking place in Bosnia, Serbia, Croatia and the former Soviet Union, bias and hate crimes are a worldwide problem. It is hoped that the recent push on college campuses to promote multicultural education, as well as the celebration of diversity, will make today's generation of college graduates well aware of the importance of tolerance and inclusion, rather than bigotry and exclusion.

Stalking

In recent years, the crime of stalking has received considerable attention. Stalking refers to an assailant's planned efforts at pursuing an intended victim. Most stalkers are males. (One notable exception is the convicted female stalker of talk show host David Letterman.) Many of these stalkers are possessive or jealous and pursue persons with whom they have had a former relationship. Some stalkers pursue people with whom they have had only an imaginary relationship.

Some stalkers have served time in prison and have waited years to "get back" at their victims. In some cases stalkers go to great lengths to locate their intended victims and frequently know their daily whereabouts. Although not all stalkers plan to batter or kill their victims, their presence and potential for violence are enough to create an extremely frightening environment for the intended victim and her family.

Fortunately, since 1990 virtually all states have enacted or tightened their laws related to stalking and have created stiff penalties for those who do stalk. In many areas, the criminal justice system is proactive in letting possible victims of stalking know, for example, when a particular inmate is going to be released. In other areas, citizens are banding together to provide support and protection for persons who may be victims of stalkers.

If you think you or someone you know is being stalked, contact the police (or local crisis intervention hotline number) to report your case and use their guidance. You can sense that you are a potential stalking victim either through the circumstances of a past relationship, or through the unusual behavior of someone who seems irrationally jealous of you or overly obsessed with you. Report a person who continues to pester you with phone calls, written notes or letters, or unwanted gifts. Report people who make

Health ACTION Guide

Tips to Help You Stick to Your Exercise Program

Sometimes it seems difficult to continue with an exercise program. Here are a few tips to keep you going.

▼ Fit your program into your daily lifestyle
▼ Exercise with your friends
▼ Incorporate music while you're active
▼ Vary your activities frequently; cross-train
▼ Reward yourself when you reach a fitness goal
▼ Avoid a complicated exercise program; keep it simple
▼ Measure your improvement (keep a log or diary)
▼ Take some time off (rest and recuperate)
▼ Keep in mind how important physical activity is to your life

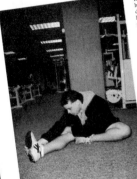

Static stretching.

DEVELOPING A CARDIORESPIRATORY FITNESS PROGRAM

Although the pronounced benefits of exercise clearly exist, we expect that readers of this book fall into some rather distinct categories: (1) those who already exercise regularly, (2) those who exercise occasionally, (3) those who do not exercise, and (4) those who would

like to start some kind of fitness program. A major limitation for readers in all groups is an uncertainty about how best to develop fitness. We ask ourselves, "Am I doing enough to develop my fitness?"; "How can I have fun and develop cardiorespiratory fitness at the same time?"; and "Am I doing things that might be dangerous?"

For persons of all ages, cardiorespiratory conditioning can be achieved through many activities. As long as the activity you choose places sufficient demand on the heart and lungs, improved fitness is possible. In addition to the familiar activities of swimming, running, cycling, and aerobic dance, today many people are participating in brisk walking, roller blading, cross-country skiing, swimnastics, skating, rowing, and even weight training (often combined with some form of aerobic activity). Regardless of age or physical limitations, you can select from a variety of enjoyable activities that will condition the cardiorespiratory system.

Many people think any kind of physical activity will produce cardiorespiratory fitness. Golf, bowling, hunting, fishing, and archery are considered forms of exercise. However, these activities would generally fail to produce positive changes in your cardiorespiratory and overall muscular fitness; they may indeed enhance your health, be enjoyable, and produce some fatigue after lengthy participation, but they do not meet the standards recently established by the American College of Sports Medicine (ACSM), the nation's premier professional organization of exercise physiologists and sport physicians.[5]

The most recent recommendations by the ACSM for achieving cardiorespiratory fitness were approved in 1990 and include five major areas: (a) mode of activity, (b) frequency of training, (c) intensity of training, (d) duration of training, and (e) resistance training. We will summarize these recommendations. Compare your existing fitness program with these standards.

Mode of Activity

The ACSM recommends the mode of activity to be any continuous physical activity that uses large muscle

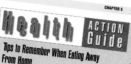

Health Action Guides
provide behavior strategies and guidelines to help you improve your health habits.

Health ACTION Guide

Tips to Remember When Eating Away From Home

Today, more than ever before, people eat more meals away from home. Many of these meals are fast food meals that are characterized by high fat density and excessive use of sweeteners. It is possible, however, to eat nutritionally while eating on the run if you follow these suggestions:

▼ Choose nutritional foods such as salads instead of french fries.
▼ At a salad bar, choose the plain vegetables; avoid mayonnaise-based salads.
▼ Order a plain hamburger without condiments; when you add your own, you control the amounts.
▼ Add lettuce and tomato to hamburgers to add vitamins, not Calories.
▼ Order plain chicken; it has fewer Calories than beef.
▼ Avoid breaded and fried foods.
▼ Choose milk or juice, not sodas or shakes.
▼ For dessert, bring a piece of fresh fruit with you.
▼ Eat a small snack at 10 AM and another at 2 PM. This kind of "grazing" can be healthier than gulping down one big, fat-filled meal at noon. ▼

nutritional benefits.[2] For years excess sugar intake was implicated in a number of major health concerns, including obesity, micronutrient deficiencies, behavioral disorders, dental caries, diabetes mellitus, and cardiovascular disease. However, with the exception of dental caries, current scientific data fail to confirm that sugar per se directly causes any of these health problems. Today, it is recommended that no more than 10% of our total Calories come from sucrose and other sweeteners.

Much of the sugar we consume is hidden—that is, sugar is a principal product we may overlook in a large number of food items. Foods such as ketchup, salad dressings, cured meat products, and canned vegetables and fruits frequently contain much hidden sugar. Corn syrup, frequently found in these items, is a very concentrated sucrose solution.

Polysaccharides are complex carbohydrates that are composed of long chains of glucose units. These long chains are better known as *starches*. They are among the most important sources for dietary carbohydrates. Starches are found primarily in vegetables, fruits, and grains. Consumption of starches helps us receive much overall nutritional benefit, since most starch sources also contain significant portions of vitamins, minerals, protein, and water. Dietary fiber is also a polysaccharide (see p. 103). Starches are nutritional "good guys."

Fats

Fats (lipids, fatty acids) are an important nutrient in our diets. Fats provide a concentrated form of energy (9 Calories per gram consumed versus 4 for carbohydrates and protein) and help give our foods high *satiety* value. The fat in our foods helps to give our foods its pleasing taste, or *palatability*. Fats also serve as carriers of fat-soluble vitamins A, D, E, and K. Without

fat, these vitamins would quickly pass through the body. Body tissues formed in part from fat retain heat.

Dietary sources of fat are often difficult to identify. The visible fats in our diet, such as butter, salad oils, and the layer of fat on some cuts of meat, represent only about 40% of the fat we consume. Most of the fat we eat is "hidden" in food because it is incorporated into the food during preparation or used to fry the food, or it is in food that we have not learned to recognize as being high in fat, such as a candy bar.

When shopping, we often notice that the fat content of some foods is reported in terms of its percentage of the product's weight. In selecting the type of milk we drink, for example, we see that milk ranges from ultralow-fat milk (½%) through low-fat milk (1% to 2%) to whole milk (3% to 4%). Skim milk contains no butter fat. Most consumers do not know, however, how much of the product's Calories are derived from fat. In the accompanying Star Box, an example of how to calculate where Calories in a food are from is provided.

nutrients (noo tree ents) elements in foods that are required for the growth, repair, and regulation of body processes.

Calories (kal oh rees) units of heat (energy); specifically, one Calorie equals the heat required to raise 1 kilogram of water 1° C.

carbohydrates (car bow high drates) chemical compounds comprising sugar (or saccharide) units; the body's primary source of energy.

satiety (suh tie uh tee) a feeling of no longer being hungry; a diminished desire to eat.

Definition boxes
feature helpful pronunciation guides for more difficult terms.

REAL LIFE REAL CHOICES

Self-Acceptance: It Starts With You

▼ Name: Keisha Saunders
▼ Age: 34
▼ University student/single parent

It's a bright, crisp, blue and gold day—the first day of the fall term at the university—and Keisha Saunders has been awake since 5:30 AM, excited and anxious as she prepares to return to school full time after 14 years. She left her bachelor's program in nursing at the end of her sophomore year to get married, and the intervening years have been full of challenges: her husband's death in a construction accident, being a single parent to her two sons while holding down a full-time job, and painstakingly building up her back-to-school fund. Cheerful, energetic, determined, and hard working, she's handled these competing demands with confidence and grace. Now her goal is to complete her bachelor's degree and then go on for a master's so

she can either teach or work as a clinical supervisor.

Keisha ticks off items on her mental list: breakfast dishes done, kittens fed, boys off to school—time to go. She glances in the mirror near the front door, and what had been mild anxiety suddenly turns to doubt and fear. I'm too old, she thinks. I don't have anything in common with these kids—the freshmen are just a few years older than Jamal (her older boy, 13). Should I try to fit in, fade into the woodwork, be the class den mother? Will the other students ignore me, make fun of me, roll their eyes when I talk in class? Will I even be older than some of the instructors? Am I making the biggest mistake of my life?

As you study this chapter, think about the challenges Keisha faces as a nontraditional student returning to school, and prepare yourself to answer the questions in **Your Turn** at the end of the chapter. ▼

Real Life Real Choices boxes
enable you to apply chapter content to real-life situations.

Learning FROM ALL Cultures

Elderly Asian-Americans

The lifestyles of many elderly Asian-Americans clearly reflect the differences between native cultures and traditions and those of their adopted country. The majority of Japanese-American, Filipino-American, and Chinese-American elderly came to America as adolescents or young adults.[2] Many of their children and grandchildren have been completely assimilated into American culture and society. Numerous instances can be found in which grandchildren (and even their parents) are unable to speak their grandparents' native language.

Many cultural traditions related to self-restraint and self-respect (including loyalty to family, respect for authority, and the importance of self-sufficiency) have been retained and reinforced by elderly Asian-Americans among family members and friends. Whether they live in the homes of their children and grandchildren or reside in Chinatowns and Koreatowns of large American cities, in their later years many elderly Asian-Americans retain membership in ethnic support groups and follow religious practices that may no longer appeal to their children. Although limited familiarity with and use of the American language may some... sense of well-being and... many elderly Asian...

For those of...

family members? If you were responsible for the delivery of health or social services to older Asian-Americans, how would you work with the...

Learning from All Cultures boxes
enable you to learn about health issues among different cultures.

Star Boxes highlight additional material to enhance the narrative.

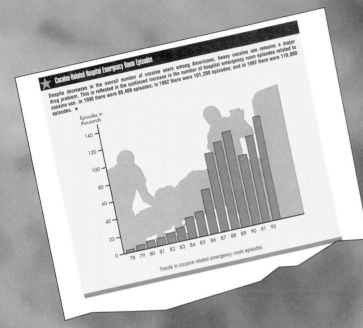

Nutritional information is now required on virtually all food products.

Serving size is set for various food products by the FDA; this is no longer left to the discretion of the manufacturer.

The percentages of Daily Food Value standards are viewed as upper limits and not as goals for diet planning.

Number of Calories from fat is listed on the new label format.

Numerous vitamin and mineral levels no longer need to be listed on the new nutitional label. Only vitamin A, vitamin C, calcium, and iron remain. The interest in or risk of deficiencies of the other vitamins and minerals is deemed too low to merit inclusion.

Ingredients listed in descending order by weight will appear here or in another place on the package.

Nutrition Facts

Serving Size 1/2 cup (114 g)
Serving Per Container 4

Amount per Serving

Calories 260
Calories from fat 120

	% Daily Value*
Total Fat 13 g	20%
Saturated Fat 5 g	25%
Cholesterol 30 mg	10%
Sodium 660 mg	28%
Total Carbohydrate 31 g	11%
Sugars 5 g	
Dietary Fiber 0 g	0%
Protein 5 g	

Figure 5-3 The new food label.

Full-color illustrations provide important visual reinforcement.

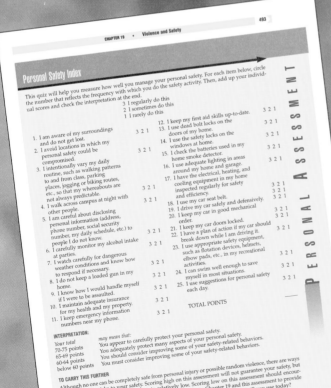

Personal Safety Index

This quiz will help you measure how well you manage your personal safety. For each item below, circle the number that reflects the frequency with which you do the safety activity. Then, add up your individual scores and check the interpretation at the end.

3 I regularly do this
2 I sometimes do this
1 I rarely do this

1. I am aware of my surroundings and do not get lost. 3 2 1
2. I avoid locations in which my personal safety could be compromised.
3. I intentionally vary my daily routine, such as walking patterns to and from class, parking places, jogging or biking routes, etc., so that my whereabouts are not always predictable. 3 2 1
4. I walk across campus at night with other people. 3 2 1
5. I am careful about disclosing personal information (address, phone number, social security number, my daily schedule, etc.) to people I do not know.
6. I carefully monitor my alcohol intake at parties. 3 2 1
7. I watch carefully for dangerous weather conditions and know how to respond if necessary. 3 2 1
8. I do not keep a loaded gun in my home. 3 2 1
9. I know how I would handle myself if I were to be assaulted. 3 2 1
10. I maintain adequate insurance for my health and my property. 3 2 1
11. I keep emergency information numbers near my phone. 3 2 1
12. I keep my first aid skills up-to-date. 3 2 1
13. I use dead bolt locks on the doors of my home. 3 2 1
14. I use the safety locks on the windows at home. 3 2 1
15. I check the batteries used in my home smoke detector. 3 2 1
16. I use adequate lighting in areas around my home and garage.
17. I have the electrical, heating, and cooling equipment in my home inspected regularly for safety and efficiency. 3 2 1
18. I use my car seat belt. 3 2 1
19. I drive my car safely and defensively. 3 2 1
20. I keep my car in good mechanical order.
21. I keep my car doors locked. 3 2 1
22. I have a plan of action if my car should break down while I am driving it. 3 2 1
23. I use appropriate safety equipment, such as flotation devices, helmets, elbow pads, etc., in my recreational activities.
24. I can swim well enough to save myself in most situations. 3 2 1
25. I use suggestions for personal safety each day. 3 2 1

TOTAL POINTS _____

INTERPRETATION:

Your total	may mean that:
70-75 points	You appear to carefully protect your personal safety.
65-69 points	You adequately protect many aspects of your personal safety.
60-64 points	You should consider improving some of your safety-related behaviors.
below 60 points	You must consider improving some of your safety-related behaviors.

TO CARRY THIS FURTHER

Although no one can be completely safe from personal injury or possible random violence, there are ways to minimize the risks to your safety. Scoring high on this assessment will not guarantee your safety, but your likelihood for injury should remain relatively low. Scoring low on this and this assessment should encourage you to consider ways to make your life more safe. Refer to Chapter 19 and this assessment to provide you with useful suggestions to enhance your personal safety. Which safety tips will you use today?

P E R S O N A L   A S S E S S M E N T

Personal Assessment boxes invite you to evaluate aspects of your own health.

Contents in Brief

1 Health: Support for Your Future, 1

UNIT ONE **Establishing a Foundation for the Years Ahead**

2 Achieving Emotional Maturity: Keys to Your Mental Health, 24
3 Stress: Managing the Unexpected, 42

UNIT TWO **The Body: Your Vehicle for Health**

4 Physical Fitness: Enhancing Work, Study, and Play, 64
5 Nutrition: The Role of Diet in Your Health, 90
6 Weight Management: Sensible Eating and Regular Exercise, 126

UNIT THREE **Products of Dependence: A Focus for Responsible Use**

7 Psychoactive Drugs: Use, Misuse, and Abuse, 160
8 Alcohol: Responsible Choices, 188
9 Tobacco Use: A Losing Choice, 214

UNIT FOUR **Diseases: Obstacles to a Healthy Life**

10 Cardiovascular Disease: Turning the Corner, 244
11 Cancer and Chronic Conditions, 268
12 Infectious Diseases: A Shared Concern, 294

UNIT FIVE Sexuality: The Person, the Partner, the Parent

13 Sexuality: Biological and Psychosocial Origins, 326
14 Sexuality: A Variety of Behaviors and Relationships, 344
15 Fertility Control: Responsible Choices for Your Future, 368
16 Sexuality: Pregnancy and Childbirth, 394

UNIT SIX Consumerism and Environment: Outside Forces Shaping Your Health

17 Consumerism and Health Care: Making Sound Decisions, 418
18 Environment: Influences From the World Around Us, 446
19 Violence and Safety: Coping in Today's Society, 476

UNIT SEVEN Growing Older: Balancing Your Future With Your Past

20 The Maturing Adult: Moving Through Transitions, 500
21 Dying and Death: The Last Transitions, 524

APPENDIXES, A-1

GLOSSARY, G-1

INDEX, I-1

CREDITS, C-1

Contents in Detail

1 Health: Support for Your Future, 1

Health Concerns of the 1990s, 2
Definitions of Health-Related Terms, 2
  A Traditional Definition of Health, 2
  Holistic Health, 3
  Health Promotion, 3
  Wellness, 4
  Empowerment, 4
  Health Objectives for the Year 2000, 5
Today's Traditional College Student, 5
Today's Nontraditional College Student, 6
Minority Students, 6
Students with Disabilities, 6
  Comfortable Language, 7
  Americans with Disabilities Act, 8
Developmental Tasks of the Young Adult
  Period, 8
  Forming an Initial Adult Identity, 8
  Establishing Independence, 8
  Assuming Responsibility, 8
  Developing Social Skills, 9
  Developing Intimacy, 10
The Role of Health, 10
The Composition of Health, 10
  Physical Dimension of Health, 11
  Emotional Dimension of Health, 11
  Social Dimension of Health, 11
  Intellectual Dimension of Health, 12
  Spiritual Dimension of Health, 12
Health: Our Definition, 12
Focus of This Textbook, 12

Personal Assessment: A Personal Profile:
  Evaluating Your Health, 13
Summary, 20

UNIT ONE — The Mind: The Foundation for the Years Ahead

2 Achieving Emotional Maturity: Keys to Your Mental Health, 24

Characteristics of an Emotionally or Mentally
  Healthy Person, 26
Emotional and Psychological Health, 26
Personality, 27
The Normal Range of Emotions, 27
  Happiness and a Sense of Humor, 28
  Self-Esteem, 28

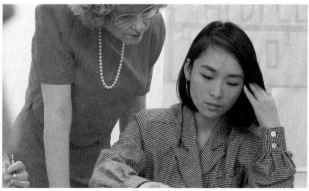

Personal Assessment: How Does My Self-Concept Compare With My Self-Ideal? 29
Depression, 30
Seasonal Affective Disorder (SAD) Syndrome, 31
Suicide, 31
Loneliness, 32
Shyness, 33
Developing Communication Skills, 33
Verbal Communication, 34
Nonverbal Communication, 34
Maslow's Hierarchy of Needs, 34
Creative Expression, 36
Spiritual/Faith Development, 36
A Plan for Enhancing Your Mental and Emotional Health, 37
Constructing Mental Pictures, 37
Accepting Mental Pictures, 37
Undertaking New Experiences, 38
Reframing Mental Pictures, 38
Emotional (or Mental) Health: A Final Thought, 39
Summary, 40

3 Stress: Managing the Unexpected, 42
Stress and Stressors, 44
Variation in Response to Stressors, 44
Generalized Physiological Response to Stressors, 45
Stressors, 45
Sensory Modalities, 45
Cerebral Cortex, 45
The Endocrine System, 45
Epinephrine, 47
Energy Release, 47
General Adaptation Syndrome, 48
Alarm Reaction Stage, 48
Resistance Stage, 48
Exhaustion Stage, 48
Intensity of Stressor, 48
Positive or Negative Stressors, 48
Inevitability of Stress, 49
Uncontrolled Stress Related to Disease States, 49
College-Centered Stressors, 49
Employment Expectations, 49
Institutional Expectations, 49
Personal Assessment: Life Stressors, 50
Financial Support, 51
Personal Expectations, 51
Family Expectations, 51
Personal Assessment: How Vulnerable Are You to Stress? 52
Time Management, 53
Cultural Conflicts, 53

Religious Faith, 53
Faculty Expectations, 54
Life-Centered Stressors, 54
Coping: Reacting to Stressors, 55
Stress Management Techniques, 56
Personality Traits, 57
A Realistic Perspective on Stress and Life, 57
Summary, 58

U N I T T W O   The Body: Your Vehicle for Health

4 Physical Fitness: Enhancing Work, Study, and Play, 64
Common Attitudes Toward Physical Fitness, 66
Components of Physical Fitness, 67
Cardiorespiratory Endurance, 67
Muscular Strength, 68
Muscular Endurance, 70
Flexibility, 70
Body Composition, 71
Developing a Cardiorespiratory Fitness Program, 72
Mode of Activity, 72
Frequency of Training, 73
Intensity of Training, 73
Personal Assessment: What Is Your Level of Fitness? 74
Duration of Training, 76
Resistance Training, 76
Warm-up Workout, Cool-down, 77
Exercise for Older Adults, 77

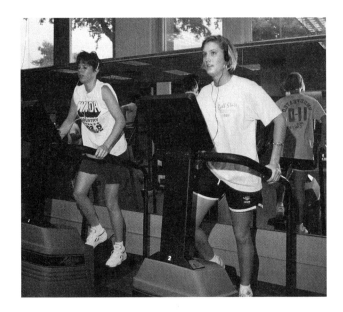

Fitness Questions and Answers, 78
  Should I See My Doctor Before I Get
    Started? 78
  What About Jumping Rope? 78
  How Important is Breast Support for
    Female Exercisers? 79
  How Beneficial is Aerobic Exercise? 79
  What are Low-Impact Aerobic
    Activities? 82
  What Is the Most Effective Fluid
    Replacement During Exercise? 82
  Why Has Bodybuilding Become So
    Popular? 82
  Can Strength Training Improve Heart
    Functioning? 82
  Where Can I Find Out About Proper
    Equipment? 82
  How Worthwhile Are Commercial Health
    and Fitness Clubs? 82
  What is Crosstraining? 83
  What are Steroids and Why Do Some
    Athletes Use Them? 83
  What Are the Two Types of Muscle Fibers
    and How Can They Affect Exercise
    Performance? 85
  Are Today's Children Physically Fit? 85
  How can Sleep Contribute to Overall
    Fitness? 85
  What Exercise Danger Signs Should I
    Watch For? 87
  What Causes Low Back Pain? 87
Summary, 87

5 Nutrition: The Role of Diet in Your Health, 90
Types and Sources of Nutrients, 92
  Carbohydrates, 92
  Fats, 93
  Tropical Oils, 95
  Proteins, 96
  Vitamins, 97
  Minerals, 100
  Water, 100
  Fiber, 103
The Food Groups, 104
  Fruits, 105
  Vegetables, 105
  Milk, Cheese, and Yogurt, 107
  Meat, Poultry, Fish, and Eggs, 107
  Breads, Cereals, Rice, and Pasta, 108
  Fats, Oils, and Sweets, 108
Fast Foods, 109
Food Exchange System, 109
Food Additives, 109

Food Labels, 111
Guidelines for Dietary Health, 113
Nontraditional Dietary Practices, 114
  Vegetarian Diets, 114
  High-Risk Dietary Practices, 117
Recommended Dietary Adjustments, 117
  Additional Milk Consumption, 117
  Additional Protein-Rich Sources, 117
  Personal Assessment: Seven-Day Diet
    Study, 118
  Additional Vitamins C and A, 120
  Additional Grain Product
    Consumption, 120
  Moderate Alcohol Consumption, 121
  Nutrient Density, 121
Nutrition and the Older Adult, 121
International Nutritional Concerns, 121
Food Technology, 122
Summary, 123

6 Healthy Weight: Sensible Eating and Regular Exercise, 126
Concern Over Body Image, 128
Overweight and Obesity Defined, 128
Determining Weight and Body
  Composition, 130
  Healthy Body Weight, 130
Body Image, 132
Origins of Obesity, 134
  Genetic Basis for Obesity, 134
  Appetite Center, 134
  Set Point Theory, 135
  Infant and Adult Feeding Patterns, 136
  Externality, 136
  Endocrine Influence, 136
  Pregnancy, 136
  Decreasing Basal Metabolism Rate, 137
  Family Dietary Practices, 137
  Inactivity, 137
Caloric Balance, 137
  Weight Loss, 137
  Weight Gain, 138
Energy Needs of the Body, 138
  Activity Requirements, 138
  Basal Metabolism, 139
  Dietary Thermogenesis, 141
  Life-Time Weight Control, 141
Weight Management Techniques, 141
  Personal Assessment: Should You Consider
    a Weight Loss Program? 142
  Dietary Alterations, 143
  Physical Intervention, 144
  Behavior Change Strategies, 147
  A Combination Approach, 149

The Weight Loss Industry, *150*
Eating Disorders, *150*
   Anorexia Nervosa, *150*
   Bulimia Nervosa, *151*
   Treatment for Eating Disorders, *152*
Undernutrition, *152*
Summary, *154*

UNIT THREE — Products of Dependence: A Focus on Responsible Use

7   Psychoactive Drugs: Use, Misuse, and Abuse, 160
Addictive Behavior, *163*
   The Process of Addiction, *163*
   Intervention and Treatment, *164*
Drug Terminology, *164*
   Dependence, *164*
   Drug Misuse and Abuse, *165*
The Dynamics of the Addictive
      Personality, *165*
   Influence of Individual Factors, *165*
   Influences of the Immediate
      Environment, *167*
   Influences within the Larger Society, *168*
Drug Impact on the Central Nervous
      System, *169*
Drug Classifications, *169*

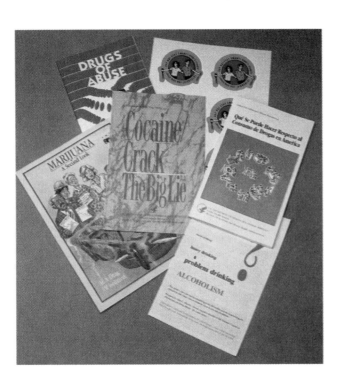

Stimulants, *169*
Cocaine, *173*
Personal Assessment: Do You Recognize
   Drug Abuse? *176*
Depressants, *177*
Hallucinogens, *177*
Cannabis, *179*
Narcotics, *180*
Inhalants, *181*
Combination Drug Effects, *181*
Society's Response to Drug Use, *181*
   Drug Testing, *182*
College and Community Support Services for
      Drug Dependence, *184*
   Treatment, *184*
   Costs of Treatment for Dependence, *184*
Personal Assessment: Nonchemical High
   Challenge, *185*
Summary, *186*

8   Alcohol: Responsible Choices, 188
Choosing to Drink, *190*
Alcohol Use Patterns, *190*
   Binge Drinking, *192*
   Uneven Distribution of Drinkers, *193*
The Nature of Alcohol Beverages, *194*
   Factors Related to the Absorption of
      Alcohol, *196*
   Blood Alcohol Concentration, *197*
   Sobering Up, *198*
   First Aid for Acute Alcohol
      Intoxication, *198*
Personal Assessment: How Do You Use
   Alcohol Beverages? *199*
Alcohol-Related Health Problems, *200*
   Fetal Alcohol Syndrome and Fetal Alcohol
      Effect, *200*
Alcohol-Related Social Problems, *202*
   Accidents, *202*
   Crime and Violence, *202*
   Suicide, *202*
Hosting a Responsible Party, *203*
Organizations Supporting Responsible
      Drinking, *203*
   Mothers Against Drunk Drivers, *203*
   Students Against Driving Drunk, *203*
   Boost Alcohol Consciousness Concerning
      the Health of University Students, *203*
   Other Approaches, *204*
Problem Drinking and Alcoholism, *204*
   Problem Drinking, *204*
   Alcohol and Driving, *204*
   Alcoholism, *206*
   Denial and Enabling, *206*

Codependence, 207
Adult Children of Alcoholics, 207
Alcoholism and the Family, 208
Helping the Alcoholic: Rehabilitation and
Recovery, 208
Twelve-Step Programs, 210
Secular Recovery Programs, 210
Women and Alcohol, 211
Alcohol Advertising, 211
Summary, 212

9 Tobacco Use: A Losing Choice, 214

Tobacco Use in American Society, 216
Use Among Adolescents, 216
The Influence of Education, 216
Personal Preferences, 217
Advertising Approaches, 217
Pipe and Cigar Smoking, 218
Tobacco Use and the Development of
Dependence, 219
Physiological Factors Related to
Dependence, 219
Personal Assessment: Test Your Knowledge
About Cigarette Smoking, 222
Psychosocial Factors Related to
Dependence, 224
Tobacco: The Source of Physiologically Active
Compounds, 225
Nicotine, 225
Carbon Monoxide, 225
Illness, Premature Death, and Tobacco
Use, 226
Cardiovascular Disease and Tobacco Use, 226
Nicotine and Cardiovascular Disease, 226
Carbon Monoxide and Cardiovascular
Disease, 226
Cancer Development and Tobacco Use, 227
Chronic Obstructive Lung Disease and
Tobacco Use, 229
Additional Health Concerns, 230
Tobacco and Caffeine Use, 230
Infertility, 230
Problem Pregnancy, 230
Breastfeeding, 231
Neonatal Health Problems, 231
Oral Contraceptives and Tobacco Use, 231
Smokeless Tobacco Use, 231
Chewing Tobacco and Snuff, 231
Involuntary (Passive) Smoking, 232
Stopping What You Started, 234
Tobacco Use: A Question of Rights, 235
Enhancing Communication Between Smokers
and Nonsmokers, 236
Summary, 237

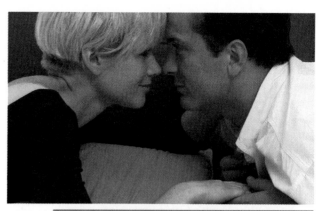

U N I T   FOUR   Diseases: Obstacles to a Health Lifestyle

10 Cardiovascular Disease: Turning the Corner, 244

Pervasiveness of Cardiovascular Disease, 246
Who Are the Potential Victims of
Cardiovascular Disease? 246
The Costs, 247
Normal Cardiovascular Function, 247
The Vascular System, 247
The Heart, 248
Heart Stimulation, 249
Blood, 249
Requirements for Overall Cardiovascular
Health, 250
Forms of Cardiovascular Disease, 250
Coronary Heart Disease, 251
Hypertension, 257
Stroke, 258
Congenital Heart Disease, 260
Rheumatic Heart Disease, 260
Related Cardiovascular Conditions, 261
Peripheral Artery Disease, 261
Congestive Heart Failure, 261
Cardiovascular Risk Factors, 261
Risk Factors for Coronary Artery Disease,
Hypertension, and Stroke, 262
Risk Factors for Congenital Heart Disease
and Rheumatic Heart Disease, 262
Personal Assessment: Take a Test for Heart
Disease, 265
Summary, 266

11 Cancer and Chronic Conditions, 268

Chronic Health Concerns, 270
Cancer: A Problem of Cell Regulation, 270
Cancer at Selected Sites in the Body, 274
Lung, 274
Breast, 274
Uterus, 276

Vagina, *278*
Prostate, *279*
Testicle, *280*
Colon and Rectum, *280*
Pancreas, *281*
Skin, *281*
The Diagnosis of Cancer, *282*
Treatment, *283*
Personal Assessment: Are You at Risk for
Skin, Breast, and Cervical Cancer? *284*
Environmental Risk for Developing Cancer
and Risk Reduction, *287*
Other Health Conditions, *288*
Diabetes Mellitus, *288*
Multiple Sclerosis, *290*
Asthma, *291*
Summary, *291*

**12 Infectious Diseases: A Shared
Concern, 294**
Infectious Diseases in the 1990s, *296*
Infectious Disease Transmission, *296*
Pathogens, *296*
Chain of Infection, *297*
Stages of Infection, *299*
Body Defenses: Mechanical and Cellular
Immune Systems, *299*
Divisions of the Immune System, *300*
Immunizations, *300*
Causes and Management of Selected
Infectious Diseases, *303*
The Common Cold, *303*
Influenza, *304*
Tuberculosis, *305*
Pneumonia, *306*
Mononucleosis, *306*
Chronic Fatigue Syndrome (CFS), *307*
Measles, *307*
Mumps, *307*
Lyme Disease, *308*
Hantavirus Pulmonary Syndrome, *308*
Toxic Shock Syndrome, *309*
Hepatitis, *310*
Acquired Immune Deficiency Syndrome
(AIDS), *310*
Sexually Transmitted Diseases, *314*
Chlamydia (Nonspecific Urethritis), *314*
Human Papillomavirus (HPV), *315*
Herpes Simplex Infections, *315*
Personal Assessment: What Is Your Risk of
Contracting a Sexually Transmitted
Disease? *316*
Syphilis, *318*
Pubic Lice, *318*
Vaginal Infections, *318*
Cystitis and Urethritis, *319*
Summary, *320*

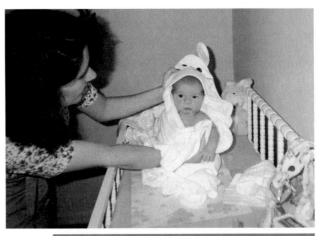

UNIT   **Sexuality: The Person, the Partner, the**
FIVE   **Parent**

**13 Sexuality: Biological and Psychosocial
Origins, 326**
The Biological Bases of Human Sexuality, *328*
Genetic Basis, *328*
Gonadal Basis, *328*
Structural Development, *328*
Biological Sexuality and the Childhood
Years, *328*
Puberty, *329*
The Psychosocial Bases of Human
Sexuality, *329*
Gender Identity, *330*
Gender Preference, *330*
Gender Adoption, *330*
Initial Adult Gender Identification, *331*
Androgyny: Sharing the Pluses, *331*
The Reproductive System, *332*
The Male Reproductive System, *332*
The Female Reproductive System, *334*
The Menstrual Cycle, *336*
Additional Aspects of Human Sexuality, *339*
Reproductive Sexuality, *339*
Genital Sexuality, *339*
Personal Assessment: Sexual Attitudes: A
Matter of Feelings, *340*
Expressionistic Sexuality, *341*
Summary, *342*

**14 Sexuality: A Variety of Behaviors and
Relationships, 344**
The Human Sexual Response Pattern, *346*
Question 1—A Predictable Response
Pattern, *347*
Question 2—Stimulus Specificity, *347*
Question 3A—Male Versus Female
Response Pattern, *347*

Question 3B—Variation: Within a Same-Sex
Group, 347
Question 3C—Variation: Within the Same
Individual, 347
Question 4—Physiological Mechanisms
Underlying the Sexual Response
Pattern, 350
Question 5—Role of Specific Organs in the
Sexual Response Pattern, 350
Patterns of Sexual Behavior, 350
Celibacy, 350
Masturbation, 350
Fantasy and Erotic Dreams, 350
Shared Touching, 350
Genital Contact, 350
Oral-Genital Stimulation, 351
Intercourse, 353
Three-Stage Dating—Mate Selection
Model, 353
Stage 1—the Marketing Stage, 353
Stage 2—the Sharing Stage, 354
Stage 3—the Behavior Stage, 354
Love, 354
Personal Assessment: How Compatible Are
You? 355
Friendship, 356
Intimacy, 356
Marriage, 357
Forms of Marriage, 357
Conflict-Habituated Marriage, 357
Devitalized Marriage, 357
Passive-Congenial Marriage, 358
Total Marriage, 359
Vital Marriage, 359
Alternatives to Marriage, 359
Divorce, 359
Singlehood, 360
Personal Assessment: If You Are Single, 361
Cohabitation, 362
Single Parenthood, 362
Sexual Orientation and Variant Sexual
Behaviors, 362
Homosexuality, 362
Bisexuality, 363
Transsexualism, 363
Variant Sexual Behaviors, 364
Commercialization of Sex, 364
Summary, 365

**15 Fertility Control: Responsible Choices for
Your Future, 368**
Birth Control Versus Contraception, 370
Reasons for Choosing to Use Birth
Control, 371
Personal Assessment: Developing Your
Personal Life Plan, 372

Theoretical Effectiveness Versus Use
Effectiveness, 373
Selecting Your Contraceptive Method, 373
Current Birth Control Methods, 373
Withdrawal, 373
Periodic Abstinence, 373
Vaginal Spermicides, 377
Condom, 378
Diaphragm, 380
Cervical Cap, 381
Contraceptive Sponge, 381
Intrauterine Device, 382
Oral Contraceptives, 382
Subdermal Implants, 384
Sterilization, 385
Abortion, 386
Personal Assessment: Which Birth Control
Method Is Best for You? 388
Summary, 391

16 Sexuality: Pregnancy and Childbirth, 394
Becoming Parents, 396
Parenting Issues for Couples, 396
Pregnancy: An Extension of the
Partnership, 397
Physiological Obstacles and Aids to
Fertilization, 397
Personal Assessment: How Do You Feel
About Parenting? 398
Pregnancy Determination, 399
Signs of Pregnancy, 400
Fetal Life, 400
Multiple Births, 401
Agents That Can Damage a Fetus, 401
Childbirth: The Labor of Delivery, 402
Determination of the Due Date, 402
Childbirth, 402
Additional Considerations Concerning
Childbirth, 406
Medications, 406
Cesarean Deliveries, 406
Breast-feeding, 406
Preparation for Birth, 406
Birth Technology, 408
Infertility, 408
A Parenting Prescription for the Early
Years, 411
Summary, 412

**UNIT SIX Consumerism and Environment: Outside
Forces Shaping Your Health**

**17 Consumerism and Health Care: Making
Sound Decisions, 418**
Health-Related Information, 420

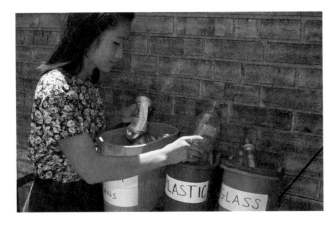

The Informed Consumer, *420*
Sources of Information, *420*
Family and Friends, *421*
Advertisements and Commercials, *421*
Labels and Directions, *421*
Folklore, *422*
Testimonials, *422*
Mass Media Exposure, *422*
Practitioners, *424*
Health Reference Publications, *424*
Reference Libraries, *424*
Consumer Advocacy Groups, *424*
Voluntary Health Agencies, *424*
Government Agencies, *424*
Qualified Health Educators, *425*
Health Care Providers, *425*
Why We Consult Health Care
Providers, *425*
Physicians and Their Training, *426*
Nonallopathic Practitioners, *427*
Restricted Practice Health Care
Providers, *427*
Nurse Professionals, *429*
Allied Health Care Professionals, *430*
Self-Care, *430*
Health Care Facilities, *431*
Patients' Institutional Rights, *432*
Health-Care Costs and Reimbursement, *432*
Health Insurance, *433*
Health Maintenance Organizations, *434*
Government Insurance Plans, *435*
National Health Care: A Solution? *436*
Health-Related Products, *437*
Prescription Drugs, *437*
Research and Development of New
Drugs, *437*
Generic Versus Brand Name Drugs, *438*
Over-the-Counter Drugs, *438*
Cosmetics, *439*
Health Care Quackery and Consumer
Fraud, *439*
Personal Assessment: Health Consumer
Skills, *440*

How to Become a Skilled Consumer, *442*
Summary, *443*

18 Environment: Influences from the World Around Us, 446

Transition to a Postindustrial Society, *448*
World Population Growth, *449*
Air Pollution, *449*
Sources of Air Pollution, *450*
Temperature Inversions, *454*
Indoor Air Pollution, *454*
Health Implications, *455*
Water Pollution, *455*
Yesterday's Pollution Problems, *455*
Today's Pollution Problem, *456*
Sources of Water Pollution, *456*
Effects on Wetlands, *458*
Effects on Health, *459*
Land Pollution, *459*
Solid Waste, *459*
Chemical Waste, *460*
Pesticides, *461*
Herbicides, *462*
Radiation, *462*
Health Effects of Radiation Exposure, *463*
Selecting Sunglasses, *463*
Electromagnetic Radiation, *463*
Nuclear Reactor Accidents and Waste
Disposal, *464*
Personal Assessment: Estimate Your
Exposure to Radiation, *465*
Radon Gas, *467*
Noise Pollution, *467*
Noise-Induced Hearing Loss, *467*
Noise as a Stressor, *467*
Personal Assessment: Are You Helping the
Environment? *470*
In Search of Balance, *472*
Summary, *473*

19 Violence and Safety: Coping in Today's Society, 476

Intentional Injuries, *478*
Homicide, *478*
Domestic Violence, *479*
Gangs and Youth Violence, *481*
Gun Violence, *483*
Bias and Hate Crimes, *483*
Stalking, *484*
Sexual Victimization, *484*
Rape and Sexual Assault, *484*
Sexual Abuse of Children, *486*
Sexual Harassment, *486*
Violence and Commercialization of Sex, *488*
Unintentional Injuries, *488*
Personal Safety, *488*
Residential Safety, *489*

Recreational Safety, *489*
Firearm Safety, *490*
Motor Vehicle Safety, *490*
Home Accident Prevention for Children
and the Elderly, *191*
Personal Assessment: Personal Safety
Index, *493*
Campus Safety and Violence Prevention, *494*
Summary, *494*

UNIT SEVEN   Growing Older: Balancing Your Future with Your Past

20   The Maturing Adult: Moving Through Transitions, 500
Aging Physically: A Process of Decline, *502*
Developmental Tasks of the Midlife
Period, *505*
Achieving Generativity, *503*
Reassessing the Plans of Young
Adulthood, *504*
The Midlife Crisis, *504*
The Joys of Midlife, *504*
Health Concerns of Midlife Adults, *505*
Sexuality and Aging, *505*
Menopause, *506*
Comorbidity, *506*
Osteoporosis, *507*
Osteoarthritis, *508*
The Elderly Years, *508*
Psychosocial Theories of Aging, *508*
Demographic Analysis of the Elderly, *509*
Quality of the Elderly Years, *509*
Why Do We Age? *510*
Tissue, Cellular, and Subcellular
Theories, *510*
Personal Assessment: What Do You Know
About Aging? *511*
Health Concerns of Elderly Adults, *513*
Comorbidity in Younger and Older Elderly
Adults, *514*

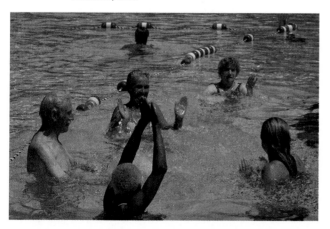

Alzheimer's Disease (Organic Brain
Syndrome), *514*
Special Concerns of Aging Adults, *515*
Health-Care Services, *515*
Housing, *515*
Transportation, *516*
Abuse, *516*
Developmental Tasks of the Elderly
Period, *517*
Accepting the Decline of Aging, *517*
Maintaining High Levels of Physical
Function, *518*
Establishing a Sense of Integrity, *518*
Summary, *521*

21   Dying and Death: The Last Transitions, 524
Personal Death Awareness, *526*
Definitions of Death, *527*
Euthanasia, *528*
Emotional Stages of Dying, *530*
Near-Death Experiences, *531*
Interacting with Dying Persons, *531*
Talking with Children About Death, *531*
Death of a Child, *531*
Hospice Care for the Terminally Ill, *532*
Grief and the Resolution of Grief, *533*
Rituals of Death, *534*
Funeral Services, *535*
Disposition of the Body, *535*
Costs, *536*
Personal Preparation for Death, *537*
Personal Assessment: Planning Your Funeral,
538
Summary, *540*

Appendix 1   Commonly Used Over-the-Counter Products, A-1

Appendix 2   First Aid, A-6

Appendix 3   A Look at Canadian Health, A-9

Appendix 4   Mental Disorders, A-16

Appendix 5   Body Systems, A-18

Glossary   G-1

Index   I-1

Credits   C-1

Understanding YOUR Health

1

Health

Support for Your Future

Have people ever warned you about your health by saying, "You'd better pay more attention to your health, because when it's gone, you'll be sorry"? If so, they were probably also telling you that without good health you cannot continue to be a productive and satisfied person.

For us to suggest that health can contribute to a productive and satisfying life is to invite the questions "What is health?" and "How does health contribute to the process of living a satisfying life?" Of course, ultimately only you can answer these two questions. We will help you answer these questions by providing a framework around which to view health. We will encourage you to study your own health as it relates to your growth and development throughout the stages of the life cycle.

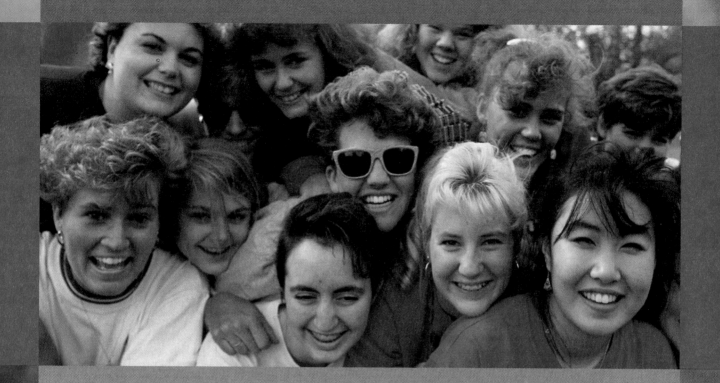

AN INTRODUCTION

The following are covered in this chapter:

▼ Increase years of healthy life to at least 65 years. (Baseline: an estimated 62 years in 1980; p. 252 in Healthy People 2000) (Note: "years of healthy life" is a summary calculation determined by age at death, years of sickness, and years of disability.)

▼ Increase to at least 50% the proportion of post-secondary institutions with institutionwide health promotion programs for students, faculty, and staff. (Baseline: at least 20% of higher education institutions offered health promotion activities for students in 1989-90; p. 256.)

▼ Increase to at least 20% the proportion of hourly workers who participate regularly in employer-sponsored health-promotion activities. (Baseline data unavailable; p. 258.)

▼ Develop and implement a national process to identify significant gaps in the nation's disease prevention and health promotion data, including data for racial and ethnic minorities, people with low incomes, and people with disabilities; and establish mechanisms to meet these needs. (Baseline: no such process existed in 1990; p. 557.)

REAL LIFE
REAL CHOICES
The Five Dimensions of Health: Meeting Personal Challenges

▼ Name: Tim Castleman
▼ Age: 20
▼ Occupation: University student

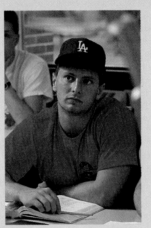

"You're the man of the family now."

The last time Tim Castleman was home on break from his university, he was browsing through his father's bookshelves and found that line in an old novel about a boy whose farmer father had died and who had to leave school to help care for his family. The story, with its dramatic overtones of duty and sacrifice, seemed quaintly remote to Tim, whose father at 47 was a successful executive pursuing a healthy lifestyle and whose death was a possibility Tim had never even thought about.

A few months later, those all-but-forgotten words played an endless refrain in Tim's mind as he stood alone in his father's study, numb with shock and grief. Just three nights earlier Tim's uncle had called him at school to choke out the story about a rainy highway, a speeding truck, a disregarded red light—and his father's instant death in a head-on collision.

Tim's family lives in an affluent suburb, not on a farm. His father was well insured and left his family comfortably provided for, so Tim hasn't had to quit school to support his mother and younger sisters.

Financial security eases many burdens, but the once bright landscape of Tim's life now seems more like a harsh desert to him. Unable to accept his father's sudden death and the end of their warm, trusting relationship, Tim let his schoolwork slide and is now at home, taking a semester off to "get himself together." A varsity track star at college, he's abandoned his daily workout and has gained 17 pounds eating snack foods and drinking beer. He goes to church each Sunday with his family but derives no comfort from the rituals; he believes that the loving God of his childhood has first punished and then deserted him. College friends call Tim to find out how he's doing and when he'll be back at school; his uncle tries hard to fill his father's place; his mother urges him to seek counseling or talk to the family's pastor.

Lonely, frightened, and bitter, Tim won't talk—or listen—to anyone. He spends most of his time alone, his mood swinging between rage and despair.

As you study this chapter, think about some positive steps Tim could take to deal with his feelings, and prepare yourself to answer the questions in **Your Turn** at the end of the chapter. ▼

HEALTH CONCERNS OF THE 1990s

As we move closer to the turn of the century, it is evident that most of us are not too far removed from a number of health issues. Heart disease, cancer, accidents, drug use, and mental health are important concerns for us, even if we are not directly affected by them. The growing problems of environmental pollution, violence, health care costs, and AIDS and other sexually transmitted diseases are becoming increasingly significant. Table 1-1 lists the twelve leading causes of death. World hunger, population control, and the threat of nuclear war represent major issues that will affect us, as well as the generations that follow.

These health concerns are not unmanageable. By the turn of the century, we hope to see advancements in the way our society successfully tackles these problems. Fortunately, we as individuals can make choices in the way we decide to live our lives. At least on a

personal level, we can decide to select a plan of healthful living. We can choose a healthful lifestyle that incorporates a sound diet, proper exercise, adequate rest, periodic medical checkups, and elimination (or moderation) of drug use, including tobacco and alcohol use. One goal of this textbook is to provide you with the information and motivation to help you select the lifestyle that will make you a happy and healthy person.

DEFINITIONS OF HEALTH-RELATED TERMS

A Traditional Definition of Health

One of the most widely recognized and most frequently quoted definitions of health is that given by the Geneva-based World Health Organization[1]:

TABLE 1-1 The 12 Leading Causes of Death*

Cause of death	Number of cases
1. Major cardiovascular diseases – *includes stroke*	929,570
2. Malignant cancers	528,470
3. Chronic obstructive lung diseases	93,840
4. Accidents and adverse effects	83,880
5. Pneumonia and influenza	76,890
6. Diabetes mellitus	51,570
7. Human immunodeficiency virus infection	33,560
8. Suicide	28,510
9. Chronic liver disease and cirrhosis	24,820
10. Homicide	24,730
11. Kidney diseases	24,110
12. Blood infections	20,040
TOTAL (including all other causes)	2,217,000

* For the 12-month period ending April 1993.

✗ Health is a state of complete physical, mental, and social well-being and not merely the absence of disease and infirmity.

This is a multifaceted view of health, with physical, mental, and social dimensions. This definition indicates that health extends beyond the structure and function of your body to include feelings, values, and reasoning. It also includes the nature of your interpersonal relationships. Furthermore, it can be implied that health can exist in the presence of disease and infirmity. You do not have to be a "picture of health" to be a productive and satisfied person. Nevertheless, for all the definition's value, one question remains unanswered: "How does health contribute to the process of living a satisfying life?"

Holistic Health

One popular description of health expands the definition supplied by the World Health Organization. **Holistic health** extends the physical, mental, and social aspects of the definition to include intellectual and spiritual dimensions. The holistically healthy person functions as a *total person*. Some experts say that holistically healthy people have reached a "high level of wellness."

Holistic health may be the broadest explanation of the composition of health. Through a holistic concept of health, we are better able to understand how a person who has a serious physical illness can also claim to be quite healthy.

At an annual meeting of the American College Health Association, a prominent group of health educators, medical professionals, and college residence hall staff professionals met to identify the most critical health issues facing college students in the 1990s.

The top five health issues for the 1990s (in order of their importance) were:

1. *Sexual health concerns,* including topics such as sexually transmitted diseases, relationship issues, unintended pregnancy, and sexual violence

2. *Substance abuse,* including a wide range of issues related to the abuse of alcohol and other drugs, tobacco, and dependency and co-dependency

3. *Mental health concerns,* including stress management, fear of failure, coping skills, complex family relationships, and depression

4. *Nutrition issues,* including healthful diets, weight management, chronic disease prevention, and eating disorders

5. *Health care services,* including financing and delivering comprehensive, low-cost health services to students and their families

Does this list of issues surprise you? Because of their importance to college students, we will cover all of these health issues in this text, as well as numerous other important concerns for today's traditional and nontraditional students. ★

Health Promotion

The term **health promotion** is frequently linked to disease prevention.[2] Health promoters believe that if you accept scientific opinion regarding health and adopt specific health-enhancing practices, you will become a healthy person. On the basis of this view of health, if you have enhanced your health, you should live longer and experience fewer health problems than the average person, and feel better than an unhealthy person.

As worthy as these outcomes are, we believe that this interpretation presents health as an end rather

holistic health a view of health in terms of its physical, emotional, social, intellectual, and spiritual makeup.

health promotion movement in which knowledge, practices, and values are transmitted to people for use in lengthening their lives, reducing the incidence of illness, and feeling better.

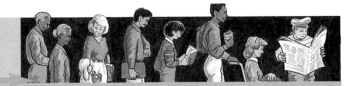

Learning FROM ALL Cultures

The Important Things in Life

What are the most important things in life for maintaining a happy and healthy existence? If any number of Americans responded to this question, the answers would vary. For some, success and happiness might mean a better job or a career change, whereas for others, contentment with oneself, family, and friends might be the answer.

The same holds true for people of other cultures. There are common experiences, however, that people from other countries consider important to their well-being. Mexico is a country with a large gap between the rich and the poor; but for the great majority of Mexicans, celebrations or "fiestas" contribute greatly to their joy of living. Religious holidays and civil events are important occasions for fiestas and can be national or local celebrations. They are generally held outdoors and last from 1 to 3 days.[13]

Chile, like Mexico, is a country of the very rich and the very poor. Regardless of economic or social status, however, most Chileans derive pride and happiness from their families, and families typically are very close. Chileans are also extremely hospitable and enjoy interacting with strangers or visitors.[14]

In the Middle East, Lebanese people are also known for their hospitality and welcome visitors and foreigners into their homes for refreshment. In fact, much of their social life revolves around sharing refreshment, particularly Arabic coffee, with friends.[15]

Although all these countries mentioned face many challenges, their people still strive for happiness and continue to participate in things that bring them joy. What things in your life do you find most important for achieving happiness? ●

than a means to an end. Indeed, living a long time, not being sick, and doing only healthful things are important, but will they assure you of growing and developing to your potential?

Wellness

Whereas *health promotion* is a term used by many in the health field, **wellness** may be the most popular health-related term of the 1990s. High-level wellness suggests an optimistic way of looking at a person's health. Wellness supports the concept that a person's health should not be judged primarily from a medical or disease standpoint, but from the standpoint of reaching or achieving human potential. Wellness is a process for the continuous self-renewal that is needed for an exciting, creative, fulfilling life.

To achieve this potential, wellness experts believe that individuals must take responsibility for their health behaviors.[3] People must understand that they have more control over their health behaviors than they might initially think. A wellness perspective encourages people to focus on the present and future and not on the past, especially when one's past is filled with negative health behaviors. Wellness discourages blaming others for our behavior.

Two wellness researchers, Brylinsky and Hoadley,[4] summarized the concept of wellness by writing:

Wellness reflects a feeling, a conscious perception, or an awareness by the whole person that his/her components

and processes are not only under control, but are also working harmoniously as a unit. Wellness also reflects a person's attitude and his/her unique response to living.

Clearly, the college campus is an ideal place to view the concept of wellness in action. College administrators and even casual observers report that today's college students seem to be embracing wellness. Students, faculty, and staff members realize the importance of health and are participating in activities designed to promote wellness. Throughout this textbook, we will encourage readers to develop the wellness lifestyle with which they feel most comfortable.

With the increased emphasis on wellness programs on many college campuses, it is not surprising to see the impact of wellness extending to many aspects of daily life, including schools and worksites.[5,6] Commonly offered wellness programs include smoking cessation, weight control, cholesterol screening, stress management, exercise, and nutrition. Many major corporations report that employee participation in wellness activities reduces health-care costs (insurance premiums) and increases employee satisfaction and productivity.[7] Indeed, you will see wellness extending beyond your college campus.

Empowerment

Within the last few years, the term *empowerment* has been recognized and discussed within the health education literature.[8] In the context of health, empowerment refers to a process in which individuals or groups

National Health Concerns

Health promotion: Identifies strategies for individual lifestyles that can positively influence one's health.
1. Physical activity and fitness
2. Nutrition
3. Tobacco
4. Alcohol and other drugs
5. Family planning
6. Mental health and mental disorders
7. Violent and abusive behavior
8. Educational and community-based programs

Health protection: Indentifies environmental or regulatory measures intended to protect large population groups.
9. Unintentional injuries
10. Occupational safety and health
11. Environmental health
12. Food and drug safety
13. Oral health

Preventive services: Identifies counseling, screening, immunization, and drug interventions in clinical settings.
14. Maternal and infant health
15. Heart disease and stroke
16. Cancer
17. Diabetes and chronic disabling conditions
18. HIV infection
19. Sexually transmitted deseases
20. Immunization and infectious diseases
21. Clinical preventive services

Surveillance and data systems: Identifies systems for data collection.
22. Surveillance and data systems

Figure 1-1 The 22 priority areas and the four major areas of concern identified in the *Year 2000 National Health Objectives.*

of people gain increasing measures of control over their health. To take control over health matters, persons or groups must learn to "liberate themselves" from a variety of sociostructural barriers and the paternalistic forces that tend to restrict health enhancement. In this sense, people learn to take charge of their lives, regardless of the current forces that discourage positive health changes. Empowered people and groups do not blame individuals or environmental realities for health conditions but focus on producing constructive change through dialogue and collaboration.

Empowerment programs have produced positive health consequences for individuals and groups that have been traditionally underserved by the healthcare system, such as the economically disadvantaged, the elderly, and minority populations. Have you seen empowerment programs working in your community? You probably have if you can identify programs in which people have organized a grassroots campaign to prevent neighborhood violence, improve childhood nutrition, promote healthy lifestyles, or prevent drug use among youth. Only when people realize that they can "make a difference" will they become empowered. We believe that your personal health

course can help you discover empowerment in your own life.

Health Objectives for the Year 2000

In 1990 Dr. Louis Sullivan (Secretary of Health and Human Services) presented a strategic plan for improving the health of the nation during the 1990s. This lengthy document is entitled *Healthy People 2000: National Health Promotion and Disease Prevention Objectives.*

Three broad goals of *Healthy People 2000* are to do the following:
▼ Increase the span of healthy life for Americans
▼ Reduce health disparities among Americans
▼ Achieve access to preventive services for all Americans

Healthy People 2000 outlines measurable health improvement targets (300 specific objectives) in 22 priority areas. (See Figure 1-1.) This report encourages the nation to move beyond an emphasis on saving lives to improving the quality of life for all. Perhaps more than any previous federal government planning document, *Healthy People 2000* stresses the importance of health promotion, health protection, and preventive services.

Understanding Your Health encourages your interest in the *Healthy People 2000* report. Each chapter begins with several of the specific objectives found in this 700-page document. Your use of the health information and health behavior suggestions in *Understanding Your Health* will help you become a part of the national push to achieve these objectives.

TODAY'S TRADITIONAL COLLEGE STUDENT

Although many terms have been used to describe the years between adolescence and adulthood, we will refer to these as the **young adult years.** The young adult period of the life cycle varies in length and in time of onset and completion. For our purposes, this period includes the traditional undergraduate years, from ages 18 to 24.

Annual statistics indicate that more than 13 million students are enrolled in U.S. colleges today. Slightly more than half of these students are women. Minority students make up approximately 20% of American college students, foreign students total nearly 3%, and

wellness a broadly based term used to describe a highly developed level of health.

young adult years segment of the life cycle from ages 18 to 24, a transitional period between adolescence and adulthood.

nearly three out of five students attend college on a full-time basis.[9]

More than half of all undergraduate college students are traditional age. This book is directed initially at these students. However, because many older students are now going to college, we will also point out a variety of life experiences and developmental tasks appropriate to these students. Certainly, the nontraditional students in our classes help our traditional-age students understand the role that health plays throughout the life cycle.

TODAY'S NONTRADITIONAL COLLEGE STUDENT

In the 1990s, more than 40% of American college students are classified as **nontraditional students.** Included in this vast overlapping group of students are part-time students, military veterans, students returning to college, single parents, adults and senior citizens, and evening students. These students enter the classroom with a wide assortment of life experiences and observations.

Many nontraditional students are trying to juggle a schedule that is very demanding. The responsibilities of managing a job, a schedule of classes, and perhaps a family, are challenging. Furthermore, doing these tasks on a limited budget adds to the difficulty. It is likely that while some students in your health class are

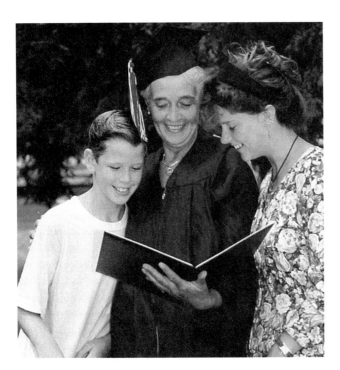

A nontraditional student achieves her goal of a college education.

especially concerned about an upcoming football game or party, others are equally worried about making the next rent payment, caring for aging parents, or finding affordable child care.

The authors strive to make this textbook meaningful for both traditional and nontraditional students. Much of the information included in this book applies to both categories of students. We do ask the nontraditional students to do two things as you read this book: (1) reflect on your own young adult years, and (2) examine your current lifestyle to see how the decisions you made as a young adult are affecting the quality of your life now. Nontraditional students may have young adult children whose lives can be observed in light of the information provided in this book.

MINORITY STUDENTS

Although enrollment patterns at colleges and universities vary, the overall number of minority students in college is increasing. Today, according to the most recent figures available, about one out of five college students is a minority student—African-Americans, Hispanics, Asians, and Native Americans represent the largest groups of minority students. These students bring a rich variety of cultural influences and traditions to today's college environment.

With multicultural student enrollment increasing on the college campus, it is important for a health textbook to consider the special health concerns of minority students. These health concerns are just starting to be more fully recognized.[10] Whenever possible, *Understanding Your Health* will address the particular needs and interests of students from ethnically diverse backgrounds. We will also point out current references and resources that may be especially important to minority students.

STUDENTS WITH DISABILITIES

Students with disabilities are a rapidly growing population on campuses. Improved diagnostic, medical, and rehabilitation procedures coupled with improved educational accommodations have opened up opportunities for these students at an increasing rate.

In addition to students who have visible disabilities, such as blindness, deafness, or a physical disability requiring use of a wheelchair, a greater number of students with "hidden" disabilities are appearing on campuses. Students with learning disabilities (including attention deficit disorders), those with psychiatric and emotional problems, and those recovering from alcohol and substance abuse are examples of this hidden group.

In the past, many people with physical disabilities could not participate in educational programs because schools did not accommodate them. Two pieces of fed-

Health ACTION Guide

Cultural Diversity at Your Campus

To help you develop some understanding of the ethnically diverse culture at your college or university, try to find the answers to these basic questions:

▼ What are the minority population figures for the community in which your college is located? Try to include figures for African-Americans, Hispanics, Asians, and Native Americans.

▼ What are the minority population figures for your college or university?

▼ Do these figures surprise you?

The following is the resource center for the federal agency whose mission is to improve the health status of minority populations in the United States. To receive information or publications, call the 800 number listed below:

Office of Minority Health (OMH)
Information Resource Center
P.O. Box 37337
Washington, DC 20013-7337
(1-800-444-6472)

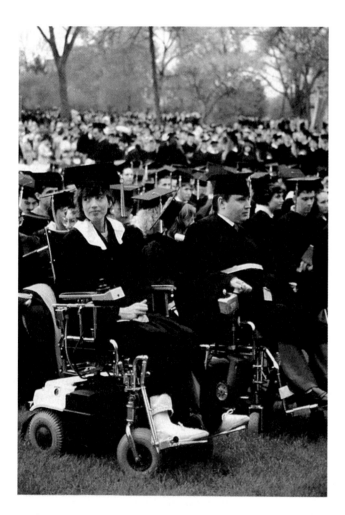

eral legislation, Section 504 of the Rehabilitation Act and the Americans with Disabilities Act (ADA), have made access to educational programs possible. These laws require institutions to examine the accessibility of services, programs, and resources.

The wheelchair figure that serves as the international access symbol means much more than just physical access to a building. It is an inclusive symbol that works toward the inclusion of people with all types of disabilities.

Comfortable Language

For most of our history, people with disabilities were labeled mainly by the medical community. Until recently, some of the terms commonly used were *invalids, victims, cripples,* and *handicapped.* Since then, many euphemisms have appeared, including physically challenged, handi-capable, inconvenienced, and differently able. Many of these terms have been unacceptable to disability activists, as they are seen as a denial of realities.

Although there is no absolutely right or wrong word choice, language does reflect attitudes. Some approaches lead to more comfortable interactions. *Disabled* is generally preferred to handicapped. Even more acceptable is "a person with a disability" (or "one who is blind," or "one who has mental retardation"), since it emphasizes the individual before the condition. Similarly, "wheelchair user" is preferable to wheelchair bound. Of course, the best approach is to get to know the individual by name. Lastly, keep in mind the term that many people with disabilities use to describe those who are not disabled: TABS—temporarily able bodied.

nontraditional students administrative term used by colleges and universities for students who, for whatever reason, are pursuing undergraduate work at an age other than that associated with the traditional college years (18-24)

Americans with Disabilities Act

The Americans with Disabilities Act (ADA) guarantees disabled people access to employment, public accommodations, transportation, public services, and telecommunications. President George Bush signed this into law on July 26, 1990.

Considered landmark legislation, ADA provides comprehensive federal civil rights protection for people with disabilities. Built upon a body of existing legislation, particularly the Rehabilitation Act of 1973 and the Civil Rights Act of 1964, the ADA states its purpose as providing "a clear and comprehensive national mandate for the elimination of discrimination against individuals with disabilities."

The ADA is not an affirmative action statute. Instead, it seeks to dispel stereotypes and assumptions about disabilities, and to assure equality of opportunity, full participation, independent living, and economic self-sufficiency for disabled people. To achieve these objectives, the law prohibits covered entities from excluding people from jobs, services, activities, or benefits based on disability. It also provides penalties for discrimination.

DEVELOPMENTAL TASKS FOR COLLEGE STUDENTS

Because *most* of today's undergraduate college students range between 18 and perhaps 40 years of age, we will present five developmental tasks that reflect this broad student range. The first four tasks (involving identity, responsibility, independence, and social skills) are especially pertinent to the more traditional-age college student. The fifth task (concerning intimacy) is probably more important for students who have moved just beyond the typical young adult years. Through the gains you make with each of these tasks, you will find yourself moving more sucessfully through your life.

However, keep in mind that many college students, regardless of their age, continue to make gains in all five developmental areas, because each person's experience and development are unique. For example, nontraditional students remind us that their identity continues to change as they see themselves progressing through college. They realize that they are not the same person they were when they started back to school. Their identities continue to develop as they learn new concepts and meet new people . . . and for this they are most pleased.

Forming an Initial Adult Identity

For most of childhood and adolescence, you were seen by adults within your neighborhood or community as someone's son or daughter. That stage has now nearly passed; both you and society are beginning to look at each other in new ways.

As an emerging adult, you probably wish to present a unique identity to society. Internally you are constructing a perception of yourself as the adult you wish to be; externally you are formulating the behavioral patterns that will project this identity to others.

We believe that the completion of this first developmental task is necessary so that you can experience a productive and satisfying life. Through your experiences in achieving an adult identity, you will eventually be capable of answering the central question of young adulthood: "Who am I?" Interestingly, many nontraditional students are also asking themselves this question as they progress through college.

Establishing Independence

In contemporary society the primary responsibility for socialization during childhood and adolescence is assigned to the family. For nearly two decades your family was the primary contributor to your knowledge, values, and behaviors. By this time, however, you should be demonstrating an interest in moving away from the dependent relationship that has existed between you and your family.

Travel, peer relationships, marriage, military service, and, of course, college have been traditional avenues for disengagement from the family. Generally your ability and willingness to follow one or more of these paths will help you to establish your independence. Your success in these endeavors will be based on your willingness to use the resources you have. You will need to draw on physical, emotional, social, intellectual, and spiritual strengths to undertake the new experiences that will bring about your independence. In a sense your family laid the foundation for the resources and experiences you will use to draw yourself away from the family's midst.

Assuming Responsibility

The assumption of increasing levels of responsibility is a third developmental task in which you are expected to progress. For adults the opportunity to assume responsibility can come from a variety of sources. You may sometimes accept responsibility voluntarily, such as when you join a campus organization or establish a new friendship. Other responsibilities are placed on you when professors assign term papers, when dating partners exert pressure on you to conform to their expectations, or when employers require that you be a consistently productive employee. In other situations you may accept responsibility for doing a particular task not for yourself but for the benefit of someone else.

As important and demanding as these areas of responsibility are, a more basic responsibility awaits the adult: the responsibility of maintaining and improving

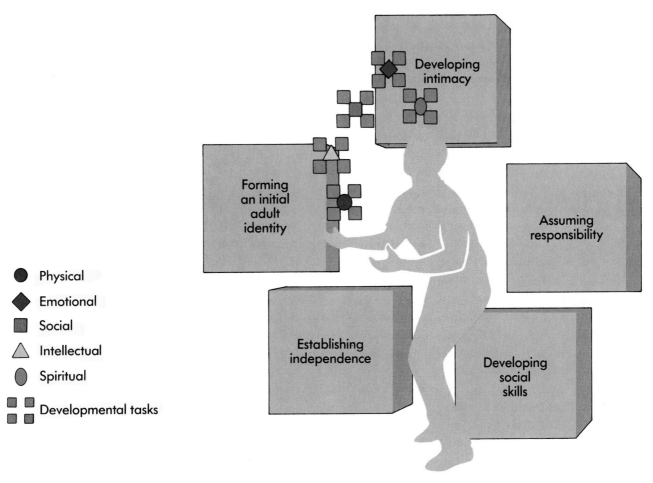

Figure 1-2 Mastery of the developmental tasks through a balanced involvement of the five dimensions will lead to your enjoying a more productive and satisfying life. The developmental tasks and the five dimensions of health are indicated throughout this book by the symbols shown below:

● Physical   ▲ Intellectual

◆ Emotional   ● Spiritual

■ Social   ▪▪ Developmental tasks

your health and the health of others. You will be challenged to be responsible for recognizing, improving, and then using the strengths that constitute your physical, emotional, social, intellectual, and spiritual makeup. At the same time you will be equally responsible for recognizing, accepting, and working within your limitations. None of the specific areas of responsibility associated with school, employment, and parenting can be undertaken with maximum effectiveness unless you make a commitment to be responsible for your own health.

▪▪ Developing Social Skills

The fourth developmental task that is a part of the young adult years is that of developing appropriate and dependable social skills. Adulthood will probably

require your "membership" in a variety of groups that range in size from a marital pair to a national political party or international corporation. These memberships will demand of you the ability to function in many different social settings and with a variety of people.

The college experience has traditionally prepared students very effectively in this regard, but the interactions in friendships, work relationships, or parenting may require that you make an effort to grow and develop beyond levels you might achieve as a result of being a college student. You will probably need to refine a variety of social skills, including communication, listening, and conflict management.

This need to interact socially will at times negatively influence your health. Examples might be the weekend

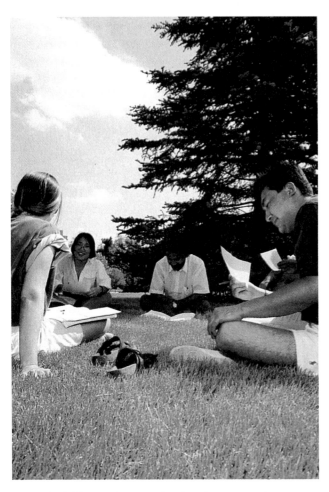

Social interaction can take place in many settings.

party that prevents you from doing well on a Monday morning examination, or the recreational or intramural activities that sometimes result in serious injury. Generally, however, social interaction contributes to your total health and is an important aid in helping you experience a productive and satisfying life.

:: Developing Intimacy

The task of developing intimacy usually presents itself to persons between young adulthood and midlife. During this time it appears developmentally important for persons to establish one or more intimate relationships. Indeed, we are looking at intimacy in its broadest sense as a deeply close, sharing relationship. Intimacy may stem from a marriage relationship or other close friendship.

People vary in their number of intimate relationships, with some having numerous intimate friends, whereas others have only one or two deep relationships. The number does not matter. From a developmental standpoint, what matters is that each person has someone with whom to share intimate thoughts, feelings, and emotions.

After becoming familiar with these developmental tasks, you should see that there is considerable overlap in the accomplishment of each task. For example, your development and refinement of social skills can enhance your independence from your family. Your willingness to accept increasing responsibility may influence your ability to develop an intimate relationship with someone.

THE ROLE OF HEALTH

Having been introduced to the five developmental tasks for most college students, you can better answer the question, "What is the *role of health* in my life?" We believe that the role of health is to assist you in mastering the developmental tasks that will make your life more satisfying and productive.

If you wanted to know about another person's health, you would probably ask, "How's your health?" However, if you asked us that question, we would respond by saying, "Our health? In relationship to what?"

We suggest that health is something that can be described meaningfully only in conjunction with a developmental task. We all have a level of health for everything we need or want to do. No one has just one level of health for all of life's many demands.

For the vast majority of today's college students, the tasks we are identifying as those likely to be accomplished with high-level health are the five developmental tasks just presented. For midlife and elderly students, the refinement of these tasks and the mastery of additional developmental tasks (see Chapter 20) will depend on your level of health.

The lack of task **mastery** because of a lowered level of health would reduce your opportunity to have a productive, satisfying life. Just as a broken leg might temporarily curtail your social activities or a catastrophic illness could alter your plans for your later life, so could a chronically low level of health reduce your ability to develop within a particular segment of the life cycle.

THE COMPOSITION OF HEALTH

Throughout this book we will contend that your health is composed of five interacting, *dynamic* dimensions. By becoming familiar with these dimensions of your health, you can more easily recognize what it is about your health that may or may not be helping you to master the developmental tasks. Fortunately, because your health is dynamic, you can modify aspects of its dimensions to make it a better tool to help you accomplish developmental tasks and live a productive, satisfying life.

Your health is not static; it cannot be stored on a shelf or given to others. The health you had yesterday

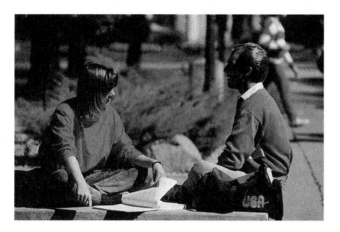

Healthy growth can occur during the college years. . .

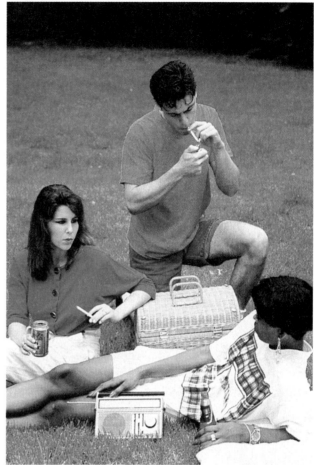

. . . as can unhealthy growth.

no longer exists. The health you aspire to have next week or next year is not guaranteed. However, scientific evidence suggests that what you do today will help determine the quality of your future health. We will now briefly consider each of the five dimensions of health so that you can more clearly see how each forms a part of your total health.

● Physical Dimension of Health

You have a number of physiological and structural characteristics that you can call on to aid you in accomplishing your developmental tasks. Among these physical characteristics are your level of susceptibility to disease, body weight, visual ability, strength, coordination, level of endurance, and powers of recuperation. In certain situations the physical dimension of your health may be the most important dimension. Perhaps this is why many authorities have for so long equated health with the design and operation of the body.

◆ Emotional Dimension of Health

You also possess certain emotional characteristics that can aid you as you grow and develop. The emotional dimension of health includes the degree to which you are able to cope with stress, remain flexible, and compromise to resolve conflict.

Your growth and development can have associated with them some vulnerability, which may lead to feelings of rejection and failure that could reduce your overall productivity and satisfaction. People who consistently try to improve their emotional health appear to lead lives of greater enjoyment than those who let feelings of vulnerability overwhelm them or block their creativity.

■ Social Dimension of Health

A third dimension of total health is that of social abilities. Whether you label these as social graces, skills, or insights, you probably have many strengths in this area. Because most of your growing and developing has been undertaken in the presence of others, you can appreciate how this dimension of your health may be a critically important factor in your life.

The social abilities of many nontraditional students may already be firmly established. Entering college may encourage them to develop new social skills that help them socialize with their traditional-age student colleagues. After being on campus for a while, nontraditional students often interact comfortably with traditional students in such diverse places as the library, the student center, and the bookstore. This interaction enhances the social dimensions of health for both types of students.

mastery when applied to growth within the young adult segment of life cycle, mastery implies becoming more self-aware, independent, responsible, and socially interactive.

▲Intellectual Dimension of Health

Your ability to process and act on information, clarify values and beliefs, and exercise your decision-making capacity ranks among the most important aspects of total health. Coping skills, flexibility, or the knack of saying the right thing at the right time may not serve you as well as does your ability to use information or understand a new idea. Certainly a refusal to grasp new information or to undertake an analysis of your beliefs could hinder the degree of growth and development your college experience can provide.

●Spiritual Dimension of Health

The fifth dimension of health is the spiritual dimension.[11,12] Although you certainly could include your religious beliefs and practices in this category, we would extend it to include your relationship to other living things, the role of a spiritual direction in your life, the nature of human behavior, and your willingness to serve others. All are important components of spiritual health.

Cultivating the spiritual side of your health may help you discover how you "fit" into this universe. You can enhance your spiritual health in a variety of ways. Many concern opening yourself to new experiences that involve nature, art, body movement, or music. Taking a walk in the woods, visiting an art museum, listening to classical music, talking with young children, writing poetry, caring for the environment, painting a picture, or pushing your body to its physical limits are just a few ways one can develop spiritual health.

HEALTH: OUR DEFINITION

By combining the role of health with the composition of health, we offer a new definition of health that we believe is unique to this book:

Health is the blending of your physical, emotional, social, intellectual, and spiritual resources as they assist you in mastering the developmental tasks necessary for you to enjoy a satisfying and productive life.

Remember that this blending of your health resources is a never-ending process. Regardless of whether you are a traditional or nontraditional student, your ability to master the tasks that await you hinges on this unique combination of health dimensions.

FOCUS OF THIS TEXTBOOK

We feel confident that this health textbook can be an important aid in your study of health and its relationship to the demands of living. By detailing valid scientific information, discussing values, and describing behavior patterns that influence health, this text can help you explore your strengths and limitations. Armed with this information, you should then be able to recognize where changes in your lifestyle may be desirable and practical and where limitations may continue to hinder your development.

Each of this book's topics, activities, and discussion questions should generate in you a recurring question:

How can I apply this new information about health to my daily life so that I can master the tasks necessary for having a productive, satisfying life?

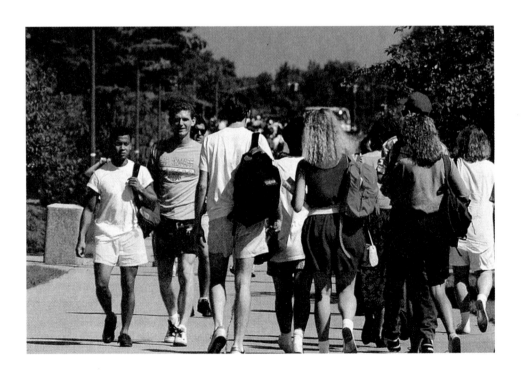

A Personal Profile: Evaluating Your Health

Your health is influenced by behaviors in a number of aspects of living. This personal health profile will help you assess these behaviors. For each statement, circle the number of the response that best describes your behavior, or how you think you will behave when confronted with a particular situation. At the end of each section, add the points received on the statements in that section and record your point total on the appropriate line. At the conclusion of the inventory you will be able to make a broad interpretation of the influence of your behaviors on your personal health status.

STRESS MANAGEMENT

1. I seek out change and accept its presence with a sense of confidence and anticipation. 3

| 1 Rarely, if ever | 2 Some of the time | 3 Most of the time | 4 Almost always |

2. I participate regularly in a physical activity that allows me to expend nervous energy. 3

| 1 Rarely, if ever | 2 Some of the time | 3 Most of the time | 4 Almost always |

3. I turn to friends for advice and assistance during periods of disruption in my life. 3

| 1 Rarely, if ever | 2 Some of the time | 3 Most of the time | 4 Almost always |

4. I periodically reevaluate my experiences with distressful events in anticipation of future events of the same type. 1

| 1 Rarely, if ever | 2 Some of the time | 3 Most of the time | 4 Almost always |

5. I seek the counsel of professional advisors when stress becomes too difficult to manage. 1

| 1 Rarely, if ever | 2 Some of the time | 3 Most of the time | 4 Almost always |

6. I seek comfort and support from my faith when faced with a difficult period of adjustment. 1

| 1 Rarely, if ever | 2 Some of the time | 3 Most of the time | 4 Almost always |

Points 16

PHYSICAL FITNESS

1. I participate in vigorous activity for approximately 30 minutes four times per week.

| 1 Rarely, if ever | 2 Some of the time | 3 Most of the time | 4 Almost always |

2. I am active during the day and prefer a more vigorous approach to work and leisure activity.

| 1 Rarely, if ever | 2 Some of the time | 3 Most of the time | 4 Almost always |

3. I do exercises specifically designed to condition my muscles and joints.

| 1 Rarely, if ever | 2 Some of the time | 3 Most of the time | 4 Almost always |

4. I enter into vigorous activity only after I am warmed up, and I warm down following vigorous activity.

| 1 Rarely, if ever | 2 Some of the time | 3 Most of the time | 4 Almost always |

PERSONAL ASSESSMENT

Continued.

PERSONAL ASSESSMENT

5. I select properly designed and well-maintained equipment and clothing for each activity.

| 1 Rarely, if ever | 2 Some of the time | 3 Most of the time | 4 Almost always |

6. I listen to my body regarding injury and fatigue, and I seek appropriate care when injured.

| 1 Rarely, if ever | 2 Some of the time | 3 Most of the time | 4 Almost always |

Points _17_

SOCIAL RELATIONSHIPS

1. I feel comfortable and confident when meeting people for the first time.

| 1 Rarely, if ever | 2 Some of the time | 3 Most of the time | 4 Almost always |

2. I establish social relationships with people of both sexes with equal ease and enjoyment.

| 1 Rarely, if ever | 2 Some of the time | 3 Most of the time | 4 Almost always |

3. I participate in a wide variety of groups, including educational, recreational, religious, and occupational groups.

| 1 Rarely, if ever | 2 Some of the time | 3 Most of the time | 4 Almost always |

4. I find the roles of leader and subordinate to be equally acceptable.

| 1 Rarely, if ever | 2 Some of the time | 3 Most of the time | 4 Almost always |

5. I seek out opportunities to become proficient at a variety of social skills.

| 1 Rarely, if ever | 2 Some of the time | 3 Most of the time | 4 Almost always |

6. I am open and accessible to others in the development of intimate relationships.

| 1 Rarely, if ever | 2 Some of the time | 3 Most of the time | 4 Almost always |

Points _17_

SPIRITUAL HEALTH

1. I find myself searching for spiritual connections in my life.

| 1 Rarely, if ever | 2 Some of the time | 3 Most of the time | 4 Almost always |

2. I can identify ways I can improve the spiritual dimension of my health.

| 1 Rarely, if ever | 2 Some of the time | 3 Most of the time | 4 Almost always |

Points _____

NUTRITION

1. I select a wide variety of foods in an attempt to eat a balanced diet.

| (1) Rarely, if ever | 2 Some of the time | 3 Most of the time | 4 Almost always |

2. I select breads, cereals, fresh fruits, and vegetables in preference to pastries, candies, sodas, and fruits canned in heavy syrup.

| 1 Rarely, if ever | 2 Some of the time | 3 Most of the time | (4) Almost always |

3. I select such foods as peas, beans, and peanut butter as my primary sources of protein while limiting my consumption of red meat and high-fat dairy products.

| (1) Rarely, if ever | 2 Some of the time | 3 Most of the time | 4 Almost always |

4. I select foods prepared with unsaturated vegetable oils while reducing my consumption of red meats, organ meats, dairy products, and foods prepared with lard or butter.

| (1) Rarely, if ever | 2 Some of the time | 3 Most of the time | 4 Almost always |

5. I limit snacking, and I select nutritious foods when I do snack.

| 1 Rarely, if ever | 2 Some of the time | 3 Most of the time | (4) Almost always |

6. I attempt to balance my caloric intake with my activity level.

| 1 Rarely, if ever | 2 Some of the time | 3 Most of the time | (4) Almost always |

Points   _15_

ALCOHOL, TOBACCO, AND DRUG USE

1. I abstain from alcohol use, or I use alcohol infrequently and in very limited amounts.

| 1 Rarely, if ever | 2 Some of the time | 3 Most of the time | (4) Almost always |

2. I avoid riding with persons who are consuming alcohol, and I drive defensively, remaining aware that other drivers may be using alcohol.

| 1 Rarely, if ever | 2 Some of the time | 3 Most of the time | (4) Almost always |

3. I avoid the use of tobacco products in all forms, including cigarettes, cigars, pipes, and smokeless tobacco products.

| (1) Rarely, if ever | 2 Some of the time | 3 Most of the time | 4 Almost always |

4. I limit my contact with others who are using tobacco, particularly when in confined spaces or when exposure would be for an extended period.

| 1 Rarely, if ever | (2) Some of the time | 3 Most of the time | 4 Almost always |

5. I take prescription drugs only in the manner prescribed, and I use over-the-counter drugs in accordance with directions.

| 1 Rarely, if ever | 2 Some of the time | 3 Most of the time | (4) Almost always |

PERSONAL ASSESSMENT

Continued.

PERSONAL ASSESSMENT

6. I refrain from using illegal drugs.

1 Rarely, if ever	2 Some of the time	3 Most of the time	4 Almost always

Points _____ 19

SAFETY

1. I attempt to identify the sources of risk or potential danger in each new setting or activity.

1 Rarely, if ever	2 Some of the time	3 Most of the time	4 Almost always

2. I learn procedures and precautions before undertaking new recreational or occupational activities.

1 Rarely, if ever	2 Some of the time	3 Most of the time	4 Almost always

3. I select appropriate equipment for all activities and maintain equipment in good working order.

1 Rarely, if ever	2 Some of the time	3 Most of the time	4 Almost always

4. I curtail my participation in activities when I am not feeling well or am distracted by other demands.

1 Rarely, if ever	2 Some of the time	3 Most of the time	4 Almost always

5. I refrain from using alcohol or drugs when engaged in potentially dangerous recreational or occupational activities.

1 Rarely, if ever	2 Some of the time	3 Most of the time	4 Almost always

6. I repair or report dangerous conditions to individuals responsible for their maintenance.

1 Rarely, if ever	2 Some of the time	3 Most of the time	4 Almost always

Points _____

SELF-CARE

1. I maintain an accurate, updated personal health history.

1 Not at all	2 To a very limited degree	3 Almost completeley	4 Completely

2. I routinely monitor my weight and blood pressure, as well as factors related to specific conditions applicable to my health.

1 Rarely, if ever	2 Some of the time	3 Most of the time	4 Almost always

3. I practice home dental health care, including brushing and flossing.

1 Rarely, if ever	2 Some of the time	3 Most of the time	4 Almost always

4. I maintain my immunization status and receive boosters when scheduled or required by specific conditions.

1 Not at all	2 To a very limited degree	3 Almost completeley	4 Completely

5. I take prescription medication through the entire course of the prescribed period of use rather than stopping use when symptoms subside.

| 1 Rarely, if ever | 2 Some of the time | 3 Most of the time | 4 Almost always |

6. I consult a reliable home-medical reference book before beginning self-care.

| 1 Rarely, if ever | 2 Some of the time | 3 Most of the time | 4 Almost always |

Points _____

Answer as Applicable

1. I routinely examine my testicles for the presence of small masses or other unusual signs.

| 1 Rarely, if ever | 2 Some of the time | 3 Most of the time | 4 Almost always |

2. I routinely examine my breasts for the presence of masses or other unusual signs.

| 1 Rarely, if ever | 2 Some of the time | 3 Most of the time | 4 Almost always |

3. I routinely receive a Pap smear test.

| 1 Rarely, if ever | 2 Some of the time | 3 Most of the time | 4 Almost always |

4. I use my birth control technique in the manner intended to maximize its effectiveness.

| 1 Rarely, if ever | 2 Some of the time | 3 Most of the time | 4 Almost always |

Points ____12____

HEREDITY

1. I can identify members of my family tree for the previous three generations.

| 1 Not at all | 2 To a limited degree | 3 Almost completeley | 4 Completely |

2. I can identify the age at death and the cause of death for all family members to whom I am genetically related for the previous three generations.

| 1 Not at all | 2 For a few but not for most | 3 For most but not for all | 4 For all |

3. I receive medical consultation for conditions for which I may have a genetic predisposition (diabetes, hypertension, etc.).

| 1 Not at all | 2 To a very limited degree | 3 Relatively continuous consultation | 4 Continuous consultation |

4. I limit my exposure to radiation and to toxic environmental pollutants.

| 1 Rarely, if ever | 2 Some of the time | 3 Most of the time | 4 Almost always |

5. I will openly share information concerning inheritance abnormalities with potential mates.

| 1 Not likely | 2 Perhaps | 3 Very likely | 4 Certainly |

PERSONAL ASSESSMENT

Continued.

PERSONAL ASSESSMENT

6. I will seek genetic counseling for known inherited conditions before having children.

1	2	3	4
Not likely	Perhaps	Very likely	Certainly

Points ___10___

SLEEP, REST, AND RELAXATION

1. I plan my daily schedule to allow time for leisure activity.

1	2	3	4
Rarely, if ever	Some of the time	Most of the time	Almost always

2. I plan my daily schedule to allow time for contemplation, meditation, or prayer.

1	2	3	4
Rarely, if ever	Some of the time	Most of the time	Almost always

3. I receive between 7 and 8 hours of sleep daily.

1	2	3	4
Rarely, if ever	Some of the time	Most of the time	Almost always

4. I refrain from using sleep-inducing over-the-counter drugs.

1	2	3	4
Rarely, if ever	Some of the time	Most of the time	Almost always

5. I curtail activities when I need to recover from illnesses and injuries.

1	2	3	4
Rarely, if ever	Some of the time	Most of the time	Almost always

6. I attempt to leave the demands of work, school, or parenting outside of my leisure or relaxation time of the day.

1	2	3	4
Rarely, if ever	Some of the time	Most of the time	Almost always

Points ___0___

HEALTH CONSUMERISM

1. I am skeptical of practitioners and clinics who advertise or offer services at rates substantially lower than those charged by reputable providers.

1	2	3	4
Rarely, if ever	Some of the time	Most of the time	Almost always

2. I have the financial resources necessary to cover the costs associated with a major illness or hospitalization.

1	2	3	4
Not at all	To a very limited degree	Almost completely	Completely

3. I am skeptical of claims that "guarantee" the effectiveness of a particular health care service or product.

1	2	3	4
Rarely, if ever	Some of the time	Most of the time	Almost always

———————————————————————————————————→

4. I accept information that is deemed valid by the established scientific community.

1	②	3	4
Rarely, if ever	Some of the time	Most of the time	Almost always

5. I pursue my rights in matters of misrepresentation or consumer dissatisfaction.

1	②	3	4
Rarely, if ever	Some of the time	Most of the time	Almost always

6. I seek additional opinions regarding diagnoses indicating a need for surgery or other costly therapies.

1	2	3	④
Rarely, if ever	Some of the time	Most of the time	Almost always

Points ___ *14*

YOUR TOTAL POINTS ___ *161*

INTERPRETATION

213-260 Behaviors are very supportive of high-level health.
164-212 Behaviors are relatively supportive of high-level health.
115-163 Behaviors are relatively destructive to high-level health.
 66-114 Behaviors are very destructive to high-level health.

TO CARRY THIS FURTHER . . .

Were you surprised at your score? Remember that this assessment provides a brief look at your health behaviors. It should help identify areas you may want to pay careful attention to as you read this book. The authors hope this assessment will serve as a positive motivator for you, regardless of your score. Remember that you can change your health behaviors. This health textbook and your instructor can get you started in the right direction. Good luck.

P E R S O N A L   A S S E S S M E N T

Summary

✔ Health can be defined in several ways.

✔ Holistic health views health in its five dimensions.

✔ Health promotion, wellness, and empowerment reflect important movements in the health field.

✔ To move successfully through life, critical developmental tasks must be achieved. Chapter 1 focused on five tasks that involve identity, independence, responsibility, social skills, and intimacy.

✔ One's health is composed of five dimensions: physical, emotional, social, intellectual, and spiritual.

✔ The authors defined health in terms of the five dimensions' ability to help one successfully complete developmental tasks.

Review Questions

1. How does the World Health Organization's definition of health differ from the definition developed in this chapter?
2. Define holistic health, health promotion, and wellness.
3. What percentages of today's college students are traditional, nontraditional, or minority students?
4. Identify the five developmental tasks for college students.
5. What is the difference between the *role* of health and the *composition* of health?
6. What is meant by "health is dynamic"?
7. What are the five dimensions of health?
8. What were the three goals of the *Healthy People 2000* report?

Think about This . . .

✔ Does your lifestyle reflect a "wellness" approach to living?

✔ To what degree does your campus reflect a multicultural community?

✔ How closely related do you think the developmental tasks of independence and responsibility are? Can you have one without the other?

✔ Which of the five dimensions of health have you developed most fully? Least fully?

REAL LIFE REAL CHOICES

YOUR TURN

▼ In which of the five dimensions of health is Tim's life lacking since his father's death?

▼ What are some ways in which Tim can improve these aspects of his health?

▼ Can friends and family be helpful to Tim in this effort? If so, in what ways?

AND NOW, YOUR CHOICES

▼ If a close friend of yours suddenly lost a parent, how would you try to help?

▼ If one of your parents died suddenly, how could your friends be most helpful to you?

References

1. World Health Organization: Constitution of the World Health Organization, *Chronicle of the World Health Organization* 1:29-43, 1947.
2. Joint Committee on Health Education Terminology: Report of the 1990 Joint Committee on Health Education Terminology, *Journal of School Health* 61(6):251-254, 1991.
3. Travis JW, Callander MG: *Wellness for helping professionals: creating compassionate cultures*, Sebastopol, Calif, 1990, Wellness Associates.
4. Brylinsky J, Hoadley M: A comparative analysis of wellness attitudes of "suicidal" and "at risk" college students, *Wellness Perspectives: Research, Theory, and Practice* 8(2):59-72, 1991.
5. Bensley LB: Schoolsite health promotion: ways of sustaining interests, *Journal of Health Education* 22(2):86-89, 1991.
6. Watts PR, et al: A university worksite health promotion and wellness education program model, *Journal of Health Education* 23(2):87-94, 1992.
7. Anderson K: Cash rewards are made to faithful few, *USA Today*, 1B, May 27, 1992.
8. Fahlberg LL, et al: Empowerment as an emerging approach in health education, *Journal of Health Education* 22(3):185-193, 1991.
9. *The nation: demographics*, Washington, DC, Sept 1990, Chronicle of Higher Education.
10. Thomas SB: Health status of the black community in the 21st century: a futuristic perspective for health education, *Journal of Health Education* 23(1):7-13, 1992.
11. Goodloe NR, Arreola PM: Spiritual health: out of the closet, *Journal of Health Education* 23(4)221-226, 1992.
12. Seaward BL: Spiritual wellbeing: a health education model, *Journal of Health Education* 22(3):166-169, 1991.
13. Rummel J: *Mexico*, New York, 1990, Chelsea House.
14. Galvin IF: *Chile: land of poets and patriots*, Minneapolis, 1990, Dillon Press.
15. Cahill MJ: *Lebanon*, New York, 1987, Chelsea House.

Suggested Readings

Cooper RK: *Health and fitness excellence—the scientific action plan*, Boston, 1990, Houghton Mifflin.

A seven-step plan for health and fitness includes chapters on stress, exercise, nutrition, body fat control, and postural vitality. Also described are ways to design a living environment and ways to develop an unlimited mind and life unity.

The good health fact book, Pleasantville, NY, 1992, The Reader's Digest Association.

This book is filled with current health facts written in an easy-to-read, question-and-answer format. Over 1000 health questions are answered. Illustrations are provided throughout. An appendix lists numerous health-related organizations.

Weil A: *Natural health, natural medicine—a comprehensive manual for wellness and self-care*, Boston, 1990, Houghton Mifflin.

One physician's approach to high-level health that emphasizes natural mechanisms. Units on preventive practices, natural treatments, and home remedies form the basis of the book.

UNIT ONE

The first unit in this textbook covers two topics that are closely linked to how we handle change in our lives. Chapter 2 discusses emotional maturity and spiritual growth, and Chapter 3 deals with stress management. As we said in Chapter 1, we believe that your personal growth closely relates to the status of your health, as seen in each of the five dimensions of health. Here are some connections between Unit 1 and the five dimensions of health.

● Physical Dimension of Health

The physical dimension of health is concerned with the structure and function of all body systems. Many of the profoundly important experiences that will shape your feelings about yourself and the value of life are made possible by a highly developed physical dimension. We experience life on the basis of our physical bodies and grow emotionally as the result. Our coping skills often involve responses that require a well-developed physical dimension of health.

◆ Emotional Dimension of Health

Unlike prehistoric humans, who primarily responded physically to confrontation, responses to stress will be largely emotional. Feelings of uneasiness arising from the demands of college, intimate relationships, parenting, or employment are the hallmarks of being stressed. Fortunately, you can cope with threatening change by using the resources associated with the emotional dimension of health. By employing your personal strengths, sense of humor, ability to be empathic, and defense mechanisms, you can persist in the face of demanding change.

■ Social Dimension of Health

Growth and development rarely take place without the influence of other people. At times, your growth and maturation can be bolstered by social relationships. When things go well with roommates, spouses, co-workers, or your own children, you begin to see how capable you are as a social person. Occasional failures in social relationships can be especially bothersome because of the stress they produce. Fortunately, these failures can remind you that emotional growth and stress-management capabilities are critical qualities that take time to develop.

▲ Intellectual Dimension of Health

Throughout your college experience and in the years to follow, intellectual resources will be called on with increasing frequency. Your ability to form creative ideas, integrate material, analyze situations, and think logically will help you function as an educated adult. More important perhaps, these resources from the intellectual dimension of health will help you to enjoy life more fully. They may be able to help you understand and better control your expanding emotional and spiritual growth, regardless of when this growth takes place. It is quite possible that during difficult times you may find the mind to be your most dependable coping source. A book, a lecture, a concert, or art may be a refuge from the stressful events of the classroom, family, or office.

● Spiritual Dimension of Health

A growing body of evidence suggests the presence of a spiritual focus in the lives of many college undergraduates. Many of today's students appear to be searching for a deeper understanding of the meaning of life. Although *you* may not feel personally pressured by the nature of your spiritual beliefs, many students do. The uncertainties arising from exploring what to believe and how to practice what you believe can create stress. One explanation for the renewed interest in the spiritual dimension of health probably stems from its value as a resource during periods of personal stress. Meditation, introspection, and prayer seem to effectively free some people from the tribulations of living in a fast-paced, sometimes uncaring world. To believe deeply in something and to act on that belief through service to others leads to personal enrichment.

The Mind

The Foundation for the Years Ahead

2

Achieving Emotional Maturity
Keys to Your Mental Health

How do you feel about yourself as a person? When you apply the multiple dimensions of health (see Chapter 1) in ways that allow you to direct your own growth, assess deeply held values, deal effectively with change, and interact in a satisfying manner with others, you will be an emotionally healthy person. As such, you will develop and maintain a positive *self-concept* and high level of *self-esteem*. Self-concept can be described as a *perception*, or mental picture, of yourself created by the interplay of beliefs, priorities, and experiences. Self-concept is also balanced by information derived from behaviors. Self-esteem is a sense of *self-acceptance* that accompanies a valid self-concept. For example, balancing marriage, employment, and parenting subsequently leads to a sense of competence. The result is both a positive self-concept and a sense of self-esteem.

Emotionally healthy people can become less emotionally healthy over time and may, in fact, develop a diagnosable emotional (or mental) illness. Information about such conditions is given in Appendix 4 of this textbook; others are addressed in this chapter.

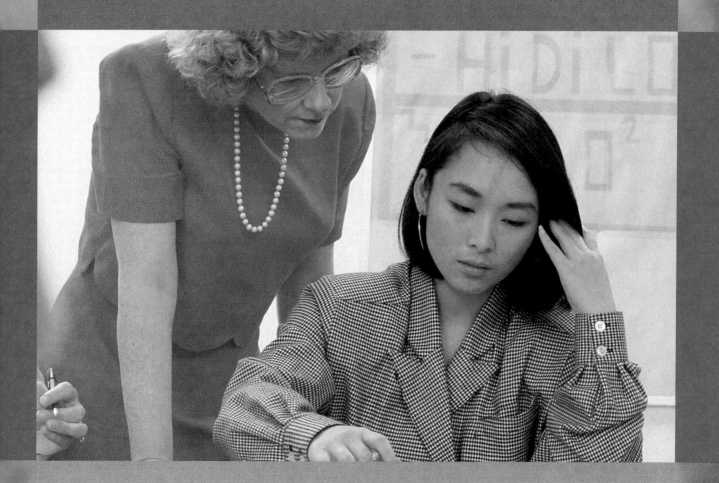

M E N T A L   H E A L T H

The following objectives are covered in this chapter:

▼ Reduce the prevalence of mental disorders (exclusive of substance abuse) among adults living in the community to less than 10.7%. (Baseline: 12.6% in 1984; p. 213.)

▼ Increase to at least 30% the proportion of people aged 18 and older with severe, persistent mental disorders who use community support programs. (Baseline: 15% in 1986; p. 215.)

▼ Increase to at least 45% the proportion of people with major depressive disorders who obtain treatment. (Baseline: 31% in 1982; p. 215.)

▼ Increase to at least 20% the proportion of people aged 18 and older who seek help in coping with personal and emotional problems. (Baseline 11.1% in 1985; p. 216.)

▼ Establish mutual help clearinghouses in at least 25 states. (Baseline: 9 states in 1989; p. 218.)

HEALTHY PEOPLE   2000 OBJECTIVES

REAL LIFE
REAL CHOICES
Self-Acceptance: It Starts With You

▼ Name: Keisha Saunders
▼ Age: 34
▼ University student/single parent

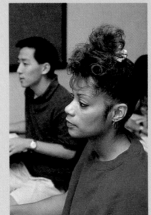

It's a bright, crisp, blue and gold day—the first day of the fall term at the university—and Keisha Saunders has been awake since 5:30 AM, excited and anxious as she prepares to return to school full time after 14 years. She left her bachelor's program in nursing at the end of her sophomore year to get married, and the intervening years have been full of challenges: her husband's death in a construction accident, being a single parent to her two sons while holding down a full-time job, and painstakingly building up her back-to-school fund. Cheerful, energetic, determined, and hard working, she's handled these competing demands with confidence and grace. Now her goal is to complete her bachelor's degree and then go on for a master's so she can either teach or work as a clinical supervisor.

Keisha ticks off items on her mental list: breakfast dishes done, kittens fed, boys off to school—time to go. She glances in the mirror near the front door, and what had been mild anxiety suddenly turns to doubt and fear. I'm too old, she thinks. I don't have anything in common with these kids—the freshmen are just a few years older than Jamal (her older boy, 13). Should I try to fit in, fade into the woodwork, be the class den mother? Will the other students ignore me, make fun of me, roll their eyes when I talk in class? Will I even be older than some of the instructors? Am I making the biggest mistake of my life?

As you study this chapter, think about the challenges Keisha faces as a nontraditional student returning to school, and prepare yourself to answer the questions in **Your Turn** at the end of the chapter. ▼

CHARACTERISTICS OF AN EMOTIONALLY OR MENTALLY HEALTHY PERSON

A more specific yardstick for measuring mental health comes from the National Mental Health Association. This group describes mentally healthy people as those who[1]:

▼ *Feel comfortable about themselves.* They are not overwhelmed by their own emotions, and they can accept many of life's disappointments in stride. They experience all of the human emotions (for example, fear, anger, love, jealousy, guilt, joy) but are not incapacitated by them.
▼ *Feel right about other people.* They feel comfortable with others and are able to give and receive love. They are concerned about the interests of other people and have relationships that are satisfying and lasting.
▼ *Are able to meet the demands of life.* Mentally healthy people respond to their problems, accept responsibility, plan ahead without fearing the future, and are able to establish realistic goals.

At times, mentally healthy people experience stress, frustrations, feelings of self-doubt, failure, and rejection. What distinguishes the mentally healthy is their resilience—their ability to recapture their sense of emotional wellness within a reasonable time.

EMOTIONAL AND PSYCHOLOGICAL HEALTH

Is there a difference between emotional and psychological health? Many people believe that there is little real difference between the terms. Rather, there is only the absence of mental illness and psychopathology.

People who believe that a difference exists would describe that difference on the basis of the focused nature of emotional health and the more global nature of psychological health. To these persons, emotional health relates to the specific (focused) responses of individuals to changing situations within their environment. These responses are subjective in origin and reflect the value orientation of the person. Defense mechanisms (see p. 33) are routinely used to soften the more painful and less acceptable of these feelings. Indeed, responses to change reflecting a sense of joy,

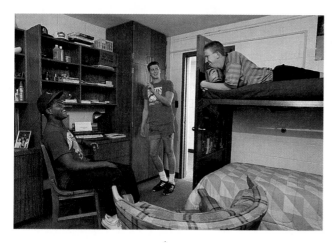

We learn about ourselves through our experiences with others.

anger, compassion, sympathy, empathy, frustration, and disappointment are familiar healthy emotions. Emotionally healthy people feel good about their responses to change, whereas those who are negative about their own feelings and their responses to change are less emotionally healthy.

In comparison to emotional health, psychological health relates to the positive and functional unfolding of the wide array of psychic traits. The extent of these traits is far too broad to be discussed in this textbook but includes the development of language, memory, perceptual processes, awareness states, and, of course, the psychophysical interfacing of the mind and body. Psychologically healthy persons deal rationally with the world, display a fully functional personality, and resolve conflict in a nondestructive manner. Psychologically healthy people use more aspects of the psyche than their feeling states.

PERSONALITY

Although difficult to define, *personality* is a familiar concept that we use to describe the emotional make-up of people, including ourselves. We routinely assign an adjective such as pleasing, destructive, or positive to define the personality of someone in an attempt to describe how we believe that person feels about life and the approach he or she takes in living life. Think about instances when you have been asked by someone to describe the personality of a friend, spouse, employer, or neighbor. Isn't it likely that you equate another's "good" personality with the existence of emotional (or mental) health?

Although there are many viewpoints concerning personality development, there is a general consensus that two factors, *innate* and *environmental*, influence the shaping of personality.[2] Innate factors most likely relate to something called *temperament*. We all know persons who are "by nature" quiet, outgoing, serious, or shy. Nothing, in our opinion, seems capable of changing these persons in the opposite direction. Even though temperament seems to have a biological basis, it still seems to play a part in how we define the emotional health of others. Some would suggest that temperament is the best means we have of observing the innate basis of personality.

Environmental factors influence the more flexible aspects of our personality—those that are layered upon basic temperament. The "up or down," "inward or outward" moods that exist on a given day, or in a given situation, can be impacted by factors as diverse as traffic congestion, weather, social relationships, family harmony, job concerns, and the financial resources that we possess. Understandably then, the personality of a classmate that you initially encounter may prove to be very different after you have had an opportunity to interact with the person over the course of several days and in a variety of settings.

THE NORMAL RANGE OF EMOTIONS

Have you known people who seem to be "up" all the time? These people appear to be confident, happy, and full of good feelings 24 hours a day. Although some people like this may exist, they are truly the exceptions. For most people, emotions are more like a roller coaster ride. At times you feel good about yourself and others; other times nothing seems to be going right. You may feel happy, sad, pleased, uncertain, confident, excited, and afraid—all in the same day or week. To an outsider, you might appear to be "moody." To

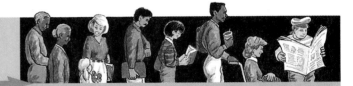

Learning FROM ALL Cultures

Humor

Humor is universal. In fact, there is no known culture in which humor is not present. People everywhere enjoy the funnier moments of everyday life. Humans all use the same elements of humor: incongruity, surprise, and local logic. Situations, however, differ from country to country, therefore making humor somewhat cultural.[15]

A nation's humor reflects its people's lives. Sexuality is a common topic for humor in Great Britain.[15] In the United States, sexual jokes are also popular, but in China and Israel, they are almost nonexistent. Israeli humor is described as aggressive

humor, humor that perhaps reflects the instability of its people's lives due to war and discrimination. This type of humor is evident in American society as we trade jokes about various groups of people, such as jokes about gays or women with blond hair. The French also are known to enjoy aggressive humor, by playfully making fun of others.[15]

A society's history, traditions, and language influence what its people find humorous. Imagine going through life without the ability to see, appreciate, and most importantly, laugh at the incongruities and surprises of our daily existence! ●

the mental health professional, you would probably appear to be normal.

Everyone, not only college students, experiences a range of emotions. This is normal and healthy. Experiencing a range of emotions is an important part of experiencing life. College students should not expect to remain calm and rational every minute of the day. They also should not expect to adjust effectively to every situation with which they are confronted. Life has its ups and downs, and the concept of the "normal range of emotions" reflects this. If there is one concept important for students to understand about mental health, it is this one.

Happiness and a Sense of Humor

Perhaps the most prized emotion to be experienced is a feeling of happiness about life; a feeling that is more likely to occur when day-to-day events are entered into with an underlying sense of humor.

Maintaining a sense of humor is now known to be a critically important component of the emotional dimension of health. People who possess this resource understand that life is not meant to be one long, boring exercise. In fact, part of the reason for living is to have fun. Life taken too seriously can be the most unhappy life imaginable.

Recognizing the humor in daily situations and occasionally being able to laugh at yourself will make you feel better not only about others, but more importantly about yourself. Others will enjoy being associated with you, and it is probable that your ability to perform physically and to recover from injuries and illnesses will be enhanced.[3] Any student-athlete that has experienced a career-threatening injury will tell

you that a positive outlook and a sense of humor were key ingredients in relation to the speed and extent of recovery.

Self-Esteem

The key to overall emotional (or mental) health may be connected to the existence of self-esteem.[4] As discussed earlier in the chapter, a *sense* of self-esteem develops as more and more information that is supportive of our self-concept accumulates. Thus we feel capable and reflect a sense of control in a wide variety of situations in which we find ourselves. We are able to get along with others, cope in stressful situations, and make contributions when we work with others. Self-esteem gives us a sense of our self-worth and may offset our self-defeating behavior patterns.

The beginning of positive self-esteem can be traced back to childhood. For those nontraditional students who are also parents, there are many ways in which your interaction with your young children imparts powerful messages about self-worth. Warm and supportive physical contact, verbal exchanges involving talking "with" rather than "to" children, and the gradual loosening of control so that more and more decisions become those of the child serve to inform children that they have competencies and are valued. Clearly, in terms of their own emerging sense of self-concept and self-esteem, children should "choose their parents very carefully."

As important as parents and others, including the peer group, are to the development of self-esteem, people become responsible for enhancing their own sense of self-esteem. The extent to which individuals wish to nurture their own self-esteem varies. Those

How Does My Self-Concept Compare With My Self-Ideal?

Below you will find a list of 15 personal attributes, each portrayed on a 9-point continuum. Mark with an X where you think you rank on each attribute. Try to be candid and accurate; these marks will collectively describe a portion of your sense of self-concept. When you are finished with the above task, go back and circle where you *wish* you could be on each dimension. These marks describe your self-ideal. Finally, in the spaces on the right, indicate the difference between your self-concept and your self-ideal for each attribute.

| Decisive | Indecisive | _____ |
| 9   8   7   6   5 | 4   3   2   1 | |

Decisive   Indecisive _____
9 8 7 6 5 4 3 2 1

Anxious   Relaxed   _____
9 8 7 6 5 4 3 2 1

Easily influenced Independent thinker _____
9 8 7 6 5 4 3 2 1

Very intelligent Less intelligent _____
9 8 7 6 5 4 3 2 1

In good physical shape In poor physical shape _____
9 8 7 6 5 4 3 2 1

Undependable Dependable _____
9 8 7 6 5 4 3 2 1

Deceitful   Honest   _____
9 8 7 6 5 4 3 2 1

A leader   A follower   _____
9 8 7 6 5 4 3 2 1

Unambitious Ambitious _____
9 8 7 6 5 4 3 2 1

Self-confident Insecure   _____
9 8 7 6 5 4 3 2 1

Conservative Adventurous _____
9 8 7 6 5 4 3 2 1

Extroverted Introverted _____
9 8 7 6 5 4 3 2 1

Physically attractive Physically unattractive _____
9 8 7 6 5 4 3 2 1

Lazy   Hardworking _____
9 8 7 6 5 4 3 2 1

Funny   Little sense of humor _____
9 8 7 6 5 4 3 2 1

TO CARRY THIS FURTHER. . .

1. Overall, how would you describe the discrepancy between your self-concept and your self-ideal (large, moderate, small, large on a few dimensions)?

2. How do sizable gaps for any of your attributes affect your sense of self-esteem?

3. Do you think that any of the gaps exist because you have had others' ideals imposed on you or because you have thoughtlessly accepted others' ideals?

4. Identify several attributes that you realistically believe can be changed to narrow the gap between your self-concept and your self-ideal and, thus, foster a well-developed sense of self-esteem.

PERSONAL ASSESSMENT

who want to take an active role in developing a more comfortable sense of self-esteem could try to meet the following objectives:

▼ *Maintain satisfying group relationships.* The best way to do this is to become affiliated with existing groups, such as social clubs, volunteer organizations, church groups, professional organizations, athletic groups, or any other group that you believe will help you feel a sense of "belonging."

▼ *Set and reach realistic goals.* Achieving their goals allows some people to feel personal power and control over themselves. In turn, this leads to improved self-confidence and further pride and motivation. The key is to make these goals realistic.

▼ *Realize your uniqueness.* The understanding and appreciation that you are indeed a unique and special person will enhance your self-esteem. Enjoy the satisfaction of a compliment when it is given to you. Take time out each day to think about your special strengths and abilities and how they differ from those possessed by others. Pat yourself on the back regularly, and remind yourself that you are a unique and special person.

▼ *Maintain contact with a mentor.* Look for certain key figures in your life who have been helpful to you and who have provided you with inspiration. These role models serve as mentors. The importance of making regular contact with your mentors should not be overlooked.

Depression

Although happiness and a sense of humor have an important, positive influence on emotional health, the full range of human emotions include some that deteriorate our overall emotional (or mental) health. *Depression* is one such mental state. Busy over-extended college students may experience it at least on occasion, and for some it may even disrupt their ability to concentrate on their studies. However, because so many people with depression can be helped, we will approach it from a positive perspective.

Depression refers to an "emotional state characterized by exaggerated feelings of sadness, melancholy, dejection, worthlessness, emptiness, and hopelessness that are inappropriate and out of proportion to reality."[5] Some of the common symptoms of depression are listed in Figure 2-1. One key to recognizing depression is the long-term presence of some of these symptoms. Everyone feels "down" or "blue" at times, but depression is characterized by a more chronic state of feeling "low."

MINOR OR SUBCLINICAL DEPRESSION

Somewhere between feeling down or blue, and being clinically depressed, exists a state of *minor* or *subclinical* depression. Regardless of whether this state lacks

Common Symptoms of Depression

Any of the following may be indications of possible depression:
- Persistent sad moods
- Feelings of hopelessness or pessimism
- Loss of interest or pleasure in ordinary activities, including sex
- Sleep and eating disorders
- Restlessness, irritability, or fatigue
- Difficulty concentrating, remembering, or making decisions
- Thoughts of death or suicide
- Persistent physical symptoms or pains that do not respond to treatment

Figure 2-1 Common symptoms of depression.

the degree of neurological dysfunction and, thus, lacks the majority of symptoms associated with major depression, or is simply missed by clinicians, it is, nevertheless, capable of causing an *amotivational* state. Hopefully for persons with this "minor" form of depression, sufficient symptoms will occur such that it can be recognized, or it will resolve itself because of a change in the environment.

MAJOR OR CLINICAL DEPRESSION

In the United States, it is estimated that approximately 25% of the adult population will experience some symptoms of depression in their lives.[6] People with depression commonly have a number of compounding problems, including difficulty with social relationships and family problems. Depression is a common factor related to many suicides.[7]

Types

According to mental-health experts, there are two main types of major or clinical depression. When depression develops after a period of difficulty, such as going through a divorce or losing a job, it is called *secondary* or *reactive depression*. However, when depression develops for no apparent reason, it is called *primary depression* and is caused by changes in brain chemistry. People with this type of depression are helped most by antidepressive drugs, whereas people with secondary depression often require counseling in addition to medications.

Collectively, secondary or reactive depression and primary depression are known as *unipolar* depression to distinguish them from *bipolar* depression. This latter form involves alternating periods of *mania* in which people are "up," followed by depressive periods during which they are very "down."

A recently recognized cause for some persons' depressive-like moods is a condition identified as *sea-*

Health ACTION Guide

Where to Go for Help with Depression

If you or a friend had concerns about depression, would you know where to search for help? Regardless of where you are—large city, suburban community, or a rural area—a variety of resources are available.

▼ Seek help from your university health center, personal physician, or community health center.
▼ Try your university mental health counseling and treatment programs.
▼ Family and social service agencies can identify mental health specialists.
▼ Check the telephone book for private psychologists or psychiatric clinics.

▼ Talk with your professor.
▼ Contact one of the organizations listed below:

The Depression/Awareness, Recognition and Treatment Program, (operated by the National Institute of Mental Health)
Room 15-C-05, 5600 Fishers Lane
Rockville, MD 20857

The National Foundation for Depressive Illness
P.O. Box 2257
New York, NY 10016

The National Mental Health Association
1021 Prince St.
Alexandria, VA 22314

The Manic-Depressive Illness Foundation
2723 P St.
Washington, DC 20007

---

sonal affective disorder. (See the following discussion.) Note its similarity to major depression, which was just described. Additionally, suicide relates to depressive states (see discussion on the right). For some, the continuing existence of an amotivational state is the basis for an eventual suicide attempt.

Through a variety of therapies, between 70% and 90% of depressed people can be helped. Therapies range from various "talking" strategies (including counseling) to the use of antidepressant drugs. Unlike the antianxiety or tranquilizer drugs that sedate, most antidepressant drugs prescribed today work by influencing neurotransmitters (chemicals released by the nervous system that help transmit impulses; see Chapter 7.) Today, four major types of antidepressant medications are in use including the *serotonin-reuptake inhibitors.* Prozac, the most frequently prescribed form of antidepressant, is a member of this classification. Many of today's antidepressant drugs produce few side effects, although some are not without controversy.[8]

Only a small percentage (about 33%) of depressed people ever seek help. This is unfortunate in light of the high rate of successful treatment.

Seasonal Affective Disorder (SAD) Syndrome

Recently, scientists have discovered that certain people may be especially vulnerable to depression on a seasonal basis. SAD is a form of depression that develops in certain persons who live in cold climates (Figure 2-2). SAD affects four times as many women as men and is characterized by weight gain, excessive lethargy and sleep, social withdrawal, loss of sex drive, and mood

swings, including feeling anxious and irritable. Although seen in adolescents, SAD more commonly begins in the young adult years.

SAD patients routinely feel much better with the coming of spring and summer, when the days are longer and the amount of sunlight increases. Fortunately, exposure to prescribed amounts of intense fluorescent light (phototherapy) helps many sufferers of SAD during the winter months. Anyone who suspects SAD or other forms of depression should seek professional assistance, perhaps through a counseling center or health center on campus.

Suicide

One of the major tragedies of our times is the high incidence of suicide. In the last year for which statistics are available (1988), 30,900 persons in the United States killed themselves.[16] Among young people (including college students), suicides follow accidents as the second leading cause of death.

What separates the potentially suicidal person from the nonsuicidal person is the degree of despair and depression experienced and the inability to cope with it. Suicidal persons tend to become overwhelmed with a range of destructive emotions, including anxiety, anger, loneliness, loss of self-esteem, and hopelessness. Suicidal persons may feel that their death is a solution to all that is afflicting them. Rarely, however, does suicide solve a problem.

In fact, college students who use suicide to resolve academic failure, difficulties with relationships, or an inability to find employment leave far greater problems for others that dwarf the original concern.

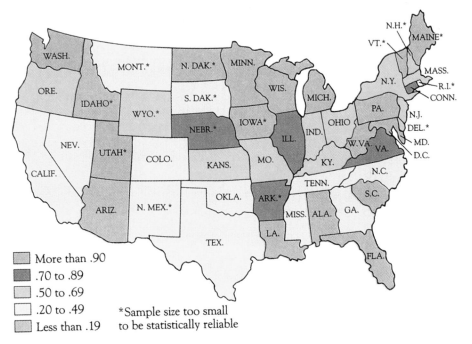

Figure 2-2 Prevalence of SAD in the United States varies with latitude. In a northern state such as Minnesota, SAD affects more than 100 people per 1000, whereas in Florida it affects fewer than six people per 100,000. (Asterisks indicate a sample that is too small to be reliable.)

★ **Warning Signs of Suicidal Behaviors**

★ **Change in appetite**

★ **Change in sleep pattern**

★ **Decreased concentration**

★ **Decreased interest in activities that were a source of pleasure**

★ **Sudden agitation or sudden slowing down in level of activity**

★ **Social withdrawal**

★ **Feelings of hopelessness, worthlessness, and self-reproach**

★ **Inappropriate or excessive guilt**

★ **Suicidal thoughts and/or talk**

★ **Making a suicide plan**

★ **Writing a suicide note**

★ **Giving away prized possessions**

★ **Recent humiliating life event**

★ **Lack of social supports**

SUICIDE PREVENTION

Many communities are recognizing the need to provide or expand suicide prevention services. Suicide prevention centers are already available in many communities. Most suicide prevention centers operate 24-hour hot lines and are staffed through volunteer agencies, mental health centers, public health departments, and hospitals. Staff members in these centers have extensive training in counseling skills required to deal with suicide-prone persons. Phone numbers for these services can be found in the telephone directory.

What signs and symptoms could indicate that a person might be considering suicide? It is recommended that we watch for the symptoms listed in the Star Box. People need professional help when they show a clustering of these suicide warning signs for more than 2 weeks.

Loneliness

Although not always associated with depression, signs of loneliness are displayed by many people who are depressed. People are said to be lonely if they "desire close personal relationships but are unable to establish them."[9] It is quite possible to feel isolated and without friends even when you are around many people in your everyday life. Feeling lonely is a common concern for many college students.

The difference between "being alone" and "feeling lonely" is important. Many people enjoy being alone

Defense Mechanisms: Protecting the Ego

Stressors, particularly when they are dealt with poorly, can challenge our self-perception, or ego. In an attempt to protect the delicate ego, we subconsciously use a variety of defense mechanisms. Many of the following will be familiar to you.

Compensation	Covering our weaknesses by emphasizing our more desirable traits; overachieving in one area to minimize our inadequacies in another
Denial	Refusing to accept the existence of something that should be obvious to us
Displacement	Redirecting our feelings about an original stressor to other persons, objects, or events
Fantasy	Escaping from reality through the use of imagination
Intellectualization	Applying intellectual operations to resolve a stressor or to protect ourselves from dealing in a more personal or emotional manner; objectivity rather than subjectivity
Isolation	Detaching ourselves emotionally from the source and resolution of a stressor
Projection	Assigning our own unacceptable feelings to another person; often our own fear or uncertainty is said to be the fear or uncertainty held by another
Rationalization	Attributing a rational explanation to our own irrational behavior or feelings
Reaction formation	Responding in a manner that is generally directly opposite to the manner in which we feel or would like to respond
Regression	Escaping from stressors by returning to more childlike, less mature responses
Repression	Suppressing uncomfortable feelings from reaching a level of consciousness; frequently we forget what we do not wish to remember

★ Now that defense mechanisms have been reviewed, are they familiar in the sense that you have on occasion employed them?

★ Are defense mechanisms innate, or are we subtly taught what they are and how to employ them in particular situations?

★ At what point is it possible that we are relying too heavily on the use of defense mechanisms?

occasionally to relax, to exercise, to read, to enjoy music, or just to think. These people can appreciate being alone, but they can also interact comfortably with others when they wish. However, when being alone or isolated is not an enjoyable experience and seeking close relationships is very difficult, then feeling lonely can produce serious feelings of rejection.

One unfortunate aspect of loneliness is that it tends to continue in people year after year, unless they take an active approach to change it. Chronically lonely people frequently cope with their loneliness by becoming consumed by their occupations or adopting habit-forming behaviors that further make them feel lonely.

The positive side of loneliness is that there are successful techniques that can help most lonely people. Counseling can help change how these people think about themselves when they interact with others. Another way involves teaching people important social skills, such as starting a conversation, taking social risks, and introducing themselves. Through social skills training, people can also learn to talk comfortably on the telephone, give and receive compliments, and even learn how to enhance their appearance. If you need help in this area, contact your campus counseling center or health center.

Shyness

Is loneliness the result of an inability to interact with others, something brought about by *shyness*? If so, why are some people so shy? Some contend that shyness is a genetically programmed component of temperament. Thus, people are shy not because they want to be shy, nor because they have been conditioned to avoid contact with others, nor because they have had unpleasant experiences with others, but rather, because they are genetically programmed to feel uncomfortable in settings involving other persons. Accordingly, they cope by avoiding such situations. Even if correct, the social skill counseling and training suggested in the discussion of loneliness can be applied to shyness. What do you think?

DEVELOPING COMMUNICATION SKILLS

Loneliness and depression, two of the more common conditions suggesting a less than optimal level of emotional health, are described earlier in the chapter. Both conditions have in common the possibility that they are the consequence of feeling uncomfortable with others. When people find it difficult to initiate or even participate in conversations with others, it is likely that they have not developed some of the communication skills with which others feel comfortable. In this section we will investigate how speaking and listening can foster improved social relationships. We will also look at the use of unspoken communication as an aid to social interaction. Remember that how you see yourself (self-concept) influences how you feel about yourself (self-esteem).

Verbal Communication

Communication between you and others can be viewed in terms of your role as sender or receiver of the spoken language. You can enhance your effectiveness as a sender of verbal information by implementing several important steps.[10]

▼ Take the time to think before speaking. Effective communication requires that you know what you want to say.

▼ Focus your words on the most important portions of your thoughts and ideas. Not every idea is as important as the central ideas that you are attempting to communicate.

▼ Speak clearly and concisely. This will aid the listener, particularly when your ideas are complex or new.

▼ Talk with, rather than at, your listener. Speaking with another person encourages the listener to share freely and comfortably with you.

▼ Start on a positive note. Even when your message may be negative, a more positive atmosphere is established when conversation begins in this manner.

▼ Seek feedback from your listener. Provide frequent intervals between your ideas to allow the listener to respond.

▼ Use other forms of communication to transmit important ideas when face-to-face conversation is not effective. Written communication or the use of a carefully selected third person is often highly effective.

Verbal communication requires that you function as skillfully as a listener, or receiver, as you do as a sender of spoken ideas. Certainly, there are skills for structuring the exchange of information. A variety of listening approaches appear below.

▼ Listen with attention. In many situations it will be important to you to hear everything that is being said.

▼ This is particularly true when you must hear and fully understand the ideas that the speaker is attempting to share.

▼ Listen selectively to what the speaker is saying. It may be the best use of your time and "listening energy" to filter out some of what is being said while

continuing to concentrate on interesting, new, or important information.

▼ On some occasions, it may be necessary to prevent a speaker from beginning or continuing a discussion. You must therefore possess the ability and willingness to tell another "That's it, our conversation is over," or "You can continue talking if you wish, but I'm not listening to what you are saying."

▼ By pretending to listen, you can accomplish a version of this same tactic. When hearing the same information over and over, it may be kinder to "listen" to the speaker without actually listening.

Nonverbal Communication

At times you share information without speaking or hearing an exchange of words. This is nonverbal communication. It is important that you recognize your nonverbal communication techniques so that you can control their impact.[11]

▼ Facial expressions often condition the receptiveness with which you will be met. Perhaps the most valuable advice is to look pleasant and happy when you are with other people.

▼ Eye contact is an important component of positive nonverbal communication. Practice by looking at yourself in the mirror, at a face on television, or at a photograph.

▼ Learn to comfortably touch others, particularly when you would want to be touched in a similar situation or setting. Touching may be the most important component of nonverbal communication. Do so, however, with care and sensitivity.

▼ Learn when the distance between you and another person is appropriate. Each person has his or her own idea of how close is too close and how far is too far.

▼ "Dress for success." We are often judged by what we are wearing in a particular setting or at a particular time. The "wrong" clothing may quickly ruin the impression you are attempting to make.

▼ Assume a posture that is in line with your verbal communication. As with dress, your body position (posture) can help or hinder the impression you are attempting to create in the mind of the person with whom you are interacting.

As with verbal communication, when nonverbal components are recognized and controlled, you will communicate more effectively.

MASLOW'S HIERARCHY OF NEEDS

In Maslow's important contribution to twentieth-century American psychological thought (the hierarchy of needs), he views emotional growth in terms of inner needs and motivation. Maslow lists motivational requirements in the following order: physiological

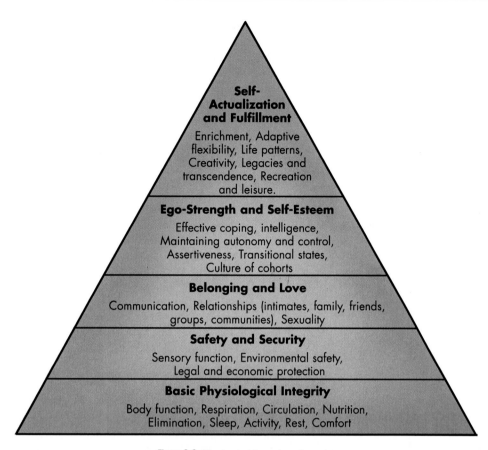

Figure 2-3 Maslow's hierarchy of needs.

needs, safety needs, belonging and love needs, esteem needs, and self-actualization needs (Figure 2-3). He distinguishes between the lower *deficiency needs* and the higher *being needs.* We do not seek the higher needs until the lower demands have been reasonably satisfied.

The healthiest and most effective people in society are those whose lives embody being values such as truth, beauty, goodness, faith, wholeness, and love. Maslow labels these as "Theory Z" people, or **transcenders. Self-actualization,** the highest level of self-development, is clearly evident in the transcender's personality. Transcenders are described as follows[12]:

▼ Transcenders have more peak or creative experiences and naturally speak the language of being values.

▼ Transcenders are more responsive to beauty, more holistic in their perceptions of humanity and the cosmos, adjust well to conflict situations, and work more wholeheartedly toward goals and purposes.

▼ Transcenders are innovators who are attracted to mystery and the unknown and see themselves as instruments for the actualization of the transpersonal being values.

▼ Transcenders tend to fuse work and play. They are

less attracted by the rewards of money and objects and more motivated by the satisfaction of being and service values.

▼ Transcenders are more likely to accept others with an unconditional positive regard, and they tend to be more oriented toward spiritual reality.

You might have noticed the similarity between transcenders and people with positive self-esteem. In following the Health Action Guide to improve self-esteem, you may also find yourself fulfilling Maslow's higher needs. If you desire to, you can become more of a transcender than you presently are.

---

transcenders (tran **send** urs) self-actualized people who have achieved a quality of being ordinarily associated with higher levels of spiritual growth.

self-actualization (self ackt **yoo** all iz **ay** shun) highest level of personality development; self-actualized persons recognize their roles in life and use personal strengths to reach their fullest potential.

CREATIVE EXPRESSION

Emotionally healthy people have a free and open approach to life. You have surely observed that they think and act positively. They also assess people and situations realistically and constructively. When you interact with emotionally healthy people, you quickly notice their flexibility in solving problems. How did these individuals become so secure, competent, and constructive? Is it possible that you too will mature in this direction? What resources will you need to help you grow in a similar fashion?

The Institute of Personality Assessment at the University of California has identified traits that characterize creative people. Assuming that **creativity** is closely related to emotional health, these traits may help describe emotionally healthy people:

▼ Creative people are intuitive and have an openness to experience. They are spontaneous and expressive and have the courage to reveal themselves. They are relatively free from fear and are not disturbed by the unknown, the mysterious, or the puzzling.

▼ Creative people are not interested in detail but in meaning and implications. They tend to be more theoretical than pragmatic in their orientation. These people have the ability to unify, synthesize, and integrate materials and experiences.

▼ Creative people are independent, self-accepting, and autonomous, yet they are not authoritarian in their attitudes. They tend to resist group work and function best when allowed to work independently in the field of their interest.

▼ Creative people are flexible. They do not use *either-or* nor *black-white* thinking but recognize that there are many ways to interpret the same situation.

▼ Creative people are governed by an internal set of values and are persistent in developing ideas and working toward goals.

You may recognize many of these characteristics as being already well developed in your personality. You may not have mastered some traits listed, and they may now appear beyond your reach. Nevertheless, you can increase your creativity if you let your high level of health help you face new challenges.

SPIRITUAL/FAITH DEVELOPMENT

A fully developed sense of self-esteem may, in the final analysis, require a knowledge and acceptance of yourself as a person of **faith.** Certainly, older adults with whom we have had contact have little difficulty sharing that they believe in something or someone greater than themselves and that this belief brings them great comfort and a sense of support. Many report that because of their personal level of faith, they do not fear death because they know that their lives have had

meaning within the context of a larger plan. Further, they would urge younger people to search for both the strength and direction in their lives that faith provides.[13]

As a resource in the spiritual dimension of health, the existence of faith provides a basis on which a belief system can mature and an expanding awareness of life's meaning can be fostered. In addition, the existence of faithfulness gives meaning (or additional meaning) to our *vocation* and assists us in better understanding the consequences of our vocational efforts. Further, faith in something (or someone) influences many of the experiences that we will seek throughout life and tempers the emotional relationships that we have with these experiences.[14]

In virtually all cultures, faith and its accompanying belief system provide individuals and groups with *rituals* and *practices* that foster the development of a sense of community—"a community of faith." In turn, the community provides the authority and guidance that nurtures the emotional stability, confidence, and sense of competence needed for living life fully.[13]

 How Does My Faith Affect My Life?

James Fowler[14] describes the nature of faith as a fundamental, universal, but infinitely varied value response within the human experience. Faith can include religious practice but also can be quite distinct. Faith is the most fundamental category in the human quest for the meaning of life. It is a developing focus of the total person that gives purpose and meaning to thoughts.

By the time people reach college age, it is possible that the maturation of their faith has placed them into a series of uncomfortable situations. These include the need to take seriously the burden of responsibility for their own commitments, lifestyles, beliefs, and attitudes. Tension and anxiety can arise because the growth of faith requires them to make personal decisions. It demands objectivity and a certain amount of independence and requires finding balances between personal aspirations and a developing sense of service to others. Finally, symbols and doctrines must be translated into personalized spiritual concepts that can then be validated on the basis of experience.

★ In light of the potential for young adults to grow in their faith, what have been your own personal experiences?

★ Would you consider yourself to be more or less "faithful" than your friends or other family members?

★ What school-related experiences have impacted most powerfully on the spiritual dimension of your health?

A PLAN FOR ENHANCING YOUR MENTAL AND EMOTIONAL HEALTH

A key to mental and emotional health rests in your interest and ability to control your own experiences. In this section, we will share a simple plan that you can use to control your experiences and, as a result, learn a great deal about yourself. Figure 2-4 shows a four-step process that continues throughout life: constructing mental pictures, accepting them, undertaking new experiences, and reframing your mental pictures. With some thought and practice, this plan can be carried out when you have the time and interest to do so.

Constructing Mental Pictures

Actively taking charge of your mental and emotional growth begins when you construct a mental picture of what you are like. This mental picture or perception should be composed of the most recent and accurate information you have about yourself. Information concerning the knowledge that is important to you, the values that you hold, and the activities in which you are competent is the material from which this picture will take shape. For example, you might envision yourself in a job interview responding to the information being given to you and the questions being asked of you.

To construct this mental picture of yourself, you will need to set aside a period of uninterrupted quiet time. This period for reflection is very important. Even in the midst of a busy schedule, most of us can "free up" several moments for a task that is important.

Before continuing to the second step in your plan for emotional development, it is important that you construct, in addition to a mental picture about *yourself*, similar mental pictures about yourself in relation to *other people* and *material objects*, including your col-

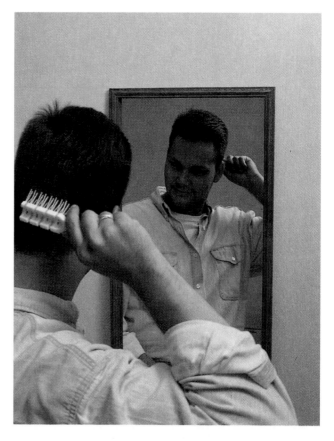

How you see yourself?

lege environment, residence, and work environment. You will then have a clearer picture of yourself and how you relate to other people and material objects. (See Figure 2-5.)

Accepting Mental Pictures

The second step of the plan involves an *acceptance* of your mental pictures. Acceptance implies a willingness on your part to honor the truthfulness of the pictures you have formed about yourself and other people. The concept of acceptance also reflects your willingness to use material objects.

As in the first step of the plan, the second stage requires time and commitment from you. Controlling your own emotional development is rarely a passive process. You must be willing to be *introspective* about yourself and the world around you.

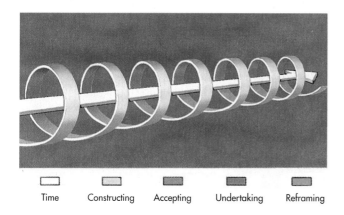

| Time | Constructing | Accepting | Undertaking | Reframing |

Figure 2-4 If you visualize the growth of the emotional dimension of your health as a four-component process, you will see the *cyclic* nature of your continued emotional growth throughout the life cycle.

creativity innovative ability; insightful capacity to solve problems; ability to move beyond analytical or logical approaches to experience.

faith the purposes and meaning that underlie an individual's hopes and dreams.

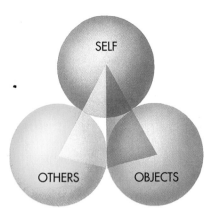

Figure 2-5 The individual interacts with the self, others, and material objects in order to grow.

Undertaking New Experiences

Of the 31 students who traveled to London, England, for one semester, 29 spent every free evening and weekend "exploring." No part of the United Kingdom was beyond their reach. Two students, however, spent nearly all their free time in the hotel room that they shared—writing letters, doing each other's hair, or watching the small television they had rented.

This story is an experience that one of us had with a group of undergraduate students. The two students who preferred the "comfort" of their small hotel room generated these questions in the minds of all who witnessed their inactivity: "Why did you bother coming to London?"; "What are you afraid of finding?"; and "Does it bother you that we do so much while you stay behind all the time?"

To mature emotionally you must progress beyond the first two steps of the prescription and test the newly formed perceptions you have constructed. This *testing* is accomplished by *undertaking a new experience* or reexperiencing something in a different way. Being in college and living away from home is certainly an example of this "new experience" for many of you.

As often as not, these new experiences do not require high levels of risk, foreign travel, or the outlay of money. They may be no more "new" than deciding to try an advanced course in a particular department, to move from the dorm into an apartment, to take a summer job that is different from your last, or to start a new friendship. The experience itself is not the end you are seeking; rather, it is a means of reaching a new "pool" of information about yourself, others, or the objects that form your material world.

Reframing Mental Pictures

If you have completed the first three steps in this plan for achieving emotional growth, the new information

Developing Your Emotional Growth

Emotional growth requires both knowing about yourself and learning from new experiences. The activities listed below can be used in support of these requirements.

★ **Keep a daily journal.** Writing down your thoughts and making note of experiences are effective tools in fostering greater self-understanding. Once written, the information that these accounts contain can be reprocessed for an even greater awareness of self.

★ **Join a support group.** Sharing experiences and feelings in the presence of people who can "stand in your shoes" creates an environment that will support your efforts to grow as a more interesting and self-directed person. Additionally, being an active participant in a support group also functions as a "new experience" through which new insights into your sense of self-worth can be gained.

★ **Take an assertiveness course.** Learning how to greet others, give and receive compliments, use "I" statements, express spontaneity, and state your feelings of disagreement are important tools in developing self-confidence. Very likely, an assertiveness course is or will be offered on your campus.

★ **Seek counseling.** Nowhere is counseling generally more available and affordable than on a college campus. Clearly, much can be learned about your sense of self and the psychological factors that have shaped it. Furthermore, growth-enhancing skills can be formulated and tested in both individual and group counseling sessions. Contact the campus health center or the psychological services center for referral to an experienced psychologist or counselor. What additional activities can you think of that would further your self-knowledge or serve as new experiences?

about yourself, others, and objects now becomes the most current source of information available for your use. Regardless of the type of new experience you have undertaken and its outcome, you are now in a position to modify the initial perceptions you constructed during the first step of this plan. You have new insights, knowledge, and perspective.

This new picture of yourself may not be too different from the perceptions it replaced. However, it will have resulted from a process that is growth oriented. By continuing to engage in this four-step process, your emotional growth will continue, and you will experience a higher level of mental health.

EMOTIONAL (OR MENTAL) HEALTH: A FINAL THOUGHT

As discussed in the introduction to Chapter 2, emotional (or mental) health is much more than the absence of clinically recognized mental illnesses. Rather, it is the resourcefulness that you are able to apply toward directing your own growth, assessing your belief and value system, and dealing effectively with change, particularly when change is unexpected and over which you will never have complete control. Emotionally healthy people possess a self-concept constructed on traits that are satisfying and also capable of contributing to the well-being of others. Consequently they experience a high level of self-esteem. The specific resources that you draw from the emotional and spiritual dimensions of your health to accomplish this will, of course, be unique to you.

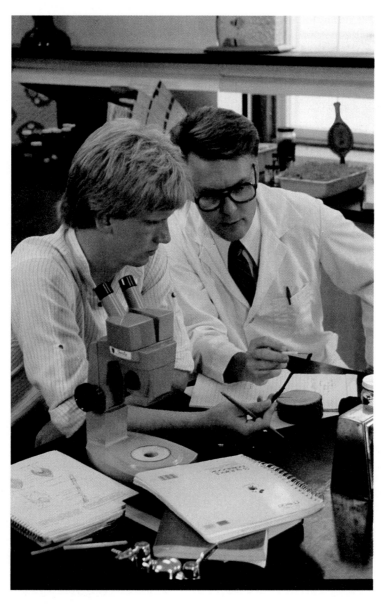

Success in meeting challenges will change how you see yourself.

Summary

- ✔ Emotional (or mental health) reflects resourcefulness that exceeds the absence of mental illness.
- ✔ A positive self-concept forms the basis of a high level of self-esteem.
- ✔ Emotionally healthy people feel comfortable about themselves and are able to meet the demands of life.
- ✔ Emotional health and psychological health are related but different concepts.
- ✔ Personality has both an innate and environmental basis.
- ✔ Happiness and a sense of humor are important resources within the emotional dimension of health.
- ✔ Depression is a commonly occurring and easily identified form of emotional illness.
- ✔ Loneliness results in the absence of adequate human contact.
- ✔ Shyness, leading to difficulty in interacting with others, may be the basis of loneliness.
- ✔ Effective skills for verbal and nonverbal communication can be learned and effectively applied.
- ✔ Creative people possess a unique outlook and approach to life.
- ✔ Faith gives meaning to life and helps structure a supportive community for the individual.
- ✔ A four-step plan can be used to foster emotional growth and maturity.

Review Questions

1. How could a person free from any diagnosable mental illness still be considered as possessing a less than high level of emotional health?
2. How do self-concept and self-esteem relate to each other?
3. What is meant by the "normal range of emotions?"
4. What makes the term *psychological health* more encompassing than the term *emotional health?*
5. What label is used to identify the innately determined aspect of personality?
6. How does a sense of humor contribute to a high level of emotional (or mental) health?
7. What are the two principal types of depression and how do they differ in terms of symptoms?
8. How could shyness contribute to a person's sense of loneliness?
9. What are several characteristics of effective verbal and nonverbal communication?
10. How does a sense of faith contribute to a high level of emotional health?
11. What steps can be taken to foster emotional maturation?

Think about This . . .

- ✔ How close do you come to meeting the characteristics of a mentally healthy person?
- ✔ Do you take yourself too seriously at times?
- ✔ Which traits of creativity have you developed within your makeup?
- ✔ Are you ready to undertake a new experience? What kind of experience will it be?
- ✔ What aspects of your personality do you sense as having been innately determined?
- ✔ In what or who do you place your deepest trust? To what extent would you describe yourself as being religious?
- ✔ How would others describe your level of self-esteem? How do their interpretations compare to your own sense of self-esteem?

REAL LIFE REAL CHOICES

YOUR TURN

▼ What kinds of risks is Keisha Saunders taking by returning to school after 14 years?

▼ Of the challenges Keisha confronts as a nontraditional student, which do you think are real and which might she be imagining or exaggerating?

▼ In what ways can Keisha's life experiences and personal qualities contribute to her success as a nontraditional student?

AND NOW, YOUR CHOICES . . .

▼ If you're a nontraditional student, imagine you're in circumstances similar to Keisha's. What would be your concerns? How do you think you would behave?

▼ If you're a traditional student, have you ever been in class with one or more nontraditional students? If so, what did you like or dislike about the experience? Why?

References

1. *Mental health 1-2-3*, National Mental Health Association: Alexandria, Va, 1992, The Association.
2. Gedo JE: The roots of personality: heredity and environment, *Harvard Medical School Health Letter* 7(1):4-6, July 1990.
3. Rose JF: Psychologic health of women: a phenomenologic study of women's inner strength, *Ad Nurs Sci*, 12(2):56, 1990.
4. Robson P: Improving self-esteem, *Harvard Medical School Mental Health Letter* 6(12):3, 1990.
5. *Mosby's medical, nursing, and allied health dictionary*, ed 4, St Louis, 1994, Mosby.
6. Johnson D, Weissman M, Klerman GL: Service utilization and social morbidity associated with depressive symptoms in the community, *JAMA* 267(11):1478, 1992.
7. Wells LA: *Psychiatric nursing*, St Louis, 1989, Warren H. Green.
8. Angier N: Eli Lilly facing million-dollar suits on its antidepressant drug Prozac, *The New York Times*, August 16, 1990, p B13.
9. Baron RA, Byrne D: *Social psychology: understanding human interaction*, ed 6, Boston, 1991, Allyn & Bacon.
10. Masters W, Johnson V, Kolodny R: *Human sexuality*, ed 4, Glenview, Ill, 1992, Harper Collins.
11. Haas A, Haas K: *Understanding sexuality*, ed 3, St Louis, 1993, Mosby.
12. Maslow AH: *The farthest reaches of human nature*, Magnolia, Mass, 1983, Peter Smith.
13. Hemenway JE (editor): *Assessing spiritual needs: a guide for caregivers*, Minneapolis, MN, 1993, Augsburg Fortress Press.
14. Fowler J: *Faith development and pastoral care*, Philadelphia, 1987, Fortress Press.
15. Ziv A, ed: *National styles of humor*, New York, 1988, Greenwood Press.
16. U.S. Dept. Health and Human Services: Annual summary of births, marriages, divorces, and deaths: United States, 1992, *Monthly Vital Statistics Report* 41(13):7, 1993.

Suggested Readings

Dowling C: *You mean I don't have to feel this way? New help for depression, anxiety, and addiction*, New York, 1992, Scribners.

This book supports a biological basis for many of the dysfunctions that occur today. Treatments appropriate for depression, eating disorders, and anxiety are discussed. The author believes that most people need professional assistance in dealing with their dysfunctions.

Kinder M: *Going nowhere fast: step off life's treadmills and find peace of mind*, New York, 1990, Prentice Hall.

As a clinical psychologist, the author believes that our struggles to be "perfect" have put many of us on a dangerous treadmill that makes an enjoyable life virtually unattainable. Real peace of mind comes from our understanding of our inner selves. The author states that it is up to us to change ourselves.

Sobel D: *The Healing Brain*, New York, 1993, Simon & Schuster.

The placebo effects (X-factor) is now recognized and used by physicians in helping patients recover from illness. Sobel traces the role of the placebo effect in earlier eras of health care and describes how it is being incorporated into modern medicine.

Yapko MD: *Free yourself from depression*, Emmaus, Pa, 1992, Rodale Press.

The author, a psychologist and hypnotist, prescribes a variety of techniques for overcoming mild depressive symptoms. The book is specific in its direction, including the use of traditional therapies, medication, and "self-help" techniques. Information on the principal causes of depression is also provided.

3

Stress

Managing the Unexpected

n the midwestern states there is a familiar saying that suggests that if you do not like the weather, "just wait a few minutes and it will change." Rapid and often unanticipated change characterizes the weather of that region. People who choose to live in that part of the country need to be prepared for dealing with such rapid climatic fluctuations.

Inasmuch as the weather is characterized by change, daily living is also influenced by change. Each person, program, and object in your immediate environment holds the potential for being threatening to you because of its ability to change. Being able to control or adjust to this threatening change can enrich your life because change is often challenging, stimulating, and rewarding. When you handle change poorly, however, your response results in a state of stress that can be disruptive to your health and unpleasant to experience.

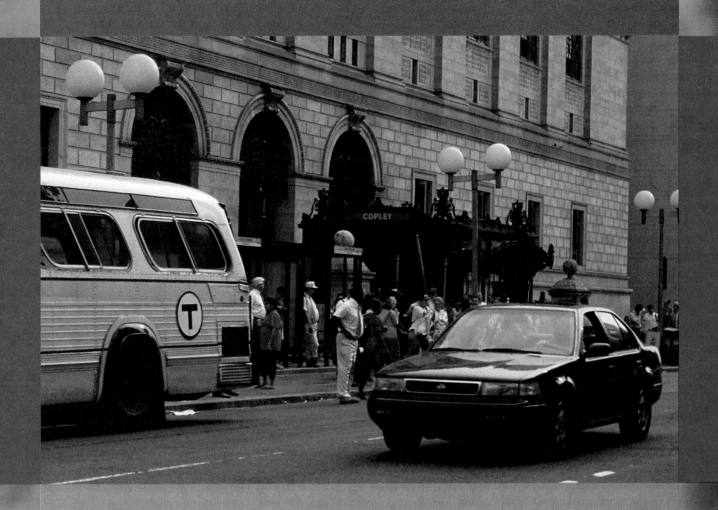

S T R E S S

The following objectives will be covered in this chapter:

▼ Reduce to less than 35% the proportion of people aged 18 and older who experience adverse health effects from stress within the past year. (Baseline: 42.6% in 1985; p. 214.)

▼ Reduce by 15% the incidence of injurious suicide attempts among adolescents aged 14 through 17. (p. 211.)

▼ Decrease to no more than 5% the proportion of people aged 18 and older who report experiencing significant levels of stress and do not take steps to reduce or control their stress. (Baseline: 21% in 1985; p. 216.)

▼ Increase to at least 40% the proportion of worksites employing 50 or more people that provide programs to reduce employee stress. (Baseline: 26.6% in 1985; p. 213.)

REAL LIFE
REAL CHOICES
School + Work + Family = Stress

▼ Name: Kate Sullivan
▼ Age: 21
▼ Occupation:
   Student/telemarketer/custodian

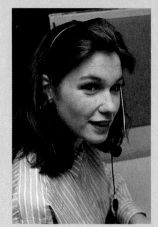

Four months from earning her bachelor's degree in social work, Kate Sullivan should be proud, happy, and excited. She'll graduate with honors from a prestigious university, and she's already been awarded a fellowship to work on her master's degree.

Kate does feel happy about her accomplishments and her future—when she has time. That's not very often, because for the last 4 years she's done very little except study and work. Although she's on a tuition scholarship, Kate must work to pay for her living expenses, as well as making payments on the used car she needs to get to and from school and her two part-time jobs.

The oldest of seven children in a single-parent family, Kate sends home half of what she earns each month. When she was small, her father died in an automobile accident and left no money or insurance. After working for more than 20 years in a fertilizer processing plant, her mother is now on Social Security disability because of damage to her lungs and skin. Kate's younger brothers and sisters aren't old enough to earn much money, and Kate wants them to concentrate on their schoolwork, so she puts in as many extra hours as she can at her two jobs.

Parties, sports, clubs, vacations—these are foreign words to Kate. All her life she's worked hard and taken on adult responsibilities, and it's never occurred to her to feel sorry for herself. Recently, however, she's had trouble concentrating on her schoolwork, and more than once she's fallen asleep in a lecture. She averages about 5 hours of sleep a night and has been waking up feeling as tired as if she's run a marathon. Concerned friends and her academic advisor urge her to ease up and take some time off to relax, but Kate is afraid that if she lets up for a minute, she'll never catch up.

As you study this chapter, think about the stressors in Kate's life and prepare yourself to answer the questions in **Your Turn** at the end of the chapter. ▼

STRESS AND STRESSORS

Almost every day on a college campus you can hear people comment about how much stress they are under. College administrators feel **stress** as they strive to maintain a positive image for their school. Department chairpersons feel pressures to maintain course enrollments. Professors may feel stress when they are assigned new courses to teach or when their journal articles are rejected. Coaches want to apply "positive stress" to the athletes to improve their performances. Certainly, for college students, the demands of school, employment, marriage, and parenting can produce feelings of distress.

Although people often use *stress* and *stressor* interchangeably, the words represent different concepts. Hans Selye,[1] the father of stress theory, described stress as "the nonspecific response of the body to any demand made on it." Stress can be viewed as a physiological and psychological response that results after one is exposed to some factor, agent, or event that forces the person to change or adapt. These factors or events that produce stress are called **stressors.** From a time standpoint, stressors always precede the development of stress. Stressors are the cause; stress is the effect.

The scientific study of stress has produced a number of general concepts that we will explore next.

Variation in Response to Stressors
Because individuals are unique, a stressor for one person might not be a stressor for another. Whereas a blizzard could prove stressful for many persons, especially the elderly and the sick, others could find the shut-in days peaceful, relaxing, and utterly enjoyable. Standing in a long line or a crowded elevator can be a stressor for some people but not for others. This variation results from the unique information that each person applies in making decisions about the seriousness of the change.[2]

Generalized Physiological Response to Stressors

Once under the influence of a stressor, people's bodies respond in remarkably similar, predictable ways. When you are confronted with an uncomfortable situation (for example, being asked to stand up in front of a group and talk), your heart rate increases, your throat becomes dry, your palms sweat, and you feel dizzy or light-headed. You may even feel sick to your stomach. It is clear that the stressor has produced these common bodily reactions. Figure 3-1 depicts this generalized response.

Stressors

For a state of stress to exist, you must first be confronted by an event, real or imagined, that you interpret as disruptive, frightening, exciting, or dangerous. On the basis of how you see it, the event becomes the stressor.

Sensory Modalities

Before you can determine if change is going to be stressful or nonstressful, it must be sensed by your *central nervous system*. With the exception of those stressors that are products of your imagination, you must hear, smell, taste, feel, or see something before it becomes real to you and thus potentially a stressor.

Cerebral Cortex

Events become stressors when, on entering the *cerebral cortex* of your brain, you define them as being stressors. By your own determination, not all events are stressors.

The Endocrine System

Your body's response to the presence of a stressor involves not only the brain and nervous system but also your *endocrine system.* The endocrine system, in conjunction with the nervous system, stimulates the body to produce the energy needed for dealing with stressors.

The process of interconnecting your nervous system and endocrine system is the task of the **hypothalamus,** a structure located deep within the brain. The hypothalamus is located immediately above the gland that plays the major role in regulating the endocrine system—the **pituitary gland.**[3]

The interplay between the hypothalamus (brain) and the pituitary gland (endocrine system) is accomplished by an exchange of nerve fibers and by the sharing of a small self-contained circulatory system. During periods of stress, communication between the hypothalamus and the pituitary gland is accomplished by the release from the hypothalamus of a chemical messenger into the blood flowing directly to the pituitary gland. This chemical stimulates the pituitary gland to produce its own powerful hormone, **adreno-corticotropic hormone (ACTH).** ACTH is then released into the bloodstream, ultimately reaching a pair of glands of the endocrine system, the **adrenal glands.**[4] ACTH works to stimulate the outer layer *(cortex)* of the adrenal glands to produce chemical substances called **corticoids.** Corticoids assist the body in acquiring energy by supporting the conversion of stored energy into usual fuel.

The hypothalamus also activates the inner core (medulla) of the adrenal gland directly through a branch of the body's autonomic nervous system. This direct contacting of the adrenal gland is responsible for the production of **epinephrine** (commonly known as **adrenaline**). Epinephrine causes most of the functional changes that occur in the body to produce the

stress physiological and psychological state of disruption caused by the presence of an unanticipated, disruptive, or stimulating event.

stressors factors or events, real or imagined, that elicit a state of stress.

hypothalamus (hype oh **thal** a muss) portion of the midbrain that provides a connection between the cerebral cortex and the pituitary gland.

pituitary gland (puh **too** it tary) "master gland" of the endocrine system; the wide variety of hormones produced by the pituitary are sent to structures throughout the body.

adrenocorticotropic hormone (ACTH) (uh **dreen** oh kore tick oh **trope** ick) hormone produced in the pituitary gland and transmitted to the cortex of the adrenal glands; stimulates production and release of corticoids.

adrenal glands (uh **dreen** ull) paired triangular endocrine glands located on the top of each kidney; site of epinephrine and corticoid production.

corticoids (**kore** tick oids) hormones generated by the adrenal cortex; corticoids influence the body's control of glucose, protein, and fat metabolism.

epinephrine (epp i **neff** rin) powerful adrenal hormone whose presence in the bloodstream prepares the body for maximal energy production and skeletal muscle response.

adrenaline (uh **dren** uh lin) common name for epinephrine.

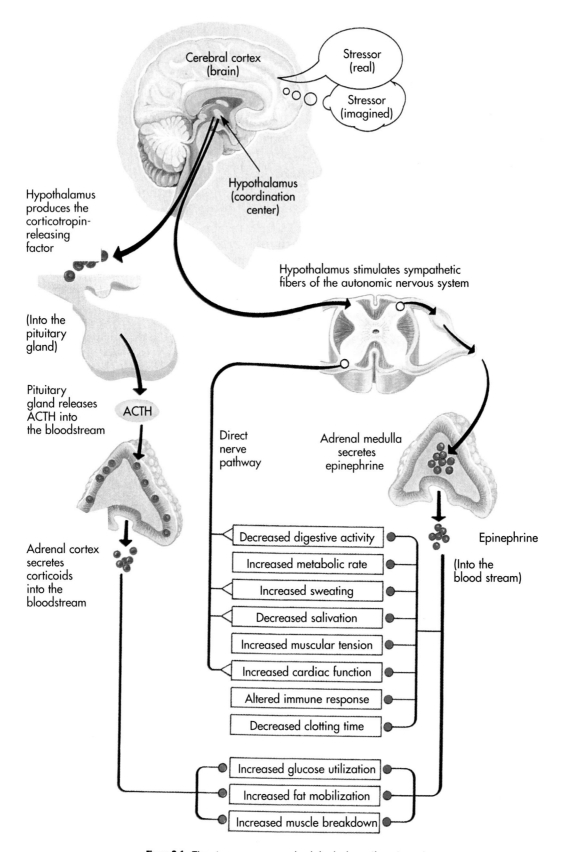

Figure 3-1 The stress response: physiological reactions to a stressor.

rapid, short-term high energy levels required in the presence of a stressor. As you can see in Figure 3-1 corticoids and epinephrine work together in freeing energy from storage.

Epinephrine

Once epinephrine is released by the adrenal gland, many of the following tissue responses can be expected.

DECREASED DIGESTIVE ACTIVITY

Because the body needs energy when a stressor must be avoided or defeated, it cannot wait for digestion to change food into glucose. Rather, the body must turn to the glucose already circulating in the blood or in a storage form within tissue. As a consequence, the entire digestive system slows down. It is not surprising that people who are under chronic stress may report gastric distress, constipation, hemorrhoids, or irritable bowel syndrome.

INCREASED METABOLIC RATE

Epinephrine will increase the **metabolic rate.** Glucose already within the system is rushed by blood circulation to the cells, where it will be combined with oxygen (oxidation) for the release of energy.

INCREASED SWEATING

To control the elevated temperatures generated by the accelerated energy production, the body sweats. The accumulated fluid forms on the skin surface, where it evaporates, thus lowering the temperature.

DECREASED SALIVATION

As a result of the overall shutdown of the digestive system, the production of saliva, a fluid that contains digestive enzymes, is also reduced. Persons who are under the influence of any type of stressor may report a "cotton-mouth" sensation.

INCREASED MUSCULAR TENSION

Twitching and tautness of the arms and legs during times of stress reflect how close to the fully contracted state the body has taken its skeletal muscles. By maintaining the muscles in this condition, the body is prepared for "fight or flight" in the shortest time.

INCREASED CARDIAC AND PULMONARY FUNCTION

During periods of stress, the heart and lungs go into high gear. Epinephrine helps increase *cardiac* and *pulmonary* function. An overall upsurge in heart output and blood pressure and the rate and depth of breathing ensure maximal oxygenation of tissue.

ALTERED IMMUNE SYSTEM RESPONSE

During periods of prolonged stress, elevated levels of adrenal hormones appear to have a destructive effect on important cells (T4-helper cells—see Chapter 12) within the immune system.[5] Infectious illnesses contracted during or shortly after long periods of stress may be directly related to the suppression of these cells that are part of the body's immune system.

DECREASED CLOTTING TIME

Unfortunately, for persons who are prone to cardiovascular and cerebrovascular diseases, blood clotting time decreases during stress. As a consequence, the tendency toward clot formation is enhanced, leading to greater risk of blocking a narrowed vessel with a blood clot.

Energy Release
INCREASED GLUCOSE USE

Because glucose is the body's most basic source of energy, an early feature of the stress response is the release of glycogen (the storage form of glucose) from its deposit sites, particularly the liver. This conversion of glycogen into usable glucose is made possible by the combined efforts of corticoids and epinephrine. Once glycogen is reconverted to glucose, the body imposes increasing demands for glucose delivery on the tissues involved in resisting the stressor.

INCREASED FAT USE

If a stressor is not eliminated promptly, the body's supply of glucose may become depleted. The body then turns to its two remaining energy reserves, fat deposits and muscle tissue (see Figure 3-1). Fat breakdown; coordinated by corticoids and epinephrine, will begin while the blood glucose level falls, resulting in the production of metabolic waste products that will eventually cause the body to turn to its most protected energy deposits, muscle tissue.

MUSCLE TISSUE BREAKDOWN AND USE

If the stressor is unusually powerful or the person's ability to deal constructively with that particular type of stressor is inadequate, energy demands will continue to the point that muscle tissue becomes involved. Fortunately, most college-related stressors are resolved long before this occurs.

Although in the short term all of the responses shown in Figure 3-1 are valuable when you confront a stressor, long-term exposure to these breakdown processes has a destructive effect on the physical component of health. Most stressors are relatively short lived, but eventually the body will shift the efforts of a prolonged "fight" to specific body systems. When this

> **metabolic rate** (met uh **bol** ick) rate or intensity at which the body produces energy.

shift occurs, the **psychosomatic disorders** associated with chronic stress begin to occur.

It is not at all uncommon to experience feelings of psychological distress in association with real or imagined stressors. Feelings of anger, fear, rage, anxiety, confusion, and depression are familiar emotional components of the stress response. At this time, however, there is no explanation for how these feelings are generated.

GENERAL ADAPTATION SYNDROME

Selye[1] described the typical physiological response to a stressor in his **general adaptation syndrome** model. Selye stated that our bodies move through three stages when we are confronted by stressors.

Alarm Reaction Stage

Once we are exposed to any event that is perceived as threatening, our bodies immediately prepare for possible confrontation. The physiological changes described in Figure 3-1 occur. These involuntary changes are controlled by hormonal and nervous system functions and, in effect, quickly prepare the body for the **fight-or-flight response.** Thus in the most primitive physiological sense, the body is prepared to allow us to expend the energy necessary to either confront or flee from the stressor.[6]

Resistance Stage

The second stage of response to a stressor, the resistance stage, reflects the body's attempt to reestablish internal equilibrium. The high level of energy seen in the initial alarm stage cannot be maintained for an extended period. The body attempts to redirect the high level of generalized response to a more manageable level. This is accomplished by reducing the production of ACTH (see p. 45), thus allowing "specificity of adaptation" to occur. Specific organ systems become the focus of the body's response, as opposed to the more generalized response of the alarm reaction stage.[6]

Exhaustion Stage

Body adaptations required through long-term exposure to a stressor often result in an overload. Specific organs and body systems that were called on during the resistance stage may not be able to resist a stressor indefinitely. Exhaustion results and ACTH levels rise when resistance cannot be continued. In extreme or chronic cases, exhaustion can become so pronounced that physiological function deteriorates. Ultimately, prolonged stress can cause death.

Intensity of Stressor

Not everyone reacts similarly to a given stressor.[7] For increasing numbers of people, cigarette smoke is a stressor, yet two nonsmokers may have different reactions to being near someone else's cigarette smoke. One person might feel only mild stress or annoyance, whereas another person could feel severe stress. Thus we might expect different behavioral responses by people exposed to the same stressor. In this example, the first person would sit quietly and continue eating, while the second person might eventually confront the smoker in a less than passive manner.

Positive or Negative Stressors

Stressors produce the same generalized physical response whether an individual perceives the stressor as positive or negative. Poor academic performance, loss of a friend, or having a wisdom tooth extracted can result in stress, just as giving birth, receiving a promotion, or starting a passionate romance can be potential stressors. In each case the impact on body systems is relatively similar.

Selye coined the word **eustress** for positive stress. Stressors that produce eustress can enhance longevity,

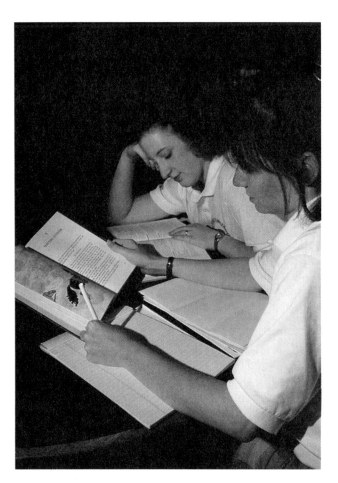

College life presents many stressors.

productivity, and life satisfaction. Examples might be the mild stress that helps you stay alert during a midterm examination, the anticipation felt on the first day of a new job, and the exhilarating stress you feel while exercising.

Selye calls harmful, unpleasant stress **distress.** Distress that goes uncontrolled can result in physical and psychological maladaptation, sickness, and even death.[8] Examples of distress are chronic pain, lack of meaningful relationships, and anxiety and depression. For some, when distress becomes overwhelming, thoughts of suicide may occur.

Inevitability of Stress

Only in death can stress be avoided. We live our lives trying to accommodate a variety of stressors—many of which we are unaware. Stress motivates us and stimulates us to action. The key to lifelong satisfaction seems to lie in our ability to accommodate myriad positive and negative stressors. Mental health professionals encourage us to identify the stress levels at which we can best function as productive, contributing, happy people.

Uncontrolled Stress Related to Disease States

If the impact of the stressor is not minimized or resolved, the effect on the human body is exhaustion. This exhaustion produces emotional and physical breakdown. Depending on the strength of the stressor and the resistance of the person, this breakdown may occur quickly or after many years.

Clearly, the effects of unresolved stress can build up. The impact builds until the body begins to break down. This breakdown leads to stress-related diseases and disorders. Among the major diseases that have some origin in unresolved stress are hypertension, stroke, heart disease, kidney disease, depression, alcoholism, and gastrointestinal disorders (ulcers, irritable bowel syndrome, and diverticulitis).[9] Other stress-related disorders are migraine headaches, allergies, asthma, hay fever, anxiety, insomnia, impotence, and menstrual irregularities. The dependency-related behaviors of cigarette smoking, overeating and undereating, and underactivity relate in part to unresolved stress. Even the immune system that protects the body from infections[10] and cancer[11] may be weakened by stress.

COLLEGE-CENTERED STRESSORS

For some people who have not attempted college coursework, the idea that college life could be stressful must seem distant. After all, even for nontraditional students, isn't college the "good life?"

For those of us who study or teach on college campuses, these perceptions are hard to understand. We know all too well that the undergraduate experience is serious because of its role in preparation for life. For the part-time, nontraditional student who comes to campus for coursework (often at night) and then returns to work, family, and community responsibility, college classes can be especially stressful.

In college and university settings, we think stressors could arise from one or more of the following areas.

Employment Expectations

For those students who believe that the major purpose of getting a college education is to prepare them for a job and a higher standard of living than that of their parents, the question of having chosen the "right" course of study is at times extremely stressful. Uncertainty about job opportunities, technical capabilities, starting salaries, and the need for a graduate degree becomes increasingly pressing when one begins to realize that college will soon end and that the world of employment (or nonemployment) awaits.

Institutional Expectations

For entry into the "community of educated people," college places demands of various types on students. Concerns centered on course selection, course withdrawal, maintaining a desired grade point average, and admission to upper division classes or graduate school are all potential stressors. For those who are just beginning the process of orchestrating a schedule of class work that will encompass eight semesters or twelve quarters or longer, the frustration arising from this responsibility can be quite stressful. Nontraditional students who are attempting to balance school with family and employment may find these expectations to be particularly stressful.

---

psychosomatic disorders (sye cho so **mat** ick) physical illnesses of the body generated by the effects of stress.

general adaptation syndrome sequenced physiological response to the presence of a stressor; the alarm, resistance, and exhaustion stages of the stress response.

fight-or-flight response the reaction to a stressor by confrontation or avoidance.

eustress (**yoo** stress) stress that adds a positive, enhancing dimension to the quality of life.

distress stress that diminishes the quality of life; commonly associated with disease, illness, and maladaptation.

PERSONAL ASSESSMENT

Which of the following events have you experienced in the past 12 months?

Life event	Point value
_____ Death of a close family member	100
_____ Jail term	80
_____ Final year or first year in college	63
_____ Pregnancy (yours or caused by you)	60
_____ Severe personal illness or injury	53
_____ Marriage	50
_____ Any interpersonal problems	45
_____ Financial difficulties	40
_____ Death of a close friend	40
_____ Arguments with your roommate (more than every other day)	40
_____ Major disagreements with your family	40
_____ Major change in personal habits	30
_____ Change in living environment	30
_____ Beginning or ending a job	30
_____ Problems with your boss or professor	25
_____ Outstanding personal achievement	25
_____ Failure in some course	25
_____ Final exams	20
_____ Increased or decreased dating	20
_____ Change in working conditions	20
_____ Change in your major	20
_____ Change in your sleeping habits	18

Life event	Point value
_____ Several day vacation	15
_____ Change in eating habits	15
_____ Family reunion	15
_____ Change in recreational activities	15
_____ Minor illness or injury	15
_____ Minor violations of the law	11

SCORE: _____

INTERPRETATION

Life events can function as stressors that influence the body through activation of the stress response. It has been suggested that an accumulation of 150 or more points in a 1-year period may lead to increased physical illness within the coming year. Of course you must remember that for a given person, certain events may be more or less stressful than the point values indicated.

TO CARRY THIS FURTHER . . .

Having completed this Personal Assessment and evaluated your responses based on the interpretation, were you surprised by the number of stress points that you generated? Are there stressors listed on the instrument that you have not encountered either in your own experiences or in those of your close friends? Have you experienced a stressor that should be added to this list? Would attending a different college or switching majors change your present level of stress?

Health ACTION Guide

Coping with Test Anxiety

Examinations have been a major part of student life for decades and will likely continue to be so. Consequently many students develop an incapacitating anxiety when preparing to take tests. Compare your current test preparation activities with the approach recommended by experts.

▼ Find a location conducive to study.
▼ Set a formal schedule for your test preparation.
▼ Keep complete resources, including class notes, background reading material, and reference texts available.
▼ Create learning aids to help you such as review questions, illustrations, outlines, definitions for technical terms, and sample test items.
▼ "Be your own best friend" by going to class, taking notes, joining and contributing to an ongoing study group, asking questions in class, and making appointments to visit with your professor to clarify material.
▼ "Be kind to yourself" by getting adequate sleep, eating balanced meals, exercising, taking time to be reflective and staying sober.

On the basis of your comparisons, do you have any greater insight as to why you might be anxious about examinations? How do your study habits compare? Remember, most colleges and universities have counseling centers that can help you with study skills and test anxiety. ▼

Financial Support

How much does a college education cost? Is it worth the money, especially at a time when loans are difficult to find and expensive to repay? Should you consider ROTC as a source of assistance in light of the fact that a military obligation awaits you after graduation? For some students these questions are not stressful, but for many students these are among the most pressing of all questions. Each registration period, each loan application, and each statement of need reintroduces these feelings of frustration and uncertainty for some college students.

Personal Expectations

While addressing the new freshmen during their orientation meeting, a college dean may tell you to shake the hands of the two people sitting next to you, because on the basis of the school's attrition rate, one will not be in your class at the end of the year. As you extend your hand to the person next to you, the reality strikes you that a hand is being extended toward you. Will you be among the students who will fail to complete the freshman year? Will you be forced to return home or to your job and explain why you are no longer at school?

Family Expectations

For many students, college is an experiment in disengagement. For 9 months each year you are given a relatively free hand at structuring your own lifestyle—being responsible for completing course requirements, establishing social relationships, and managing your own time.

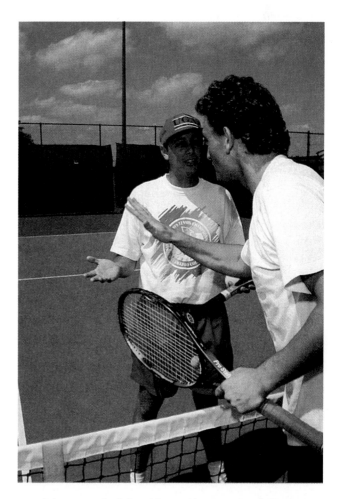

Interpersonal relationships can be a source of stress.

PERSONAL ASSESSMENT

How Vulnerable Are You to Stress?

A wide variety of situations can function as stressors that influence us physically and psychologically. This assessment will help to identify situations that could be stressful and to determine your overall vulnerability to stress. Use the following scoring system for each situation below:

1 = Always (yes)
2 = Almost always
3 = Most of the time
4 = Some of the time
5 = Never (no)

Situation	Score
I get the appropriate amount of sleep my body needs to function.	_____
I exercise to the point of perspiration at least twice a week.	_____
I do not smoke, or I smoke less than half of a pack of cigarettes a day.	_____
I regularly attend club or social activities.	_____
I have one or more friends to confide in about personal matters.	_____
I am able to vent my feelings when angry or worried.	_____
I am able to organize my time effectively.	_____
I drink fewer than three cups of coffee (or tea or cola drinks) a day.	_____
I take quiet time for myself during the day.	_____
I do not procrastinate; I get things done right away.	_____
Before a test I go to bed the same time I normally would.	_____
I live at home (with my family or spouse) while attending school.	_____
I try not to let other people's problems become my own.	_____
(If sexually active) I practice safer sex.	_____
The people closest to me are supportive of my goals.	_____
I have money to meet recreational expenses.	_____

Situation	Score
I am attending college by choice.	_____
I rarely compare myself with my friends.	_____
I do not hold a job and go to school full time.	_____
My grade point average is set only for personal satisfaction.	_____
I do not plan on going on to higher levels of education.	_____

SCORING

Your Total Points _____ − 20 = _____ Final Score

INTERPRETATION

30-49 Points = Vulnerable to stress
50-75 Points = Seriously vulnerable to stress
76-105 Points = Extremely vulnerable to stress

TO CARRY THIS FURTHER . . .

Having completed this Personal Assessment and the interpretation based on your responses, is the "stress status" indicated by your score compatible with your feelings regarding your vulnerability to stress? Have you identified the specific behaviors that need alteration to reduce your level of vulnerability to stress?

Learning FROM ALL Cultures

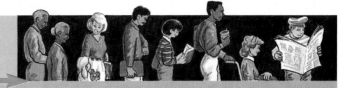

Reducing Stress

Many of us are looking for ways to reduce stress in our lives, whether we do it by exercising, reading self-help books, doing relaxation exercises, or seeing a therapist. Is peace of mind illusive, or is it achievable in today's society?

Stress is experienced by many people regardless of culture. The Lebanese purchase "worry beads" and handle them for periods of time to help them deal with anger or anxiety. If one were to visit Lebanon, the clicking of beads might be a common sound.[15]

Perhaps we can learn from the Far Eastern cultures and their ways of dealing with stress. Eastern people seem to understand the concept of inner peace, and they work and practice to develop it. Many Japanese,

through self-discipline and training, learn to block out outside disturbances and stressors. This practice is described as achieving tranquility.[16]

Tranquility does not come naturally to the Japanese. It is learned through very specific exercises. The exercises consist of three levels: stillness of the body, breathing, and the center of being. It is not known exactly how these exercises originated, but it has been suggested that they are derived from the practices of Buddhist monks and Shinto priests.[16]

For the Japanese the idea of tranquility seems to be a way of life and a goal to achieve. Does one have to be of the Eastern culture to understand the concept of tranquility, or is it a practice that those of us from Western society can learn and internalize?

If these responsibilities seem difficult, then you may be stressed by the feeling that you are not capable of doing what others expect you to be able to do. For many, this "disengagement shock" is the most pressing stressor that they will face. For some, the adjustment will be too great and they will return to their families or to work before making further educational decisions. For nontraditional students, family expectations may come from spouses or children who are counting on you to do well in school.

Time Management

As suggested above, the productive use of time is a significant problem for many college students either because of the poor use of "free time" associated with a typical school day, or because of the added demands of marriage, employment, and parenting. Even the minutes lost on a daily basis to commuting, waiting in campus lines, athletic practice, and hanging out with friends can make quality time for school work in short supply. Ultimately, however, it becomes an issue of priorities and the management of time so that sufficient time is available for meeting academic demands.

Although there is no single "best approach" to managing time, most experts suggest that the following would be helpful:

▼ Keep a log of how you use your time for 1 week. Check about each half hour to see what you are doing.

▼ Analyze your records, and eliminate those activities that take too much time.

▼ Once the eliminations have been made, divide your time into blocks so that related activities can be

scheduled together. There should be a block for each major area of responsibility applicable to you. Examples might include academics, employment, recreation, and socialization.

▼ Schedule specific activities within each block of time. Attempt to conclude activities that you have started.

▼ Reassess your time management activities occasionally, and make adjustments when necessary.[12]

Cultural Conflicts

For many persons, the culture of which they are a part does not assign great value to formal education, particularly a college education. Breaking away from a family that believes that little can be attained by "more" education or departing a neighborhood characterized by poverty, gangs, crime, and drug abuse will challenge even the most resourceful persons. Fortunately, as colleges and universities become more experienced in meeting the needs of these students, greater sensitivity on the part of faculty, staff, and fellow students, in combination with support programs, is making these transitions easier. It is necessary, however, for students to join the institution in searching out and finding each other so that these resources can be used effectively in reducing the stress of attaining a higher education.

Religious Faith

Consider this scenario: By the end of your first semester at college you no longer attend religious services. You become an agnostic by the middle of the second semester, and by the end of your first year in college you are a confirmed atheist.

As ridiculous as this scenario may sound, it could be the anticipated "falling from grace" imagined by some as they see you leave the security of their home for life on the "radical" college campus. A current twist to this theme is that of your being captured by one of the religious cults. Interfaith dating may represent an even more common religion-oriented stressor.

Questions about religion can become a part of your educational experience and be the source of uncertainty and stress. Higher education is designed to challenge your knowledge, values, and practices so that they may serve you better in the future. Many will find their religious beliefs challenged.

Faculty Expectations

Faculty members consider the college classroom a very real part of the world. It is an arena in which they experience success or failure. It is one of their major means of achieving a sense of contribution. Most professors take their teaching seriously, and they expect you to pursue your studies with equal seriousness. Should you disregard this academic reality, stressors could occur in the form of poor grades or weak employment recommendations. Indeed, faculty expectations can be a major stressor for students.

Education in a college or university setting is never passive. It will nearly always demand active participation and effort and at times may demand more than you believe you are capable of giving. Not surprisingly, it is frequently the source of many stressors.

LIFE-CENTERED STRESSORS

For many people, day-to-day living provides stressors that must be confronted and resolved. Although these stressors might differ from those associated with college, these life-centered stressors hold the same potential for causing physical and psychological distress.

When adults were asked to identify the causes of their stress, not surprisingly, many familiar factors surfaced.

▼ **Cost of living:** From necessities to luxury items, the cost of goods and services can easily exceed our financial resources. Particularly for older students with children, rent to pay, and a limited earning ability, the cost of living can be a powerful stressor.

▼ **Loss of property:** When a home, business, or farm is lost as the result of natural disaster, vandalism, or accident, a sense of chronic stress may result. The devastating 1993 floods in the Midwest became a source of stress for tens of thousands of people (see p. 459).

▼ **Being too busy:** We can often experience short and long periods of time that ask more of us than we have time to give. Single parents who are also college students find that the lack of time is constant. The day seems too short for all that needs to be done.

▼ **Money concerns:** We can be confused and concerned about the complexity of contracts, estates, taxes, loans, and investments.

 Headaches

An estimated 45 million Americans suffer from headaches. If you have chronic headache symptoms or symptoms that are especially bothersome, you should seek medical help. Headaches can result from many causes. The three most common categories follow:

TENSION

Description   A dull constricting pain centered in the hatband region. Pain may be on both sides of the head and extend down the neck to the shoulders. Produced by stress, eye strain, muscle tension, sinus congestion, temporomandibular joint (TMJ) dysfunction, nasal congestion, or caffeine withdrawal.

   Treatment   Nonnarcotic pain relievers, muscle relaxants, relaxation exercises, massage.

   Prevention   Preventive relaxation exercises, certain antidepressant medications.

MIGRAINE

Description   Throbbing pain on one side of the head, usually preceded by visual disturbances. Sensitivity to lights and sounds; nausea and dizziness. More common in women. May be triggered by a number of causes. Can last from a few hours to 2 days.

   Treatment   Rest in a quiet, dark place. Nonnarcotic pain relievers. Ergot compounds (prescription medications).

   Prevention   Avoidance of certain foods, perhaps including red wines, other alcoholic beverages, ripened cheeses, chocolate, cured meats, and MSG (monosodium glutamate). In some cases, prescription medications are recommended.

CLUSTER

Description   Focused, intense pain near one eye; often producing a red and teary eye, as well as a runny nose. Headaches occur daily for weeks or months. They mainly affect men and last up to 2 hours.

   Treatment   Oxygen and/or ergot compounds during the headache.

   Prevention   Avoidance of alcohol and nitrite-containing foods. Various prescription medications, including antidepressants, steroids, ergotlike compounds, or heart-regulating drugs. ★

Health ACTION Guide

Tips for the Computer

Tips for reducing stress at a computer workstation:

▼ Be sure that the computer's air vents are unobstructed and free of dust.

▼ Eyes should be level with the top of the screen.
▼ Position the terminal to avoid glare.
▼ Use a document holder positioned close to and at the same level as the screen.
▼ Keep your back and neck erect with your upper arms perpendicular to the floor.
▼ Keep your forearms and wrists as close to horizontal as possible.
▼ Position your feet flat on the floor, or use a footrest.

▼ **Relaxation:** At times we can consciously know that relaxation is in our best interest but are unable to do so.

▼ **Family illness:** Many of us eventually may experience family illnesses involving spouses, children, or aging parents. Middle aged, nontraditional students in particular may find that having children and older parents, both of whom may need care, can be very stressful.

▼ **Personal illness:** Often without notice, we can be confronted by our own illnesses, leading to fear, apprehension, and inconvenience.

Although the above concerns were given by people in 1986, it is our belief that most would still be high on a list of stressors given today. Today, of course, we would need to add personal safety. As random, senseless killings escalate on the streets, at worksites, and in homes, many would claim this as a significant source of stress also.

COPING: REACTING TO STRESSORS

Because the effects of stress are cumulative, now is the time to examine your stress-related behaviors. This fact is difficult for some people to accept. For most persons, life won't get any easier once their college days are over. Just ask an older, nontraditional student in your class! The pressures of employment, finances, and family all seem to make life more difficult and more complicated. Obviously the best time to learn how to cope with your stress is now—before faulty habits have turned to dependencies and the long-term effects of stress have started to damage your health.

The keys to coping with stressors are found in the ways we choose to live. Traditional methods of handling stress that have been both simple to accomplish and socially supported have included all of the *negative dependency behaviors* (smoking, excessive drinking, overeating), withdrawal from the stressor, and attacking stress through direct confrontation. Although they may be effective in the short term, these coping methods ultimately may produce additional stress.

Efforts to develop appropriate and effective coping skills in today's world are in some regards more difficult than in the past. No longer is it socially acceptable to escape stressors through negative dependency behaviors, withdrawal, or aggressiveness. The emphasis now is on lifestyle management techniques that are not only effective, but also supportive of overall health, social relationships, and the environment.

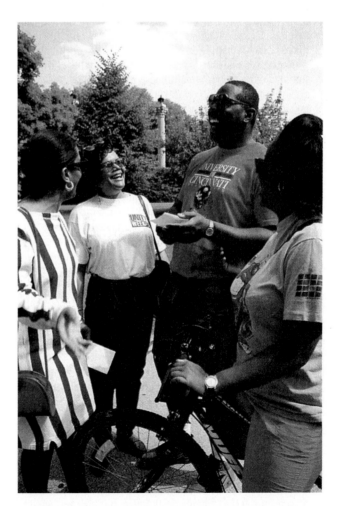

Periods of reduced stress are vital for mental health.

Certainly, the existence of a variety of effective coping skills would be encompassed in the currently popular concept of *hardiness*. Hardy people respond to change effectively, not only because they have developed approaches to encourage change in their lives (see Chapter 2), but also because they have mastered coping strategies that work when change is imposed from outside.

STRESS MANAGEMENT TECHNIQUES

Experts in stress management indicate that the most successful methods of coping with distress include self-hypnosis, relaxation, quieting, transcendental meditation, biofeedback, exercise, and yoga. Each of these techniques is described in the box below.

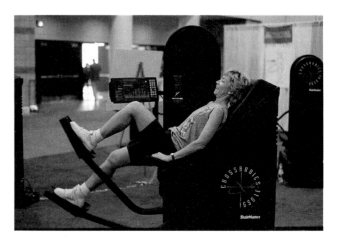

Exercise is an excellent way to reduce stress.

★ Tension Reduction: Taking Control of Stress

SELF-HYPNOSIS

Techniques for increased awareness, mental relaxation, and enhanced self-directedness are taught by trained professionals to people capable of being hypnotized. The techniques, which can be learned in one lesson, are self-administered on a daily basis in sessions lasting 10 to 20 minutes. Unqualified practitioners frequently sell their services through newspaper advertisements. Professional organizations such as psychological or psychiatric societies can recommend qualified therapists.

RELAXATION

Relaxation is based on a technique developed by Herbert Benson, M.D., through which one learns to quiet the body and mind. Relaxation technique centers on exhalations and allowing the body to relax while sitting in a comfortable position. The technique can be learned in a single session but requires a commitment to making time to practice. Relatively effective for most people, the technique is described in Dr. Benson's book, *The Relaxation Response.*

QUIETING   — deep breathe count to 10

A set of specific responses, for example, striving for a positive mental state, an "inner smile," and a deep exhalation with the tongue relaxed and the shoulders relaxed, is used immediately upon sensing the onset of stress. This technique can be done at any time; it is easily learned and supplies immediate feelings of being "on top of stress." The technique can be learned from *QR: The Quieting Reflex* by Charles Stroebel, MD, PhD.

TRANSCENDENTAL MEDITATION

Transcendental meditation allows the mind to transcend thought effortlessly when the person recites a "mantra," or a personal word, twice daily for 20 minutes. TM is a seven-step program that usually costs between $250 and $400 to learn. TM centers are listed in the telephone directory under Transcendental Meditation.

BIOFEEDBACK

A system is learned for monitoring and subsequently controlling specific physiological functions such as heart rate, respiratory rate, and body temperature. Training with an experienced instructor and appropriate monitoring instruments will require weekly sessions that last 1 hour or longer over a period of 12 or more weeks. When used with other tension reduction techniques, biofeedback provides concrete reinforcement of stress-reduction goals. For more information, contact the Biofeedback Society of America, 4301 Owens Street, Wheat Ridge, CO 80033.

EXERCISE

There is a wide variety of movement activities intended to reduce stress, expend energy, promote relaxation, and provide enjoyment through social contact. Running, jogging, lap swimming, walking, rope skipping, biking, stair climbing, and aerobic workouts are all excellent ways to burn the energy produced by the stress response. Equipment needs, facilities, and required skills vary. Three to four sessions per week at a half-hour duration per session are sufficient for most people. Many health and fitness clubs offer exercise programs.

YOGA

An ancient exercise program for the mind and body, yoga can be learned from a qualified instructor in approximately 1 to 3 months. Yoga is practiced on a daily basis in a quiet setting in sessions of 15 to 45 minutes. It can alter specific physiological functions, enhance flexibility, and free the mind from immediate involvement with stressors. Many good yoga books and classes are available. ★

Whether a particular coping technique is effective for you will not be known until you have participated in such for an adequate period of time.

Personality Traits

Can personality play a role in making people more or less prone to stress? If so, what outlook on life is now considered the most stress-producing? The answer to this latter question has changed over the past two decades.

The initial, and still widely recognized, theory describing personality's role in fostering stress was that of Type A and Type B personalities developed by cardiologists Friedman and Rosenman. In this model, time-dependence ("hurry sickness") was related to high levels of stress and, eventually, to heart disease.

Effective Coping: Stress and Exercise

The energy produced by the stress response is most easily reduced through physical activity. In fact, coping by engaging in an exercise program during stressful situations closely resembles how our ancestors used the energy of their stress response—by fighting or fleeing.

The following list identifies physical activities that you can use to cope with stress during your lunch hour or before or after school or work. Describe your experience with each, including when, where, how long, and with whom you engaged in this activity. Also identify the health benefits you received. For those activities you have not yet tried, identify what would be necessary to make them more attractive to you.

★ Walking (power, leisure):

★ Jogging:

★ Running (5 mph +):

★ Aerobic Activities (stair stepping, dance, rowing, etc.):

★ Biking (12-15 mph +):

★ Racquet Sports (squash, racquetball, tennis):

★ Bowling:

★ Weight Training (power, body building):

★ Golf (with/without cart):

The authors believed that slowing down was so important to reducing stress and preventing heart disease that they advanced many familiar recommendations, including such suggestions as follow:

▼ Listen quietly when others are talking. Do not try to finish the sentences of others or interrupt with speed-up phrases such as "Yes, yes."

▼ Move more slowly. Walk at a slower pace, and drive less aggressively.

▼ Take time to offer sincere thanks to others. Don't just grunt. Speak in full sentences while looking directly at the faces of those you are thanking.

Today, the concept of time-dependency as being the most influential personality trait associated with high levels of stress has given way to concern over high levels of anger and cynicism. Anger is the intense feeling of rage and fury that accompanies unexpected change. For those people who, for whatever reasons, seem to be always angry, the stress put on the body is detrimental to both physical and emotional health.[13] The term *angry heart* has been coined to describe a condition too frequently seen in people who have experienced a heart attack.

Closely akin to anger is cynicism, the second personality trait that fosters high levels of stress. This trait is associated with deeply held dislike and distrust of others and their ideas. People who are cynics have nothing to say that is good about others. They are, perhaps, profoundly angry about their relationships with others, and can only express this feeling by being super-critical. Regardless, cynicism, like anger, places the body under chronic stress and erodes the physical and emotional well-being of the cynic.

Time-dependency techniques can be developed to slow Type A people down. In contrast, anger and cynicism seem more deeply ingrained and therefore less easily altered. Perhaps the only effective treatment for the chronically angry or cynical person is either a profoundly moving personal experience that truly changes their outlook on life or counseling to get in touch with the reasons underlying their negative outlook on life.

A Realistic Perspective on Stress and Life

Although in theory life should be stressless, reality dictates otherwise. Therefore it is desirable that we approach life with a tough-minded optimism that provides a sense of hope and anticipation, as well as an understanding that life will never be without stress. The development of this realistic approach to today's fast-paced demanding lifestyle may best be achieved by fostering many of the perspectives listed below.[14]

▼ Do not be surprised by trouble. Anticipate problems and see yourself as a "problem solver."

▼ Search for solutions. Act on a partial solution, even when a complete solution seems distant.

▼ Take control of your own future. Set out to accomplish all the items that are on your agenda. Do not view yourself as a victim.

▼ Move away from negative thought patterns. Do not extend or generalize difficulties from one area into another.

▼ Rehearse success. Do not disregard the possibility of failure. Rather, focus on those things that are necessary and possible to ensure success.

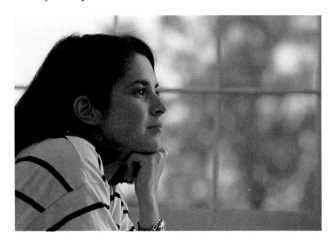

Envisioning success.

▼ Accept the unchangeable. The direction your life takes is only in part the result of your own doing. Cope as effectively as possible with those events over which you have no direct control.

▼ Live each day well. Combine activity, contemplation, and a sense of cheerfulness with the many things that must be done each day. Celebrate special occasions.

▼ Act on your capacity for growth. Undertake new experiences and then extract from them new information about your own interests and capacities.

▼ Allow for renewal. Make time for yourself, and take advantage of opportunities to pursue new and fulfilling relationships. Foster growth of your spiritual nature.

▼ Tolerate mistakes. Both you and others will make mistakes. Recognize that these can cause anger, and learn to avoid feelings of hostility.

With a realistic and positive outlook on life, less coping time will be required for living a satisfying and productive life. Change, in all aspects of life, is inevitable. In the presence of high-level health, change should be anticipated, nurtured, and then incorporated into the maturing sense of yourself.

Summary

✔ Stress is the physiologic and emotional response to the presence of a stressor. Stressors are events that generate the stress response.

✔ An intricate interplay involving the brain, nervous system, and endocrine system results in a series of physiological changes that prepare the body to respond to stressors.

✔ Critical to the stress response are the sensory modalities, the cerebral cortex, the hypothalamus, the adrenal glands, the hormone ACTH, corticoids, and epinephrine.

✔ The general adaptation syndrome consists of three distinct stages: alarm, resistance, and exhaustion.

✔ The stress response mobilizes energy for the fight/flight response.

✔ Distress and eustress reflect similar physiological responses but different emotional interpretations.

✔ Uncontrolled stress can lead to a variety of illnesses.

Since the effects of stress are cumulative, stress-related health problems can develop slowly.

✔ The college experience can generate stressors from several different areas, including finances and institutional and personal expectations, and cultural expectations.

✔ Time management can provide an effective solution for lowering the stress level of many college students.

✔ Day-to-day living is routinely the source of many types of stressors.

✔ A variety of coping techniques can be easily learned and may prove to be beneficial in reducing stress.

✔ Chronic feelings of anger and cynicism can be central to feelings of stress.

✔ An optimistic outlook on life may protect some people from the potentially damaging effects of stressors.

Review Questions

1. Differentiate between stress and stressors.
2. How do distress and eustress differ? In what way are they similar?
3. In what predictable manner does the stress response unfold? What is the role of the endocrine system? What portions of the nervous system play important roles in the unfolding of the stress response? How do the digestive and cardiovascular systems contribute to the flight/fight response?
4. What are the three stages of Selye's general adaptation syndrome?
5. What are several of the more familiar health conditions attributed to chronic unresolved stress? To what extent are the effects of stress cumulative?
6. In what way does the college experience contribute to the stress level of students?
7. What techniques can be applied toward more effective time management?
8. What life experience do typical Americans report as being most stressful?
9. In what manner do anger and cynicism contribute to stress? How has the popular Type A/Type B theory of time-dependency changed in regard to the cause of stress?
10. What coping techniques have proven helpful when used on a regular basis?
11. What traits characterize the optimistic lifestyle?

Think about This . . .

✔ Can you remember a stressful experience you recently had in which your body responses clearly followed the pattern of Selye's general adaptation syndrome? How long did you remain in each of the specific stages?
✔ If the body's response to stressors is similar for both distress and eustress, how do we learn to distinguish between the two?
✔ Do you have a realistic perception about the potential stressful nature of life?

✔ Which dimension of your health (physical, emotional, social, intellectual, or spiritual) do you most frequently rely on when you are confronted with a stressful situation)?
✔ If you believe that the enhancement of your stress management skills will be important to you in the future, which of the suggested approaches to coping with stress could you most comfortably develop? When can you start to develop these skills?

REAL LIFE REAL CHOICES

YOUR TURN

▼ What are the sources of stress in Kate Sullivan's life?
▼ Does Kate have any choice about the structure and pace of her life?
▼ Do you agree or disagree with Kate that she can't afford to take time to relax?

AND NOW, YOUR CHOICES. . .

▼ If you were in Kate's circumstances, what, if anything, would you do differently? The same? Why?
▼ What kinds of stresses are you under, and how do you deal with them?

References

1. Selye H: *Stress without distress*, New York, 1975, New American Library.
2. King M, Stanley G, Burrows G: *Stress: theory and practice*, Philadelphia, 1987, WB Saunders.
3. Moffett D, Moffett SB, Schauf CL: *Human physiology: foundations and frontiers*, St Louis, 1993, Mosby.
4. Thibodeau GA, Patton K: *Human body in health and disease*, St Louis, 1992, Mosby.
5. O'Leary A: Stress, emotion, and human immune function, *Psychol Bull* 108(3):353-363, 1990.
6. Girdano D, Everly G: *Controlling stress and tension*, ed 3, Englewood Cliffs, NJ, 1989, Prentice-Hall.
7. Selye H: *Selye's guide to stress research*, vol 3, New York, 1983, Von Nostrand Reinhold.
8. Julius M, et al: Anger-coping types, blood pressure, and all causes of mortality: a follow-up in Tecumseh, Michigan (1971-1983), *Am J Epidemiol* 124:220-233, 1986.
9. McGinnis J: *Medicine for the layman: behavioral patterns and health*, US Department of Health and Human Services, NIH Pub No 85-2682, Washington, DC, 1986, US Government Printing Office.
10. Tyrrell DJ, Smith AP: Psychological stress and susceptibility to the common cold, *New Engl J Med* 325(9):606-613, 1991.
11. Kune S: Stressful life events and cancer (editorial), *Epidemiology*, 4(5):395-397, 1993.
12. Buchert W: A key to managing time: planning and discipline, *USA Today* 9A, April 16, 1990.
13. Almada SJ, et al: Neuroticism and cynicism and risk of death in middle-aged men: the Western Electric Study, *Psychosom Med* 53(2):165-175, 1991.
14. McGinnis L: *The power of optimism*, New York, 1990, Harper & Row.
15. Cahill MJ: *Lebanon*, New York, 1987, Chelsea House.
16. Durekheim K: *The Japanese cult of tranquility*, York Beach, Maine, 1991, Samuel Weiser.

Suggested Readings

Davidson J: *Breathing space: living and working at a comfortable pace in a sped-up society*, New York, 1991, MasterMedia Limited.

Why are we moving so fast in today's world? According to the author, technological advances, such as the computer and the fax machine, have caused us to be pressed for time and thus in a leisure squeeze. Suggestions are given for making the most beneficial use of our remaining leisure time.

Goleman D: *Mind/body medicine, how to use your mind for better health*, Yonkers, NY, 1993, Consumer Reports Books.

What are the effects of thoughts and emotions on health (or disease)? Explains this question in easily understood terms, as well as providing approaches to use the mind in the prevention and healing of diseases.

Dienstfrey H: *Where the mind meets the body*, New York, 1992, Harper-Collins.

Describes a wide variety of topics relating to the mind and body interface. Includes Type A behavior, relaxation, biofeedback, imagery, and hypnosis. Timely coverage in light of the government's recent decision to fund research into "alternative" aspects of health care.

Weinstein W: *Managing stress*, Bellingham, Wash, 1991, Self-Counsel Press, Inc.

Provides a detailed description of the role of relaxation in stress management: muscle tensing and relaxing, as well as deep breathing, are important components of total relaxation.

The information you have mastered in Unit 1 will be helpful to you as you work on the five developmental tasks this book addresses. Remember that the role of health is to assist you in completing the developmental tasks that will allow you to have a satisfying and productive life.

Forming an Initial Adult Identity

You may have noticed that we have qualified the adult self-identity concept as initial, or tentative. This suggests an identity that is temporary—one that can evolve over time. The idea that further changes in your identity are possible (even probable) can lead to feelings of uncertainty, confusion, and stress. However, we believe that as you increasingly come to grips with your evolving identity, you will find new opportunities for growth, creativity, and service. In many ways this personal growth and development can be an exciting experience. High-level emotional health encourages the formation of your emerging identity. Through healthful introspection and reflection, you learn a great deal about the person you are becoming. By exploring the ways you handle stressful situations, you learn even more about yourself. Indeed, interest in your emotional and spiritual makeup will serve you throughout life as you repeatedly ask "Who am I?"

Establishing Independence

This major developmental task is represented by your steady movement away from a dependent relationship with family and friends. For nontraditional students it may be represented by a sim-

ilar pulling back from a spouse, limited employment opportunities, or parenting. Regardless, to progress toward independence you must be successful in dealing with people, institutions, programs, and yourself. Establishing independence is a developmental progression in which emotional health can play an extremely supportive role.

Your emotional maturity is a major factor in determining the rate at which you progress toward independence. Stress will probably be produced in those who progress too slowly or too rapidly in their search toward independence. For those who move toward relative independence at a rate soundly based on their needs and health resources, this search will produce eustress. Enjoy the journey.

Assuming Responsibility

Although an adult of any age may lack an adequately developed sense of responsibility, it is in the young adult years that significant progress in that direction is expected. To whom is one most responsible? We take the position that primary responsibility during the young adult years must be to yourself. For example, mastery of all five of the developmental tasks is your responsibility. Parents, faculty, and friends cannot force you to take charge of your own development; your growth in confidence, self-respect, and insight gained through new experiences rests in your own hands. Fortunately, this is the way most students want it.

Developing Social Skills

Since the costs of making

friends and keeping friendships can sometimes be high, we would like to introduce someone who can be helpful in your search for improved social interaction—a mentor. For the purposes of this book, a mentor is a person slightly older than you (8 to 15 years older) who functions not as a peer nor as a parent substitute, but as an exemplar, counselor, and a person capable of sharing your aspirations. The process of identifying potential mentors within an occupational, educational, or recreational setting cannot be prescribed. Potential mentors need not be of your own sex, nor do they necessarily need to hold a position significantly higher than yours.

It is through mentor relationships that some will find the most pleasurable social, occupational, and professional rewards. With your mentor you will sense a more deeply focused relationship against which to evaluate initial successes and failures. Your mentor will listen, demand, share, critique, and counsel as you progress in this challenging period of life.

Developing Intimacy

To develop intimacy, you must be willing and able to extend your identity to others in an open manner. Intimacy is almost always accompanied by feelings of vulnerability as well as the possibility of rejection. Consequently, stress and intimacy usually go together. Effective coping skills are important resources to develop in any relationship, especially an intimate one. Think of intimate relationships as new experiences which will help to shape your life.

UNIT TWO

The second unit is composed of three chapters whose topics are especially important to today's college students: physical fitness, nutrition, and weight management. We think these are interesting topics for students because most students tell us that they want to stay in good physical condition, eat well, and maintain a desirable weight. We discuss the upcoming content in terms of our philosophy that health is composed of five interacting dimensions.

● Physical Dimension of Health

Many health experts indicate that fitness, nutrition, and weight management are interrelated. How well our bodies work depends on what we eat and how we exercise. Since most of us need some degree of fitness just to complete our daily activities, we can appreciate the value of an appropriate exercise program. Healthy bodies can avoid costly repairs and bounce back more quickly from illness and injury.

◆ Emotional Dimension of Health

When you start a fitness program or begin to monitor food consumption behavior, you learn about your level of motivation and commitment. Undoubtedly, you will be challenged, but the mental and emotional rewards for your efforts can be monumental. Students who are conscientious about maintaining their fitness levels, food consumption habits, and body weight seem to bubble with enthusiasm. There must exist some intrinsic, emotional rewards that go hand in hand with eating properly and being physically fit.

■ Social Dimension of Health

The social dimension of health is closely related to the content in Chapters 4, 5, and 6. Exercising with others offers opportunities for social interaction. Combined with most forms of group fitness activities are varying amounts of listening, sharing, and counseling by the participants. For college students of all ages, university facilities, commercial health clubs, local YMCAs and YWCAs, and competitive events provide social settings where they can improve social skills.

There is little question that food, like alcohol, can function as a "social lubricant." Food brings and holds people together. Kitchens and restaurants become meeting places, picnics and barbecues reunite scattered families and friends, and even supermarkets have served as contact points for eligibles. Food may also serve as a potentially dangerous agent that can hinder our social relationships. Intake of food that results in a significant deviation from desirable weight can make interactions with family members, friends, and employers more strained. Thus we may become hindered in social developments regardless of our stage in the life cycle.

▲ Intellectual Dimension of Health

Whether being physically fit, eating well, and maintaining an appropriate weight level have much effect on your intellectual functioning is a question that could be debated. Anecdotal evidence suggests that people do feel mentally sharper after exercise. Our students claim that they can study more efficiently after their workouts. As professors, we are able to teach with more enthusiasm, interest, and clear thinking when we are in good physical condition. People deprived of adequate exercise and nutrition may suffer intellectual impairment. Good fitness, a sound diet, and reasonable weight management will help you be able to enjoy the widest range of new experiences. These new experiences can lead to improved intellectual functioning. This thought is inherent in our "Plan for Enhancing Your Mental and Emotional Growth" in Chapter 2.

● Spiritual Dimension of Health

Throughout this text we emphasize that a major dimension of your spiritual growth takes the form of service to others. Physical fitness, good nutrition, and weight management can enhance your ability to serve others. You can better live your faith and assist others in bringing meaning into their lives when you feel the drive that results from a well-conditioned, adequately nourished body.

The Body
Your Vehicle for Health

4

Physical Fitness

Enhancing Work, Study, and Play

When your day begins early in the morning, then you go to class or work or immerse yourself in family activities, and your day does not end until after midnight, you must be physically fit. Even a highly motivated college student must have a conditioned, rested body to maintain such a schedule.

When you have this level of conditioning, you will not only be capable of meeting the demands of your college schedule, but you will also master your developmental tasks with greater ease. Like many, you may find the psychological benefits as rewarding as the physical benefits.

Fortunately, the health benefits of fitness can come from regular participation in moderate exercise, such as brisk walking or dancing.[1] You do not have to be a top-notch athlete to receive the health benefits of physical activity.

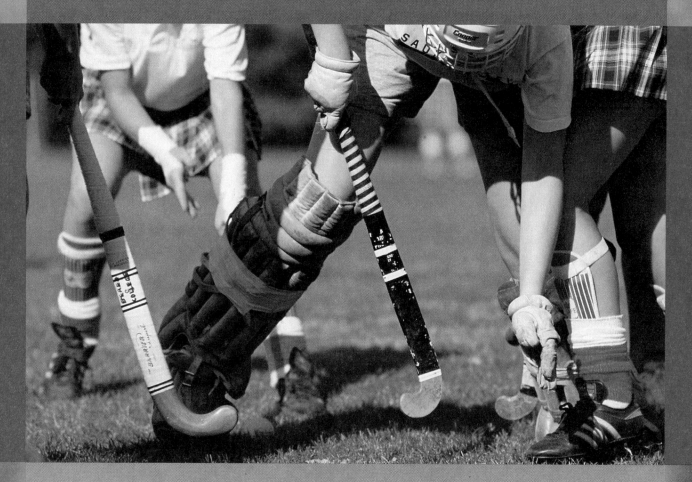

F I T N E S S

The following objectives are covered in this chapter:

▼ Increase to at least 30% the proportion of people aged 6 and older who engage regularly, preferably daily, in light-to-moderate physical activity for at least 30 minutes per day. (Baseline: 22% of people aged 18 and older were active for at least 30 minutes 5 or more times per week and 12% were active 7 or more times per week in 1985; p. 97.)

▼ Reduce to no more than 15% the proportion of people aged 6 and older who engage in no leisure-time physical activity. (Baseline: 24% for people aged 18 and older in 1985; p. 99.)

▼ Increase to at least 20% the proportion of people aged 18 and older who engage in vigorous physical activity that promotes the develop-

ment and maintenance of cardiorespiratory fitness 3 or more days per week for 20 or more minutes per occasion. (Baseline: 12% for people aged 18 and older in 1985; p. 98.)

▼ Increase to at least 40% the proportion of people aged 6 and older who regularly perform physical activities that enhance and maintain muscular strength, muscular endurance, and flexibility. (Baseline data unavailable in 1991.)

▼ Increase the proportion of worksites offering employer-sponsored physical activity and fitness programs. (Baseline: 14% for small companies [50-99 employees] and 54% for large companies [more than 750 employees] in 1985. Target goals: 20% for small companies and 80% for large ones; p. 103.)

REAL LIFE
REAL CHOICES
The Fitness Imperative: A Matter of Life and Health

▼ Name: Jack Wozniak
▼ Age: 44
▼ Occupation: sales representative
▼ Physical characteristics: 5'11", 182 lb

No caffeine. No alcohol. No smoking. No red meat. No rich desserts. No road trips. Plenty of fruits and vegetables; plenty of rest; moderate daily exercise.

To Jack Wozniak, a hard-charging, fun-loving embodiment of the Type A personality, that list of restrictions sounded like the last chapter in the book of his life. A successful sales representative for a plastics manufacturer, Jack spent 8 months out of each year on the road. At his last annual checkup his blood pressure had risen to 175 over 85, and he grudgingly admitted to his concerned physician that 18 years of rushing for the red-eye, wining and dining prospects, and sleeping in strange beds were taking their toll. Factor in no exer-

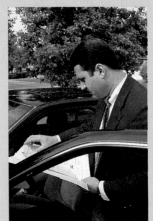

cise, a two-pack-a-day smoking habit, and a passion for beer and corn chips, and you're looking at a disaster waiting to happen.

It did. One morning Jack was battling rush-hour traffic to the airport to catch a plane for Dallas. He never made it. When he woke up, he found himself in a cardiac-care unit, hooked up to more wires and flashing dials than the space shuttle. Not even 45, he'd suffered a massive heart attack, and his doctor was offering him a stark choice: maintain your lifestyle and die, or follow a new regimen and (maybe) live.

As you study this chapter, think about a healthy approach to exercise for someone of Jack's personality type and lifestyle, and prepare yourself to answer the questions in **Your Turn** at the end of the chapter. ▼

COMMON ATTITUDES TOWARD PHYSICAL FITNESS

Recently we were told by a student that setting aside time for improving his physical fitness would be a total misuse of his time. He assured us that he would be no better served by a fitness program than by learning to play bridge. College and preparation for a career were his only priorities.

This student perceived being physically fit as an end rather than the means we know it to be. His opinion is one of the many feelings, pro or con, that people hold about their personal involvement in a physical fitness program.

Many people, including college students of all ages, spend little time in pursuit of physical fitness. Certainly some of these individuals may have physical limitations that make activity extremely difficult, and others may be engaged in time-consuming activities that until finished do not permit opportunities for recreation. However, what about the majority who could do much more but do so little? Does one of the following statements sound like you?

"I know it's important, but I just don't have time right now."

"I'm already fit, and with my schedule, I'll have no difficulty staying that way."

"I should do more than I do, but I just don't have the facilities and I don't get much support from others."

"Exercise makes me feel gross. Even when I shower, I get to my next class wet, sticky, and probably smelling like a locker room."

Unlike these people who have made no commitment to fitness, you may have made a commitment to a physical fitness program that might be rather narrow in scope. If one of the following comments fits you, perhaps you are failing to see the broader values of maintaining a high level of physical fitness.

"Everyone in the dorm runs. That's why I run."

"For every 3500 Calories I can `burn' during exercise, I'll lose a pound of fat. I have only 10 pounds more to drop before vacation."

"This weekend will be cool and overcast. Saturday looks like a good day for a personal record."

"Some people say I have a fear of death. Really, I just want to live a long time."

If you see your own attitude represented by one of these comments, your reason for valuing fitness may be shortsighted. We suggest that you reexamine your approach to fitness and its ability to positively influence other aspects of your life.

Ask yourself, "What could I achieve if I were really in top physical condition?" Because fitness levels are

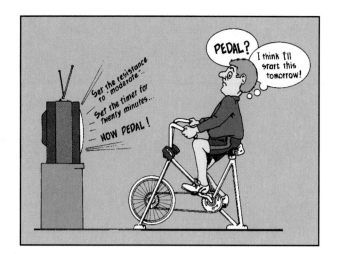

easily observed and can be measured, you can quickly start to see the person you are capable of becoming. Progress and accomplishment can be seen almost daily. Keep in mind, however, that all people are different and some may progress faster than others.

Your increase in physical activity can help the nation achieve its Healthy People 2000 Objectives and in the final analysis, although fitness will not guarantee you a longer life, it can help you enjoy the years you have.

COMPONENTS OF PHYSICAL FITNESS

Physical fitness is achieved when "the organic systems of the body are healthy and function efficiently so as to resist disease, to enable the fit person to engage in rigorous tasks and leisure activities, and to handle situations of emergency."[2] The number of components of physical fitness may vary; here we will discuss cardiorespiratory endurance, muscular strength, muscular endurance, flexibility, and body composition. These components are targeted in the Healthy People 2000 Objectives.

Cardiorespiratory Endurance

If you were limited to improving only one area of physical fitness, which would you choose—muscular strength, muscular endurance, or flexibility? Which would a dancer choose? Which would a marathon runner select? Which would an expert recommend?

The experts, exercise physiologists, would say that another fitness dimension is of greatest importance. These research scientists regard enhancement of your heart, lung, and blood vessel function to be the most important focal point for a physical fitness program. **Cardiorespiratory endurance** forms the foundation for whole-body fitness.

Cardiorespiratory endurance increases your capacity to sustain a given level of energy production for a prolonged period. Development of cardiorespiratory endurance helps your body work longer and at greater levels of intensity.

Your body cannot always produce the energy needed for long-term activity. Certain activities require performance at a level of intensity that will outstrip your cardiorespiratory system's ability to transport oxygen efficiently to contracting muscle fibers. When the oxygen demands of the muscles cannot be met, a phenomenon called **oxygen debt** occurs. Any activity that must continue beyond the point at which oxygen debt begins will require a form of energy production that does not depend on oxygen.

This oxygen-deprived form of energy production is called **anaerobic** (without oxygen) **energy production,** the type of energy production regularly found in many intense, short-duration activities. Rope climbing, weight lifting for strength, and sprinting are short-duration activities that quickly cause muscle fatigue. These kinds of activities are generally considered anaerobic activities.

If you usually work or play at lower intensity but for a longer duration, you have developed an ability to maintain **aerobic** (with oxygen) **energy production.** As long as your body can meet its energy demands in this oxygen-rich mode, you will not experience conversion to anaerobic energy production. Thus you will not find fatigue an important factor in determining whether you can continue to participate. Marathon runners, serious joggers, distance swimmers, bikers, and aerobic dancers can persist in their activities because of their highly developed aerobic fitness. These aerobically fit people take in, transport, and use oxygen in the most efficient manner possible.

---

cardiorespiratory endurance (car dee oh **ress** pur uh tory) ability of the heart, lungs, and blood vessels to process and transport oxygen required by muscle cells so that they can contract over a period of time.

oxygen debt physical state that occurs when the body can no longer process and transport sufficient amounts of oxygen for continued muscle contraction.

anaerobic energy production (an err oh bick) body's production of energy when needed amounts of oxygen are not readily available.

aerobic energy production (err oh bick) body's production of energy when the respiratory and circulatory systems are able to process and transport sufficient amounts of oxygen to muscle cells.

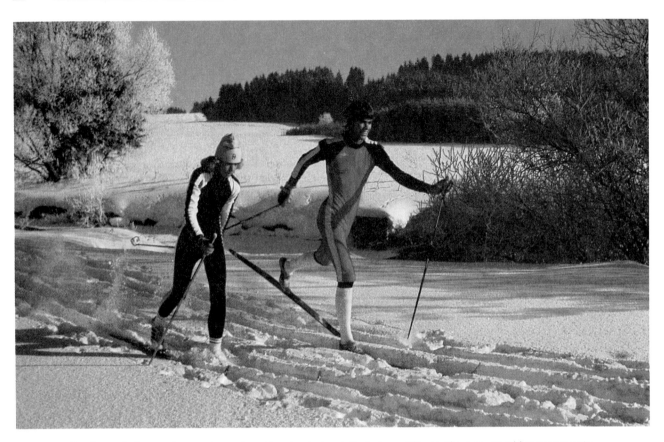

Cardiorespiratory endurance is produced by physical activity that provides continuous, repetitive movements.

Besides allowing you to participate in activities such as those mentioned, aerobic conditioning (cardiorespiratory endurance conditioning) may also provide you with certain structural and functional benefits that may extend into other dimensions of your life. These recognized benefits (see the box on p. 69) have received considerable documented support. Some data suggest that aerobic fitness increases life expectancy,[3] and reduces the risk of developing cancers of the colon, breast, uterus, cervix and ovaries.[4]

Muscular Strength

Muscular strength is essential for your body to accomplish any *work*. Your ability to maintain posture, walk, lift, push, and pull are familiar examples of the constant demands you make on your muscles to maintain or increase their level of *contraction*. The stronger you are, the greater will be your ability to contract muscles and maintain a level of contraction sufficient to complete tasks.

Many of the undertakings associated with being a college student require more than a minimal level of strength. Walking across campus, climbing stairs, and participating in physical education courses and intramural sports will maintain your strength. Occasionally your body's performance—or lack of performance—when you try to move furniture, lift weights, or sprint

to catch a bus will remind you of the importance of developing more than minimal levels of muscle strength and tone.

Muscular strength can best be improved by training activities that use the **overload principle.** By overloading, or gradually increasing the resistance (load, object, or weight) your muscles must move, you can increase your muscular strength. The following three types of training exercises are based on the overload principle.

In **isometric** (meaning "same measure") **exercises,** the resistance is so great that your contracting muscles cannot move the resistance object at all. Thus your muscles contract against immovable objects, usually in increasingly greater efforts (see Figure 4-1). Isometric exercises, because of the difficulty of precisely evaluating the training effects, are not generally used as primary developers of muscular strength and can be dangerous for people with hypertension.

Progressive resistance exercises, also called *isotonic* or "same-tension" exercises, are currently the most popular type of strength-building exercises. Progressive resistance exercises are represented by the use of traditional free weights (dumbbells and barbells), as well as Universal and Nautilus machines. Devotees of progressive resistance exercise use various muscle groups to move (or lift) specific fixed resistances or

★ Structural and Functional Benefits of Cardiorespiratory (Aerobic) Fitness

Aerobic fitness can help you:

★ Complete your daily activities with enjoyment

★ Strengthen your heart muscle and make it more efficient

★ Increase your proportion of high-density lipoproteins

★ Increase the capillary network in your body

★ Improve collateral circulation

★ Control your weight

★ Stimulate bone growth

★ Cope with stressors

★ Ward off infections

★ Improve the efficiency of your other body systems

★ Bolster your self-esteem

★ Achieve self-directed fitness goals

★ Reduce negative dependency behaviors

★ Sleep better

★ Recover more quickly from common illnesses

★ Meet other people with similar interests

★ Receive lowered insurance premiums

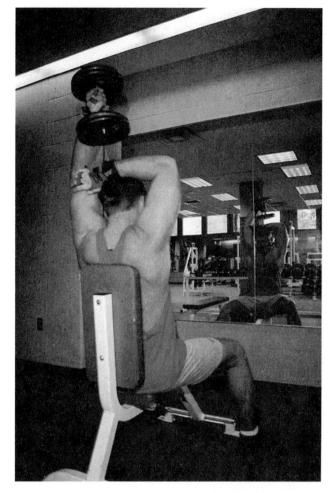

Muscular strength.

muscular strength the ability to contract skeletal muscles to engage in work; the force that a muscle can exert.

overload principle principle (often used in training programs to increase muscular strength) whereby a person gradually increases the resistance load that must be moved or lifted; this principle also applies to other types of fitness training.

isometric exercises (**eye** so **met** rick) muscular strength training exercises that use a resistance so great that the resistance object cannot be moved.

progressive resistance exercises muscular strength training exercises that use traditional barbells and dumbells with fixed resistances.

isokinetic exercises (**eye** so kin **et** ick) muscular strength training exercises that use machines to provide variable resistances throughout the full range of motion.

weights. Although during a given repetitive exercise the weight resistance remains the same, the muscular contraction effort required varies according to the joint angles in the *range of motion*.[2] The greatest effort is required at the start and finish of the movement.

Isokinetic (meaning "same motion") **exercises** employ mechanical devices that provide resistances that consistently overload muscles throughout the entire range of motion. The resistance will move only at a preset speed regardless of the force applied to it. For the exercise to be effective, a user must apply maximal force.[2] Currently believed to be the most effective form of exercise to promote the strength of specific muscle groups, isokinetic training requires elaborate, expensive equipment. Thus the use of isokinetic equipment may be limited to certain athletic teams, diagnostic centers, or rehabilitation clinics. Common isokinetic machines are Cybex, Orthotron, and Mini-gym.

The concept of *specificity* is of key importance. Specificity refers to the fact that by using carefully con-

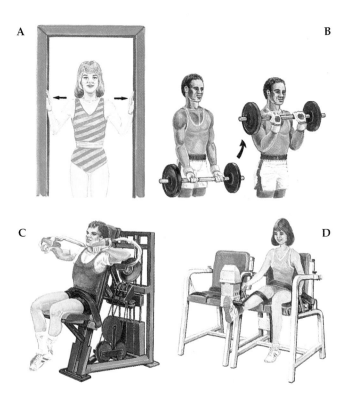

Figure 4-1 Three types of training exercises to improve muscular strength. **A,** Isometric exercise. **B** and **C,** Progressive resistance exercises. **D,** Isokinetic exercise.

trolled exercises, muscular strength can be precisely increased for a particular task or series of skills. In most cases, specificity helps you accomplish particular goals. However, specificity can also create problems when muscle strength is highly developed in one part of the body and neglected in another part. In such a situation the risk of injury can be great. People should strive for appropriate, proportional balances of muscular strength throughout the body. Specificity applies to all components of fitness, not just muscular strength. Each fitness component responds to the specific demands made on it.

Muscular Endurance

Muscular endurance is a component of physical fitness associated with strength. When muscles contract and their individual muscle fibers shorten, energy is required. Energy production requires that oxygen and nutrients be delivered by the circulatory system to the muscles. Following the transformation of these products into energy by individual muscle cells, the body must remove the potentially toxic waste by-products.

Amateur and professional athletes often wish to increase the muscular endurance of specific muscle groups associated with their sports activities. They achieve such muscular endurance by using exercises that gradually increase the number of repetitions of a given movement. Muscular endurance is not the physiological equivalent of cardiorespiratory endurance. For example, a world-ranked distance runner with highly developed cardiorespiratory endurance and extensive muscular endurance of the legs may not have a corresponding level of muscular endurance of the abdominal muscles.

Flexibility

The ability of your joints to move through their natural range of motion is a measure of your **flexibility.** This fitness trait, like so many other aspects of structure and function, differs from point to point within your body and between different people. Not every joint in your body is equally flexible (by design), and over the course of time use or disuse will alter the flexibility of a given joint. Certainly sex, age, genetically determined body build, and current level of physical fitness will affect your flexibility. You may not be as flexible as a gymnast nor as inflexible as a person with arthritis, but certain inborn characteristics will influence your level of flexibility throughout life.

Your ability or inability to move easily during physical activity will be a constant reminder that aging and inactivity are the foes of flexibility. Failure to use joints regularly will quickly result in a loss of elasticity in the connective tissue and shortening of muscles associated

Muscular endurance.

with the joints. Benefits of flexibility include improved balance, posture, athletic performance, and reduced risk of low back pain.

As seen in a young gymnast, flexibility can be highly developed and maintained with a program of activity that includes regular stretching. Stretching also helps reduce the risk of injury. Athletic trainers generally prefer **static stretching** to **ballistic stretching** for people who wish to improve their range of motion. Guidelines for stretching are given in the box below.

★ Guidelines for Stretching

The following precautions should serve as guidelines to reduce the possibility of injury during stretching:

★ Warm up using a slow jog or fast walk before stretching vigorously.

★ Stretch only to the point where you feel tightness or resistance to your stretching. Stretching should not be painful.

★ Be sure to continue normal breathing during a stretch. Do not hold your breath.

★ Use caution when stretching muscles that surround painful joints. Pain is an indication that something is wrong—it should not be ignored.

Body Composition

Body composition refers to the "makeup of the body in terms of muscle, bone, fat, and other elements."[2] Of particular interest to fitness experts are percentages of body fat and fat-free weight. Health experts are especially concerned about the large numbers of people in our society who are overweight and obese. Increasingly, cardiorespiratory fitness programs are recognizing the importance of a person's body composition and are including strength training exercises to help reduce body fat. (See Chapter 6 for further information about body composition, health effects of obesity, and weight management.)

muscular endurance the ability of a muscle or a muscle group to function over time; supported by the respiratory and circulatory systems.

flexibility ability of joints to function through an intended range of motion.

static stretching (**stat** ick) the slow lengthening of a muscle group to an extended level of stretch; followed by holding the extended position for a recommended time period.

ballistic stretching (buh **list** ick) a "bouncing" form of stretching in which a muscle group is lengthened repetitively to produce multiple quick, forceful stretches.

Health ACTION Guide

Tips to Help You Stick to Your Exercise Program

Sometimes it seems difficult to continue with an exercise program. Here are a few tips to keep you going:

▼ Fit your program into your daily lifestyle
▼ Exercise with your friends
▼ Incorporate music with your activity
▼ Vary your activities frequently; cross-train
▼ Reward yourself when you reach a fitness goal
▼ Avoid a complicated exercise program; keep it simple
▼ Measure your improvement (keep a log or diary)
▼ Take some time off (rest and recuperate)
▼ Keep in mind how important physical activity is to your life

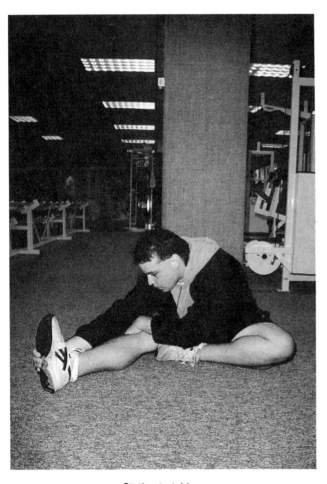

Static stretching.

DEVELOPING A CARDIORESPIRATORY FITNESS PROGRAM

Although the pronounced benefits of exercise clearly exist, we expect that readers of this book fall into some rather distinct categories: (1) those who already exercise regularly, (2) those who exercise occasionally, (3) those who do not exercise, and (4) those who would like to start some kind of fitness program. A major limitation for readers in all groups is an uncertainty about how best to develop fitness. We ask ourselves, "Am I doing enough to develop my fitness?"; "How can I have fun and develop cardiorespiratory fitness at the same time?"; and "Am I doing things that might be dangerous?"

For persons of all ages, cardiorespiratory conditioning can be achieved through many activities. As long as the activity you choose places sufficient demand on the heart and lungs, improved fitness is possible. In addition to the familiar activities of swimming, running, cycling, and aerobic dance, today many people are participating in brisk walking, roller blading, cross-country skiing, swimnastics, skating, rowing, and even weight training (often combined with some form of aerobic activity). Regardless of age or physical limitations, you can select from a variety of enjoyable activities that will condition the cardiorespiratory system.

Many people think any kind of physical activity will produce cardiorespiratory fitness. Golf, bowling, hunting, fishing, and archery are considered forms of exercise. However, these activities would generally fail to produce positive changes in your cardiorespiratory and overall muscular fitness; they may indeed enhance your health, be enjoyable, and produce some fatigue after lengthy participation, but they do not meet the standards recently established by the American College of Sports Medicine (ACSM), the nation's premier professional organization of exercise physiologists and sport physicians.[5]

The most recent recommendations by the ACSM for achieving cardiorespiratory fitness were approved in 1990 and include five major areas: (a) mode of activity, (b) frequency of training, (c) intensity of training, (d) duration of training, and (e) resistance training. We will summarize these recommendations. Compare your existing fitness program with these standards.

Mode of Activity

The ACSM recommends the mode of activity to be any continuous physical activity that uses large muscle groups and can be rhythmic and aerobic in nature. Among the activities that generally meet this requirement are continuous swimming, cycling, aerobic dancing, basketball, cross-country skiing, roller blading, step training (bench aerobics), hiking, walking, rowing, stair climbing, dancing, and running. Endurance games and activities such as tennis, racquetball, and handball are fine, as long as you and your partner are skilled enough to keep the ball in play; walking after the ball will do very little for you. Riding a bicycle is a good activity, if you keep pedaling. Coasting through a residential neighborhood will do little to improve fitness. Softball and football are generally less than sufficient continuous activities—especially the way they are played by weekend athletes.

Regardless of which continuous activity you select, it should also be enjoyable. Running is not for everyone—despite what some accomplished runners will say! Find an activity you enjoy. If you need others around you to have a good time, corral a group of friends to join you. Vary your activities to keep from becoming bored. You might cycle in the summer, run in the fall, swim in the winter, and play racquetball in the spring.

Frequency of Training

Frequency of training refers to the number of times per week a person should exercise. The ACSM recommends three to five times per week. For most people, participation in fitness activities more than five times each week does not significantly improve their level of conditioning. Likewise, an average of only two workouts each week does not seem to produce a measureable improvement in cardiorespiratory conditioning. Thus although you may have a lot of fun cycling twice each week, do not expect to see a significant improvement in your cardiorespiratory fitness level.

Intensity of Training

How much effort should you put into an activity? Should you run quickly, jog slowly, or swim at a comfortable pace? Must a person sweat profusely to achieve fitness? These questions all refer to **intensity** of effort.

The ACSM recommends that healthy adults participate in their fitness activity at an intensity level of between 60% and 90% of their maximum heart rate (calculated by subtracting your age from 220). This level of intensity is called the **target heart rate (THR).** This rate refers to the minimum number of times your heart needs to contract (beat) each minute to have a positive effect on your heart, lungs, and blood vessels. This improvement is called the *training effect.* Intensity of activity below the THR will be insufficient to make a significant improvement in your fitness. Intensity below the THR will still help you expend calories and thus lose weight, but it will probably do little to make you

How to Calculate Your Target Heart Rate

The target heart rate (THR) is the recommended rate for increasing cardiorespiratory endurance. To maintain a training effect, you must sustain activity at your THR. To find your THR, subtract your age from 220 (the maximum heart rate) and multiply by .60 to .90. Here are two examples:

For a 20-year-old person (wanting a THR of 80% of maximum)

Maximum heart rate:
220 − 20 = 200
200 × .80 = 160
THR = 160 beats per minute

For a 40-year-old person (wanting a THR of 65% of maximum)

Maximum heart rate:
220 − 40 = 180
180 × .65 = 117
THR = 117 beats per minute

more aerobically fit. Intensity that is significantly above your THR will in all likelihood cause you to become so fatigued that you will be forced to stop the activity before the training effect can be achieved.

Choosing a particular THR between 60% and 90% of your maximum heart rate depends on your initial level of fitness. If you are already in relatively good physical shape, you might want to start exercising at 75% of your maximum heart rate. A well-conditioned person may decide to select a higher THR for his or her intensity level. On the other hand, a person with a low fitness level will still be able to achieve a training effect at the lower THR of 60% of maximum.

In the box above, the younger person would need to select a continuous and enjoyable activity and participate in this activity for an extended period while working at a THR of 160 beats per minute. The older person in the example would need to function at a THR of 117 beats per minute to achieve a positive training effect.

Determining your heart rate is not a complicated procedure. You need to find a location on your body where an artery passes near the surface of the skin. Pulse rates are quite difficult to determine by touching veins, which are more superficial than arteries. Two easily accessible sites for determining heart rate are the

frequency number of times per week one should exercise to achieve a training effect.

intensity level of effort put into an activity.

target heart rate (THR) number of times per minute the heart must contract to produce a training effect.

PERSONAL ASSESSMENT

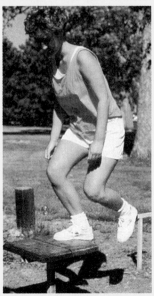

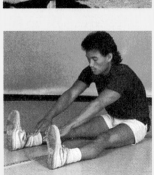

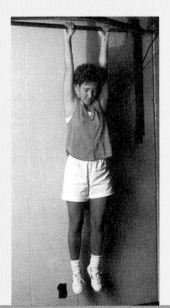

You can determine your level of fitness in 30 minutes or less by completing this short group of tests based on the National Fitness Test developed by the President's Council on Physical Fitness and Sports. If you are over 40 years old or have chronic medical disorders such as diabetes or obesity, check with your physician before taking this or any other fitness test. You will need another person to monitor your test and keep time.

THREE-MINUTE STEP TEST

Aerobic capacity. Equipment: 12-inch bench, crate, block, or step ladder; stopwatch. Procedure: face bench. Complete 24 full steps (both feet on the bench, both feet on the ground) per minute for 3 minutes. After finishing, sit down, have your partner find your pulse within 5 seconds and take your pulse for 1 minute. Your score is your pulse rate for 1 full minute.

Scoring Standards (Heart Rate for 1 Minute)

Age	18-29		30-39		40-49		50-59		60+	
Sex	F	M	F	M	F	M	F	M	F	M
Excellent	<80	<75	<84	<78	<88	<80	<92	<85	<95	<90
Good	80-110	75-100	85-115	78-109	88-118	80-112	92-123	85-115	95-127	90-118
Average	>110	>100	>115	>109	>118	>112	>123	>115	>127	>118

SIT AND REACH

Hamstring flexibility. Equipment: yardstick; tape. Between your legs, tape the yardstick to the floor. Sit with legs straight and heels about 5 inches apart, heels even with the 15-inch mark on the yardstick. While in a sitting position, slowly stretch forward as far as possible. Your score is the number of inches reached.

Scoring Standards (Inches)

Age	18-29		30-39		40-49		50-59		60+	
Sex	F	M	F	M	F	M	F	M	F	M
Excellent	>22	>21	>22	>21	>21	>20	>20	>19	>20	>19
Good	17-22	13-21	17-22	13-21	15-21	13-20	14-20	12-19	14-20	12-19
Average	<17	<13	<17	<13	<15	<13	<14	<12	<14	<12

ARM HANG

Upper body strength. Equipment: horizontal bar (high enough to prevent your feet from touching the floor); stopwatch. Procedure: hang with straight arms, palms facing forward. Start watch when subject is in position. Stop when subject lets go. Your score is the number of minutes and seconds spent hanging.

Scoring Standards (Minutes and Seconds)

Age	18-29		30-39		40-49		50-59		60+	
Sex	F	M	F	M	F	M	F	M	F	M
Excellent	>1:30	>2:00	>1:20	>1:50	>1:10	>1:35	>1:00	>1:20	>:50	>1:10
Good	:46-1:30	1:00-2:00	:40-1:20	:50-1:50	:30-1:10	:45-1:35	:30-1:00	:35-1:20	:21-:50	:30-1:10
Average	<:46	<1:00	<:40	<:50	<:30	<:45	<:30	<:35	<:21	<:30

CURL-UPS

Abdominal and low back strength. Equipment: stopwatch. Procedure: Lie flat on upper back, knees bent, shoulders touching the floor, arms extended above your thighs or by your sides, palms down. Bend knees so that feet are flat and 12 inches from the buttocks. Curl up by lifting head and shoulders off the floor, sliding hands forward above your thighs or the floor. Curl down and repeat. Your score is the number of curl-ups in 1 minute.

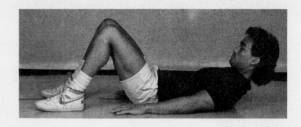

Scoring Standards (Number in 1 Minute)

Age	18-29		30-39		40-49		50-59		60+	
Sex	F	M	F	M	F	M	F	M	F	M
Excellent	>45	>50	>40	>45	>35	>40	>30	>35	>25	>30
Good	25-45	30-50	20-40	22-45	16-35	21-40	12-30	18-35	11-25	15-30
Average	<25	<30	<20	<22	<16	<21	<12	<18	<11	<15

PUSH-UPS (MEN)

Upper body strength. Equipment: stopwatch. Assume a front-leaning position. Lower your body until chest touches the floor. Raise and repeat for 1 minute. Your score is the number of push-ups completed in 1 minute.

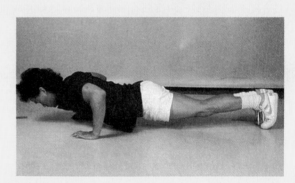

Scoring Standards (Number in 1 Minute)

Age	18-29	30-39	40-49	50-59	60+
Excellent	>50	>45	>40	>35	>30
Good	25-50	22-45	19-40	15-35	10-30
Average	<25	<22	<19	<15	<10

PUSH-UPS (WOMEN)

Upper body strength. Equipment: stopwatch. Assume a front-leaning position with knees on the floor, feet raised, and hands under shoulders. Lower your chest to the floor, raise, and repeat. Your score is the number of push-ups completed in 1 minute.

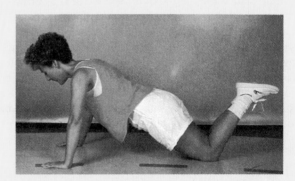

Scoring Standards (Number In 1 Minute)

Age	18-29	30-39	40-49	50-59	60+
Excellent	>45	>40	>35	>30	>25
Good	17-45	12-40	8-35	6-30	5-25
Average	<17	<12	<8	<6	<5

TO CARRY THIS FURTHER . . .

Note your areas of strengths and weaknesses. To improve your fitness, become involved in a fitness program that reflects the concepts discussed in this chapter. Talking with fitness experts on your campus might be a good first step.

PERSONAL ASSESSMENT

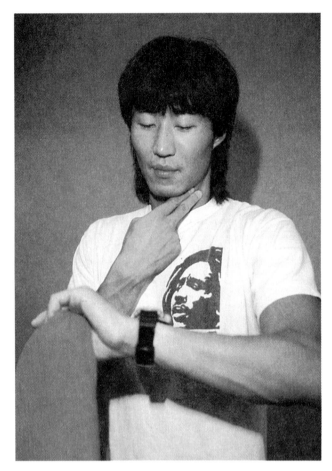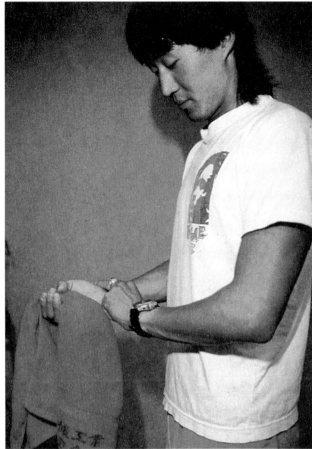

The pulse rate can be measured at the carotid artery (left) or at the radial artery (right).

carotid artery (one on either side of the Adam's apple at the front of your neck) and the *radial artery* (on the inside of your wrist, just above the base of the thumb).

You should practice placing the front surface of your index and middle fingertips at either of these locations and feeling for a pulse. Once you have found a regular pulse, look at the second hand of a watch. Count the number of beats you feel in a 10-second period and multiply this number by 6. This number will be your heart rate. With a little practice you can become very proficient at counting your heart rate.

Duration of Training

The ACSM recommends that the **duration** should be between 20 and 60 minutes of continuous aerobic activity. Generally speaking, the duration can be on the shorter end of this range for athletic people whose activities use a high intensity of training (80% to 90% of maximum heart rate). Those who utilize activities with a lower range of itensity (60% to 70% of maximum) should maintain that activity for a longer time. Thus a fast jog and a moderate walk will require different levels of duration to accomplish the training effect. The fast jog might be maintained for 25 minutes, whereas

the brisk walk should be kept up longer—perhaps 50 minutes.

Resistance Training

Recognizing the important point that overall body fitness includes muscular fitness, the ACSM now recommends resistance training in its current standards. The ACSM suggests participation in strength training of moderate intensity at least two times a week. This training should help develop and maintain a healthy body composition—one with an emphasis on fat-free weight. The goal of resistance training is not to improve cardiorespiratory endurance, but to improve overall muscle strength and tone. For the average person, resistance training with heavy weights is not recommended because it can induce a sudden and dangerous increase in blood pressure.

The resistance training recommended includes one set of 8 to 12 repetitions of 8 to 10 exercises. These exercises should be geared to the body's major muscle groups (that is, legs, arms, shoulders, trunk, and back) and should not focus on just one or two body areas. Isotonic (progressive resistance) or isokinetic exercises are recommended (see pp. 68-70). For the typical per-

Health ACTION Guide

Safety Precautions

To avoid injury during strength training exercises, you should employ the following safety precautions:

▼ Warm up appropriately

▼ Use proper lifting techniques
▼ Always have a spotter if you are using free weights
▼ Do not hold your breath during a lift
▼ Avoid single lifts of very heavy weights
▼ Before using a machine (such as Nautilus, Universal, or Cybex), be certain you know how to use it correctly
▼ Seek advice for training programs from experts
▼ Work within your limitations; avoid "showing off"

son, resistance training activities should be done at a moderate to slow speed, should employ the full range of motion, and should not impair normal forced breathing. With just one set recommended for each exercise, resistance training should not be too time consuming.

Warm-up, Workout, Cool-down

Each training session consists of three basic parts: the warm-up, the workout, and the cool-down.[2] The *warm-up* should last between 10 and 15 minutes. During this period, slow, gradual, comfortable movements related to the upcoming activity should be started, such as walking or slow jogging. All body segments and muscle groups should be exercised as you gradually increase your heart rate. Near the end of the warm-up period, the major muscle groups should be stretched. This preparation helps protect you from muscle strains and joint sprains.

Warm-up is a fine time to socialize with others. Furthermore, you can mentally prepare yourself for your activity or think about the beauty of the morning sky, the changing colors of the leaves, or the friends you will meet later in the day. You may even enjoy contemplating the vigor of the activity you are about to undertake. Mental warm-ups can be as beneficial for you psychologically as physical warm-ups are physiologically.

The second part of the training session is the *workout*. This is the part of the session that involves improving muscular strength and endurance, cardiorespiratory endurance, and flexibility. Workouts can be tailor-made, but they should follow the ACSM guidelines discussed earlier in this chapter.

The third important part of each fitness session is the *cool-down*. This consists of a 5- to 10-minute session of relaxing exercises (such as slow jogging, walking, and stretching).[6] This allows your body to cool and return to a resting state. Cool-down periods help reduce muscle soreness.

Exercise for Older Adults

An exercise program designed for younger adults may be inappropriate for older persons, particularly for those over age 50. Special attention must be paid to matching the program to the interests and abilities of the participants. The goals of the program should include both social interaction and physical conditioning.

★ A Revised Program for Fitness?

A number of health professionals have recently begun to urge the American public to consider the health benefits of less directed physical activity than that prescribed by the American College of Sports Medicine. These fitness experts believe that people shy away from physical activity because they are afraid that a fitness program requires too much effort and commitment.

One major aspect of this revised approach is the belief that the 20 to 60 minutes of physical activity does not have to be accomplished all at once. People can accumulate their minutes in segments over the course of a day. For example, raking leaves for 15 minutes, brisk walking for 10 minutes at lunch, and dancing for 10 minutes can produce health benefits if done on most days.

Opponents of this "kinder, gentler" approach to fitness are concerned that people already exercising regularly may slack off and actually reduce their current fitness levels. Opponents also believe that, without a prescription for exercise, the public will fool itself into thinking that it is much more active than it really is.

Which approach would be better for you? Do you wish to follow prescribed fitness guidelines, such as those given by the ACSM? Or do you believe that a lifestyle that incorporates short-term fitness activities throughout the day is a better approach for you? ★

duration length of time one needs to exercise at the THR to produce the training effect.

Older adults, especially those with a personal or family history of heart problems, should have a physical examination before starting a fitness program. Included in this examination should be a stress cardiogram,[7] blood pressure check, and an evaluation of joint functioning. It is a good idea for participants to learn how to monitor their own cardiorespiratory status during exercise.

Well-designed fitness programs for older adults will have activities that begin slowly, are monitored frequently, and are geared to the enjoyment of the participants. The professional staff coordinating the program should be familiar with the signs of distress (excessively elevated heart rate, nausea, breathing difficulty, pallor, and pain) and must be able to perform cardiopulmonary resuscitation (CPR). Periods of warm-up and cool-down should be included. Activities to increase flexibility are beneficial in the beginning and ending segments of the program. Participants should wear comfortable clothing and appropriate shoes, and should be mentally prepared to enjoy the activities.

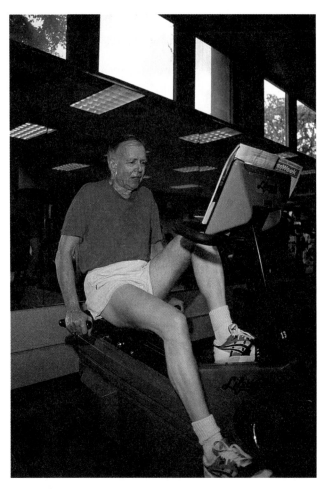

Exercise at any age is important to the cardiorespiratory system.

A program designed for older adults will largely conform to the ACSM criteria specified earlier in this chapter. However, except for certain very fit older athletes (such as runners and triathletes), the THR should not exceed 120 beats per minute. Also, because of possible joint, muscular, or skeletal problems, certain activities may have to be done in a sitting position. Pain and discomfort should be reported immediately to the fitness instructor.

Fortunately, properly screened older adults will rarely have health emergencies during a well-monitored fitness program. Like their youthful counterparts, many older adults find fitness programs socially enjoyable, physically beneficial, and—occasionally—addictive.

FITNESS QUESTIONS AND ANSWERS

Along with the five necessary elements to include in your fitness program, many additional issues should be considered when you start a fitness program.

Should I See My Doctor Before I Get Started?

This issue has probably kept thousands of people from ever beginning a fitness program. The hassle and expense of getting a comprehensive physical examination are excellent alibis for people who are not completely sold on the idea of exercise. A complete examination, including *blood analysis*, a *stress test*, a *cardiogram, serum lipid analysis,* and *body fat analysis,* is a valuable tool for developing some baseline physical data for your medical record.

Is this examination really necessary? Most exercise physiologists do not think so. The value of these measurements as safety predictors is questioned by many professionals. A good general rule of thumb to follow would be to undergo a physical examination if (1) you have an existing medical condition (diabetes, obesity, hypertension, heart abnormalities, or arthritis, for example), or (2) you are age 30 or over and have not pursued vigorous activity for at least 5 years, or (3) you smoke.

What About Jumping Rope?

For most people jumping rope is a skill that takes a long time to develop well. Yet we hear claims that jumping rope only 10 minutes a day can make you fit. Jumping rope is not generally a good choice of activity unless you are already in good physical condition or are a member of an organized rope jumping program. The average person strains too hard to keep the jumping and rope maneuvering in synchronization. Thus the novice jumper quickly becomes fatigued and must stop.

Contrast this picture with that of a well-conditioned welterweight boxer. He is already in top cardiorespira-

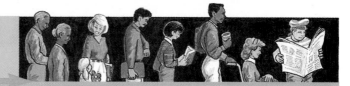

Learning FROM ALL Cultures

Keeping Fit

It is not uncommon in the United States for men and women to take time out of their day to go to an aerobics class, jog for several miles, or play a few games of racquetball. This practice is not unique to Americans. The people of Japan are also showing an interest in fitness and sport, and commercialized sports facilities are rapidly developing. Japanese women, especially, are participating in fitness activities. Many women who are housewives participate in activities such as aerobic exercise, jazz, yoga, and Chinese martial arts; these activities are taught through programs at the sports centers.[13]

In China, one would not see commercialized sports centers, but there is an emphasis on physical fitness and sport. The emphasis comes from the government. For students in primary and secondary school, there are two required physical education classes per week,

each 50 minutes long. For adult workers, participation in exercise is also encouraged. In offices and factories, employees take 10-minute exercise breaks in the mornings and afternoons. Physical activities may include calisthenics and even eye exercises.[14]

Fitness seems to have gained in popularity since many people now recognize the benefits. It is interesting to note a German visitor's observation of the fitness habits of a number of Americans. He observed that Americans get in their cars and drive to their fitness clubs, exercise, and then drive back to work or home. Merely walking to their destinations and forgetting the club seemed to make more sense to him!

Knowing how important fitness is to good health, think about your own daily routine. What kinds of exercise and activities do you do to enhance your fitness? ●

---

tory condition and has developed excellent rope jumping skills. Thus he could keep the continuous activity going at his THR for the required 30 minutes. He would not become fatigued to the point of stopping. This athlete is so fit that he could even conduct an interview while he exercised.

Unless you too are already in good physical condition and have the requisite skills, you should not consider rope jumping as your only fitness activity.

How Important Is Breast Support for Female Exercisers?

Because of the violent up-and-down and lateral breast movement that can occur with jumping and running activities, it is important that women wear bras that fully support their breasts. This is especially important for large-breasted women. A good support bra can reduce discomfort and distraction during physical activity. Also, adequate support reduces damage to the Cooper's ligaments. Damage to these ligaments can cause premature sagging of the breasts.

Another problem that female exercisers may face is a condition called runner's nipples. This is an abrasion caused by the constant friction from the jogger's shirt. A good bra prevents this, as well as a condition called bicyclist's nipples, in which the nipples become painful because of the combination of sweat evaporation and wind chill.[6]

Christine E. Haycock, MD, has researched sports bras and believes that the ideal sports bra depends on a woman's weight and breast size, her physical activity, and what feels comfortable. She believes that any sports bra should be made with (a) breathable material, (b) a minimal amount of elastic, (c) no seams over the nipple area, (d) comfortable support under the breast that prevents the bra from rising during activity, and (e) nonelastic straps that prevent the shoulder straps from slipping off during activity.[8]

How Beneficial Is Aerobic Exercise?

One of the most popular fitness approaches is aerobic exercise, including aerobic dancing. Many organizations sponsor classes in this form of continuous dancing and movement. The rise in popularity of televised and videotaped aerobic exercise programs reflects the enthusiasm for this form of exercise. Because some extravagant claims are made for the value of these programs, the wise consumer should observe at least one session of the activity before enrolling. Discover for yourself whether the program meets the criteria outlined earlier in this chapter: mode of activity, frequency, intensity, duration, and resistance training.

In the mid 1990s, street dancing has fast become one of the most popular aerobic exercises. Popularized by rap music, classic funk, and the growth of vigorous "Street Jam" dancing in music videos, street dancing is

Choosing an Athletic Shoe

AEROBIC SHOES

When selecting shoes for aerobic dancing, J. Lynn Reese, president of J. Lynn & Co. Endurance Sports, Washington, DC, advises the following:

★ Check the width of the shoe at the widest part of your foot. The bottom of the shoe should be as wide as the bottom of your foot; the uppers shouldn't go over the sides.

★ Look for leather or nylon uppers. Leather is durable and gives good support, but it can stretch. Nylon won't stretch and gives support, but it's not as durable. Canvas generally doesn't offer much support.

★ Look for rubber rather than polyurethane or black carbon rubber soles. Treads should be fairly flat in the forefoot. If you're dancing on carpet, you can go with less tread; if you're dancing on gym floors, you may need more grab.

COURT SHOES

What's more important when choosing a tennis shoe? Jack Groppel, technical editor of *World Tennis* magazine and associate professor of Bioengineering, University of Illinois, offers this list:

★ Cushioning. Cushioning is especially important in the heel counter.

★ Side support. Side support, also called *lateral* and *medial* support, is also important.

★ Back-of-heel fit. Try on the shoe, and then put your little finger in behind the heel. It should fit snugly.

★ Toe box (top front of shoe). Make sure the toe box isn't too tight or too loose.

★ Traction. Keep in mind the surface you play on most often. Rubber gives better traction than synthetic materials such as polyurethane but is less durable.

When buying shoes for racquetball, Doug Richie, podiatrist, Seal Beach, California, advises the following:

★ Choose side-to-side support over flexibility and cushioning.

★ Choose a heavy shoe with lots of support.

★ The tread should be relatively smooth—compatible with hardwood surfaces.

★ Choose the brushed cotton jersey sock over terry liners.

RUNNING SHOES

Need new running shoes? Here's advice from Jeff Galloway, former Olympic runner, founder and president of Phidippides International aerobic sports stores, headquartered in Atlanta.

★ Take time to shop, and find a knowledgeable salesperson. Good advice is crucial.

★ Check the wear pattern on your old shoes to see whether you have floppy or rigid feet. Floppy-footed runners wear out their soles on the outside and inside edges; rigid-footed runners wear out soles predominantly on the outside edges. Floppy-footed runners can sacrifice cushioning for support; rigid-footed runners can sacrifice support for cushioning.

★ Know your feet, whether they're curved or straight and whether you have high arches or are flat footed. The shoe should fit the shape of your foot.

AEROBIC SHOES

Flexibility: More at ball of foot than running shoes; sole is firmer; less flexible than court shoes or running shoes

Cushioning: More than court shoes; less than running shoes

Uppers: Most are leather or leather-reinforced nylon

Heel: Little or no flare

Soles: Rubber if you are dancing on wood floors; polyurethane for other surfaces

Tread: Should be fairly flat, especially on forefoot; may also have "dot" on the ball of the foot for pivoting

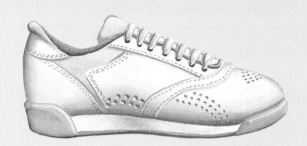

COURT SHOES

Flexibility: Flexible at ball of foot

Cushioning: Less than running shoes

Uppers: Usually nylon mesh or nylon; leather; no canvas

Heel: Not flared (flared heels reduce side-to-side support)

Soles: For tennis, flat; usually polyurethane—more durable for tennis courts; for racquetball, rounded (to allow quicker side-to-side movement); usually rubber—less durable because wood courts are slicker and don't wear down shoes as fast

Tread: Much flatter than running shoes; may have tread pattern designed around ball of foot where the foot pivots

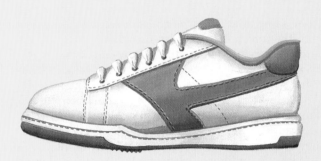

RUNNING SHOES

Cushioning: More than court shoes, especially at heel

Heel: Flare gives foot broader, more stable base

Soles: Usually carbon-based for longer wear

Tread: "Waffle" or other deep-cut tread for grip on many surfaces ★

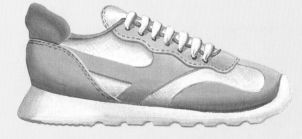

viewed as an excellent method of having fun and developing cardiorespiratory fitness. Street dancing was even introduced to fitness experts at the 1991 AAH-PERD National Convention in San Francisco.

What Are Low-Impact Aerobic Activities?

Because long-term participation in some aerobic activities (for example, jogging, running, aerobic dance, and rope skipping) may cause damage to the hip, knee, and ankle joints, many fitness experts are promoting low-impact aerobic activities. Low-impact aerobic dance, swimnastics, brisk walking, and bench aerobics are examples of this kind of fitness activity. Participants still conform to the principal components of a cardiorespiratory fitness program. THR levels remain the same as in high-impact activities.

The main difference between low- and high-impact aerobic activities is in the use of the legs. Low-impact aerobics do not require having both feet off the ground at the same time. Thus weight transfer does not occur with the forcefulness seen in traditional, high-impact aerobic activities. In addition, low-impact activities may include exaggerated arm movements and the use of hand or wrist weights. All of these variations are designed to increase the heart rate to the THR without damaging the joints of the lower extremities. Low-impact aerobics are excellent for people of all ages, and they may be especially beneficial to older adults.

With 7 million participants, in-line skating (rollerblading) has been reported as the fastest growing participant activity in 1990-91.[9] This low-impact activity has similar cardiorespiratory and muscular benefits as running, but without the pounding effect which running can produce.[10] Rollerblading does require important safety equipment: sturdy skates, knee and elbow pads, wrist supports, and a helmet.

What Is the Most Effective Fluid Replacement During Exercise?

Despite all the advertising hype associated with commercial fluid replacement products, for an average person involved in typical fitness activities, water is still the best fluid replacement available. The availability and cost are unbeatable. However, when activity is prolonged and intense, commercial sport drinks may be preferable to water because they contain electrolytes (that replace lost sodium and potassium) and carbohydrates (that replace depleted energy stores).[11] Regardless of the drink you choose, it is recommended that you drink fluids at frequent intervals throughout your activity.

Why Has Bodybuilding Become So Popular?

It is true that *bodybuilding* has increased significantly in popularity in recent years. The reasons for this growth are many. Bodybuilders often start lifting weights to get into better shape—to improve muscle tone. They may just want to look healthier and feel stronger. Once they realize that they can alter the shape of their bodies, they find that bodybuilding offers challenges that—through hard work—are attainable. Bodybuilders also report enjoying the physical sensations (the "pump") that results from a good workout. The results of their efforts are clearly visible and measurable. Some bodybuilders become involved in competitive events to test their advancements.

Perhaps we should dispel a few myths about bodybuilding. Are bodybuilders strong? The answer is emphatically—yes! Will muscle cells turn into fat cells if weightlifting programs are discontinued? *No*, muscle cells are physiologically incapable of turning into fat cells. Will women develop bulky muscles through weight training? *No*, they can improve muscle strength and tone, but unless they take steroids, their muscle mass cannot increase like men's muscle mass. Is bodybuilding socially acceptable? *Yes*, for many people. Just observe all the health clubs that cater to weightlifters and bodybuilders.

Can Strength Training Improve Heart Functioning?

Yes. Cardiovascular improvement has been seen among people who lift weights, especially those who use light weights repetitively.

Where Can I Find Out About Proper Equipment?

College students are generally in an excellent setting to locate people and resources that can provide helpful information about equipment. Contacting physical education or health education faculty members who have an interest in your chosen activity might be a good start. Most colleges also have a number of clubs that specialize in fitness interests—cycling, hiking, and jogging clubs, for example. Attend one of their upcoming meetings. Such clubs are often looking for new members.

Sporting goods stores and specialized stores (for runners, tennis and racquetball players, and cyclists) are convenient places to obtain information. Employees of these stores are usually knowledgable about sports and equipment (see the box on p. 80).

How Worthwhile Are Commercial Health and Fitness Clubs?

The business in health and fitness clubs is booming. Fitness clubs offer activities ranging from free weights to weight machines to step walking to general aerobics. Some clubs have saunas and whirlpools and lots of frills. Others have course offerings that include wellness, smoking cessation, stress management, time management, dance, and yoga. The atmosphere at most clubs is friendly, and people are encouraged to "have a good time while working out."

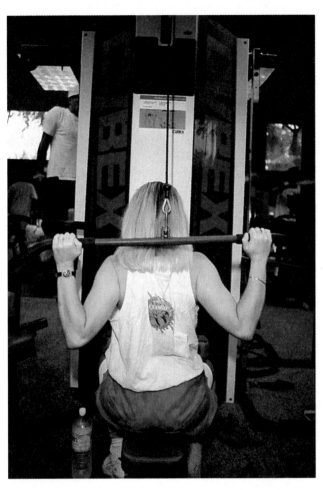

Bodybuilding improves muscle tone and makes you look healthier and feel stronger.

If your purpose in joining a fitness club is to improve your cardiorespiratory fitness, measure the program offered by the club with the American College of Sports Medicine standards. If your primary purpose in joining is to meet people and have fun, request a trial membership to see if you like the environment.

Before signing a contract at a health club or spa, do some careful questioning. Find out how long the business has been established, ask about the qualifications of the employees, contact some members for their observations, and request a thorough tour of the facilities. You might even consult your local Better Business Bureau for additional information. Finally, make certain you read and understand every word of the contract.

What Is Crosstraining?

Crosstraining is the use of more than one aerobic activity to achieve cardiorespiratory fitness. For example, runners may use swimming, cycling, or rowing to pe-

riodically replace running in their training routines. Crosstraining allows certain muscle groups to rest and injuries to heal. Also, crosstraining provides a refreshing change of pace for the participant. You will probably enjoy your fitness program more if you vary the activities. And your enjoyment will make it more likely that the Healthy People 2000 Objectives can be achieved.

What Are Steroids and Why Do Some Athletes Use Them?

Steroids are drugs that can be legally prescribed by physicians for a variety of health conditions, including certain forms of anemia, inadequate growth patterns, as an aid in recovery from surgery of burns, or for chronic debilitating diseases. **Anabolic steroids** are drugs that function like the male sex hormone *testosterone.*[12]

Anabolic steroids are used by athletes who hope to gain weight and increase muscle size and strength, power, endurance, and aggressiveness. Over the last few decades, numerous bodybuilders, weightlifters, track athletes, and football players have chosen illegal steroid use and ignored the health risks. Anabolic steroids can be taken orally or by injection.

The use of steroids is highly dangerous because of serious, life-threatening side effects and adverse reactions. These effects include heart problems, certain forms of cancer, liver complications, and even psychological disturbances. The side effects on female steroid users are as dangerous as those on men. Figure 4-2 shows the adverse effects of steroid use.

Steroid users have developed a terminology of their own. Anabolic steroids are called *roids* or *juice. Roid rage* refers to an aggressive, psychotic response to chronic steroid use. *Stacking* is a term that describes the use of multiple steroids at the same time.

Many organizations that control athletic competition (NCAA, The Athletics Congress, the National Football League, and the International Olympic Committee) have banned steroids and are testing athletes for illegal use. The recent death of pro football player Lyle Alzado highlighted the serious threats from steroid use. Fortunately, athletes finally seem to be getting the message and are steering clear of steroids.

---

anabolic steroids (ann uh **bol** ick) drugs that function like testosterone to produce increases in weight, strength, endurance, and aggressiveness.

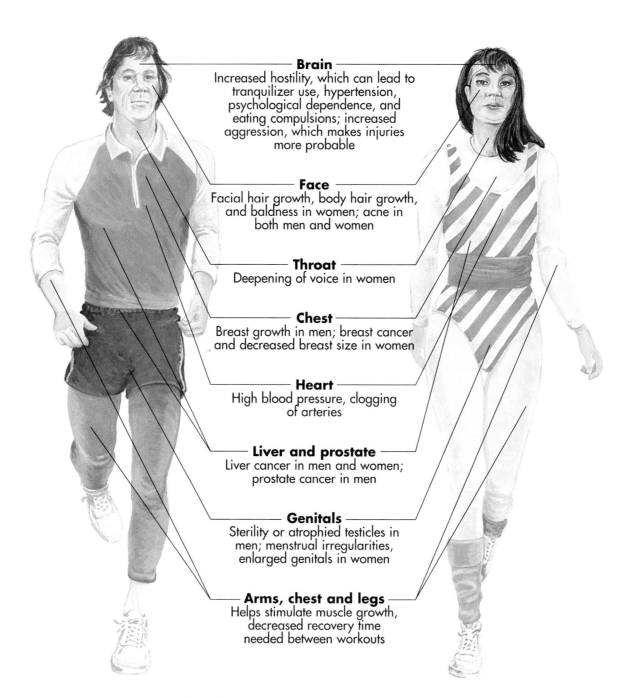

Brain
Increased hostility, which can lead to tranquilizer use, hypertension, psychological dependence, and eating compulsions; increased aggression, which makes injuries more probable

Face
Facial hair growth, body hair growth, and baldness in women; acne in both men and women

Throat
Deepening of voice in women

Chest
Breast growth in men; breast cancer and decreased breast size in women

Heart
High blood pressure, clogging of arteries

Liver and prostate
Liver cancer in men and women; prostate cancer in men

Genitals
Sterility or atrophied testicles in men; menstrual irregularities, enlarged genitals in women

Arms, chest and legs
Helps stimulate muscle growth, decreased recovery time needed between workouts

Figure 4-2 Adverse effects of steroids on parts of the body.

What Are the Two Types of Muscle Fibers and How Can They Affect Exercise Performance?

Through a *needle biopsy procedure,* two basic types of fibers (muscle cells) can be seen in human muscle. These fibers are the **fast-twitch (FT)** and **slow-twitch (ST) fibers.** The high enzyme activity in FT fibers makes these fibers better suited for high-intensity activity, whereas the greater aerobic capacity of ST fibers makes them better suited for endurance-type activities.

People inherit varying proportions of these fiber types. People with greater percentages of FT fibers than ST fibers have a greater capacity for anaerobic activities. Those having a greater percentage of ST fibers than FT fibers seem more capable of endurance activities.

Although FT fibers cannot be converted to ST fibers, some research suggests that with proper exercise training, FT fibers are capable of developing some properties of ST fibers. One example of the application of this knowledge is in track and field, where increasing numbers of middle-distance runners are redirecting their training methods and finding great success at full-length marathons. ST fibers appear to be less able to develop the properties of FT fibers. Thus it is doubtful that marathon runners can be trained to be first-class sprinters. Indeed, it seems that we are born with predispositions to certain kinds of athletic activities.

Are Today's Children Physically Fit?

The answer to this question has major implications for achieving success on some of the Healthy People 2000 Objectives presented at the start of this chapter. Unfortunately, major research studies published in the last 10 years have indicated that U.S. children and teenagers lead very sedentary lives. Children ages 6 to 17 score extremely poorly in the areas of strength, flexibility, and cardiorespiratory endurance. In many cases, parents have been shown to be in better shape than their children.

This information challenges educators and parents to emphasize the need for strenuous play activity. Television watching and parental inactivity were implicated as major culprits in these studies. For students reading this text who are parents or grandparents of young children, what can you do to encourage more physical activity and less sedentary activity?

How Can Sleep Contribute to Overall Fitness?

Although sleep may seem the opposite of exercise, sleep is an important adjunct to a well-planned exercise program (see the box on the right). In fact, sleep is so vital to health that people who are unable to sleep sufficiently (those with insomnia) or who are deprived of sleep experience deterioration in every dimension of their health. Fortunately, exercise is frequently associated with improvements in sleeping.

★ **To Help You Sleep . . .**

Can we work at being better sleepers? The answer is yes. There are many activities that when done at the appropriate time will aid you in your quest for sound sleep.

ACTIVITIES FOR THE DAY

Schedule. Maintain a consistent schedule of daily activities; a disrupted day makes sleeping difficult.

Physical activity. Regular vigorous activity promotes sleep; exercising too near bedtime, however, can make you too energized to sleep soundly.

Eating. A large meal taken late in the evening interferes with sleeping; avoid large late-night snacks as well.

Alcohol use. A single drink in the evening may be relaxing, but too many drinks during the day make sleeping difficult.

CNS stimulants. Coffee, tea, soft drinks with caffeine, and some medications can disrupt normal sleeping patterns.

Worry. Problems and concerns should be put behind you by the time you retire; practice leaving your concerns at the office or in the classroom.

Rituals. A ritualistic "winding down" over the course of the evening promotes sleep; watching television, listening to music, and reading during the evening are excellent ways to prepare the body for sleep.

ACTIVITIES FOR THE END OF THE DAY

Bathing. For many people, a warm bath immediately before retiring promotes sleep.

Yoga. The quiet, relaxing exercises of yoga promote sleep by slowing the body's activity level.

Snack or nightcap. A light snack of foods high in L-tryptophan (eggs, tuna, and turkey) and a glass of milk will help you fall asleep.

Muscular relaxation. Alternating contraction and relaxation of the large muscles of the extremities aids the body in falling asleep.

Imaging. Quieting images can distract the mind, thus allowing sleep to occur more easily.

Fantasies. Escape into fantasies slows the mind and facilitates the onset of sleep.

Breathing. Slow, deep breaths set a restful rhythm the body can "ride" into sleep.

Thinking. By envisioning yourself as sleeping soundly, you may actually fall asleep more quickly.

fast-twitch (FT) fibers type of muscle cell especially suited for anaerobic activities.

slow-twitch (ST) fibers type of muscle cell especially suited for aerobic activities.

Health ACTION Guide

The Power Nap

Rarely do college students get the amount of sleep they really need. This may be especially true for older students who are parents of young children, students who are employed, and students who are involved in numerous extracurricular activities, such as student government or athletics. College students should aim for 8 to 10 hours of sleep each night. If this amount of sleep cannot be achieved, students might want to consider the value of afternoon napping to catch up on sleep debt. A short nap of about an hour in the afternoon (a "power nap") can be quite refreshing and valuable to overall performance. Experts recommend that a nap be short—never longer than 2 hours, since too much afternoon sleep might disrupt or delay one's nighttime sleep. ▼

Sleep is by no means a simple turning off of the body and mind, as some might imagine it to be. Rather, sleep reflects a progression of changes in the electrical activity of the brain. Through the course of the 6 to 8 hours of sleep per night that most adults achieve, the frequencies and intensities of electrical impulses being transmitted through the brain change in a cyclic and repetitive manner. When recorded on an *electroencephalogram (EEG)*, activity patterns suggest two major states of sleep—**rapid eye movement (REM) sleep** and **slow wave (SW) sleep.** Slow wave sleep, a period producing primarily low frequency–high intensity delta waves, and REM sleep, in which dreaming predominates, recycle completely approximately every 90 minutes.

The value of sleep is expressed in a variety of positive changes in the body. Dreaming is thought to play a valuable role in supporting the emotional dimension of health. Problem-solving vignettes that occur during dreams seem to afford some carry-over value in actual coping experiences. A variety of changes in physiological functioning, particularly a deceleration of the cardiovascular system, occur while you sleep. The familiar feeling of being well rested is an expression of the mental and physiological rejuvenation you feel after a good night's sleep.

The amount of sleep needed varies among people. In fact, for any person, sleep needs vary according to activity level and overall state of health. As we become older, the need for sleep appears to decrease from the 8 or so hours young adults require. Elderly people routinely sleep less than they did when they were younger. This decrease may be offset by the short naps older people may take during the day. For all persons, however, periods of relaxation and daydreaming generate electrical activity patterns that help regenerate the mind and body just as sleep does.

What do you hope to achieve with your fitness program?

rapid eye movement (REM) sleep dream stage of sleep characterized by twitching movements of the eyes beneath the eyelids.

slow wave (SW) sleep stage of sleep characterized by minimal dream activity.

What Exercise Danger Signs Should I Watch For?

The human body is an amazing piece of equipment. It functions well whether or not you are conscious of its processes. It also delivers clear signals when something goes wrong.

You should monitor any sign that seems abnormal during or after your exercise. "Listen to your body" is a good rule for self-awareness. The following are some common signs to monitor:

▼ A delay of over 1 hour in your body's return to a fully relaxed, comfortable state after exercise.
▼ Difficulty in sleep patterns. Although it is not uncommon for a beginner to experience sleep difficulties during the early stages of fitness development, continued problems may indicate overexertion. Reduce the intensity or frequency of your workouts for a while. Avoid exercising too close to bedtime.
▼ Any noticeable breathing difficulties or chest pains. Exercise at your THR should not initiate these problems. Any problems should be referred to a physician.
▼ Persistent joint and muscle pains. Starting to exercise after years of inactivity will naturally bring on some muscle soreness and joint discomfort. However, these should be temporary problems. Listen to your body. Any lingering joint or muscle pain might signal a problem. Seek the help of an athletic trainer, physical therapist, or your physician.
▼ Unusual changes in urine composition or output. Marked color change in your urine could signal possible kidney or bladder difficulties. Drink plenty of water before, during, and after your activity.
▼ Anything of an unusual nature that you notice after starting your fitness program. Some examples are headaches, nosebleeds, fainting, numbness in an extremity, or hemorrhoids. Such occurrences are extremely unusual. Fear of developing these difficulties should not deter you from starting a fitness program. These risks are minimal—and the benefits far outnumber the risks.

What Causes Low Back Pain?

A common experience for adults is the sudden onset of low back pain. Each year 10 million adults develop this condition to such a degree that they miss work, lose sleep, and generally feel incapable of engaging in day-to-day activities. Eighty percent of all adults who have this condition will experience these effects two to three times per year.

Although low back pain can reflect potentially serious health problems, most low back pain results from mechanical (postural) causes. As uncomfortable as low back pain is, the problem is usually self-correcting within a week or two. The services of a physician, physical therapist, or chiropractor are not generally required after an initial visit.

By engaging in regular exercise, such as swimming, walking, and bicycling, and by paying attention to your back during bending, lifting, and sitting, you can minimize the occurrence of this uncomfortable and incapacitating condition.

Summary

✔ Physical fitness allows one to avoid illness, perform routine activities, and respond to emergencies.
✔ The health benefits of exercise can be achieved through regular, moderate exercise.
✔ Fitness is composed of five components: cardiorespiratory endurance, muscular strength, muscular endurance, flexibility, and body composition.
✔ The American College of Sports Medicine's program for cardiorespiratory fitness has five components: mode of activity, frequency of training, intensity of training, duration of training, and resistance training.
✔ The target heart rate refers to the number of times per minute the heart must contract to produce a training effect.
✔ Training sessions should take place in three phases: warm-up, workout, and cool-down.
✔ Fitness experts are concerned about the lack of fitness in today's youth.
✔ Street dancing, step aerobics, and in-line skating reflect currently popular aerobic activities.
✔ Steroid use, crosstraining, fluid replacement, bodybuilding, and proper sleep are important topics for college students interested in fitness.

Review Questions

1. Identify a few of the common reasons people give for not participating in a regular fitness program. Identify a few of the reasons people do participate in a regular fitness program.
2. Identify the five components of fitness described in this chapter. Explain how each dimension relates to physical fitness.
3. Describe the various methods used to promote muscular strength.
4. What do the principles of overload and specificity mean in regard to training programs used to develop fitness?
5. What is the difference between anaerobic and aerobic energy production? What types of activities are associated with anaerobic energy production? With aerobic energy production?
6. List some of the benefits of aerobic fitness.
7. Identify the ACSM's five components of an effective cardiorespiratory program. Explain the important aspects of each component.
8. Under what circumstances should you see a physician before starting a physical fitness program?
9. Describe some of the negative consequences of anabolic steroid use.
10. How can people improve their sleeping habits?

Think about This . . .

✔ What are your attitudes toward physical fitness? Do you participate in a regular physical fitness program? Why or why not?
✔ Does your present level of fitness allow you to effectively carry out the activities your schedule demands? Are there things that you would like to do but cannot because of your current level of fitness?
✔ Describe your own level of fitness, taking into consideration cardiorespiratory endurance, strength, and flexibility.
✔ After determining your own target heart rate (THR), calculate the THR for a parent or older friend. Talk to these people about starting their own fitness program. Be ready to help with encouragement and accurate information. They may look to you as a role model for their own health.

✔ Design a personal physical fitness plan for yourself, taking into consideration all of the dimensions of body structure and function and the five components of an effective fitness program described in this chapter. What are the chances that you will continue this program after college?

REAL LIFE
REAL CHOICES

YOUR TURN

▼ Would exercise have been beneficial to Jack in his pre-heart attack days? Why or why not?
▼ What kinds of exercise might Jack find enjoyable and healthful? What kinds of exercise do you think he should avoid?
▼ Before Jack begins a program of moderate exercise, what tests will his physician want him to undergo?

AND NOW, YOUR CHOICES . . .

▼ Do you exercise regularly? If so, how do you benefit from your exercise routine? What happens when you don't exercise?
▼ If you don't exercise regularly, what are your reasons? What forms of exercise do you think you would enjoy doing several times a week?

References

1. Blair SN: Exercise and health, *Sports Science Exchange* 3(29):1-6, 1990.

2. Prentice WE: *Fitness for college and life*, ed 4, St Louis, 1994, Mosby.

3. Fit, fitter, fittest, *Harvard Medical School Health Letter* 15(4):2, 1990.

4. Simon HB: Can you run away from cancer? *Harvard Medical School Health Letter* 17(5):5-7, 1992.

5. American College of Sports Medicine: Position statement on the recommended quantity and quality of exercise for developing and maintaining fitness in healthy adults, *Med Sci Sports Exerc* 22(2):265-274, 1990.

6. Arnheim DD, Prentice WE: *Principles of athletic training*, ed 8, St Louis, 1993, Mosby.

7. What is an exercise stress test? *The Johns Hopkins Medical Letter: Health After 50*, 3(10):6-7, 1991.

8. Lack of support can cause health problems, *USA Today*, 6D, Mar 30, 1987.

9. New skates rolling along, *USA Today*, C1, June 12, 1992.

10. Glashow J: Cross training with in-line skates, *Running and Fit-News*, American Running and Fitness Association, 9(12):1, 1991.

11. Loosli AR: Athletes, food and nutrition, *Food and Nutrition News* 62(3):15-18, 1990.

12. Mishra R: Steroids and sports are a losing proposition, *FDA Consumer* 25(7):25-27, 1991.

13. Saeki T: Sports in Japan. In Wagner E, editor: *Sport in Asia and Africa: a comparative handbook*, New York, 1989, Greenwood Press.

14. Rizak G: Sport in the People's Republic of China. In Wagner E, editor: *Sport in Asia and Africa: a comparative handbook*, New York, 1989, Greenwood Press.

Suggested Readings

Cooper KH: *Kid fitness*, New York, 1991, Bantam Books.
Responding to the crisis over the fitness of American youth, Dr. Kenneth Cooper (the "Father of Aerobics") encourages parents to get involved in their kids' fitness. Parents can show children that being active can be fun. Cooper provides many suggestions for activities to improve endurance and lower body fat.

Prentice WE: *Fitness for college and life*, ed 4, St Louis, 1994, Mosby.
Highly recommended, a comprehensive textbook that covers all aspects of fitness and wellness. Particularly well written coverage of strength training and stretching activities. Author's unique background as a scholar, athletic trainer, and physical therapist adds to the validity of this book.

Rippe JM: *Dr. James Rippe's Complete Book of Fitness Walking*, Englewood Cliffs, NJ, 1991, Prentice Hall.
From the "Father of the Walking Movement," this book is an excellent primer for people who wish to achieve fitness through walking. Rippe carries the reader through an entire program of walking. Includes sections on starting a program, injury prevention, weight loss, special concerns for women, the older adult, walking during pregnancy, and cardiac rehabilitation.

5

Nutrition

The Role of Diet in Your Health

Although other aspects of nutrition are important, the *nutrients* are the elements in food that are required for the energy, growth, and repair of the body, as well as regulation of body processes. Nutritionists indicate that our bodies require seven nutrients.* From the standpoint of the physical dimension of health, all seven nutrient categories are essential. Serious nutritional deficiencies could occur if they are neglected. Despite Madison Avenue's preference for protein, vitamins, and fiber, your body also requires carbohydrates, fats, minerals, and water for sound nutritional health.

*Since most of our water intake comes through beverages rather than from food, some nutritionists *do not* consider water a nutrient, even though it is essential for life.

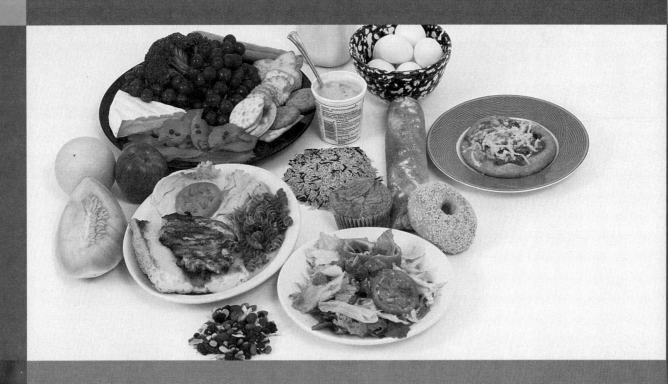

N U T R I T I O N

The following objectives are covered in this chapter:

▽ Reduce dietary fat to an average of 30% of Calories or less and average saturated fat intake to less than 10% of Calories among people aged 2 and older. (Baseline: 36% of Calories from total fat and 13% from saturated fat for people aged 20 through 74 in 1976-80; 36% and 13% for women aged 19 through 50 in 1985; p. 117.)

▽ Increase complex carbohydrates and fiber-containing foods in the diets of adults to 5 or more daily servings for vegetables (including legumes) and fruits and to 6 or more daily servings for grain products. (Baseline: 2 ½ servings of vegetables and fruits and 3 servings of grain products for women aged 19 through 50 in 1985; p. 118.)

▽ Reduce iron deficiency to less than 3% among children aged 1 through 4 and among women of childbearing age. (Baseline: 9% of children aged 1 through 2; 4% of children aged 3 through 4, and 5% for women aged 20 through 44 in 1976-80; p. 122.)

▽ Increase to at least 85% the proportion of people aged 18 and older who use food labels to make nutritious food selections. (Baseline: 74% read labels to make food selections in 1988; p. 124.)

▽ Increase to at least 5000 brand items the availability of processed food products that are reduced in fat and saturated fat. (Baseline: 2500 items reduced in fat in 1986; p. 125.)

REAL LIFE REAL CHOICES

Diet and Lifestyle: Finding a Healthy Balance

▼ Names: Vincent and Angela Martinelli
▼ Ages: 64 and 61
▼ Ethnic background: Italian
▼ Occupation: Restaurant owners
▼ Physical characteristics: Vincent: 5′9″, 189 lb.
  Angela: 5′2″, 143 lb.

Does anyone really know how many kinds of pasta there are in the world? If you want an expert opinion, the people to ask are Vincent and Angela Martinelli, the owners of a popular market and deli in their city's lively Italian neighborhood.

Martinelli's Fine Foods was started by Vincent's father in the 1920s, and Vincent began helping out when he was 5 years old. When his father died in the early 1950s, Vincent and Angela took over. Now in their sixties, they're beginning to talk about retiring and turning the business over to their daughter and her husband.

A family business like Martinelli's isn't a nine-to-five proposition. For more than 40 years, Vincent and

Angela have routinely worked 12 to 14 hours a day, 6 days a week—at the same time raising five children and putting them through college. Their hectic, stressful schedule has left them little time for leisure, and they're looking forward to taking life easier when they retire.

Both Vincent and Angela enjoy cooking—and eating—the delicious dishes they offer for sale in the deli and for catered parties. Their favorite is fettucine carbonara, which features pasta in cream sauce with bacon. At a recent checkup, the Martinellis' physician found that Vincent's serum cholesterol level is elevated to the point where heart disease is a concern; and Angela, who has a family history of hypertension, is taking in as much as 3000 milligrams of sodium per day.

As you study this chapter, think about some steps Vincent and Angela can take to adopt a healthier lifestyle, and prepare yourself to answer the questions in **Your Turn** at the end of the chapter. ▼

TYPES AND SOURCES OF NUTRIENTS

We will discuss the familiar carbohydrates, fats, and proteins first. These are the three nutrients that provide our bodies with **Calories**.* These Calories are either used quickly by our bodies in energy metabolism or are stored in the form of glycogen or adipose tissue. The other nutrient groups, not sources of *energy* for the body, are discussed later in this chapter.

Carbohydrates

Carbohydrates are various combinations of sugar units, or saccharides. The body uses carbohydrates primarily for energy. Each gram of carbohydrate contains 4 Calories. Since the average person requires approximately 2000 Calories per day and about 60% of our Calories come from carbohydrates, we obtain 1200 Calories per day from carbohydrates.[1]

Carbohydrates occur in three forms depending on the number of saccharides (sugar) units that make up the molecule. Carbohydrates that contain only one saccharide unit are classified as monosaccharides, those with two units are disaccharides, and those with more than two are polysaccharides. Monosaccharides and disaccharides are more commonly called *sugars,*

whereas polysaccharides are referred to as *starches.* Today it is recommended that about 50% of our total Caloric intake should come from starches and only 10% from sugars.

Monosaccharides are the simplest sugar units. Four forms of monosaccharides exist: glucose, fructose, galactose, and an infrequently found form, mannose. Of these, *glucose* is the most important monosaccharide; it makes up the blood sugar used as the body's primary source of energy. It is almost the sole source of energy for the brain and nervous system. Glucose, also known as dextrose, is found in vegetables, honey, molasses, fruits, and syrup. *Fructose*, also called levulose, is another monosaccharide that provides a source of simple sugar. This simple sugar is most often derived from fruits and berries.

Disaccharides are sugars composed of two monosaccharides, one of which is always a glucose unit. *Sucrose* is perhaps the most widely recognized disaccharide source; it is better known as table sugar. Sucrose is a combination of a glucose and a fructose molecule. Other disaccharides include *maltose,* derived from germinating cereals, and lactose, the carbohydrate found in human and animal milk.

The average adult American now ingests approximately 125 pounds of sucrose each year—usually in colas, candies, and pastries, which offer few additional

*Calorie with a capital C refers to kilocalorie (kcal), which is the accepted scientific expression of the energy value of a food.

Health ACTION Guide

Tips to Remember When Eating Away From Home

Today, more than ever before, people eat more meals away from home. Many of these will be fast food meals that are characterized by high fat density and excessive use of sweeteners. It is possible, however, to eat nutritionally while eating on the run if you follow these suggestions:

▼ Choose nutritional foods such as salads instead of french fries.
▼ At a salad bar, choose the plain vegetables; avoid mayonnaise-based salads.
▼ Order a plain hamburger without condiments; when you add your own, you control the amounts.
▼ Add lettuce and tomato to hamburgers to add vitamins, not Calories.
▼ Order plain chicken; it has fewer Calories than beef.
▼ Avoid breaded and fried foods.
▼ Choose milk or juice, not sodas or shakes.
▼ For dessert, bring a piece of fresh fruit with you.
▼ Eat a small snack at 10 AM and another at 2 PM. This kind of "grazing" can be healthier than gulping down one big, fat-filled meal at noon.

nutritional benefits.[2] For years excess sugar intake was implicated in a number of major health concerns, including obesity, micronutrient deficiencies, behavioral disorders, dental caries, diabetes mellitus, and cardiovascular disease. However, with the exception of dental caries, current scientific data fail to confirm that sugar per se directly causes any of these health problems. Today, it is recommended that no more than 10% of our total Calories come from sucrose and other sweeteners.

Much of the sugar we consume is hidden—that is, sugar is a principal product we may overlook in a large number of food items. Foods such as ketchup, salad dressings, cured meat products, and canned vegetables and fruits frequently contain much hidden sugar. Corn syrup, frequently found in these items, is a very concentrated sucrose solution.

Polysaccharides are complex carbohydrates that are composed of long chains of glucose units. These long chains are better known as *starches*. They are among the most important sources for dietary carbohydrates. Starches are found primarily in vegetables, fruits, and grains. Consumption of starches helps us receive much overall nutritional benefit, since most starch sources also contain significant portions of vitamins, minerals, protein, and water. Dietary fiber is also a polysaccharide (see p. 103). Starches are nutritional "good guys."

Fats

Fats (lipids, fatty acids) are an important nutrient in our diets. Fats provide a concentrated form of energy (9 Calories per gram consumed versus 4 for carbohydrates and protein) and help give our foods high **satiety** value. The fat in our foods helps to give our foods its pleasing taste, or *palatability*. Fats also serve as carriers of fat-soluble vitamins A, D, E, and K. Without

fat, these vitamins would quickly pass through the body. Body tissues formed in part from fat help us retain heat.

Dietary sources of fat are often difficult to identify. The visible fats in our diet, such as butter, salad oils, and the layer of fat on some cuts of meat, represent only about 40% of the fat we consume. Most of the fat we eat is "hidden" in food because it is incorporated into the food during preparation or used to fry the food, or it is in food that we have not learned to recognize as being high in fat, such as a candy bar.

When shopping, we often notice that the fat content of some foods is reported in terms of its percentage of the product's weight. In selecting the type of milk we drink, for example, we see that milk ranges from ultralow-fat milk (½%) through low-fat milk (1% to 2%) to whole milk (3% to 4%). Skim milk contains no butter fat. Most consumers do not know, however, how much of the product's Calories are derived from fat. In the accompanying Star Box, an example of how to calculate where Calories in a food are from is provided.

---

nutrients (**noo** tree ents) elements in foods that are required for the growth, repair, and regulation of body processes.

Calories (**kal** oh rees) units of heat (energy); specifically, one Calorie equals the heat required to raise 1 kilogram of water 1° C.

carbohydrates (car bow **high** drates) chemical compounds comprising sugar (or saccharide) units; the body's primary source of energy.

satiety (suh **tie** uh tee) a feeling of no longer being hungry; a diminished desire to eat.

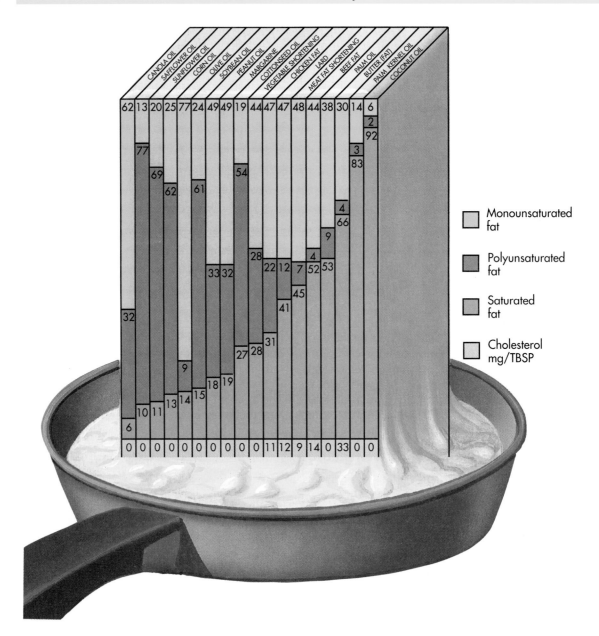

Figure 5-1 Comparison of dietary fats. (Fatty acid content normalized to 100%.)

Later in this chapter, recommendations regarding the role of fat as a source of Calories in a healthful diet are discussed.

Every type of dietary fat is made up of a combination of three forms of fat (saturated, monounsaturated, and polyunsaturated) based on chemical composition. Today, consumers need to pay attention to the amount of each type of fat in dietary fat because of the role that each form plays in heart disease (see Chapter 10). **Saturated fats** in particular need to be carefully limited in a modern healthy diet.

Saturated fats are found in abundance in animal products such as meats, dairy products, lard, and eggs.

Saturated fats consumed in excess have been accused of promoting a wide variety of cardiovascular diseases.

Fortunately, the replacement of saturated fats with monounsaturated and polyunsaturated fats and oils appears to lower blood cholesterol levels and reduce the risk of heart disease.[3] Vegetable oils tend to be low in saturated fats, with the exception of the tropical oils (coconut, palm, and palm kernel oils). Monounsaturated fats are found in high quantities in olive oil, peanut oil, and sesame oil. Polyunsaturated fats are especially prevalent in safflower oil, sunflower oil, and corn oil (Figure 5-1).

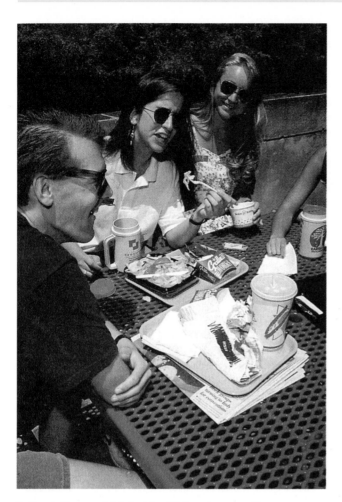

Eating patterns established in childhood can continue throughout life.

Tropical Oils

Although all cooking oils (and fats such as butter, lard, margarine, and shortening) have the same number of Calories by weight (9 Calories per gram), some oils contain high percentages of saturated fats. *All oils and fats contain varying percentages of saturated, monounsaturated, and polyunsaturated fats.* Saturated fats are known to elevate blood cholesterol levels and increase the chances of developing heart disease (see Chapter 10). The tropical oils—coconut, palm, and palm kernel—contain much higher percentages of saturated fats than do other cooking oils.[4] Coconut oil is 92% saturated fat (see Figure 5-1).

Tropical oils can be found in numerous brands of snack foods, crackers, cookies, nondairy creamers, and breakfast cereals. Realizing that the American public is beginning to avoid foods containing tropical oils, some food companies are starting to replace inexpensive tropical oils with more healthful alternatives.[5] Do you check for tropical oils on the ingredient labels of the foods you select?

★ Candy: A Hidden Source of Fat

Candies are much higher in fat, including tropical oils, than most people think. The percentage of Calories from fat for each of the top 10 selling candies is listed below:

Candy	Calories from fat (%)
Hershey's Milk Chocolate Bar with Almonds	56
Reese's Peanut Butter Cups	55
Hershey's Milk Chocolate Bar	50
Kit Kat	48
M&Ms Peanut	47
Snickers	45
M&Ms Plain	43
Nestle Crunch	43
Butterfinger	39
Milky Way	35

High blood levels of **triglycerides** and **cholesterol** (fat-related substances in alcohol form) have also been reported to be risk factors in the development of cardiovascular disease (see Chapter 10). Cholesterol is a necessary constituent of all animal tissue and is synthesized by our own bodies from carbohydrate and fat sources. Considerable evidence suggests that increased intake of saturated fats may increase triglyceride and serum (blood) cholesterol levels.[6] However, after extensive investigation, the relationship between intake of dietary cholesterol and serum cholesterol levels remains unclear.[7] High-cholesterol foods include whole milk, shellfish, animal fat, and egg yolk. Acceptable fat substitutes are only now coming into the market[8] (see the box on p. 96).

saturated fats (**satch** you ray ted) fats that are difficult for the body to use; these are fats in solid form at room temperature; primarily animal fats.

triglycerides (try **gliss** er ides) fats made up of glycerol units, each having three fatty acid molecules; high blood levels are associated with increased risk of cardiovascular disease.

cholesterol (kol **es** ter all) a primary form of fat found in the blood; lipid material manufactured within the body, as well as derived through dietary sources.

Low-Calorie Fat Substitutes

Newly developed products containing fat substitutes (Simplesse, Simple Pleasures, Olestra, and Trailblazer) are now available, or will soon be available. By combining high-protein sources such as egg whites and milk through a process called microparticulation, or by constructing new undigestible molecules, food technologists are able to restructure the configuration of protein to resemble that of fat. These new products contain no cholesterol and have 80% fewer Calories than similar products made with fat. Because fat substitutes tend to be unstable when heated, they are being used in foods such as ice cream, salad dressing, cheese spreads, and yogurt. Whether significant health benefits can be derived from these products remains to be seen. ★

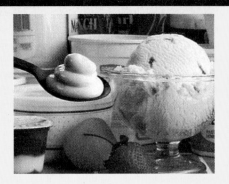

Proteins

The term *protein* is derived from a word meaning "first importance." **Proteins** are manufactured in every living cell; they are composed of chains of **amino acids.** Amino acids are the "building blocks" from which the body constructs its own protein. Twenty amino acids are used in various combinations to build the protein required for physiological processes to continue in a healthy manner.

The human body obtains amino acids from two sources—it obtains them by breaking down protein from food to make building blocks from outside sources, and it attempts to manufacture building blocks within its cells. The later process is less than fully successful because only 11 of the necessary 20 amino acids can be built by the body. The nine amino acids than *cannot* be built by the body are called *essential amino acids* (indispensable amino acids) because they must be obtained from outside the body through the protein in food. The 11 amino acids that the body *can* make itself are called *nonessential amino acids* (dis-

pensable amino acids) because the body does not have to rely solely on food protein to obtain these building blocks.[8]

In terms of food sources of amino acids, foods can be classified into one of two types depending on whether they can supply the body with the important essential amino acids or not. *Complete protein foods* contain all nine essential amino acids within their protein and are of animal origin (milk, meat, cheese, and eggs). The *incomplete protein foods* do not contain all of the essential amino acids and are of plant origin (vegetables, grains, and legumes—peas or beans, including chickpeas, butter beans, and tofu). Fortunately, it is possible to combine various sources of incomplete protein foods to achieve complete sources. Many of us do this already when we combine peanut butter and break, milk and cereal, and macaroni and cheese.

Protein serves primarily to promote growth and maintenance of body tissue. However, when Calorie intake falls, protein will be broken down for glucose.

Health ACTION Guide

Reducing Fat Intake

A newly developed procedure is available for removing fat, including saturated fat and cholesterol, from meat. The following washing technique reduces the fat content of ground beef, pork, or lamb.

▼ Heat a pint to a quart of vegetable oil to 176° F.
▼ Add 2 lb of ground meat or poultry; stir until oil

starts to boil. Cook, with oil barely bubbling, 5 to 10 minutes.
▼ Strain meat and oil, saving oil; pour a cup or two of boiling water over meat, remove the meat and add the water to oil.
▼ Refrigerate this liquid (oil plus water) for an hour; skim off congealed fat. Pour the remaining liquid back onto the meat.

Although effective in lowering fat content by as much as 65%, this technique may be too complicated and time-consuming for today's lifestyles. A concerted effort to eat less meat would lower dietary fat as effectively. ▼

Calculating Calories from Carbohydrate, Fats, and Protein

To calculate the percentage of Calories in a food item that are supplied by carbohydrate, fat, and proteins, you need to know only the number of grams of each. For example, if a food item has 10 grams of carbohydrate, 6 grams of fat, and 3 grams of protein, calculate the percent of Calories:

STEP ONE

1. Multiply grams of carbohydrate by 4 to obtain Calories supplied by carbohydrate: $10 \times 4 = 40$ C
2. Multiply grams of fat by 9 to obtain Calories supplied by fat: $6 \times 9 = 54$ C
3. Multiply grams of protein by 4 to obtain Calories supplied by protein: $3 \times 4 = 12$ C
4. Add Calories from all sources to obtain Total Calories: 106 C

STEP TWO

1. Divide carbohydrate Calories by Total Calories to determine percent of Calories supplied by carbohydrate: $\frac{40}{106} = 37.7\%$
2. Divide number of fat Calories by Total Calories to determine percent of Calories supplied by fat: $\frac{54}{106} = 50.9\%$
3. Divide number of protein Calories by Total Calories to determine percent of Calories supplied by protein: $\frac{12}{106} = 11.3\%$

INTERPRETATION

This particular food item obtains half of its Calories from fat, slightly over one third of its Calories from carbohydrate, and only about one tenth of its Calories from protein. ★

This loss of protein can impede growth and repair of tissue. From this, we can see that adequate carbohydrate intake prevents protein from serving as an energy source.[8] Protein also is a primary component of enzyme and hormone structure; it helps maintain the *acid-base balance* of our bodies, and serves as a source of energy (4 Calories per gram consumed). Nutritionists recommend that 15% of our caloric intake be from protein. Malnutrition in the world's underdeveloped countries in often seen in the protein deficiency disease called *kwashiorkor*. This disease is rarely seen in countries that have an abundant supply of protein.

Vitamins

Vitamins are organic compounds that are required in small amounts for normal growth, reproduction, and maintenance of health. Vitamins differ from carbohydrates, fats, and proteins because they do not provide Calories or serve as structural elements for our bodies. Vitamins serve as *coenzymes*. By facilitating the action of **enzymes,** vitamins help initiate a wide variety of body responses, including energy production, use of minerals, and growth of healthy tissue.

Discovered just after the turn of the twentieth century, vitamins can be classified as *water soluble* (capable of being dissolved in water) or *fat soluble* (capable of being dissolved in fat or lipid tissue). Water-soluble vitamins include the B-complex vitamins and vitamin C. Most of the excess of these water-soluble vitamins is eliminated from the body during urination. The fat-soluble vitamins are A, D, E, and K. Excessive intake of these vitamins causes them to be stored in the body in the adipose tissue or fat. It is therefore possible to consume and retain too many of these vitamins, particularly A and D. Table 5-1 shows that all of the fat-soluble vitamins hold the potential for toxicity if taken in amounts that far exceed recommended daily allowances (RDAs). Most toxicity results from the use of supplements by adults or through excessive food intake of particular sources in very small children. When toxicity develops, the condition is referred to as **hypervitaminosis.**

The extent to which toxicity from water-soluble vitamins can occur is somewhat open to debate. As seen in Table 5-2, some of the water-soluble vitamins (Niacin, B-6, and C) have been associated with toxic effects when taken in megadoses. For adults, intake of this level would occur only through the excessive use of supplements.

proteins compounds composed of chains of amino acids; primary components of muscle and connective tissue.

amino acids (uh **meen** oh) "building blocks" of protein; manufactured by the body or obtained from dietary sources.

vitamins organic compounds that facilitate the action of enzymes.

enzymes (**enn** zymes) organic substances that control the rate of physiological reactions but are not altered in the process.

hypervitaminosis (hi **purr** vi ta min **oh** sis) excessive accumulation of vitamins within the body; associated with the fat-soluble vitamins.

TABLE 5-1   Summary of the Fat-Soluble Vitamins, Their Functions, Deficiency Conditions, and Food Sources

Vitamin	Major functions	Deficiency symptoms	People most at risk	Dietary sources	RDA	Toxicity symptoms
Vitamin A (retinoids) and pro-vitamin A (carotenoids)	1. Vision, light, and color 2. Promotes growth 3. Prevents drying of skin and eyes 4. Promotes resistance to bacterial infection	1. Night blindness 2. Xerophthalmia 3. Poor growth 4. Dry skin (keratinization)	People in poverty, especially preschool children (still very rare)	Vitamin A Liver Fortified milk Provitamin A Sweet potatoes Spinach Greens Carrots Cantaloupe Apricots Broccoli	Females: 800 RE* (4000 IU†) Males: 1000 RE* (5000 IU†)	Fetal malformations, hair loss, skin changes, pain in bones
Vitamin D (chole-calciferol and ergo-calciferol)	1. Facilitates absorption of calcium and phosphorus 2. Maintains optimum calcification of bone	1. Rickets 2. Osteomalacia	Breastfed infants, elderly shut-ins	Vitamin D-fortified milk Fish oils Tuna fish Salmon	5-10 micrograms (200-400 IU)	Growth retardation, kidney damage, calcium deposits in soft tissue
Vitamin E (tocopherols, tocotrienols)	1. Antioxidant: prevents breakdown of vitamin A and unsaturated fatty acids	1. Hemolysis of red blood cells 2. Nerve destruction	People with poor fat absorption (still very rare)	Vegetable oils Some greens Some fruits	Females: 8 Alpha-tocopherol equivalents Males: 10 Alpha-tocopherol equivalents	Muscle weakness, headaches, fatigue, nausea, inhibition of vitamin K metabolism
Vitamin K (phylloquinone and menaquinone)	1. Helps form prothrombin and other factors for blood clotting	1. Hemorrhage	People taking antibotics for months at a time	Green vegetables Liver	60-80 micrograms	Anemia and jaundice

*RE, Retinol equivalents.
†IU, International units.

Because water-soluble vitamins dissolve rather quickly in water, you should be cautious in the preparation of fresh fruits and vegetables. One precaution is to avoid overcooking fresh vegetables. The longer fresh vegetables are steamed or boiled, the more water-soluble vitamins will be lost. Even soaking sliced fresh fruit or vegetables can result in the loss of vitamin C and B-complex vitamins. You may wish to drink (or use in baking) any water in which fresh vegetables were boiled or steamed.

To ensure an adequate vitamin intake, do not rely on bottled vitamins sold in grocery stores or health food stores. The best way is really the simplest and least expensive way: eat a variety of foods. Unless there are special circumstances, such as pregnancy, infancy, or an existing health problem, virtually everyone in our society who eats a reasonable well-rounded diet consumes appropriate levels of all vitamins.

In spite of the availability of vitamin-rich foods, not all people eat a balanced diet based on a variety of

TABLE 5-2 Summary of the Water-Soluble Vitamins, Their Functions, Deficiency Conditions, and Food Sources

Name	Major functions	Deficiency symptoms	People most at risk	Dietary sources	RDA or ESADDI	Toxicity
Thiamin	Coenzyme involved with enzymes in carbohydrate metabolism; nerve function	Beriberi; nervous tingling, poor coordination, edema, heart changes, weakness	People with alcoholism, people in poverty	Sunflower seeds, pork, whole and enriched grains, dried beans, peas, brewer's yeast	1.1-1.5 milligrams	None possible from food
Riboflavin	Coenzymes involved in energy metabolism	Inflammation of mouth and tongue, cracks at corners of the mouth, eye disorders	Possibly people on certain medications if no dairy products consumed	Milk, mushrooms, spinach, liver, enriched grains	1.2-1.7 milligrams	None reported
Niacin	Coenzymes involved in energy metabolism, fat synthesis, fat breakdown	Pellagra, diarrhea, dermatitis, dementia	People in severe poverty where corn is dominant food, people with alcoholism	Mushrooms, bran, tuna, salmon, chicken, beef, liver, peanuts, enriched grains	15-19 milligrams	Flushing of skin at >100 milligrams
Pantothenic acid	Coenzyme involved in energy metabolism, fat synthesis, fat breakdown	Using an antagonist causes tingling in hands, fatigue, headache, nausea	People with alcoholism	Mushrooms, liver, broccoli, eggs; most foods have some	4-7 milligrams	None
Biotin	Coenzyme involved in glucose production, fat synthesis	Dermatitis, tongue soreness, anemia, depression	People with alcoholism	Cheese, egg yolks, cauliflower, peanut butter, liver	30-100 micrograms	Unknown
Vitamin B-6, pyridoxine and other forms	Coenzyme involved in protein metabolism, neurotransmitter synthesis, hemoglobin synthesis, many other functions	Headache, anemia, convulsions, nausea, vomiting, flaky skin, sore tongue	Adolescent and adult women, people on certain medications, people with alcoholism	Animal protein foods, spinach, broccoli, bananas, salmon, sunflower seeds	1.8-2 milligrams	Nerve destruction at doses >100 milligrams
Folate (folic acid)	Coenzyme involved in DNA synthesis	Megatoblastic anemia, inflammation of tongue, diarrhea, poor growth, mental disorders	People with alcoholism; pregnant women; people taking certain medications	Green leafy vegetables, orange juice, organ meats, sprouts, sunflower seeds	180-200 microgram	None, nonprescription vitamin dosage is controlled by FDA
Vitamin B-12 (cobalamins)	Coenzyme involved in folate metabolism, nerve function	Macrocytic anemia, poor nerve function	Elderly, because of poor absorption; vegans	Animal foods, especially organ meats, oysters, clams (B_{12} not naturally in plant foods)	2 micrograms	None
Vitamin C (ascorbic acid)	Collagen synthesis, hormone synthesis, neurotransmitter synthesis	Scurvy: poor wound healing, pinpoint hemorrhages, bleeding gums, edema	People with alcoholism; elderly men living alone	Citrus fruits, strawberries, broccoli, greens	60 milligrams	Doses >1-2 grams cause diarrhea and can alter some diagnostic tests

foods. Also, recent studies suggest that a somewhat higher intake of vitamins A, C, and E for adults, and folicin before and during pregnancy might have a positive effect in reducing the risk of developing cancer, atherosclerosis, birth defects, and depressed levels of HDL cholesterol (see Chapter 10).[9-11] To date, these findings have not been translated into specific recommendations, but they are drawing increased interest on the part of both the scientific community and the general public.[12] Apparently, it is the antioxidation-properties of vitamins A, C, and E that most keenly interests health experts (see Chapter 20—free radical formation).

At the same time that many health experts are reconsidering recommendations concerning additional consumption of vitamins, the Food and Drug Administration (FDA) implemented strict new requirements on the labeling of *food supplements* regarding unsubstantiated claims* for the cure or prevention of disease.[13] Not surprisingly, the manufacturers of these products attempted to curtail this action by strongly suggesting to consumers that this action means that vitamins will be taken off the over-the-counter (OTC) market and become prescription "drugs." Today, the sale of food supplements (vitamins, minerals and amino acids) is a huge industry in this country, with 75 million Americans using *dietary aids* at an annual cost of more than $1.5 billion. (See Table 5-3.)

---

*Before such a claim can be made for a particular dietary aid, there must be substantial scientific agreement supporting the claim.

TABLE 5-3   Sales of Most Popular Vitamins*

Vitamin	Amount of sales
Multivitamins	$1.2 billion
Vitamin C	$350 million
Vitamin E	$275 million
B Complex	$260 million

*1992 sales figures.

Minerals

Nearly 5% of the body is composed of inorganic materials, the *minerals*. Minerals function primarily as structural elements (seen in teeth, muscles, hemoglobin, and hormones.) They are also critical in the regulation of a number of body processes, including cell membrane permeability, muscle contraction, heart function, blood clotting, protein synthesis, and red blood cell synthesis. Approximately 21 minerals have been recognized as being essential minerals for human health.[8]

Macronutrients are those minerals that are seen in relatively high amounts in our body tissues. Examples of macronutrients are calcium, phosphorus, sulfur, sodium, potassium, and magnesium. Examples of *micronutrients,* those minerals seen in relatively small amounts in body tissues, include zinc, iron, copper, selenium, and iodine. Although micronutrients (**trace el-**ements) are required only in small quantities, they are still essential for good health. (See Tables 5-4 and 5-5 for listings of minerals and their functions.) As with vitamins, the safest, most appropriate way in which to receive a sufficient amount of all necessary minerals is to eat a balanced diet.

Water

Water may well be our most essential nutrient,* since without water most people would die from **dehydration** effects in less than a week. We could survive for weeks and even years without some of the essential minerals and vitamins. More than half our body weight comes from water. Water provides the medium for nutrient and waste transport and temperature control and plays a key role in nearly all of our body's biochemical reactions. A familiar indicator of inadequate fluid intake is strained, uncomfortable bowel movements.

*See p. 90 regarding the classification of water as a nutrient.

> **trace elements** minerals whose presence in the body occurs in very small amounts; micronutrient elements.
>
> **dehydration** (dee high **dray** shun) abnormal depletion of fluids from the body; severe dehydration can lead to death.

TABLE 5-4   Summary of Water and the Macronutrients (Major Minerals)

Name	Major functions	Deficiency symptoms	People most at risk	RDA or minimum requirement	Nutrient dense dietary sources	Results of toxicity
Water	Medium for chemical reactions, removal of waste products, perspiration to cool the body	Thirst, muscle weakness, poor endurance	Infants with a fever, elderly in nursing homes	1 milliliter per Calorie burned*	As such and in foods	Probably occurs only in mental disorders: headache, blurred vision, convulsions
Sodium	A major ion of the extracellular fluid; nerve impulse transmission	Muscle cramps	People who severely restrict sodium to lower blood pressure (250-500 milligrams/day)	500 milligrams	Table salt, processed foods	High blood pressure in susceptible individuals

*An approximation; best to keep urine volume greater than 1 liter (4 cups).

TABLE 5-4   Summary of Water and the Macronutrients (Major Minerals)—cont'd

Name	Major functions	Deficiency symptoms	People most at risk	RDA or minimum requirement	Nutrient dense dietary sources	Results of toxicity
Potassium	A major ion of intracellular fluid; nerve impulse transmission	Irregular heart beat, loss of appetite, muscle cramps	People who use potassium-wasting diuretics or have poor diets, as seen in poverty and with alcoholism	2000 milligrams	Spinach, squash, bananas, orange juice, other vegetables and fruits, milk	Slowing of the heart beat; seen in kidney failure
Chloride	A major ion of the extracellular fluid; acid production in stomach; nerve transmission	Convulsions in infants	No one, probably, when infant formula manufacturers control product quality adequately	700 milligrams	Table salt, some vegetables	High blood pressure in susceptible people when combined with sodium
Calcium	Bone and tooth strength; blood clotting; nerve impulse transmission; muscle contractions; cell regulation	Poor intake increases the risk for osteoporosis	Women in general, especially those who constantly restrict their energy intake and consume few dairy products	800 milligrams (older than 24 years old)	Dairy products, canned fish, leafy vegetables, tofu, fortified orange juice	Very high intakes may cause kidney stones in susceptible people
Phosphorus	Bone and tooth strength; part of various metabolic compounds; major ion of intracellular fluid	Probably none; poor bone maintenance possible	Elderly consuming very nutrient-poor diets; possibly total vegetarians and those with alcoholism	800 milligrams (older than 24 years old)	Dairy products, processed foods, fish, soft drinks	Hampers bone health in people with kidney failure; poor bone mineralization if calcium intakes are low
Magnesium	Bone strength; enzyme function; nerve and heart function	Weakness, muscle pain, poor heart function	People on thiazide diuretics, women in general	Men: 350 milligrams Women: 280 milligrams	Wheat bran, green vegetables, nuts, chocolate	Causes weakness in people with kidney failure
Sulfur	Part of vitamins and amino acids; drug detoxification; acid-base balance	None	No one who meets their protein needs	None	Protein foods	None likely

*An approximation; best to keep urine volume greater than 1 liter (4 cups).

TABLE 5-5   Summary of Key Micronutrients (Trace Minerals)

Mineral	Major functions	Deficiency symptoms	People most at risk	RDA or ESADDI	Nutrient dense dietary sources	Results of toxicity
Iron	Part of hemoglobin and other key compounds used in respiration; used for immune function	Low serum iron levels, small, pale red blood cells, low blood hemoglobin values	Infants, preschool children, adolescents, women in child-bearing years	Men: 10 milligrams Women: 15 milligrams	Meats, spinach, seafood, broccoli, peas, bran, enriched breads	Toxicity is seen in children who consume 200-400 milligrams in iron pills and in people with hemochromatosis; in this latter case people over-absorb iron
Zinc	Over 200 enzymes need zinc, including enzymes involved in growth, immunity, alcohol metabolism, sexual development, and reproduction	Skin rash, diarrhea, decreased appetite and sense of taste, hair loss, poor growth and development, poor wound healing	Vegetarians, women in general, the elderly	Men: 15 milligrams Women: 12 milligrams	Seafoods, meats, greens, whole grains	Reduces iron and copper absorption; can cause diarrhea, cramps, and depressed immune function
Selenium	Part of antioxidant system	Muscle pain, muscle weakness, heart disease	Unknown	55-70 micrograms	Meats, eggs, fish, seafoods, whole grains	Nausea, vomiting, hair loss, weakness, liver disease
Iodide	Part of thyroid hormone	Goiter, poor growth in infancy when mother is deficient in pregnancy	None in America, as salt is usually fortified	150 micrograms	Iodized salt, white bread, saltwater fish, dairy products	Inhibition of function of the thyroid gland
Copper	Aids in iron metabolism; works with many enzymes, such as those involved in protein metabolism and hormone synthesis	Anemia, low white blood cell count, poor growth	Infants recovering from malnutrition, people who use overzealous supplementation of zinc	1.5-3 milligrams	Liver, cocoa, beans, nuts, whole grains, dried fruits	Vomiting, nervous system disorders

TABLE 5-5 Summary of Key Micronutrients (Trace Minerals)—cont'd

Mineral	Major functions	Deficiency symptoms	People most at risk	RDA or ESADDI	Nutrient dense dietary sources	Results of toxicity
Fluoride	Increases resistance of tooth enamel to dental caries	Increased risk of dental caries	Areas where water is not fluoridated and dental treatments do not make up for this lack of fluoride	1.5-4 milligrams	Fluoridated water, toothpaste, dental treatments, tea, seaweed	Stomach upset, mottling (staining) of teeth during development
Chromium	Enhances blood glucose control	High blood glucose levels after eating	People on total parenteral nutrition and perhaps elderly people with noninsulin-dependent diabetes mellitus	50-200 micrograms	Egg yolks, whole grains, pork	Caused by industrial contamination, not dietary excess
Manganese	Aids action of some enzymes, such as those involved in carbohydrate metabolism	None in humans	Unknown	2-5 milligrams	Nuts, rice, oats, beans	Unknown in humans
Molybdenum	Aids action of some enzymes	None in humans	Unknown	75-250 micrograms	Beans, grains, nuts	Unknown in humans

Most people seldom think about the importance of an adequate intake of water and fluids. Adults require about 6 to 10 glasses a day, depending on their exercise level and environment. People who drink beverages that tend to dehydrate the body (tea, coffee, and alcohol) should increase their water consumption. Of course, we also obtain needed fluids from fruits, vegetables, fruit/vegetable juices, milk, and noncaffeinated soft drinks. The latter are important sources of fluids because of the tendency of Americans to consume more of these beverages than they do water.

Fiber

Although not considered a nutrient by definition, **fiber** is an important component of sound nutrition. Fiber consists of plant material that is not digested but rather moves through the digestive tract and out of the body. Cereal, fruits, and vegetables all provide us with dietary fiber.

Fiber can be classified into two large groups on the basis of whether solubility. *Insoluble* fibers are those that can absorb water from the intestinal tract. By absorbing water, the insoluble fibers give the stool bulk and decrease the time it takes the stool to move through the digestive tract. In contrast, *soluble* fiber turns to a "gel" within the intestinal tract and in so doing binds to liver bile, which has cholesterol attached. Thus the soluble fibers may be valuable in removing (lowering) blood cholesterol levels.[14] Also, since foods high in soluble fiber are generally low in sugar and saturated fats, fiber may indirectly contribute to keep-

plant material

fiber (fī ber) cellulose-based plant material that cannot be digested; found in cereal, fruits, and vegetables.

ing blood sugar low and reduce the risk of colon cancer associated with diets high in saturated fats.[15]

In recent years attention has been directed toward three forms of soluble fiber—oat bran, psyllium (from the weed plantain), and rice bran—in terms of their ability to lower blood cholesterol levels. The sale of products containing oat bran, such as cereals and baked goods, has increased greatly since 1987. Psyllium use, in the form of laxatives such as Metamucil, Konsyl, and Mondame, has also increased.

Although earlier studies were contradictory regarding the effectiveness of soluble fiber in lowering cholesterol levels, today it appears that oat bran is effective in lowering cholesterol levels by five to six points in persons whose initial cholesterol levels are moderately high.[16] To accomplish this reduction, a daily consumption of oat bran equaling a large bowl of oat bran cold cereal or three or more packs of instant oatmeal would be necessary. Of course, oatmeal can be eaten as a cooked cereal or used in other foods such as hamburgers, pancakes, or meatloaf. The role of psyllium and rice bran in lowering cholesterol levels is less well established.*

THE FOOD GROUPS

As already mentioned, the most effective way to take in adequate amounts of nutrients is to eat a **balanced diet,** that is, to eat a diet that includes selections from several food groups (see Table 5-7). Over the past several decades, various grouping patterns have identified five, seven, four, and now (again) five food groups

*A 1993 Canadian study substantiated the effectiveness of oat bran and psyllium in lowering cholesterol, but suggested that the amount consumed would need to be 50 grams per day to achieve a 5% lowering. This is about three times the current daily intake of fiber.

TABLE 5-6a Adult Recommended Dietary Allowances,* Revised 1989

Category	Age (years)	Weight† (kg)	(lb)	Height† (cm)	(in)	Protein (g)	Vitamin A (µg RE)‡	Vitamin D (µg)§	Vitamin E (mg α-TE)‖	Vitamin K (µg)
Males	15-18	66	145	176	69	59	1000	10	10	65
	19-24	72	160	177	70	58	1000	10	10	70
	25-50	79	174	176	70	63	1000	5	10	80
	51+	77	170	173	68	63	1000	5	10	80
Females	15-18	55	120	163	64	44	800	10	8	55
	19-24	58	128	164	65	46	800	10	8	60
	25-50	63	138	163	64	50	800	5	8	65
	51+	65	143	160	63	50	800	5	8	65
Pregnant						60	800	10	10	65
Lactating	1st 6 Months					65	1300	10	12	65
	2nd 6 Months					62	1200	10	11	65

*The allowances, expressed as average daily intakes over time, are intended to provide for individual variations among most normal persons as they live in the United States under usual environmental stresses. Diets should be based on a variety of common foods in order to provide other nutrients for which human requirements have been less well defined. See text for detailed discussion of allowances and of nutrients not tabulated.
†Weights and heights of reference adults are actual medians for the U.S. population of the designated age, as reported by NHANES II. The use of these figures does not imply that the height-to-weight ratios are ideal.

TABLE 5-6b Estimated Safe and Adequate Daily Dietary Intakes of Selected Vitamins and Minerals for Adults*

Vitamins		Trace element†				
Biotin (µg)	Pantothenic acid (mg)	Copper (mg)	Manganese (mg)	Fluoride (mg)	Chromium (mg)	Molybdenum (µg)
30-100	4-7	1.5-3.0	2.0-5.0	1.5-4.0	50-200	75-250

*Because there is less information on which to base allowances, these figures are not given in the main table of RDA and are provided here in the form of ranges of recommended intakes.
†Because the toxic levels for many trace elements may be only several times the usual intake, the upper levels for the trace elements given in this table should not be habitually exceeded.

from which selections were to be made. Today, the five food group format outlines five groups for which recommendations are established and an additional sixth group (fats, oils, and sweets) for which no specific recommendations exist. Table 5-7 summarizes the major nutrients each food group supplies.

Fruits

Two to four daily servings from the fruit group are recommended for an adult. The important function of this group is to provide vitamin A, vitamin C, complex carbohydrates, and fiber in our diets. The American Cancer Society indicates that this food group may play an important role in the prevention of certain forms of cancer. Included foods are citrus fruits and fruit juices. At least one serving high in vitamin C should be eaten daily.

Vegetables

Three to five servings from the vegetable group are recommended for an adult. As with the fruit group, the important function of this group is to provide vitamin A, vitamin C, complex carbohydrates, and fiber. The American Cancer Society states that this food group may also play an important role in the prevention of some cancers. Foods included in this group are dark green, yellow, and orange vegetables, canned or cooked vegetables, and tossed salads. At least one serving of dark green, yellow, or orange vegetable containing fat-soluble vitamin A should be consumed

balanced diet diet featuring food selections from each food group.

Water-soluble vitamins							Minerals						
Vitamin C (mg)	Thiamin (mg)	Riboflavin (mg)	Niacin (mg NE)¶	Vitamin B₆ (mg)	Folate (μg)	Vitamin B₁₂ (μg)	Calcium (mg)	Phosphorus (mg)	Magnesium (mg)	Iron (mg)	Zinc (mg)	Iodine (μg)	Selenium (μg)
60	1.5	1.8	20	2.0	200	2.0	1200	1200	400	12	15	150	50
60	1.5	1.7	19	2.0	200	2.0	1200	1200	350	10	15	150	70
60	1.5	1.7	19	2.0	200	2.0	800	800	350	10	15	150	70
60	1.2	1.4	15	2.0	200	2.0	800	800	350	10	15	150	70
60	1.1	1.3	15	1.5	180	2.0	1200	1200	300	15	12	150	50
60	1.1	1.3	15	1.6	180	2.0	1200	1200	280	15	12	150	55
60	1.1	1.3	15	1.6	180	2.0	800	800	280	15	12	150	55
60	1.0	1.2	13	1.6	180	2.0	800	800	280	10	12	150	55
70	1.5	1.6	17	2.2	400	2.2	1200	1200	320	30	15	175	65
95	1.6	1.8	20	2.1	280	2.6	1200	1200	355	15	19	200	75
95	1.6	1.7	20	2.1	260	2.6	1200	1200	340	15	16	200	75

‡Retinol equivalents. 1 retinol=1 μg retinol or 6 μg B-carotene.
§As cholecalciterol. 10 μg cholecalciferol=400 IU of vitamin D.
‖α-Tocopherol equivalents. 1 mg d-α tocopherol=1 α-TE.
¶1 NE (niacin equivalent) is equal to 1 mg of niacin or 60 mg of dietary tryptophan.

TABLE 5-6c Estimated Sodium, Chloride, and Potassium Minimum Requirements of Healthy Persons*

Age	Weight (kg)*	Sodium (mg)*†	Chloride (mg)*†	Potassium (mg)‡
10-18	50.0	500	750	2000
>18§⁾	70.0	500	750	2000

*No allowance has been included for large, prolonged losses from the skin through sweat.
†There is no evidence that higher intakes confer any health benefit.
‡Desirable intakes of potassium considerably exceed these values (~3500 mg for adults).
§No allowance included for growth. Values for those below 18 years assume a growth rate at the 50th percentile reported by the National Center for Health Statistics and averaged for males and females.

TABLE 5-7   **Guide to Daily Food Choices—a Summary**

Food group	Serving	Major contributions	Foods and serving size*
Milk, yogurt, and cheese	2 (adult†) 3 (children, teens, young adults, and pregnant or lactating women)	Calcium Riboflavin Protein Potassium Zinc	1 cup milk 1 ½ oz cheese 2 oz processed cheese 1 cup yogurt 2 cups cottage cheese 1 cup custard/pudding 1 ½ cups ice cream
Meat, poultry, fish, dry beans, eggs and nuts	2-3	Protein Niacin Iron Vitamin B_6 Zinc Thiamin Vitamin B_{12}‡	2-3 oz cooked meat, poultry, fish 1-1 ½ cups cooked dry beans 4 T peanut butter 2 eggs ½-1 cup nuts
Fruits	2-4	Vitamin C Fiber	¼ cup dried fruit ½ cup cooked fruit ¾ cup juice 1 whole piece fruit 1 melon wedge
Vegetables	3-5	Vitamin A Vitamin C Folate Magnesium Fiber	½ cup raw or cooked vegetables 1 cup raw leafy vegetables
Bread, cereals, rice, and pasta	6-11	Starch Thiamin Riboflavin§ Iron Niacin Folate Magnesium‖ Fiber‖ Zinc‖	1 slice of bread 1 oz ready-to-eat cereal ½-¾ cup cooked cereal, rice, or pasta
Fats, oils, and sweets		Foods from this group should not replace any from the other groups. Amounts consumed should be determined by individual energy needs.	

This is a practical way to turn the RDA into food choices. You can get all essential nutrients by eating a balanced variety of foods each day from the food groups listed here. Eat a variety of foods in each food group, and adjust serving sizes appropriately to reach and maintain desirable weight.

*May be reduced for children's servings.
†≥25 years of age.
‡Only in animal food choices.
§If enriched.
‖ Whole grains especially.

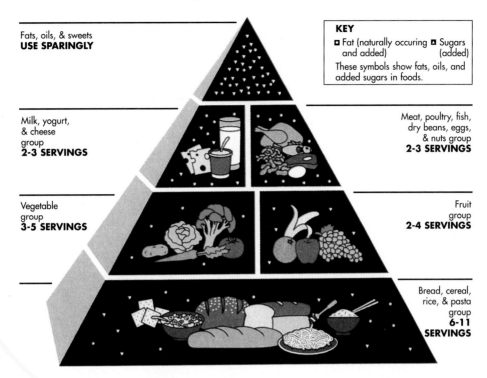

Figure 5-2 The USDA's Food Guide Pyramid.

KEY
- Fat (naturally occuring and added)
- Sugars (added)

These symbols show fats, oils, and added sugars in foods.

Fats, oils, & sweets
USE SPARINGLY

Milk, yogurt, & cheese group
2-3 SERVINGS

Meat, poultry, fish, dry beans, eggs, & nuts group
2-3 SERVINGS

Vegetable group
3-5 SERVINGS

Fruit group
2-4 SERVINGS

Bread, cereal, rice, & pasta group
6-11 SERVINGS

every other day. **Cruciferous vegetables** such as broccoli, cabbage, brussels sprouts, and cauliflower may be especially helpful in the prevention of certain forms of cancer.[17]

Milk, Cheese, and Yogurt

The milk, cheese, and yogurt group contributes two primary nutritional benefits: high-quality protein and calcium (required for bone and tooth development). Foods included in this group are whole milk, low-fat milk, yogurt, cheese, and ice cream. The adult recommendation is 2 to 3 cups of milk or two to three equivalent servings from this group each day. For teenagers the recommendation is 4 cups of milk each day. Recently, some physicians have begun recommending that premenopausal women consume three to four servings from this group to provide maximal protection from osteoporosis (see Chapter 20).

Because of the general concern over saturated fat, cholesterol, and additional calories, low-fat milk products are recommended in place of high-fat milk products. Both low-fat and high-fat dairy products provide similar nutritional benefits. Table 5-8 presents a nutritional comparison of dairy products.

Meat, Poultry, Fish, and Eggs

Our need for daily selections from the protein-rich meat, poultry, fish, and eggs group is based on our daily need for protein, iron, and the B vitamins. Meats include all red meats (beef, pork, and game), fish, and poultry. Meat substitutes include eggs, cheese, dried peas and beans (legumes), and peanut butter. The current recommendation for adults is 4 ounces total per day, preferably in two to three servings. However, some nutrition specialists suggest one serving per day (or every other day), with use of legumes as a protein supplement. If you select a food that fits into both the meat and the milk categories, be careful to include that food in only one of those categories for that particular day. Also, be certain that meat and fish are fresh, stored appropriately, and cooked adequately to prevent the possibility of serious food-borne infections.

The fat content of meat varies considerably. Some forms of meat yield only 1% fat, whereas others may be as high as 40% fat. Poultry and fish are generally significantly lower in overall fat than are red meats. Interestingly, the higher the grade of red meats, the more fat will be marbled throughout the muscle fiber and the higher will be its caloric value. Most of us prefer high-grade steaks because they appear to be more lean, but just the opposite is true. Indeed, the higher grade steak usually tastes better, but that is because of the presence of a higher fat content.

cruciferous vegetables (crew **sif** er us) vegetables that have flowers with four leaves in the pattern of a cross. *broccoli, cauliflower*

TABLE 5-8   **A Nutritional Comparison of Familiar Dairy Products**

Product	Calories	Carbohydrate (g)	Fat (g)	Saturated fat(g)	Cholesterol (mg)	Protein (g)	Calcium (mg)
Milk							
Whole (3.3% fat) 1 cup	150	11	8	6.1	33	8	291
Low-fat (2% fat) 1 cup	120	12	5	2.9	18	8	297
Low-fat (1% fat) 1 cup	100	12	3	1.6	10	8	300
Non-fat (skim) 1 cup	85	12	Trace	0.3	4	8	302
Buttermilk 1 cup	100	12	2	1.3	9	8	285
Dried 1 cup	245	35	Trace	0.3	12	24	837
Milk beverages							
Chocolate milk (3.3% fat) 1 cup	210	26	8	5.3	31	8	280
Chocolate flavored 6 oz water+1 oz powdered milk	100	22	1	0.6	1	3	90
Milk desserts							
Ice cream (11% fat) 1 cup	270	32	14	8.9	59	5	176
Ice milk (4% fat) 1 cup	185	29	6	3.5	18	5	176
Sherbet (2% fat) 1 cup	270	59	4	2.4	14	2	103
Yogurt							
Whole milk, plain 8 oz container	140	11	7	4.8	29	8	274
No fat, plain 8 oz container	125	16	Trace	0.3	4	13	452
Low-fat, fruit flavored 8 oz container	230	43	2	1.6	10	10	345
Cream							
Half and half							
1 cup	315	10	28	17.3	89	7	254
1 Tbsp	20	1	2	1.1	6	Trace	16
Sour cream							
1 cup	495	10	48	30	102	7	268
1 Tbsp	25	1	3	1.6	5	Trace	1

Meats are generally excellent sources of iron. Iron is present in much greater amounts in red meats and organ meats (liver, kideny, and heart) than in poultry and fish. Iron plays a critically important role in hemoglobin synthesis on red blood cells and, thus, is an important contributor to physical fitness (Chapter 4) and overall cardiovascular health (Chapter 10).

Breads, Cereals, Rice, and Pasta

The nutritional benefit from the bread, cereal, rice, and pasta group lies in its contribution of B-complex vitamins and energy (in the form of Calories) to our diet. Some nutritionists believe that the use of foods from this group promotes protein intake, since many foods in this group are prepared as complete-protein foods: macaroni and cheese, cereal and milk, and bread and meat sandwiches.

Six to eleven servings daily from this group are recommended. Several daily servings of any **enriched** or whole-grain bread or cereal are recommended. Milling of cereal grains into flour tends to deplete the flour of important nutrients, including fiber, vitamin B_6, vitamin E, magnesium, and various trace elements. The process of enrichment returns only four of these nutrients: thiamine, niacin, riboflavin (all B vitamins), and the mineral iron.

Fortunately, *whole-grain flour* is a healthful alternative for most consumers, since few, if any, nutrients are lost in the milling process. The *cereal germ,* the fiber, and additional nutrients are not destroyed.

Fats, Oils, and Sweets

Where do such items as beer, butter, candy, colas, cookies, corn chips, and pastries fit into a food group pattern? Today they are included under the label "fats, oils, and sweets." Most of the items mentioned contribute relatively little to healthful nutrition other than providing additional Calories (generally from sucrose) and significant amounts of salt and fat. As you will see in Chapter 10, persons who are salt-sensitive must reduce their salt intake as a step in preventing the development of high blood pressure. It is not surprising that many of these items are referred to collectively as *junk foods*. Of course, if particular food items, such as cookies, are made from high-quality flour and contain raisins and nuts, you can receive some nutritional benefit from consuming such goodies (see the discussion of nutrient density on p. 121).

Understandably, the processed-food industry encourages this empty-Calorie approach to eating. Many vending machines are filled with relatively expensive junk foods. Indeed, advertising for nonnutritious foods overwhelmingly exceeds advertising for nutritious foods. Although it is difficult to recall a television commercial for lettuce, broccoli, or green beans, we can all recite advertising slogans for our favorite soft drink, alcoholic beverage, breakfast snack, or candy bar. It takes a lot of willpower to say "no" to the foods in this group.

FAST FOODS

Fast foods are convenience foods usually prepared in walk-in or drive-through restaurants. In contrast to that of junk foods, the nutritional value of fast foods can vary considerably (see the box on p. 110). As can be seen in the *Calories from fat (%)* column, **fat density** remains a serious limitation of fast foods. In comparison to the recommended standard (25% to 30% of total calories from fat) depicted in Figure 5-5, p.114, 40% to 50% of the Calories in fast foods are made up of fats. The recent conversion from animal fat to vegetable oil for frying (to reduce cholesterol levels) did not alter the fat-dense nature of these foods items. In fact, some nutritionists contend that the vegetable oil formula used by the major fast food companies is hydrogenated vegetable shortening and not liquid vegetable oil as they advertise.[18] If so, this shortening contributes fat in a molecular configuration (trans-fatty acids) that is very difficult for the body to metabolize.

On the more positive side, fast food restaurants have broadened their menus to include whole-wheat breads and rolls, salad bars, lower-fat meats, and low-fat milk products. Many of the larger fast food restaurants provide nutritional information for consumers. Unlike junk foods, fast foods may be reasonably nutritious, but to rely on these foods as a primary source of nutrition—as many college students and busy families do—is both unwise and expensive. You can, however, learn to practice a more nutritionally sound approach to eating even with a diet that relies heavily on fast foods.

FOOD EXCHANGE SYSTEM

The American Dietetic Association has recently developed a food classification system designed to aid per-

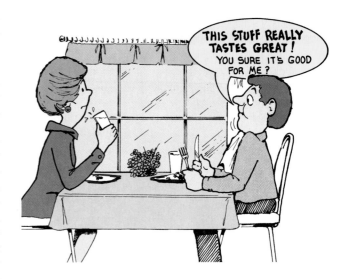

sons who wish to control the caloric and fat content of their diets. This food exchange list is available from the ADA.* By selecting the appropriate types and amounts of foods from each of the six categories of food, people will achieve nutritional balance and better control of fat and Calorie intake.

FOOD ADDITIVES

The lament about the "good old days" is certainly applicable to our current food supply. Today many people believe that the food they consume is dangerously compromised by intentionally and unintentionally introduced **food additives.**

The presence of additives in the food supply is not a totally modern occurrence. Salt, spices, and the chemicals imparted during the smoke curing of meats have altered the food supply since the dawn of recorded history. In addition, naturally occurring *biological toxins* and the foreign materials once added to food by processors made yesterday's food far less than pure and natural. Because of extensive federal regulation, it is doubtful whether the approximate 2800 food

*To receive a food exchange list, send $2.00 to The American Dietetic Association, 430 N. Michigan Ave., Chicago, IL 60611.

---

enriched the process of returning to foods some of the nutritional elements (B vitamins and iron) removed during processing.

fat density percentage of a food's total Calories that are derived from fat; above 30% reflects higher fat density.

food additives chemical compounds that are intentionally or unintentionally added to our food supply.

Facts about Fast Foods

Are you stopping at a fast food restaurant today? Consider these points before you do: (1) Will this be an extra meal, or have I planned for it as a part of my food intake for the day? (2) Can fast foods be part of a balanced diet? (3) Do I realize how fat-dense this meal will be? If you answer yes to these questions, then you are practicing responsible, healthful nutrition planning.

Food	Calories	Protein (g)	Carbohydrate (g)	fat (g)	Calories from fat (g)	Cholesterol (mg)	Sodium (mg)
Hamburgers							
McDonald's hamburger	263	12.4	28.3	11.3	38.6	29.1	506
Dairy Queen single hamburger w/cheese	410	24	33	20	43.9	50	790
Hardee's ¼ pound cheeseburger	506	28	41	26	46.2	61	1950
Wendy's double hamburger, white bun	560	41	24	34	54.6	125	575
McDonald's Big Mac	570	24.6	39.2	35	55.2	83	979
Burger King Whopper sandwich	640	27	42	41	57.6	94	842
Jack in the Box Jumbo Jack	485	26	38	26	48.2	64	905
Chicken							
Arby's chicken breast sandwich	592	28	56	27	41.0	57	1340
Burger King chicken sandwich	688	26	56	40	52.3	82	1423
Dairy Queen chicken sandwich	670	29	46	41	55.0	75	870
Church's Crispy Nuggets (one; regular)	55	3	4	3	49.0	—	125
Kentucky Fried Chicken Nuggets (one)	46	2.82	2.2	2.9	56.7	11.9	140
Fish							
Church's Southern fried catfish	67	4	4	4	53.7	—	151
Long John Silver's Fish & More	978	34	82	58	53.3	88	2124
McDonald's Filet-O-Fish	435	14.7	35.9	25.7	53.1	45.2	799
Others							
Hardee's hot dog	346	11	26	22	57.2	42	744
Jack in the Box taco	191	8	16	11	51.8	21	406
Arby's roast beef sandwich (regular)	350	22	32	15	38.5	39	590
Hardee's roast beef sandwich	377	21	36	17	40.5	57	1030
French fries							
Arby's french fries	211	2	33	8	34.1	6	30
McDonald's french fries (regular)	220	3	26.1	11.5	47.0	8.6	109
Wendy's french fries (regular)	280	40	35	14	45.0	15	95
Shakes							
Dairy Queen	710	14	120	19	24.0	50	260
McDonald's							
Vanilla	352	9.3	59.6	8.4	21.4	30.6	201
Chocolate	383	9.9	65.5	9	21.1	29.7	300
Strawberry	362	9	62.1	8.7	22.3	32.2	207
Soft Drinks							
Coca-Cola Classic	144	—	38	—	—	—	14
Coca-Cola	154	—	40	—	—	—	6
Diet Coke	0.9	—	0.3	—	—	—	16
Sprite	142	—	36	—	—	—	45
Tab	1	—	1	—	—	—	30
Diet Sprite	3	—	0	—	—	—	9

Fast foods can be a part of a balanced diet, especially since many companies are reformulating their products in the direction of better nutrition. However, you should remember that fast foods do have limitations, including their low calcium content, low vitamin A and C levels, and high Calorie content. Plan carefully for your fast food intake, remembering to eat a wide variety of all foods from each of the basic five food groups.

★ Examples of the Food Groups

These illustrations represent examples of foods from each of the food groups. Choose foods from each of the first five groups. Avoid the last group whenever possible. ★

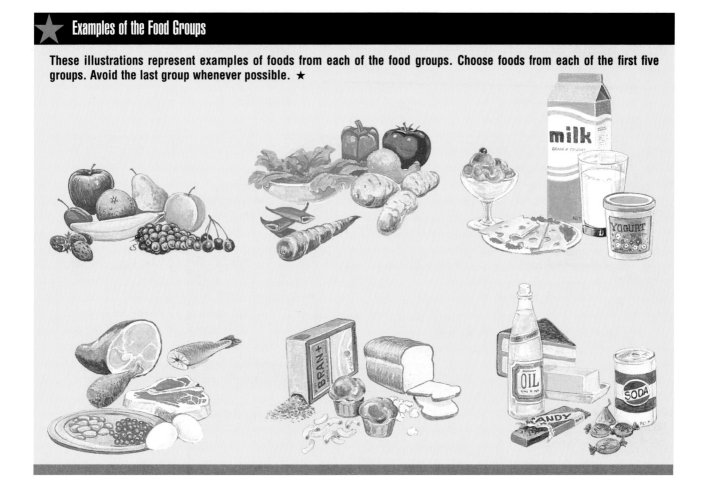

additives that can be *intentionally* used or the 10,000 substances that could be *incidentally* introduced during production or preparation pose a significant health threat.[2,19] What is clear, however, is that if we wish to live in an urban setting, work outside the home, insist on convenience, and escape the limitations imposed by the seasonal nature of many foods, we will likely have to accept the presence of a considerable number of food additives.

Today's food processors add chemical compounds to the food supply for several reasons that they believe we, the consumers, support. Compounds are added to food to (1) maintain the nutritional value of the food, (2) maintain the food's freshness by preventing changes in its color, flavor, and texture, (3) contribute to the processing of the food by controlling its texture, acidity, and thickness, and (4) make the food more appealing to the consumer by enhancing its flavor and standardizing its color. Market research apparently indicates that consumers will continue to accept these alterations regardless of what we might say about our desire that they not occur.

The Food Additives Amendment (1958) and the Color Additive Amendments (1960) to the federal Food, Drug and Cosmetic Act (1938) require that new additives to the food supply be safe for human con-

sumption. The process through which the manufacturer must go to gain approval is lengthy and expensive. Even compounds that have long been considered to be "generally recognized as safe" by experts are now undergoing reevaluation through modern laboratory technology. It is to be hoped that all truly harmful additives will soon be identified and removed from the food supply.

FOOD LABELS

Since 1973, food manufacturers have been required by the Food and Drug Administration (FDA) to provide nutritional information (labels) on products to which one or more additional nutrients have been added or for which some nutritional claim has been made. Despite the presence of these labels, there was concern about whether the public could understand the labels as they appeared and whether additional information was required. Accordingly, the FDA, in consultation with individual states and public interest groups, developed new labeling regulations. Newly devised labels began appearing on food during May, 1993. The newly adopted label is shown in Figure 5-3. Specific types of information contained on the new label are highlighted. Additionally, newly developed defini-

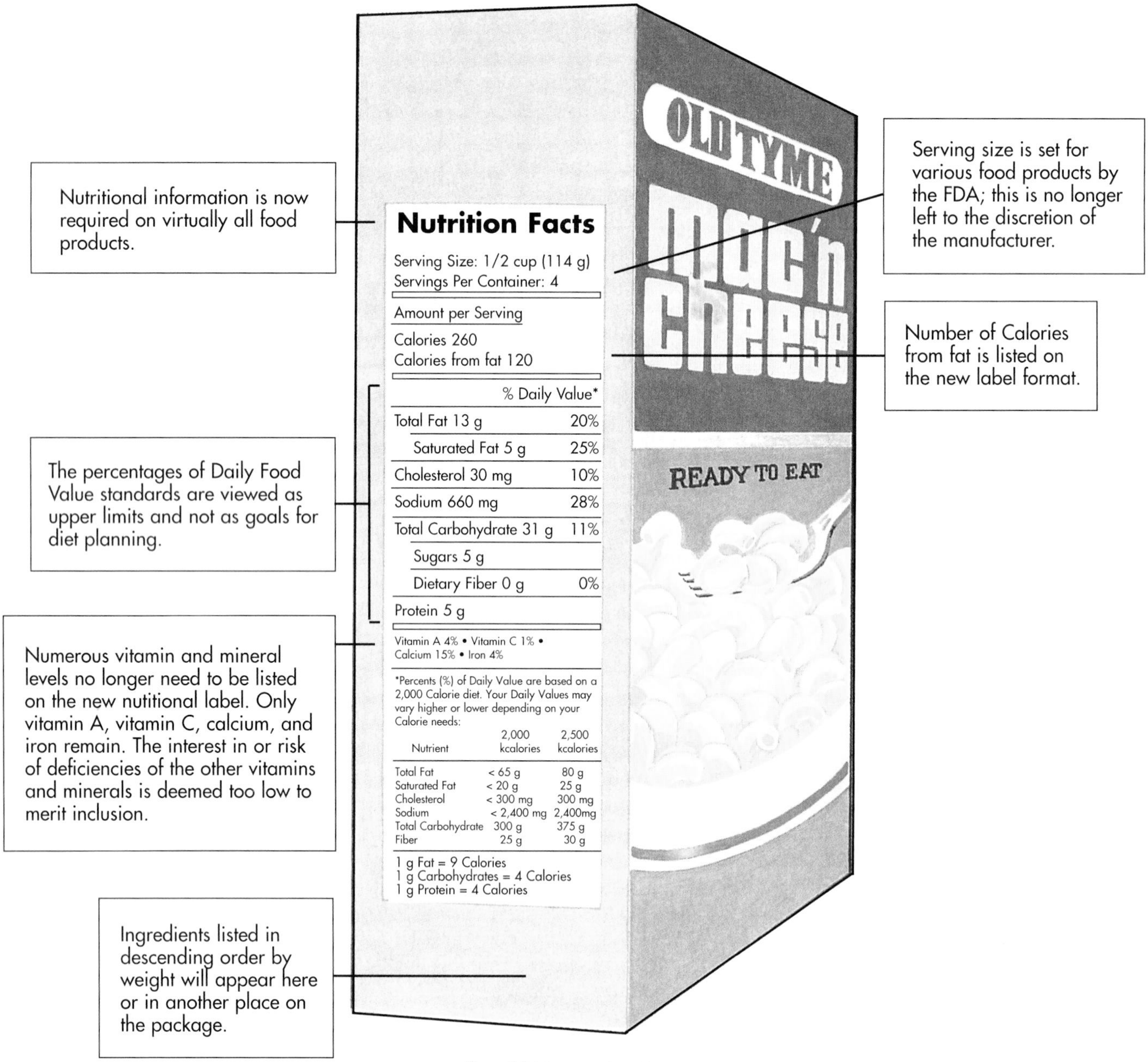

Nutritional information is now required on virtually all food products.

Serving size is set for various food products by the FDA; this is no longer left to the discretion of the manufacturer.

Number of Calories from fat is listed on the new label format.

The percentages of Daily Food Value standards are viewed as upper limits and not as goals for diet planning.

Numerous vitamin and mineral levels no longer need to be listed on the new nutitional label. Only vitamin A, vitamin C, calcium, and iron remain. The interest in or risk of deficiencies of the other vitamins and minerals is deemed too low to merit inclusion.

Ingredients listed in descending order by weight will appear here or in another place on the package.

OLD TYME

mac'n Cheese

READY TO EAT

Nutrition Facts

Serving Size: 1/2 cup (114 g)
Servings Per Container: 4

Amount per Serving	
Calories 260	
Calories from fat 120	

	% Daily Value*
Total Fat 13 g	20%
Saturated Fat 5 g	25%
Cholesterol 30 mg	10%
Sodium 660 mg	28%
Total Carbohydrate 31 g	11%
Sugars 5 g	
Dietary Fiber 0 g	0%
Protein 5 g	

Vitamin A 4% • Vitamin C 1% •
Calcium 15% • Iron 4%

*Percents (%) of Daily Value are based on a 2,000 Calorie diet. Your Daily Values may vary higher or lower depending on your Calorie needs:

Nutrient	2,000 kcalories	2,500 kcalories
Total Fat	< 65 g	80 g
Saturated Fat	< 20 g	25 g
Cholesterol	< 300 mg	300 mg
Sodium	< 2,400 mg	2,400mg
Total Carbohydrate	300 g	375 g
Fiber	25 g	30 g

1 g Fat = 9 Calories
1 g Carbohydrates = 4 Calories
1 g Protein = 4 Calories

Figure 5-3 The new food label.

Nutrient Definitions

- *Free:* an amount that is "nutritonally trivial" and unlikely to have a physiological consequence
- *Calorie free:* fewer than 5 calories a serving
- *Sugar free: less than 0.5 grams per serving*
- *Sodium free* and *salt free:* less than 5 milligrams of sodium per serving
- *Fat free: less than 0.5 grams of fat per serving, providing that it has no added fat or oil ingredient*
- *Low fat:* 3 grams or less of fat per serving per 100 grams of the food
- *Low in saturated fat:* may be used to describe a food that contains 1 gram or less of saturated fat per serving and not more than 15% calories from saturated fat
- *Cholesterol free:* less than 2 milligrams of cholesterol per serving and 2 grams or less saturated fat per serving
- *Low in cholesterol:* 20 milligrams or less per serving and per 100 grams of food and 2 grams or less of saturated fat per serving

Figure 5-4 Nutrient claim definitions.

tions for nutritionally related terms are shown in Figure 5-4.

Proposals for the labeling of raw foods, including fresh produce, meat, and seafoods are now being studied. Concern for consumer protection stems from recent disclosures regarding meat inspection, undercooking of hamburgers, and the risk of contaminated seafood. Although specific guidelines are not now in place, many suppliers of raw foods have adopted versions of the United States Department of Agriculture's guidelines in response to consumer concern. The USDA's proposed guidelines are shown in the Health Action Guide below.

It is hoped that these new labeling regulations will make it possible for us to be even more effective in our efforts to eat in a healthy manner. In the final analysis, however, the consumer must want to eat more healthfully or the labels will contain only wasted information.

GUIDELINES FOR DIETARY HEALTH

For decades the American public has received dietary guidelines from a variety of professional and governmental groups. In each case the intent has been to foster changes in dietary practices that were intended to reduce the risk of developing chronic diseases and enhance the overall nutritional health of the public. In most cases these guidelines have been generated by concerns over the actual dietary practices of the public as compared with those practices that should be followed on the basis of scientific understanding (Figure 5-5).

Although dietary guidelines of one type or another have been issued on numerous occasions, the Dietary Guidelines for Americans represent the most current and widely disseminated guidelines. The newest version appeared in 1990 as the third edition of *Nutrition and Your Health: Dietary Guidelines for Americans.*[20] As presently constructed, these guidelines are directed to Healthy Americans 2 years of age and older and to the health professionals who can influence the public dietary practices. Information contained within these guidelines was extracted from a variety of sources, including the Surgeon General's Report on Nutrition and Health. The most recent dietary guidelines are shown in Figure 5-6.

Beyond the simply stated guidelines, the most recent report contains new information pertaining to specific modifications applicable to most Americans and some applicable to specific groups of persons appears in the Health Action Guide on page 116.

Table 5-9 shows how healthful dietary changes can lead to reduced chances of developing certain major diseases.

Whether the newest Dietary Guidelines for Americans will be more fully implemented than their predecessors remains to be seen. Regardless, the vast majority of Americans could move much closer toward meeting these guidelines.

Health ACTION Guide

USDA's Safety Tips for Proper Handling of Meat

▼ Keep meat refrigerated or frozen
▼ Thaw meat in refrigerator or microwave

▼ Keep raw meat separate from other foods
▼ Wash working surfaces, utensils, and hands after use
▼ Cook meat thoroughly
▼ Refrigerate leftovers within 2 hours of cooking

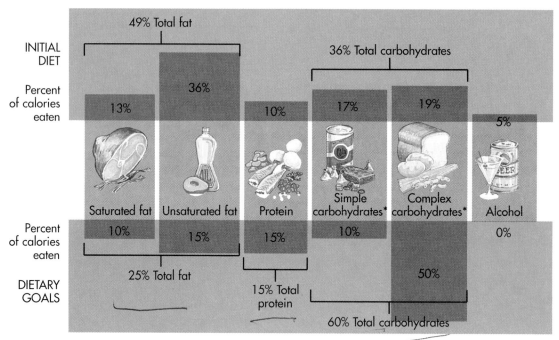

*Estimates based on Senate Select Subcommittee on Nutrition and Health data (circa 1970).
**Some versions of the Dietary Goals use ranges rather than specific values:
Fats   25%-30%
Protein   12%-15%
Carbohydrate   58%-60%

Figure 5-5 Where do your Calories come from? This figure compares our present sources of Calories with the sources that are currently recommended by nutritionists. (See p. 91 for current fat consumption.)

Nutrition and Your Health: Dietary Guidelines for Americans—1990

- Eat a variety of foods.
- Maintain healthy weight.
- Choose a diet low in fat, saturated fat, and cholesterol.
- Choose a diet with plenty of vegetables, fruits, and grain products.
- Use sugars only in moderation.
- Use salt and sodium only in moderation.

Figure 5-6 The current dietary guidelines.

NONTRADITIONAL DIETARY PRACTICES

Nutritionists have shared with us their concerns about some of the dietary practices observed among young adults because they realize that dietary practices established during the college years may continue throughout life. Their recommendations are made with full knowledge that the demands of life will continue to force some compromises in the adoption of dietary patterns.

It is not uncommon to pursue some form of nontraditional diet. Vegetarian diets, weight-reduction diets, and over-reliance on *fast foods* represent some of these nontraditional diet approaches. Most nutritionists believe that these diets need not be discontinued or avoided, but they should be undertaken with care and with insight because of potential nutritional limitations.

Vegetarian Diets

A *vegetarian diet* relies on plant sources for all or the vast majority of the nutrients needed by the body. Vegetarian diets encompass a continuum from diets that allow some animal sources of nutrients to those that not only exclude animal sources but also are restrictive even in terms of the plant sources of nutrients permitted. We will briefly describe three vegetarian diets, beginning with the least restrictive in terms of food sources.

OVOLACTOVEGETARIAN DIET

Depending on the particular pattern of consuming eggs *(ova)* and milk *(lacto)* or using one but not the other, **ovolactovegetarianism** can be an extremely sound approach to healthful eating during the entire course of the adult years. Ovolactovegetarian diets

TABLE 5-9 Convergence of Recommendations*

Change in diet:	Reduce fats	Control calories	Increase starch† and fiber	Reduce sodium	Control alcohol
Reduce risk of:					
Heart disease	✔	✔		✔	
Cancer	✔	✔	✔		✔
Stroke	✔	✔		✔	✔
Diabetes	✔	✔	✔		
Gastrointestinal disease‡	✔	✔	✔		✔

*To reduce the risk of diseases or their complications.
†Starch refers to complex carbohydrates provided by fruits, vegetables, and whole grain products.
‡Primarily gallbladder disease (fat), diverticular disease (fiber), and cirrhosis (alcohol).

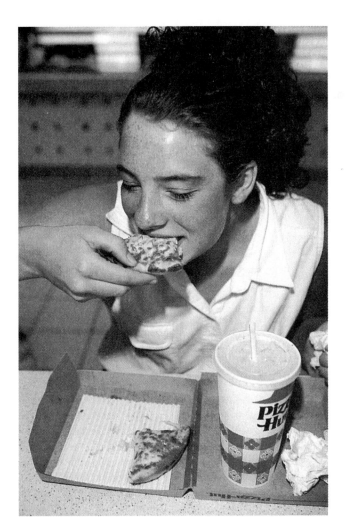

Pizza is a fast food commonly consumed by college students.

provide the body with the essential amino acids and limit the high intake of fats seen in more conventional diets. The exclusion of meat as a protein source lowers the total fat intake, while the consumption of milk or eggs allows for an adequate amount of saturated fat to remain in the diet. The consistent use of vegetable products as the primary source of nutrients supports the current dietary recommendations for an increase in overall carbohydrates, an increase in complex carbohydrates, and an increase in fiber.

Meatlike products composed of *textured vegetable protein* are available in supermarkets. Nonmeat bacon strips, hamburger patties, and link sausage can be used by people who want to restrict their meat intake. Soybeans are a primary source of this textured vegetable protein.

Two relatively minor concerns associated with some ovolactovegetarian diets are those of zinc deficiency and the overuse of a wide variety of **food supplements.** Because of zinc's role in the body's use of iron, ovolactovegetarians may need to take this mineral in supplement form. The general use of large quantities of food supplements may be harmful or, at best, unnecessary.

LACTOVEGETARIAN DIET

Persons who include dairy products in their diet—but no other animal products, such as eggs—are *lactovegetarians.* As with the ovolactovegetarian diet, there is little risk associated with this dietary pattern.

---

ovolactovegetarian diet (oh voe **lack** toe veg a **ter** ee in) diet that exludes the use of all meat but does allow the consumption of eggs and dairy products.

food supplements nutrients taken in addition to those obtained through the diet; includes powdered protein, vitamins, and mineral extracts.

Health ACTION Guide

Dietary Recommendations

ISSUES FOR MOST PEOPLE:

Your nutritional health could probably be enhanced if you implement the practices described here.

▼ **Fats and cholesterol:** Reduce consumption of fat (especially saturated fat) and cholesterol. Choose foods relatively low in these substances, such as vegetables, fruits, whole grain foods, fish, poultry, lean meats, and low-fat dairy products. Use food preparation methods that add little or no fat.

▼ **Energy and weight control:** Achieve and maintain a desirable body weight. To do so, choose a dietary pattern in which energy (caloric) intake is consistent with energy expenditure. To reduce energy intake, limit consumption of foods relatively high in Calories, fats, and sugars and minimize alcohol consumption. Increase energy expenditure through regular and sustained physical activity.

▼ **Complex carbohydrates and fiber:** Increase consumption of whole-grain foods and cereal products, vegetables (including dried beans and peas), and fruits.

▼ **Sodium:** Reduce intake of sodium by choosing foods relatively low in sodium and limiting the amount of salt added in food preparation and at the table.

▼ **Alcohol:** To reduce the risk of chronic disease, drink alcohol only in moderation (no more than two drinks a day), if at all. Avoid drinking any alcohol before or while driving, operating machinery, taking medications, or engaging in any other activity requiring judgment. Avoid drinking alcohol while pregnant.

ISSUES FOR SOME PEOPLE:

If your nutritional needs fall into one of the groups listed, you should implement the following recommendations.

▼ **Fluoride:** Community water systems should contain fluoride at optimal levels for prevention of tooth decay. If such water is not available, use other appropriate sources of fluoride.

▼ **Sugars:** Those who are particularly vulnerable to dental caries (cavities), especially children, should limit their consumption and frequency of use of foods high in sugars.

▼ **Calcium:** Adolescent girls and adult women should increase consumption of foods high in calcium, including low-fat dairy products.

▼ **Iron:** Children, adolescents, and women of childbearing age should be sure to consume foods that are good sources of iron, such as lean red meats, fish, certain beans, and iron-enriched cereals and whole grain products. This issue is of special concern for low-income families.

VEGAN VEGETARIAN DIET

A **vegan vegetarian diet** is one in which not only meat but also other animal products, such as milk, cheese, and eggs, are removed from the diet. When compared with the ovolactovegetarian diet, the vegan diet requires a higher level of nutritional understanding to avoid malnourishment.

When plants represent the body's only source of nutrients, several difficulties can occur. The novice vegan will need to be particularly alert for these difficulties. One potential difficulty is that of obtaining all of the essential amino acids. Since a single plant source does not contain all the essential amino acids, the vegan dieter must learn to consistently employ a *complementary* diet. By carefully combining various grains, seeds, and legumes, amino acid deficiency can be prevented. This diet probably should not be used by children, pregnant women, and **lactating** mothers.

In addition to the potential difficulty with amino acid deficiency, the vegan dieter could experience some difficulty in maintaining the necessary intake of vitamin B_{12}. Possible ramifications of inadequate B_{12} intake include depression, anemia, back pain, and menstrual irregularity. Vegan dieters often have difficulty maintaining adequate intakes of iron, zinc, and calcium.[2] Calcium intake must be monitored closely by the vegan dieter. In addition, vitamin D deficiencies can occur. Supplements and daily exposure to sunshine will aid in maintaining adequate levels of this vitamin.

A final area of potential difficulty for the vegan dieter is that of an insufficient caloric intake because of the *satiation* resulting from the *voluminous* nature of the diet. Early satiation caused by a large amount of fiber may lower carbohydrate intake to the point that protein stores (muscle mass) are used for energy.

Because of its nutritional limitations, many nutritionists do not recommend the vegan vegetarian diet, even for adults. They suggest that unless undertaken for reasons closely related to emotional, spiritual, or philosophical beliefs, the total exclusion of animal products seems to accomplish little from a nutritional-health point of view that cannot be accomplished through ovolactovegetarianism. Clearly, the ovolactovegetarian diet is much less likely to lead to malnutrition than is the vegan diet.

High-Risk Dietary Practices

Whereas the health benefits and relatively low risks of vegetarianism make those diets attractive, the diets in the following discussion hold the potential for serious health risks.

MACROBIOTIC DIET

At the extreme end of the vegetarian continuum is the **macrobiotic diet.** One form of this diet is the Zen macrobiotic diet. Characterized by an almost total dependence on brown rice as the source of nutrients, this diet moves the individual through progressive stages—each of which gradually removes undesirable foods until little remains other than brown rice. So potentially harmful is this limited approach to nutrition (with deficiencies in vitamin C, calcium, and high-quality protein) that it is not recommended.[1] Regardless of the spiritual benefits or curative properties often claimed for the diet by its practitioners, any diet that prevents the body from meeting its nutritional needs is an unhealthful approach to eating.

UNBALANCED AND FAD DIETS

After vegetarian diets, a second area of concern about collegiate dietary practices is that associated with an **unbalanced diet** to achieve or maintain weight loss. An unbalanced diet might consist of a *single food* (like pizza) or food selections from just one or two of the five main food groups. Whether you eat only grapefruit, bananas, avocados, or some other "special foods," the point remains the same: a diet lacking variety and balance generally cannot provide you with all of the needed nutrients.

Nutritionists at our university continue to inform us that young adults, for some reason, tend to adopt these very unbalanced diets more frequently than other adults. Noticing the poor dietary practices of a friend or roommate should prompt you to look carefully at your own dietary practices (see the box on pp 118–119). Make certain that your own dietary pattern is not more unbalanced than you might have suspected.

RECOMMENDED DIETARY ADJUSTMENTS

In addition to the dietary patterns just discussed, nutritionists also recommend certain modifications in the diets of young adults. These modifications include the following six considerations.

Additional Milk Consumption

Because of the tendency for aging women to develop a loss in bone mass density, a condition called *osteoporo-*

sis, it is recommended that adult women increase their dairy product intake to achieve the equivalent of four servings. This additional intake provides needed calcium, which may prevent the incidence of hip, wrist, and vertebral fractures when these women become older adults. Excessive caloric and fat intake can be controlled by using skim milk or low-fat yogurt and by decreasing the daily intake of all fats. For students who do not like dairy products or who are allergic to milk, calcium supplements are an alternative. Of course, the other nutritional benefits from the milk group cannot be obtained through calcium supplements. (Osteoporosis is discussed further in Chapter 20.)

Additional Protein-Rich Sources

Nutritionists recommend that to maintain iron stores within the body to replace any iron lost during menstruation, women who menstruate should include 3 ounces of red meat in their diets 3 or 4 times per week. Iron obtained from red meat (called *heme iron*) is iron in its most *biologically available* form. A general lowering of fat intake will allow this small inclusion of red meat to be undertaken without increasing overall fat intake or adding Calories.

Vegetarians can obtain adequate amounts of iron only if they carefully structure their diets to include appropriate vegetables, fruits, and grain products. Some excellent vegetable sources of iron are lettuce, endive, beets, tomatoes, spinach, green peas, green beans, legumes, and broccoli. Good fruit sources of iron are apricots, cantaloupe, dates, prunes, and raisins. Enriched or whole-grain breads and cereals are also good iron sources. Products prepared in iron cookware will often contain higher amounts of iron than those prepared in other forms of cookware. Milk products contain little iron.

Iron supplements may help provide needed iron. However, you might wish to consult a physician before taking iron supplements. Supplements alone do not provide the additional benefits found in the protein-rich food group, and they may cause severe digestive complications.

---

vegan vegetarian diet (**vay** gan) vegetarian diet that excludes the use of all animal products, including eggs and dairy products.

lactating (**lack** tate ing) breastfeeding nursing.

macrobiotic diet (mack row bye **ott** ick) vegetarian diet composed almost entirely of brown rice.

unbalanced diet diet lacking adequate representation from each of the food groups.

PERSONAL ASSESSMENT

A primary requirement for good nutrition is a balanced diet. A variety of food selections can be made to form the basis of this diet.

For a 7-day period, assign yourself the points indicated when each area is met. Record your points in the appropriate column for each day. Total your daily and weekly points. Negative points for junk food consumption should be subtracted from your daily and weekly totals.

Food	Points	Maximum score	Daily score						
			M	T	W	T	F	S	S
Milk and milk products		30							
One cup of milk or equivalent	10								
Second cup of milk	10								
Third cup of milk	10								
Protein-rich foods		25							
One serving of egg, meat, fish, poultry, cheese, dried beans, or peas	15								
One or two additional servings of egg, meat, fish, poultry, or cheese	10 each								
Fruits and vegetables		30							
One serving of green or yellow vegetables	10								
One serving of citrus fruit, tomato, or cabbage	10								
Two or more servings of other fruits and vegetables, including potatoes	5 each								
Breads and cereals		15							
Four or more servings of whole-grain or enriched cereals or breads	5 each								
Junk foods (or negative point value foods)									
Sweet rolls	−5								
Fruit pies	−5								
Potato chips, corn chips, or cheese curls	−5								
Candy	−5								
Nondiet sodas	−5								
		100							

Point record

Weekly point total   _____
Negative point total   _____
Adjusted weekly point total   _____

Interpretation

600-700	Excellent dietary practices
450-599	Adequate dietary practices
300-449	Marginal dietary practices
Below 300	Poor dietary practices

TO CARRY THIS FURTHER . . .

1. On which day of the week was it most difficult for you to eat a balanced diet? Why? _____

_____

_____

2. Approximately what percent of your total points was from foods purchased in a restaurant? _____

_____

_____

3. Approximately how much money did you spend on food during this 7-day period? _____

_____

_____

4. How much time do you estimate that you spent eating during this 7-day period? _____

_____

_____

5. Was this a typical 7-day period in terms of the types of food eaten? If no, describe how a more typical

7-day period would appear. _____

_____

_____

6. Your instructor may prepare a dietary profile of the class against which you can evaluate your personal

7-day diet assessment. _____

_____

_____

PERSONAL ASSESSMENT

Health ACTION Guide

Making Healthful Food Choices

It is very likely that you can improve your dietary health and reduce the risk of developing heart disease and cancer by implementing the following practices.

EAT MORE HIGH-FIBER FOODS

▼ Choose dried beans, peas, and lentils more often.
▼ Eat whole-grain breads, cereals, and crackers.
▼ Eat more vegetables—raw and cooked.
▼ Eat whole fruit in place of drinking fruit juice.
▼ Try other high-fiber foods, such as oat bran, barley, brown rice, or wild rice.

EAT LESS SUGAR

▼ Avoid regular soft drinks. One 12-ounce can has 9 teaspoons of sugar!
▼ Avoid eating table sugar, honey, syrup, jam, jelly, candy, sweet rolls, fruit canned in syrup, regular gelatin desserts, cake with icing, pie, or other sweets.
▼ Choose fresh fruit or fruit canned in natural juice or water.
▼ If desired, use sweeteners that don't have any Calories, such as saccharin or aspartame, instead of sugar.

USE LESS SALT

▼ Reduce the amount of salt you use in cooking.
▼ Avoid adding additional salt to food at the table.
▼ Eat fewer high-salt foods, such as canned soups, ham, sauerkraut, hot dogs, pickles, and foods that taste salty.
▼ Eat fewer convenience and fast foods.

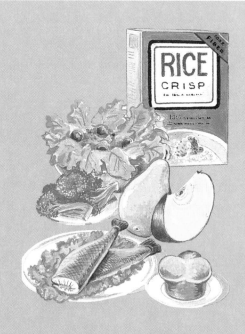

EAT LESS FAT

▼ Eat smaller servings of meat. Eat fish and poultry more often. Choose lean cuts of red meat.
▼ Prepare all meats by roasting, baking, or broiling. Trim off all fat. Limit addition of sauces or gravy. Remove skin from poultry.
▼ Avoid fried foods. Avoid adding fat when cooking.
▼ Eat fewer high-fat foods such as cold cuts, bacon, sausage, hot dogs, butter, margarine, nuts, salad dressing, lard, and solid shortening.
▼ Drink skim or low-fat milk.
▼ Eat less ice cream, cheese, sour cream, cream, whole milk, and other high-fat dairy products.

Additional Vitamins C and A

Foods chosen from the fruits group and the vegetables group on a regular basis should include those that are good sources of vitamins C and A. The inclusion of additional vitamin C in the diet will assist in the absorption of iron from bread, cereal, and eggs. For the woman of reproductive age, iron stores are an important consideration, since iron is a component of the hemoglobin found in red blood cells that are lost during menstruation.

In addition to the recommendation concerning vitamin C, larger servings of fruits and vegetables, particularly the dark green vegetables, are recommended. By increasing intake in this food group, desirable increases in **folacin** and vitamin A can be achieved. Folacin's role in intrauterine development and in preventing **macrocytic anemia** makes its increased presence in the diet of critical importance. High levels of carotenes found in dark green vegetables aid in the production of vitamin A, a necessary fat-soluble vitamin.

Additional Grain Product Consumption

The dietary guidelines for Americans recommend that 60% of your total Calories come from carbohydrates. Increasing the quantity of whole-grain breads and cereals in your diet can make sure this 60% recommendation is met.

Moderate Alcohol Consumption

The risks and benefits of alcohol use are discussed at length in Chapter 8. However, because so many adults consume alcohol, we should indicate here that heavy use of alcoholic beverages can have a major impact on nutritional status.

Alcohol provides a significant amount of empty Calories. This can be a major concern for alcohol users who wish to control weight. Also, the overuse of alcohol can rob the body of its ability to absorb other nutrients successfully, may prevent you from consuming a healthy diet, and is associated with a wide variety of diseases, including cancer and liver complications. From a health standpoint, moderation in the use of alcohol makes a lot of sense.

Nutrient Density

For numerous college students, the consideration of nutrient density may prompt certain dietary adjustments. The *nutrient density* of a food item relates to its ability to supply proportionally more of the RDA (for select vitamins and minerals) than it does daily calorie requirements. Foods with a high nutrient density are better choices than those that supply only **empty Calories.** For example, a bag of potato chips or a bottle of beer has a much lower nutrient density than either a taco or a slice of pizza. Choosing to eat foods with high nutrient density is especially important for persons who are trying to limit caloric intake.

NUTRITION AND THE OLDER ADULT

Nutritional needs change as adults age. Age-related alterations to the structure and function of the body are primarily responsible for this. Included among the changes that alter nutritional requirements and practices are changes in the teeth, salivary glands, taste buds, oral muscles, gastric acid production, and peristaltic action. Older adults can find food less tasteful and harder to chew. Chronic constipation resulting from changes in gastrointestinal tract function can also decrease interest in eating.

The progressive lowering of the body's basal metabolism is another factor that eventually influences dietary patterns of older adults. As energy requirements fall, the body gradually senses the need for less food. This gradual recognition of lower energy needs results in a lessened food intake and "loss of appetite" in many elderly people. Because of this decreased need for calories, nutrient density—the nutritional value of food per Calories supplied—is an important factor for the elderly.

Besides the physiological factors that influence dietary patterns among the elderly, there are psychosocial factors that alter the role of food in the lives of many older adults. Social isolation, depression,

chronic alcohol consumption, loss of income, transportation limitations, and housing restrictions are factors in lifestyle patterns that can alter the ease and enjoyment associated with the preparation and consumption of food.[21]

INTERNATIONAL NUTRITIONAL CONCERNS

Whereas nutrition-related concerns in this country are centered on overnutrition, including fat density and excessive caloric intake, the main concern in many areas of the world is the limited quantity and quality of food. Reasons for these problems are numerous, including diverse factors such as the limitations imposed by weather, the availability of arable land, religious practices, political unrest, war, social infrastructure, and material and technology shortages. Underlying virtually all of these, however, is unabated population growth.

In an attempt to increase the availability of food to countries whose demand for food outweighs their ability to produce it, a number of steps have been suggested. Included among these are:

▼ Increasing the yield of land currently under cultivation
▼ Increasing the amount of land under cultivation
▼ Increasing animal production on land not suitable for cultivation
▼ Using water (seas, lakes, and ponds) more efficiently for the production of food
▼ Developing unconventional foods through the application of technology
▼ Improving nutritional practices through education

Little progress is being made despite impressive technological breakthroughs related to agriculture and food technology (such as "miracle" rice, disease-resistant high-yield corn, and soybean-enhanced infant

folacin (**foe** la sin) folic acid; a vitamin of the B-complex group; used in the treatment of nutritional anemia.

macrocytic anemia (mac roe **sittick** uh **knee** mee a) form of anemia in which large red blood cells predominate, but in which total red blood cell count is depressed.

empty Calories Calories obtained from foods that lack most other important nutrients.

foods), the efforts of governmental programs, and the support of the Food and Agricultural Organization of the United Nations and the United States Department of Agriculture. Particularly in Third World countries in which fertility rates are two to four times higher than those of the United States, annual food produc-

Health ACTION Guide

Remember These Important Points

▼ Reach and maintain a reasonable weight
▼ Increase daily activity
▼ Moderate food serving sizes
▼ Avoid skipping meals

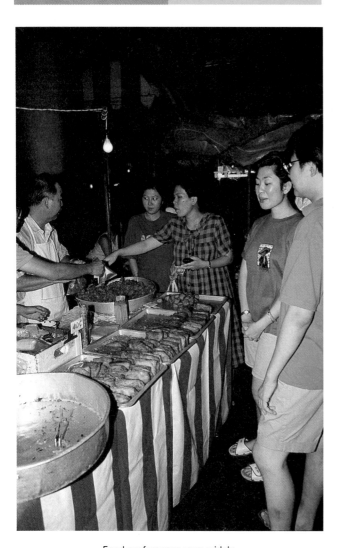

Food preferences vary widely.

★ A Comparison of Dietary Practices

Dietary practices differ among various areas of the world. This simple concept is clearly demonstrated when comparing dietary patterns seen in China with those of the West. These differing patterns then influence the prevalence of health problems. Notice in the data presented below that the average cholesterol difference could be explained on the basis of dietary practices. It is likely that the limited consumption of meat and the heavy consumption of vegetables gives China an advantage in "heart health."

Dietary intake	China	West
Total protein	64.1 g	91.0 g
Plant protein	60.0 g	27.0 g
Complex carbohydrates	371.0 g	120.0 g
Fat as a percent of total Calories	14.5%	38.8%
Cholesterol	127 ml/100 ml	212 ml/100 ml

tion would have to increase from 2.7% to 3.9% to alleviate the problems. If population growth and food production are not altered in these countries, unmet needs will continue to be common.

FOOD TECHNOLOGY

For most of this century the food supply of this country and the world has been improved through advances in agricultural practices, including selective breeding leading to the development of disease-resistant plants and more productive animals. Today, however, genetic engineering is on the threshold of creating plants and animals with properties never before possible. For example, gene-alteration of food could result in new vegetables, grains, and fruits such as the following:

▼ Tomatoes with Antarctic flounder genes that reduce freeze damage.
▼ Tomatoes with bacteria genes to keep them from ripening too fast.
▼ Tofu with cattle genes that make it taste like beef.
▼ Potatoes with chicken genes that impart a chicken flavor.

Whether gene-alteration can impact the severe malnutrition seen in many areas of the world remains to be seen. Regardless, its development suggests that much might be accomplished through technological advances.

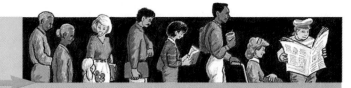

Learning FROM ALL Cultures

A Variety of Diets

Do you eat to live or live to eat? Maybe it depends on what day it is! We do know that to stay healthy we need to eat a variety of good foods.

What we eat reflects our culture. In the United States we have "American" food, such as hamburgers and corn on the cob. Because of the variety of ethnic groups in this country, foods from other cultures are also enjoyed by many. In fact, it would be difficult to identify the staple food of the American diet.

People in other countries often consume those particular foods that are most abundant. Corn, for example, is the main ingredient in food for most Mexicans, and it is eaten in a variety of forms. Beans, or frijoles, are another staple food found in the Mexican diet. There are many varieties of beans, and they are commonly eaten with rice and hot peppers. The Mexican diet is basically a healthy one, but there is not enough food to feed all the people, especially the poorest peasants.[22]

Corn and beans are also popular in Chile and are often included in the average diet. Because the fishing is good along Chile's coast, fish and seafood dishes are commonly served too.[23]

Seafood is also enjoyed by many Canadians. Fishing is an important industry to northern Canadian natives. Some Indian groups have a long history of commercial fishing. Salmon and cod have been caught and sold by the Inuit of Labrador for many years, and fish were sold to the Gold Rush miners by the Yukon Indians. Fisheries run by native Canadians are operational today through government assistance and provide fish to northern and southern parts of the country.[24]

Can you identify food choices in your own diet that are commonly found in other cultures? ●

Summary

✔ Carbohydrates, fat, and protein supply the body with Calories.

✔ The complexity of carbohydrates differs on the basis of their molecular makeup, with sugars being the least and starches the most complex.

✔ Fat plays important roles in nutritional health beyond serving as the body's primary site for the storage of excessive Calories.

✔ Protein supplies the body with amino acids that subsequently provide the body with the material needed to construct its own protein.

✔ Vitamins serve as catalysts for the body and are found in either water-soluble or fat-soluble forms.

✔ Minerals are incorporated into various tissues of the body and also participate in regulatory functions within the body.

✔ Adequate water and fluids are required by the body on a daily basis and are obtained from a variety of food sources including beverages.

✔ Fiber is undigestible plant material and can be found in two forms, water-soluble and water-insoluble.

✔ Six food groups are currently identified, although only five have been given as a recommendation regarding the needed number of daily servings.

✔ Fast foods should play a limited role in daily food intake because of their high fat density, as well as their high levels of sugar and sodium.

✔ Food additives enhance the overall quality of our food supply and the convenience of its use.

✔ New food labels provide considerably more information for the consumer than did labels used previously.

✔ Current dietary recommendations focus on the role of fat, saturated fat, starch, and sodium in health and disease.

✔ Ovolactovegetarianism, lactovegetarianism, vegan vegetarianism, and macrobiotic diets represent different forms of vegetarianism.

✔ A variety of factors contribute to malnourishment in many areas of the world.

✔ As people age, the quality (nutritional density) of their food must improve to offset the age-related tendency to need fewer Calories.

✔ Gene-alteration is a new technology that holds the possibility of making significant alterations in many familiar food sources.

Review Questions

1. Define the term *nutrient*.
2. Identify the six essential nutrients and explain their contributions to the growth, repair, and regulation of the body.
3. What roles does fat play in nutritional health besides serving as the body's primary storage site for excessive Calories?
4. What is the principal role of protein in the body?
5. Which vitamins are water soluble and which are fat soluble? What is our most current perception regarding the need for vitamin supplementation?
6. What roles do minerals play in the body? What is a trace element?
7. What are the two principal forms of fiber, and how do each of them contribute to health?
8. Identify each of the five food groups. What makes up the additional sixth food group?
9. Explain the nutritional benefit of each food group and the recommended daily adult serving minimums.
10. Define a *vegetarian diet*. Explain the difference between an ovolactovegetarian, lactovegetarian, and a vegan vegetarian diet. Which one poses more potential nutritional problems? In what ways?
11. What are the current dietary recommendations regarding fat, saturated fat, starches, and sodium intake?
12. Identify some general modifications recommended in the diets of young adults and the reasoning behind each.
13. What is nutritional density, and how does it relate to the aging process?

Think about This . . .

✔ Is it more economical to buy a generic brand of cereal and take a generic multivitamin than to buy a highly supplemented, but more expensive, brand name of cereal?

✔ What nutrients are missing from your diet?

✔ Do your possible roles in parenting, employment, and home management compromise your ability to eat healthfully?

✔ Analyze your diet in terms of the recommendations made by *Nutrition and Your Health: Dietary Guidelines for Americans*.

✔ Consider your own dietary practices, as well as those of your friends. Are sound nutritional guidelines being followed?

✔ Would you say that you live to eat or eat to live?

✔ What are the most immediate changes that need to be made in your diet?

REAL LIFE REAL CHOICES

YOUR TURN

▼ What is serum cholesterol? How can Vincent Martinelli modify his diet to lower his serum cholesterol level while still enjoying some tasty Italian specialties?

▼ What are some dietary sources of sodium? How can Angela Martinelli reduce her sodium intake?

▼ Can you design a nutritious, healthy meal featuring a popular Italian specialty like pizza or pasta?

AND NOW, YOUR CHOICES . . .

▼ What are your favorite specialty or ethnic foods? Do you consider them healthy or unhealthy? Why?

▼ How do you think your eating habits would change if you worked in a deli, bakery, or ice cream shop?

References

1. Guthrie H: *Introductory nutrition,* ed 7, St Louis, 1989, Mosby.
2. Wardlaw G, Insel P, Seyler M: *Contemporary nutrition: issues and insights,* St Louis, 1994, Mosby.
3. Dremon D, et al: The effects of polyunsaturated fat vs. monounsaturated fat on plasma lipoproteins, *JAMA* 263:2462-2466, 1990.
4. Cooking oils: into the frying pan, *Harvard Medical School Health Letter* 13(1):4-5, 1987.
5. Elliott S: Food firms reduce fats in products, *USA Today* 1D, Jan 17, 1989.
6. United States Department of Health and Human Services: *The Surgeon General's report on nutrition and health,* DHHS Publ. No. 88-50210. Washington, DC; 1988, US Government Printing Office.
7. Addis P: Coronary heart disease: an update with emphasis on dietary lipid oxidation products, *Food & Nutrition News* 62(2):7-14, 1990.
8. Wardlaw G, Insel P: *Perspectives in nutrition,* St Louis, 1993, Mosby.
9. Rimm EB, et al: Vitamin E consumption and the risk of coronary heart disease in men, *New Eng J Med* 328(20)1450-1456, 1993.
10. Leary WE: Vitamins cut cancer in China study, *The New York Times,* Sept 15, 1993.
11. Czeizel AE, Dudas I: Prevention of the first occurrence of neural-tube defects by periconceptional vitamin supplementation. *New Eng J Med* 327(26):1832-1835, 1992.
12. Food and Nutrition Board, Commission on Life Science, National Research Council: *Diet and health: implications for reducing chronic disease risk/Committee on Diet and Health,* Washington, DC, 1989, National Academy Press.
13. Food labeling: Health claims and label statements: antioxidant vitamins and cancer, *Federal Register* 58(3):2622-2660. United States Government Printing office, Washington, DC, January 6, 1993.
14. Neiman DC, Butterworth DE, Nieman CN: *Nutrition,* Dubuque, Iowa, 1990, William C Brown.
15. Fiber: essential to a healthy diet, *Worldview* 3((3):1-5, 1991.
16. Ripsin CM, et al: Oat products and lipid lowering: a metaanalysis, *JAMA* 267(24):3317-3325, 1992.
17. American Cancer Society: *Cancer facts and figures—1992,* Atlanta, 1992, The Association.
18. Hellmich N: Fast-food fries under fire again for unhealthy fat, *USA Today,* October 21, 1993, p 1A.
19. Office of the Federal Register National Archives and Research Administration, *Code of federal regulations: food and drugs,* 21 (Parts 170 to 199):417-420, April 1, 1991.
20. US Department of Agriculture and US Department of Health and Human Services, *Nutrition and your health: dietary guidelines for Americans,* ed 3, Home Garden Bulletin no 232, Washington, DC, 1990, US Government Printing Office.
21. Williams SR, Worthington-Roberts B: *Nutrition throughout the life cycle,* St Louis, 1992, Mosby.
22. Rummel J: *Mexico,* New York, 1990, Chelsea House.
23. Galvin IF: *Chile: land of poets and patriots,* Minneapolis, 1990, Dillon Press.
24. Crowe K: *A history of the original peoples of northern Canada,* Montreal, 1991, McGill-Queen.

Suggested Readings

Carper J: *The food pharmacy guide to good eating,* New York, 1991, Bantam Books.

Recommendations for health and a longer life through healthful eating are central to this book. The author provides 22 guidelines that should all be followed in selecting and preparing food, as well as recipes for low-fat, low-cholesterol and low-sodium meals. Disease prevention and health promotion are stressed.

Connor SJ, Connor WE: *The new American diet system,* New York, 1991, Simon & Schuster.

A book of tested recipes intended to move Americans in the direction of lowered fat (low saturated fat) diets. Some recipes are new, while others are modifications of recipes known to most Americans.

Shaevitz MH: *Lean & mean: the no hassle, life-extending weight loss program for men,* New York, 1993, GP Putnam's Sons.

An excellent resource for anyone trying to lose weight or, more importantly, maintain a high level of health. Stresses high complex-carbohydrates, low-fat, limited alcohol consumption, and regular aerobic activity. Provides "how-to" information for food consumption away from home.

6

Healthy Weight

Sensible Eating and Regular Exercise

You are probably aware that many people in our society think *obesity* is a serious health concern. Physicians counsel their patients about the need to maintain a desirable weight. People from virtually all backgrounds diet, participate in weight control programs, or engage in physical activity to lose weight, gain weight, or maintain their present weight. Yet most people are above their desirable weight, and a significant number of adults (25% to 50%) are classified as obese.[1] In a society that has an abundance of high-quality food and a vast array of labor-saving devices, *overweight* is almost the rule rather than the exception.

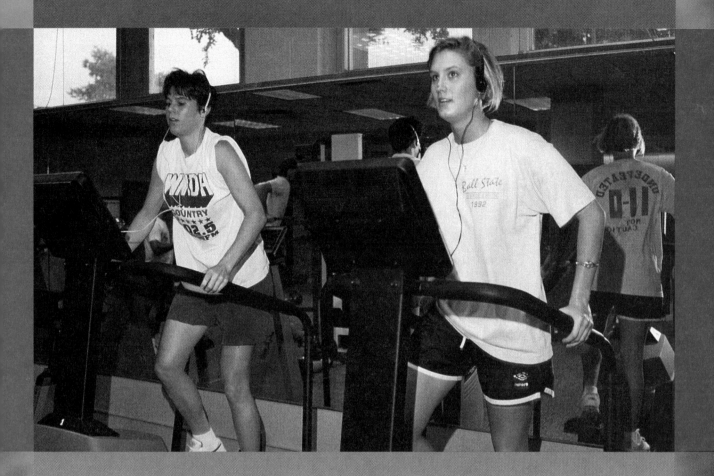

WEIGHT MANAGEMENT

The following objectives are covered in this chapter:

▽ Reduce overweight to a prevalence of no more than 20% among people aged 20 and older and no more than 15% among adolescents aged 12 through 19. (Baseline: 26% for people aged 20 through 74 in 1976-80, 24% for men and 27% for women; 15% for adolescents aged 12 through 19 in 1976-80; p. 96.)

▽ Increase to at least 50% the proportion of overweight people aged 12 and older who have adopted sound dietary practices combined with regular physical activity to attain an appropriate body weight. (Baseline: 30% of overweight women and 25% of overweight men for people aged 18 and older in 1985; p. 100.)

▽ Increase to at least 90% the proportion of restaurants and institutional food-service operations that offer identifiable low-fat, low-calorie food choices, consistent with the "Dietary Guidelines for Americans." (Baseline: About 70% of fast-food and family restaurant chains with 350 or more units had at least one low-fat, low-calorie item on their menu in 1989, p. 125.)

▽ Increase to at least 50% the proportion of worksites with 50 or more employees that offer nutrition education or weight-management programs for employees. (Baseline: 17% offered nutrition education activities and 15% offered weight-control activities in 1985; p. 128.)

HEALTHY PEOPLE 2000 OBJECTIVES

▼ Name: Kate Donnelly
▼ Age: 28
▼ Occupation: Newspaper reporter
▼ Physical characteristics: 5'4", 147 lb.

Yo-yos can be fun to play with—but when you feel like *you're* the one at the end of the string, it stops being a game.

That's how Kate Donnelly has felt most of her life. The fourth in a boisterous family of nine children, Kate realized in grade school that she wasn't slender and small boned like her mother and older sisters, but stocky and sturdy like the women on her father's side of the family, who tended to gain weight easily. She wasn't really fat, and she wasn't a junk-food junkie, but she definitely wasn't slim. She was wearing "miss" size clothes when she was 12— the ultra-slender styles of the junior department were not for her.

Kate's close, warm family didn't pressure her to lose weight or shape up. She pressured herself—by constantly comparing herself to friends, classmates, and her sisters; by devouring teen magazines that showed ultrathin types wearing body-hugging leg-

gings, leotards, and minis that looked like doll clothes; and by blaming herself for being lazy and self-indulgent.

Starting in junior high, Kate tried every fad diet she could find. She fasted; she even sent away for some "miracle fat-burning" pills she saw advertised in the back of a magazine. Every time, the results were the same: she lost weight—sometimes a substantial amount—and then she quit the diet and regained what she'd lost, sometimes even more.

Now a successful newspaper reporter, Kate's still on the yo-yo. And it still doesn't work. She often feels tired, depressed, unmotivated—and sometimes angry because her efforts to lose weight are never more than temporarily successful. She avoids exercise because she "knows" she'd look terrible in bright, form-fitting bodywear.

As you study this chapter, think about some steps Kate can take to improve her situation from both a psychological and physical standpoint, and prepare yourself to answer the questions in **Your Turn** at the end of the chapter. ▼

CONCERN OVER BODY IMAGE

When the body is supplied with more energy than it can expend, a predictable response is seen—the storage of excess energy in the form of body fat. This progressive accumulation of **adipose tissue** can eventually result in obesity.

Most people, including some professionals, believe that any weight above desirable is clearly associated with serious health problems. However, the current consensus is that being mildly to moderately overweight may not be as closely associated with serious health problems as once thought. There is, however, little question that severe or morbid obesity is closely associated with several serious health problems.

Among the health problems caused by or complicated by excess body fat (obesity) are increased surgical risk, hypertension, various forms of heart disease, type II diabetes mellitus, several forms of cancer, deterioration of joints, complications during pregnancy, gallbladder disease, and an overall increased risk of mortality. Table 6-1 provides additional information about the contribution of obesity to these conditions. Among the health dangers associated with more extensive obesity are high blood pressure, stroke, heart disease, gallstones, diabetes mellitus, and overall mortality.[2]

For our image-conscious population, however, there is little debate about overweight being undesirable. All too often, advertisements tell us that being overweight can make our lives unpleasant, particularly when it interferes with our ability to conform to certain stereotypical body image perceptions (such as being tall and thin with clear muscular definition). Unfortunately, today's lean but muscular version of the "ideal" body is a very demanding standard to meet. In fact, the average actress and model is thinner than 95% of the female population, the average model weighing 23% less than the average woman. Pictures of film and television stars of past decades show that a heavier body with a softer, less muscular appearance was more acceptable than it is now.

There has traditionally been little media attention paid to being **underweight,** yet the **body image** problems experienced by some extremely thin people are equally stressful.

OVERWEIGHT AND OBESITY DEFINED

The most prevalent forms of malnutrition in the more affluent countries of the world are overweight and obesity. Most of us think of malnourishment as a shortage of certain types of essential nutrients. In developing countries, food deprivation forms the basis of mal-

TABLE 6-1 Health Problems Associated With Excess Body Fat

Health problems	Partially attributed to:
Surgical risk	Increased anesthesia needs and greater risk of wound infections
Pulmonary disease	Excess weight over lungs
Adult-onset diabetes mellitus (NIDDM)	Enlarged fat cells, which then poorly bind insulin and also poorly respond to the message insulin sends to the cell
Hypertension	Increased miles of blood vessels found in the fat tissue; however, no validated cause is yet known
Coronary heart disease	Increases in serum cholesterol and triglyceride levels, as well as a decrease in physical activity
Bone and joint disorders	Excess pressure put on knee, ankle, and hip joints
Gallbladder stones	An increase in cholesterol content of bile
Skin disorders	The trapping of moisture and microbes in fat folds
Various cancers	Estrogen production by fat cells; animal studies suggest excess energy intake encourages tumor development
Shorter stature (in some forms of obesity)	An earlier onset of puberty
Pregnancy risk	More difficult delivery and increased anesthesia needs (if used)
Early death	A variety of risk factors for diseases listed above

The greater the degree of obesity, the more likely and the more serious these health problems generally become. They are much more likely to appear in people who are greater than twice their desirable body weight.

nutrition. However, malnutrition can also be a disease of plenty. Because our food supply exceeds the needs of our population, we are able to eat more than is required for healthful living. We consume more Calories than we expend. We become overweight and may become obese.

How can we tell the difference between overweight and obesity? Nutritionists have traditionally said that obesity is apparent when fat accumulation produces a body weight that is more than 20% above an ideal or **desirable weight.** People are said to be overweight if their weight is between 1% and 19% above their desirable weight. The more people increase their weight above their desirable weight the more likely they are to be labeled obese.

The term *obesity* requires further delineation. When persons are between 20% and 40% above desirable weight, their obesity is described as *mild* (about 90% of all obese people), whereas excessive weight in the 41% to 99% above desirable range is defined as *moderate obesity* (9%) and weight of 100% or more above desirable is defined as *severe* or *morbid* obesity (< 1%).

Being most familiar with the weight guidelines used in the past, most clinicians and the general public continue to use standard height/weight tables to determine the extent to which scale weight exceeds desirable weight and, thus, the existence of mild, moderate, or severe obesity. However, other more precise techniques are now available that can be used to determine body composition. In the next section of this chapter, several of those techniques, including waist/hip ratio *(healthy body weight)*, body mass index, hydrostatic weighing, skin fold measurements, and electrical impedance are described.

How prevalent is obesity? Recent estimates indicate that about 34% of the adult population is moderately overweight to obese.[3] This high percentage may surprise you, because among college students, most are not this heavy. Most obesity is seen in the older age groups, and more than 50% of these people may be overweight if not actually obese. Obesity, although perhaps genetically and behaviorally determined early in life, often takes many years to develop fully. A daily caloric surplus of only 10 Calories yields 10 unwanted pounds of fat in 10 years; 20 or 30 years of con-

obesity (oh **bee** sit ee) condition in which a person's excess fat accumulation results in a body weight that exceeds desirable weight by 20% or more.

overweight condition in which a person's excess fat accumulation results in a body weight that exceeds desirable weight by 1% to 19%.

adipose tissue (**add** ih pose) tissue comprised of fibrous strands around which specialized cells designed to store liquified fat are ordered.

underweight condition in which body weight is below desirable weight.

body image our subjective perception of how our body appears.

desirable weight weight range deemed appropriate for persons of a specific sex, age, and frame size.

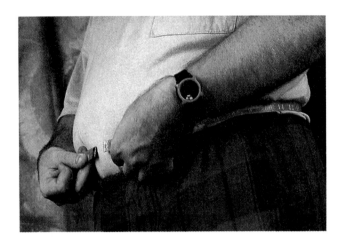

A daily surplus of 10 Calories yields 10 unwanted pounds in 10 years.

sistent excess food intake or gradually declining activity can easily result in obesity.

As you read in Chapter 5, some foods are considered very healthful—lean meats, fresh fruits and vegetables, and low-fat dairy products, for example. However, the overconsumption of even high-quality foods will contribute to a **positive caloric balance.** The key to sustaining a specific weight (as you will soon read) is to maintain a balance between energy intake and energy expenditure. The key to taking weight off and keeping it off is exercise and dietary control; in other words, eat healthfully and exercise on a regular basis.

DETERMINING WEIGHT AND BODY COMPOSITION

Height/Weight Tables

The familiar "1983 Metropolitan Life Insurance Height and Weight Table" can be the basis for determining whether one's scale weight is below, at, or above desirable for his or her gender, height, and frame size (see Table 6-2). Many clinicians and the majority of the public turn to this table (or 1985 versions issued by the federal government) to assess body weight. However, the use of these tables is no longer considered the best way to determine if body weight is acceptable, mainly because they use only scale weight in their assessment. Important factors such as waist measurement, body composition, and age are not included, and thus these tables are being gradually replaced by other assessment techniques. The concept of healthy body weight is, in fact, becoming the standard around which more and more clinicians are determining the possible health-related consequences of body weight.

TABLE 6-2   1983 Metropolitan Life Insurance Height and Weight Table

Height	Small frame	Medium frame	Large frame
Men*			
5'2"	128-134	131-141	138-150
5'3"	130-136	133-143	140-153
5'4"	132-138	135-145	142-156
5'5"	134-140	137-148	144-160
5'6"	136-142	139-151	146-164
5'7"	138-145	142-154	149-168
5'8"	140-148	145-157	152-172
5'9"	142-151	148-160	155-176
5'10"	144-154	151-163	158-180
5'11"	146-157	154-166	161-184
6'0"	149-160	157-170	164-188
6'1"	152-164	160-174	168-192
6'2"	155-168	164-178	172-197
6'3"	158-172	167-182	176-202
6'4"	162-176	171-187	181-207
Women†			
4'10"	102-111	109-121	118-131
4'11"	103-113	111-123	120-134
5'0"	104-115	113-126	122-137
5'1"	106-118	115-129	125-140
5'2"	108-121	118-132	128-143
5'3"	111-124	121-135	131-147
5'4"	114-127	124-138	134-151
5'5"	117-130	127-141	137-155
5'6"	120-133	130-144	140-159
5'7"	123-136	133-147	143-163
5'8"	126-139	136-150	146-167
5'9"	129-142	139-153	149-170
5'10"	132-145	142-156	152-173
5'11"	135-148	145-159	155-176
6'0"	138-151	148-162	158-179

*Weights at ages 25 to 59, based on lowest mortality. Weight in pounds according to frame (in indoor clothing weighing 5 lb, shoes with 1" heels).
†Weights at ages 25 to 59, based on lowest mortality. Weight in pounds according to frame (in indoor clothing weighing 3 lb, shoes with 1" heels).

Healthy Body Weight

How can a *healthy body weight* be determined? Today, this process is most appropriately undertaken by using the weight guidelines that are contained in the newly issued Dietary Guidelines for Americans.[4] This assessment involves the conversion of two body measurements, the abdominal circumference and the hip circumference, into a ratio that can then be applied to weight ranges for people of particular ages and heights. Female "healthy weight" is near the lower end of each weight range, whereas male "healthy

TABLE 6-3 Healthy Weight: Recommended Weight Guidelines

Height without shoes	Weight without clothes	
	19-34 years	35 years and over
5'	97-128	108-138
5'1"	101-132	111-143
5'2"	104-137	115-148
5'3"	107-141	119-152
5'4"	111-146	122-157
5'5"	114-150	126-162
5'6"	118-155	130-167
5'7"	121-160	134-172
5'8"	125-164	138-178
5'9"	129-169	142-183
5'10"	132-174	146-188
5'11"	136-179	151-194
6'	140-184	155-199
6'1"	144-189	159-205
6'2"	148-195	164-210
6'3"	152-200	168-216
6'4"	156-205	173-222
6'5"	160-211	177-228
6'6"	164-216	182-234

weight" is at the higher end of each weight range. (See Table 6-3.)

To use these newly established weight ranges, the following procedure must be performed:

▼ Measure around your waist near your navel while you stand relaxed, not pulling in your stomach.
▼ Measure around your hips, over the buttocks where hips are the largest.
▼ Divide the waist measure by the hip measure. A 25-inch waist and 36-inch hips equal .69, which is well within the healthful range. The ratio should be less than .80 for women and less than .90 for men.

Women with a *waist-to-hip ratio (WHR)* of less than .80 are generally found to have a body weight that falls within the range appropriate for their age and height; men with a WHR of less than .90 will also probably fall within the range that is appropriate for their age and height. It is recommended that persons with a waist-to-hip ratio at or above 1.00 should attempt to lose weight. When weight loss is attempted, according to these guidelines, it should occur no faster than $\frac{1}{2}$ to 1 pound per week.

The stimulus for the development of this assessment procedure is the growing concern over the relationship between the amount of fat in the central abdominal cavity *(upper body obesity)* and the develop-

ment of several serious health problems. In addition to an unacceptably high waist-to-hip ratio, a protruding stomach and/or high blood pressure indicate a need to lose weight. Certainly people who exhibit all three of these signs are most in need of weight loss. Interestingly, this "spare tire" pattern of fat distribution is most frequently seen in men and is most likely influenced by the action of *testosterone*, the male sex hormone.

In comparison to the upper body distribution seen in men, women more often demonstrate an excessive accumulation of fat in the hips and upper legs. This *lower body obesity* is less closely associated with chronic health problems such as cardiovascular disease and diabetes mellitus (Type II). However, few people would describe this "pear-shaped" appearance as being in line with today's perception of body image.

Perhaps the most important contribution made by the Dietary Guidelines for Americans assessment procedure is its allowance for increasing age as a factor that influences body weight. For persons older than 35 years of age, some of the "demand" to maintain a youthful appearance (including lower weight) has been lifted.

BODY MASS INDEX

A second important and relatively new procedure for assessing healthy body weight is the use of the **body mass index (BMI)** or Queteletindex (QI). The body mass index is an expression of the relationship of body weight (expressed in kilograms) to height (expressed in meters) for both men and women.[5] The BMI does not calculate body composition (fat versus lean tissue) or consider the degree of fat accumulated within the central body cavity, nor is it adjusted for age. It is, nevertheless, widely used in determining obesity. A BMI greater than 27.8 for men and 27.3 for women reflects a state of obesity. Figure 6-1 shows how to calculate body mass index.

An alternative method of determining the BMI is to employ a **nomogram** such as that in Figure 6-2. Like the formula for calculating the BMI, the nomogram requires information pertaining to both weight and height.

positive caloric balance caloric intake greater than caloric expenditure.

body mass index (BMI) numerical expression of body weight based on height and weight.

nomogram (no ma gram) graphic means for finding an unknown value.

Calculating BMI

To determine your body mass index (BMI):
1. Divide your weight in pounds by 2.2 to convert it to kilograms.

$$A = weight (kg) = your\ weight\ (lb) \div 2.2$$

2. Multiply your height in inches by 2.54 and divide by 100 to convert height to meters.

$$B = height\ (m) = your\ height\ (inches) \times 2.54 \div 100$$

3. Muliply B by B to get your height (in meters) squared.

$$C = height\ (m) \times height\ (m)$$

4. Divide A by C to determine BMI.

$$BMI = weight\ (kg) \div height^2\ (m)$$

EXAMPLE: 176-lb person, 72 inches (6 feet) tall

1. $A = 176 \div 2.2 = 80$

2. $B = \dfrac{72 \times 2.54}{100} = \dfrac{182.88}{100} = 1.83$

3. $C = 1.83 \times 1.83 = 3.35$

4. $BMI = \dfrac{80}{3.35} = 23.88$

Figure 6-1 Calculating body mass index.

TABLE 6-4   Desirable Body Mass Index in Relation to Age

Age-group (years)	BMI (kg/m²)
19-24	19-24
25-34	20-25
35-44	21-26
45-54	22-27
55-65	23-28
>65	24-29

Once the BMI has been obtained, its relationship to desirable body mass indexes can be determined using Table 6-4.

ELECTRICAL IMPEDANCE

Electrical impedance is a newly developed method to test for body composition. This method, which uses fairly expensive equipment and computer software, measures electrical resistance as small currents of electricity are directed through human tissue. Electrodes are attached to the arm and leg. Because fat tissue resists the passage of electrical current much more than muscle tissue does, a electrical impedance can accurately calculate the percentage of body fat. Fortunately, electrical impedance measurements are painless. Additional techniques including *computerized axial tomography (CAT) scans, magnetic resonance imaging (MRI), infrared light transmission* and *neutron activation* may become common ways to measure body composition in the future.[5]

SKINFOLD MEASUREMENTS

Skinfold measurements provide a relatively precise indicator of body fat percentage. Skinfold measurements rely on constant-pressure **calipers** to measure the thickness of the layer of fat beneath the skin's surface. This layer is called subcutaneous fat. Skinfold measurements of subcutaneous fat are taken at several key places on the body (see Figure 6-3). Measurements of skinfold thickness can then be used to establish the percentage of body fat.

Young adult men normally have a body fat percentage of between 10% and 15%. The normal range for young adult women is 20% to 25%.[6] When a man's body fat percentage exceeds 25% and a woman's body fat percentage exceeds 30%, they are classified as obese. The relatively higher percentage of fat found in women is related to the female biological role of childbearer and **lactator.**

Once the percentage of body fat has been calculated, a relatively simple conversion can be made to determine desired body weight. Figure 6-4 will allow you to assess your own body composition.

HYDROSTATIC WEIGHING

Hydrostatic, or underwater, **weighing** is a precise method that determines the relative amounts of fat and lean body mass that make up body weight. A person's percentage of body fat is determined by comparing the underwater body weight with the body weight out of the water. Expensive equipment and trained technicians make the use of this method impractical for the average person.

BODY IMAGE

Despite the numerous ways in which obesity can be determined, the simplest method may be to look at yourself in the mirror. The old saying, "Mirrors don't lie," speaks for itself. For many large people, this method is fairly accurate and certainly inexpensive. Unless a person is very muscular or has retained an excessive amount of water, the reflection in the mirror should be a good indicator of weight. Although this simple method does not allow a person to pinpoint a body fat percentage, the person should be able to visually determine whether he or she is obese.

However, for many heavy people, it can be difficult to be objective. They may not accurately judge their bodies and may perceive themselves as obese. Their imagined *body image* and their actual appearance are markedly different. The ability to accurately perceive one's own appearance (body image) is particularly difficult for persons with anorexia nervosa (see page 150).

For many people, it is important to appear a certain way. This desired body image may or may not be compatible with their inherited body type or their ability to gain or lose weight. Nevertheless, they try to achieve the "look" that they have in mind.

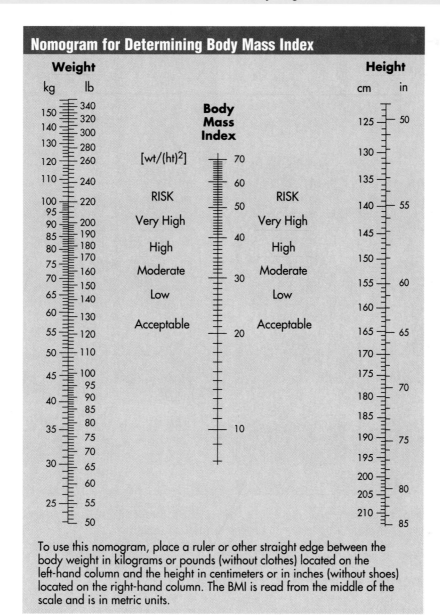

Nomogram for Determining Body Mass Index

Weight

kg   lb

Body Mass Index

$[wt/(ht)^2]$

RISK

Very High

High

Moderate

Low

Acceptable

Height

cm   in

RISK

Very High

High

Moderate

Low

Acceptable

To use this nomogram, place a ruler or other straight edge between the body weight in kilograms or pounds (without clothes) located on the left-hand column and the height in centimeters or in inches (without shoes) located on the right-hand column. The BMI is read from the middle of the scale and is in metric units.

Figure 6-2

In the body image that appears popular for today's women, hips, waist, and shoulders line-up in a manner to suggest a vertical line. The traditional emphasis on an "hour glass" figure, with a small waist and large chest, has given way to a more angular, athletic appearance, somewhat similar to the body build of many young men. As is true for women, the scale weight, WHR, and body composition of many men do not align with the body they wish to possess.

Whether the body image desired is reasonably obtained seems unimportant to many people. For some, hours may be spent each week in weight rooms, and food intake will be reduced or increased dramatically in a quest for the desired body image. For those who are ultimately unsuccessful, disappointment and frustration can result.

electrical impedance (im **peed** ence) method to test for the percentage of body fat using harmless electrical current.

skinfold measurement measurement to determine the thickness of the fat layer that lies immediately beneath the skin.

calipers (**kal** ip ers) device to measure the thickness of a skinfold from which percent body fat can be calculated.

lactator (**lack** tate or) woman who is producing breast milk.

hydrostatic weighing (hi dro **stat** ick) weighing the body while it is submerged in water.

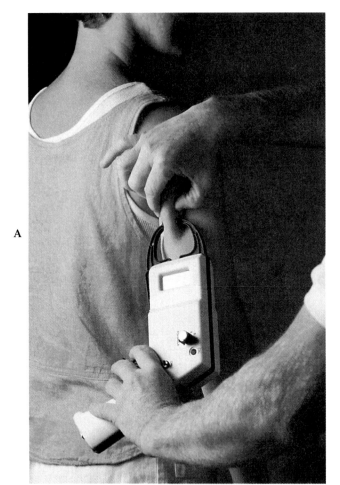
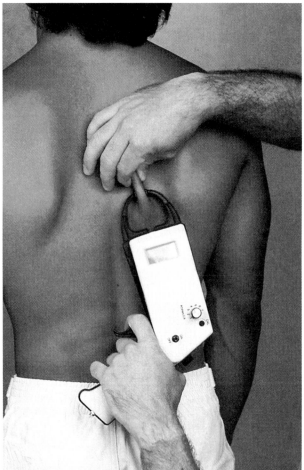

Figure 6-3 Body fat determination using skinfold calipers. Skinfold measurements are used in equations that calculate body density and the percentage of body fat. **A,** Triceps. **B,** Subscapular.

ORIGINS OF OBESITY

Experts continue to question the origins of obesity. As might be expected, the numerous theories focus on factors within the individual, as well as from the environment. If a definitive cause is ever identified, it will be comprised of an interplay of genetic, metabolic, psychological, and environmental factors. However, until such a discovery, it is safe to assume that obesity is a complex condition whose cause involves a variety of factors. No two obese persons will have gained their excessive weight in exactly the same manner or for the same reasons.

Genetic Basis for Obesity

Based on studies involving both identical and fraternal (nonidentical) twins, raised together and separately, it has been demonstrated that both environment and genetics influence obesity. In some cases the role of inherited tendencies toward excessive weight appears to be almost solely responsible for the amount and distribution of body fat. For example the "apple" shape associated with fat storage in males and the "pear" shape seen in females is strongly influenced by genetic factors.[7] In terms of other similarities or differences in body fat disposition, the role of genetics is clearly limited. At the present scientists are uncertain whether a gene or genes on a single chromosome or genes on multiple chromosomes are responsible for the genetic contribution to obesity, or why this may be a more powerful force for some than for others.

Appetite Center

Building on the neurophysiological basis of obesity proposed by Mayer,[8] a center for the control of eating was postulated and subsequently identified within the central nervous system. This appetite center is found within the brain's hypothalamus and is responsible for the regulation of both hunger and satiety. Although the exact mechanisms by which the appetite center operates are not fully understood, this center is thought to continuously monitor the body's stores of glucose, amino acids, and free fatty acids, and stimulates

Calculating Percentage of Body Fat and Desirable Body Weight

The triceps skinfold is measured over the right arm triceps muscle (back of the upper arm) halfway between the elbow and the tip of the shoulder (see Figure 6-3, *A*).

1. Instruct the subject to let the arm hang limply at the side.
   Grasp the skinfold parallel to the vertical axis of the arm.
   Lift the skinfold away from the arm and be sure that no muscle tissue is caught in the fold.
2. Place the contact surfaces of the calipers ½ inch (12 mm) below the fingers. Release the lever arm on the caliper and allow pressure from the instrument to bring the two sides together. The caliper pointer then indicates the skinfold thickness in millimeters (mm). Repeat and record the measurement two or three times; then record the average of these measurements.

The subscapular (below the shoulder blade) measurement site is approximately ½ inch below the inferior angle of the scapula in line with the natural cleavage lines of the skin (see Figure 6-3, *B*).

1. Have the subject stand erect with shoulders thrust backward and arms at the sides. The point of the scapula (shoulder blade) located toward the spine should be obvious. Mark this point and then measure ½ inch below it and place a mark that will be the measurement site.
2. Standing behind the subject, use the thumb and index fingers and grasp the skinfold in the natural cleavage line (along an imaginary line from the elbow to the neck). Lift the skinfold away from the scapula and shake it to be sure no muscle tissue is caught in the fold.
3. Use the caliper to measure as described previously.

With the measurements for the triceps and the subscapular skinfolds, percentage of body fat can be easily calculated using the following equations:

Women: Percent body fat = 0.55 (A) + 0.31(B) + 6.13
Where A = triceps skinfold (mm)
B = subscapular skinfold (mm)
Men: Percent body fat = 0.43(A) + 0.58(B) + 1.47
Where A = triceps skinfold (mm)
B = subscapular skinfold (mm)

Once the percentage of body fat has been calculated, it becomes relatively simple to determine a desired body weight.

To calculate desirable body weight, fill in the blanks below:
1. Present weight _____ lb
2. Present percentage body fat (as determined in previous activity) _____ %
3. Desired body fat _____ %
4. Percent body fat to be lost _____ % (no. 2 − no. 3)
5. Pounds to be lost _____ lb (no. 4 × no. 1)
6. Desired weight _____ lb (no. 1 × no. 5)

Calculated desirable weight will often need to be increased by 3 to 5 pounds if either of the following situations is present: (1) The person has been sedentary or is involved in training to build muscle mass (therefore an allowance must be made for an increase in muscle mass) or (2) the person is growing.

Figure 6-4 Assess your body composition.

hunger (desire to eat) and satiety (desire to stop eating) accordingly.[9]

In people predisposed to obesity, it is possible that the monitoring of body stores is less sensitive than that found in those who are better able to maintain weight within desirable limits. Further, some believe that dieting alters our ability to accurately gauge satiety. Thus, once dieting has stopped, a newly decreased awareness of satiety allows us to overeat and begin gaining weight back.

Set Point Theory

Current theories suggest that the appetite center possesses a genetically programmed **set point.**[10] According to the set point theory, the body knows when it is near its "best" weight. Attempts to lower weight below the set point are met with physiological resistance.

In fact, heavy people trying to lose weight often report that their efforts are virtually fruitless after they reach a certain weight. Perhaps it is impossible to achieve a weight level that is below the level your body was physiologically designed to carry, unless, of course, caloric intake is restricted to starvation levels.

Because the body appears to resist the wholesale loss of weight, an adjustment in basal metabolism rate (BMR) (see p. 139) has been suggested as a possible reason for a weight plateau. Starvation or dieting results in a lowering of the energy needs of the body,

> **set point** genetically programmed range of body weights beyond which a person finds it difficult to gain or lose additional weight.

thus allowing the body to retain fat.[10] This protective adjustment in BMR is referred to as **adaptive thermogenesis.**

Although this starvation response is widely reported, recent research suggests that it might be only a temporary scaling back of the BMR.[11] Particularly for people on a very low–Calorie diet, such as those administered in some hospital-supervised programs, their BMR may move upward again after being depressed during the initial weeks of the program.

Infant and Adult Feeding Patterns

Many **bariatricians** categorize obesity according to the way in which feeding patterns seem to produce it. Two general feeding patterns are related to two forms of obesity: hypercellular and hypertrophic obesity.

The first of these patterns involves infant feeding. It is believed by many that the number of fat cells that a person has will be initially determined during the first 2 years of life. Through the process of *lipogenesis*, babies who are overfed during their early years will develop a greater number of adipose cells than babies who receive a balanced diet of appropriate, infant-sized portions. Overfed babies, especially those with a family history of obesity, will tend to develop **hypercellular obesity.**

When these children grow into adulthood, they will have more adipose cells, which potentially can be filled with excess energy in the form of fat. Many researchers now believe that these fat cells drive the body's metabolic processes in the direction of a positive caloric balance (more than is needed for immediate energy requirements) and a filling of these cells.

Armed with the knowledge that overfeeding can contribute to future obesity, parents of newborns and small children are faced with a potentially troubling problem: how to "fat-proof" a child without crossing the fine line into undernourishment. Physicians consistently recommend a balanced diet, appropriate-sized servings, low-fat milk after the age of 1 year, cereals low in sugar, and regular physical activity. The use of these approaches is a good prescription for sound growth and development and the prevention of hypercellular obesity.

Although the origins of hypercellular obesity are most often associated with infancy, the development of excessive fat cells can begin later in life. The years of late childhood and pubescence are also times during which children are susceptible to developing excessive fat cells. For adults, weight gain leading to a body weight that is 75% or more above the desirable level can also stimulate an increase in fat cell number and thus move them toward hypercellular obesity.

A second type of obesity that has its origins in a different eating pattern is called **hypertrophic obesity.** This form of obesity is related to a long-term, positive caloric balance that often starts shortly after the tradi-

tional undergraduate college years. Over a period of years, established fat cells increase in size—up to 150% of their empty size—to accommodate excess food intake.

Hypertrophic obesity is generally associated with excessive fat around the waist (central body cavity) and is thought to contribute to conditions such as diabetes mellitus (noninsulin dependent diabetes, or type II diabetes), excessive levels of fat in the blood, high blood pressure, and heart disease.[10] In our society, hypertrophic obesity becomes evident during middle age—a time when our physical activity declines but our food intake remains constant.

Externality

Studies have demonstrated that many obese people have highly developed levels of sensitivity to the outside world.[1] They can be said to have a high degree of externality. Thus in comparison with those of nonobese people, the eating behaviors of some obese people may be more controlled by external stimuli such as a clock, a food advertisement or commercial, or the smell of food. These external cues trigger an eating response. Consequently, high levels of externality can make it very difficult for an obese person to adjust to a controlled diet.

Endocrine Influence

For a number of years, people believed that obesity was the result of "glandular" problems. Often the thyroid gland was said to be underactive, thus preventing the person from "burning up" food. Obesity supposedly resulted from a condition over which the individual had no control.

Today it is known that only a few obese people have an endocrine dysfunction of the type that would result in obesity. Clinicians report that no more than 3% to 5% of the obesity they observe is the result of **hypothyroidism.**

Pregnancy

During a normal pregnancy, approximately 75,000 additional Calories are required to support the development of the fetus and the formation of *maternal supportive tissues* and to fuel the elevated maternal metabolism rate. In addition, the woman will develop approximately 9 extra pounds of adipose tissue, which will be used as an energy source during lactation. In total, the typical woman enters childbirth having gained approximately 28 pounds over her pregnancy weight. Early prenatal care should include specific information about both diet and fitness activities for the appropriate weight gain during pregnancy.

Ideally, after the birth of the baby, the mother will display a weight gain of only 2 to 3 pounds over her prepregnancy weight. This small amount of additional weight will normally be lost by the end of the sixth to eighth month after the birth of the baby.[12] Some women experience an overall decrease in weight after pregnancy because of their concerted efforts to improve on their prepregnancy weight status.

In those women who do experience a significant weight gain as the result of having been pregnant, it is likely that their weight gain during pregnancy was excessive. For the majority of women, however, pregnancy and resultant obesity do not have to go hand in hand.

Decreasing Basal Metabolism Rate

The human body's requirement for energy to maintain basic physiological processes decreases progressively with age. This change reflects the loss of muscle tissue with age in both men and women. This loss of muscle mass eventually alters the ratio of lean body tissue to fat. Thus as the proportion of fat increases, the energy needs of the body are more strongly influenced by the lower metabolic needs of fat cells.[13] This excess energy must then be stored in the fat cells of the body.

Although on a short-term basis little adjustment needs to be made to maintain weight, weight gain can be significant over time if adjustments are not made. A gradual decrease in caloric intake or a conscious effort to expend more Calories can be effective in preventing the gradual onset of obesity.

Family Dietary Practices

The family subtly but effectively instructs its children on many topics; information, value stances, and diverse skills are passed from one generation to the next. Food preferences and dietary practices are among the many areas of instruction for which the family assumes responsibility. In some families the lessons are taught as though they were outlined from a nutrition textbook, whereas for others the patterns taught are destined to lead to a life of malnourishment, including obesity. Between-meal snacking, large serving sizes, multiple servings, and high-Calorie meals can lead to obesity. For busy families, the tendency to rely on fat-dense foods, including fast foods and other convenience foods, becomes the basis for excess weight gain.

Not only do family behavioral practices contribute to obesity, but just as important, they can also play a constructive role in the weight loss achieved by obese children. Research suggests that when parents are trained to reinforce their children during the weight-loss programs, the children experience maximal success.

Inactivity

When experts in the field of weight management are asked to identify the single most encompassing reason to explain the prevalence of obesity in today's society, they are almost certain to respond, "Inactivity." People of all ages tend to do less and therefore expend fewer Calories than did their ancestors only a few generations ago. Automation in the workplace, labor-saving devices in the home, the inactivity associated with watching television, and general disdain for sweating are but a few of the changes that account for this inactivity.

As weight gain fostered by inactivity occurs, not only does weight gain occur but the body is also progressively deprived of its most efficient way to reduce fat stores. Thus inactivity is a double-edged sword that promotes the development of a problem, while depriving individuals of a mechanism that would efficiently resolve the problem.

CALORIC BALANCE

As previously mentioned, any Calories consumed beyond those that are used by the body are converted to fat stores. We gain weight when our energy input exceeds our energy output. Conversely, we lose weight when our energy output exceeds our energy input (Figure 6-5). The basic formula is quite simple and can be analogous to a seesaw or lever with a fulcrum at the center-point. Weight remains constant when caloric input and caloric output are identical. In such a situation, our bodies are said to be in *caloric balance*.

Weight Loss

During periods of reasonable physical activity (often in the spring and summer months), we tend to have greater energy expenditures than energy inputs; thus we lose weight. Attempts to lose weight by increasing caloric expenditure through exercise can seem discouraging though when monitoring loss by means of scale weight. The inability to lower scale weight, even with a new commitment to activity, is most likely the result of muscular development fostered by the exercise program. Because muscle tissue weighs more than

adaptive thermogenesis (**thur** mo **gen** a sis) physiological response of the body to adjust its metabolic rate to the presence of food.

bariatrician (barry a **trish** an) physician who specializes in the study and treatment of obesity.

hypercellular obesity (high per **cell** you lar) form of obesity seen in individuals who possess an abnormally large number of fat cells.

hypertrophic obesity (high per **trowe** fick) form of obesity in which fat cells are enlarged, but not excessive in number.

hypothyroidism (high **po** thigh **roid** is um) condition in which the thyroid gland produces an insufficient amount of its hormone, thyroxin.

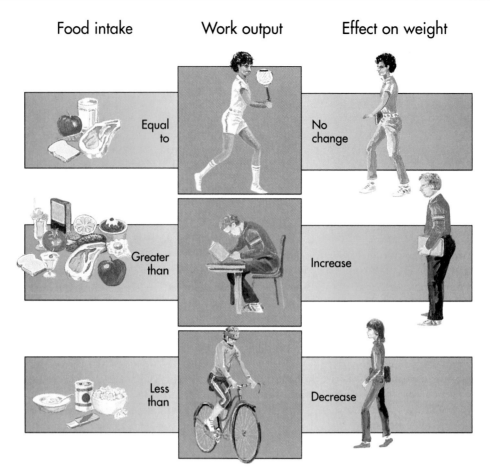

Food intake	Work output	Effect on weight
Equal to		No change
Greater than		Increase
Less than		Decrease

Figure 6-5 Caloric balance: caloric input equals caloric output, some of which comes from physical activity.

fat, scale loss is minimal, even though body composition has changed in direction toward a leaner body. Obviously, weight loss can also occur when we are dieting or not eating because of illness.

Regardless of the mechanisms through which weight loss has occurred, it is now recognized that repeated weight loss followed by weight gain (see yo-yo dieting on p. 149) is associated with health problems, including higher mortality rates.[14]

Weight Gain

Some people want to gain weight: the desire to weigh more to fill out the frame, look better in particular types of clothing, or "bulk-up" for athletic events stimulates some people to gain weight. Weight gain, of course, reflects a positive caloric balance and should be possible by increasing food intake and participating in an exercise program designed to develop muscular strength. We can also unintentionally gain weight when we are less active than usual.

For those whose thinness is pronounced and for whom weight gain has been very difficult, a genetic predisposition to thinness is probably the principal limiting factor. When a person is thin by nature and has an extremely sensitive thermogenesis mechanism, weight gain is difficult (see the Health Action Guide on p. 149 for weight management tips).

ENERGY NEEDS OF THE BODY

What are our energy needs? How many Calories should we consume (or expend) to achieve our ideal weight? There is no one answer for everyone. Although there are some ballpark estimates for college-age men (2500 to 3300 Calories) and women (approximately 2500 Calories), we all vary in our specific energy needs.[15] These needs are based on three factors: (1) the person's activity requirements, (2) the person's basal metabolism, and (3) the thermic effect of food.

Activity Requirements

The caloric *activity requirements* of each individual vary in direct proportion to the amount of daily physical work completed. Sedentary office workers will require a smaller daily caloric intake than will construction workers, lumberjacks, or farm workers. Even within a

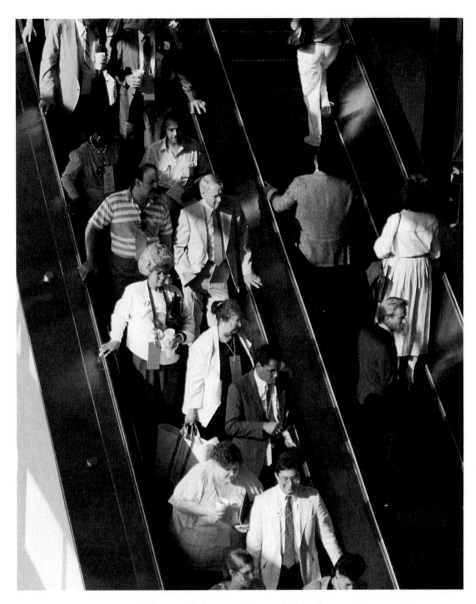

We search for ways to remain inactive.

given general job type, the amount of caloric expenditure will vary according to the physical effort required. A police officer who walks a neighborhood beat will usually expend many more Calories than the typical police dispatcher or equestrian or motorcycle officer.

Physical activity that occurs outside the occupational setting also adds to caloric needs. Sedentary office workers may be quite active in their recreational pursuits. Active employees may spend their off-hours lounging in front of the television. You must closely examine the total amount of work or activity expended by an individual to accurately estimate that person's caloric requirements. Physical activity uses between 20% and 40% of caloric intake. See Table 6-5 for a breakdown of caloric expenditures for various recreational pursuits.

Basal Metabolism

Of the three factors that determine caloric need, the basal metabolism uses the highest proportion (50% to 70%) of the total Calories required by each person. Expressed as a **basal metabolism rate (BMR),** the basal metabolism reflects the minimum amount of energy the body requires to carry on all vital functions. We seldom consciously think of our blood circulation, respiration, glandular and brain activity, cellular me-

> **basal metabolism rate (BMR) (bay** zil) amount of energy (in Calories) the body requires to maintain basic functions.

TABLE 6-5   Calories Expended During Physical Activity

To determine the Calories you have spent in an hour of activity, simply multiply the *Calories per hour per pound* column by your weight (in pounds). For example, after an hour of archery, a 120-pound person will have expended 209 Calories; a 160-pound person, 278 Calories; and a 220-pound person, 383 Calories.

Activity	Calories/hour/pound	Activity	Calories/hour/pound
Archery	1.74	Marching (rapid)	3.84
Basketball	3.78	Painting (outside)	2.10
Baseball	1.86	Playing music (sitting)	1.08
Boxing (sparring)	3.78	Racquetball	3.90
Canoeing (leisure)	1.20	Running (cross-country)	4.44
Climbing hills (no load)	3.30	Running	
Cleaning	1.62	11 min 30 sec per mile	3.66
Cooking	1.20	9 min per mile	5.28
Cycling		8 min per mile	5.64
5.5 mph	1.74	7 min per mile	6.24
9.4 mph	2.70	6 min per mile	6.84
Racing	4.62	5 min 30 sec per mile	7.86
Dance (modern)	2.28	Scrubbing floors	3.00
Eating (sitting)	0.60	Sailing	1.20
Field hockey	3.66	Skiing	
Fishing	1.68	Cross-country	4.43
Football	3.60	Snow, downhill	3.84
Gardening		Water	3.12
Digging	3.42	Skating (moderate)	2.28
Mowing	3.06	Soccer	3.54
Raking	1.44	Squash	5.76
Golf	2.34	Swimming	
Gymnastics	1.80	Backstroke	4.62
Handball	3.78	Breaststroke	4.44
Hiking	2.52	Free, fast	4.26
Horseback riding		Free, slow	3.48
Galloping	3.72	Butterfly	4.68
Trotting	3.00	Table tennis	1.86
Walking	1.14	Tennis	3.00
Ice hockey	5.70	Volleyball	1.32
Jogging	4.15	Walking (normal pace)	2.16
Judo	5.34	Weight training	1.90
Knitting (sewing)	0.60	Wrestling	5.10
Lacrosse	5.70	Writing (sitting)	0.78

tabolism, muscle tone, and body temperature as activities that require large amounts of fuel in the form of Calories, but these functions do require energy. Even when you are totally relaxed or sleeping, these vital body functions continue to expend Calories.

Your basal metabolism is variable. Clearly your BMR changes with age. For both males and females the BMR is relatively high at birth and continues to increase until the age of 2. Except for a slight rise at puberty, your BMR will gradually decline throughout your lifetime. A variety of other variables also affect BMR, including body composition (muscular bodies are associated with higher BMRs), physical condition (fit people have higher BMRs), sex (males have 5% higher BMRs), hormone secretions (people with exces-

sively active thyroid and adrenal glands have higher BMRs), sleep (BMRs are about 10% lower during sleep), pregnancy (a 20% increase in BMR is typical, especially in the last trimester), body temperature (a 1° rise in body temperature increases BMR about 7%), and environmental temperature (deviations above and below 78° F result in increased BMRs).[1,13]

The most important variables related to BMR are aging, body composition, activity level, and caloric intake. For example, you fail to recognize that BMR declines with aging, you might fail to adjust food intake accordingly and weight gain will occur. Also, for those who are thinner, the presence of lean tissue favors a higher basal metabolic rate with greater resistance to weight gain. Finally, an increase in your physical ac-

Calculating BMR

The basal metabolism rate (BMR) reflects the amount of energy in Calories (C) that your body requires to maintain basic functions. The formula below can be used to calculate your approximate basal metabolism rate.

$$\text{BMR per day} = 1C \times \frac{\text{body weight (lb)}}{2.2} \times 24$$

EXAMPLE: 150-lb person

$$\text{BMR per day} = 1C \times \frac{150}{2.2} \times 24$$

$$= 1C \times 68.2 \times 24$$

$$= 1636.8\ C$$

This person would need approximately 1637 Calories to maintain the body at rest for an entire day. Activity of any kind, of course, elevates the requirement for Calories.

NOTE: A woman's BMR would be approximately 5% lower than that of a man of the same age.

Figure 6-6 Calculate your basal metabolism rate (BMR).

tivity will foster a faster BMR that contributes to weight loss. In contrast, in those with above average levels of body fat, BMR rates are lower, thus providing the body with excess Calories that will be stored as fat. If you restrict your caloric intake through dieting, your BMR will drop to a lower level, making weight loss increasingly harder to achieve. Use the formula in Figure 6-6 to determine your BMR and the approximate number of Calories it requires.

Dietary Thermogenesis

Formerly called the specific dynamic effect of food, or *dietary thermogenesis,* the *thermic effect* of food represents the energy our bodies require for the digestion, absorption, and transportation of food. This energy breaks the electrochemical bonds that hold complex food molecules together, resulting in smaller nutrient units that can be distributed throughout the body. This energy need is in addition to activity needs and basal metabolism needs. Estimates are that the thermic effect of food represents about 10% of our total energy needs.[16] Some nutritionists now consider the thermic effect of food merely a component of overall basal metabolism. This lack of distinction is understandable, since the digestive process does represent a vital body function. Thus some professionals categorize total energy needs into just two components—activity needs and basal metabolism needs.

Life-Time Weight Control

Obesity and frequent fluctuation in weight are clearly associated with higher levels of morbidity and mortality. Therefore, it is clear that maintenance of weight and body composition at or near optimum levels is

highly desirable. Although you may believe that this is a difficult goal to achieve, it is not unrealistic when begun early in life and from a starting point at or near optimum levels. You will need to draw upon resources from each dimension of your health to maintain a lifestyle that fosters the maintenance of optimum weight and body compositions. Keys to your success will include:

▼ **Exercise** Caloric expenditure through regular exercise, including cardiovascular exercises and strength training, is a key to maintaining optimum weight and body composition. Dietary approaches alone cannot replace the contributions of regular physical exercise to caloric expenditure and metabolic rate increase.

▼ **Dietary modification** Meals planned around foods low in total fat and saturated fat and high in complex carbohydrates will play a major role in your ability to maintain optimum weight and body composition. Fresh fruits, vegetables, pastas, and, occasionally, lean meat such as skinless chicken and baked fish should be regular food choices.

▼ **Lifestyle support** Not only must you be committed to a lifestyle featuring regular physical activity and careful food choices, but you must build a support group that will encourage you in these endeavors. Inform family, friends, classmates, and co-workers about your intent to rely on them for support and encouragement. Perhaps you will eventually serve as a model for their involvement in a similar process.

▼ **Problem solving** You will certainly need to reevaluate your current approach to dealing with stressors. Replace any reliance on food as a coping mechanism with nonfood options such as exercise or talking with friends or family members. Additionally, your personal reward system may need to be reviewed to decrease the use of food as a reward for work that is well done.

▼ **Redefinition of health** Your ability to think about health in a manner that recognizes the importance of proactivity (see Chapter 2) and involvement, rather than simply not becoming sick or incapacitated, is important.

Assuming you are at an acceptable weight and body composition at this time, the lifestyle choices just suggested will make a significant contribution to the absence of a "weight problem" during your adult years. Aging will, of course, exert its effects to some degree upon your weight and body composition, but the damaging influences of poor dietary practices and a sedentary lifestyle will not be present.

WEIGHT MANAGEMENT TECHNIQUES

For those who are already overweight adults, the need to reduce weight to attain their optimum weight and body composition will require intervention that in

P E R S O N A L   A S S E S S M E N T

Before undertaking a program it is important to look at your past experiences and feelings about weight loss. Perhaps in doing so you might decide that you would do better with other alternatives besides dieting. Answer each of the following items with a "True" or "False" as it applies to you!

_____ 1. I am frustrated about my inability to stick to a diet.

_____ 2. I feel I have less self-control than most dieters.

_____ 3. Most of the times I try to lose weight, I lose control and go off my diet.

_____ 4. When I try to develop a habit of regular exercise, something always interferes, and I stop.

_____ 5. Exercise seems to be an ordeal to me.

_____ 6. I often feel tired during the day.

_____ 7. My weight has gone up and down several times when I go on and off diets.

_____ 8. My body seems to be getting thicker in the middle over the years.

_____ 9. My weight seems to be increasing over the years.

_____ 10. I find myself thinking about food more than I should.

_____ 11. I find myself thinking about my weight all through the day.

_____ 12. I feel there is probably no hope for my weight problem.

_____ 13. Sometimes I lose control and really binge on food.

_____ 14. I use food to make myself feel better when I am angry, nervous, or depressed.

_____ 15. Some people reject me as a friend because I am too heavy.

_____ 16. My social life is limited because of my weight.

_____ 17. My sex life is limited because of my weight.

_____ 18. Other people think I am unattractive because of my weight.

_____ 19. I put a lot of effort into wearing clothes that tend to cover up my weight problem.

TO CARRY THIS FURTHER . . .

For those items that you answered as True, consider these recommendations:

Items 1, 2, and 3: Rather than "going on a diet," why not try to reduce your fat intake by avoiding fried food and foods with added fat. Eat more low-fat foods, and make certain that your dairy products are low-fat and your meats are lean.

Items 4, 5, and 6: You need a gradual but regular exercise program. Check around your community, and identify a reputable program that has a proven success rate in helping others who have had a weight problem.

Items 7, 8, and 9: These items indicate the development of a weight problem that could truly be damaging your health. These are reasons for being serious about weight loss that goes beyond appearance.

Items 10, 11, 12, 13, and 14: You may be into "living to eat" rather than "eating to live." Now is the time to give serious thought about what is important in your life, other than appearance-related needs.

Items 15, 16, and 17: Work at forming new relationships. Seek out people who are capable of looking beyond your physical appearance for those attributes that they will find to be attractive in you.

Items 18 and 19: As for 15 to 17, assess your current relationships. Put your efforts into relationships with people who seem capable of looking "into" you, rather than only "at" you.

some ways may be different from the total lifestyle approach just described. However, upon reaching a more healthful weight and body composition, maintenance of that status will depend on adopting the lifestyle changes described. Remember that weight loss followed by weight gain may be less healthful (and certainly more frustrating) than maintaining body weight, even at levels above desirable.

Weight loss occurs when energy taken into the body is less than that demanded by the body for physiological maintenance and voluntary activity. A number of approaches to weight loss can be pursued.

Dietary Alterations

A diet that reduces the Calories entering the body is the most common approach to what seems to be a national obsession with weight loss. The selection of foods included in the diet and the amount of food that can be consumed are the two factors that distinguish the wide range of diets currently available. Unfortunately, dieting alone usually does not result in long-term weight loss. In fact, whether managing their diets by themselves or following the advice of one of the widely recognized weight loss programs, the majority of dieters regain at least two thirds of their lost weight within 2 years after their initial loss.[17]

BALANCED DIETS SUPPORTED BY PORTION CONTROL

For nutritional health, a logical approach to weight loss and subsequent management of that loss is to establish a nutritionally sound balanced diet (low fat, low saturated fat, and high complex carbohydrate) that controls portions. This approach is best undertaken with nutritionists and physicians who are knowledgeable in diet management. After a study of your day-to-day energy needs, they can establish a diet designed to produce a gradual loss. A working understanding of portion size can be achieved using diet scales or through a nutrition education program in which realistic models of food servings are used.

A balanced diet—portion control approach to weight loss reflects a nutritionally sound program that has some probability for success without the negative feature of forcing you to adapt to a restrictive approach to eating. People have extreme difficulty adjusting to a diet that presents them with uncommon foods. To people who need to lose weight, dieting is often bad enough without feeling that they must be deprived of foods that satisfy their emotional needs.

FAD DIETS

People use a variety of fad diets in an attempt to achieve weight loss within a short time. With exceptions, these approaches are both ineffective and potentially unhealthful. In addition, some require far greater expense than would be associated with weight loss or management techniques using portion control and

regular physical activity. The pros and cons of a variety of popular diet plans are presented in Table 6-6.

LOW-CALORIE FOODS AND CONTROLLED SERVING SIZES

Recently a variety of familiar foods in a reduced-calorie form have been developed. By lowering the carbohydrate content with the use of nonnutritive sweeteners or reducing the fat content of the original formulations, manufacturers have given us "lite" versions of many food products. An additional aid to selecting lower calorie and lower fat foods is the newly required food label described in Chapter 5. For the first time terms such as "lite" and "low fat" that are used on food labels have been defined by the FDA and are now used in a consistent manner.

An even more recent addition to the diet arsenal has been the portion-controlled serving of food. Initially marketed as "single-serving" sizes, many familiar brands are now available in premeasured lunch or dinner servings. It is possible to find a fairly wide selection of attractively prepared frozen entrees with fewer than 300 Calories each.

CONTROLLED FASTING

In cases of extreme obesity, some patients are placed on a *complete fast* in a hospital setting. The patient is maintained on only water, electrolytes, and vitamins. Weight loss is profound, because the body is quickly forced to begin **catabolizing** its fat and muscle tissues.

Complete fasting is such an extreme approach to weight loss that it must be done in an institutional setting so the patient can be closely monitored. Sodium loss, a negative nitrogen balance, and potassium loss are particular concerns.

Today some people regularly practice short periods of modified fasting. Solid foods are removed from the diet for a number of days. Fruit juices, water, supplements, and vitamins are used to minimize the risks described in association with total fasting. However, unsupervised short-term fasting can be dangerous and is not generally recommended.

SELF-HELP WEIGHT REDUCTION PROGRAMS

In virtually every area of the country a person can find at least one version of the popular, reputable weight reduction programs that are often operated commercially. Popularized by Weight Watchers, these programs currently feature a format consisting of (1) a well-balanced diet emphasizing portion control and low-fat, low–saturated fat, and high-complex carbohydrate foods, (2) realistic weight loss goals to be at-

> **catabolism** (ka **tab** oh liz um) metabolic process of breaking down tissue for the purpose of converting it into energy.

TABLE 6-6   Diets—Past, Present, and Future

Type of diet	Advantages	Disadvantages	Examples
High-protein, low-carbohydrate diets			
Usually include all the meat, fish, poultry, and eggs you can eat Occasionally permit milk and cheese in limited amounts Prohibit fruits, vegetables, and any bread or cereal products	Rapid initial weight loss because of diuretic effect Very little hunger	Too low in carbohydrates Deficient in many nutrients—vitamin C, vitamin A (unless eggs are included), calcium, and several trace elements High in saturated fat, cholesterol, and total fat Extreme diets of this type could cause death Impossible to adhere to these diets long enough to lose any appreciable amount of weight Dangerous for people with kidney disease Weight lost, which is largely water, is rapidly regained Expensive Unpalatable after first few days Difficult for dieter to eat out	Dr. Stillman's Quick Weight Loss Diet Calories Don't Count by Dr. Taller Dr. Atkin's Diet Revolution Scarsdale Diet Air Force Diet
Low-calorie, high-protein supplement diets			
Usually a premeasured powder to be reconstituted with water or a prepared liquid formula	Rapid initial weight loss Easy to prepare—already measured Palatable for first few days Usually fortified to provide recommended amount of micronutrients Must be labeled if >50% protein.	Usually prescribed at dangerously low Calorie intake of 300 to 500 Cal Overpriced Low in fiber and bulk—constipating in short amount of time	Metracal Diet Cambridge Diet Liquid Protein Diets Last Chance Diet Oxford Diet
High-fiber, low-calorie diets			
	High satiety value Provide bulk	Irritating to the lower colon Decreases absorption of trace elements, especially iron Nutritionally deficient Low in protein	Pritikin Diet F Diet Zen macrobiotic Diet
Protein-sparing modified fats			
<50% protein: 400 Cal	Safe under supervision High-quality protein Minimize loss of lean body mass	Decreases BMR Monotonous Expensive	Optifast Medifast
Premeasured food plans			
	Provide prescribed portion sizes—little chance of too small or too large a portion Total food programs Some provide adequate Calories (1200) Nutritionally balanced or supplemented	Expensive Do not retrain dieters in acceptable eating habits Preclude eating out or social eating Often low in bulk Monotonous Low long-term success rates	Nutri-System Carnation Plan

tained over a realistic time period, (3) encouragement from supportive leaders and fellow group members, (4) emphasis on regular physical activity, and (5) a weight management program (follow-up program).

These programs offer a reasonable, effective, noninstitutional approach to weight loss for people who cannot or will not participate in an activity program. However, as already discussed, participation levels can decline steadily in these programs and initial weight loss is largely regained within 2 years.[17] They are costly when compared with self-directed approaches, especially when the program markets its own food products.

Physical Intervention

A second approach to weight loss involves techniques and products designed to alter the basic patterns of eating. These techniques range from those that are self-selected and self-applied to those that must be administered within an institutional setting by highly trained professionals.

APPETITE SUPPRESSANTS

One of the fondest wishes of overweight people is to lose the desire to eat—to actually have the feeling that food is not interesting or attractive. Today a variety of appetite suppressants are marketed in an attempt to achieve this for the dieter.

Pills, capsules, and candies containing sugar can be purchased that generate a short-term elevation in the body's blood glucose level. When the hypothalamus senses this elevated glucose level, the satiety center is triggered, causing the appetite to decrease. Since the active ingredient is usually some form of sugar, a piece of candy would probably accomplish the same result. These over-the-counter products are relatively harm-

TABLE 6-6   Diets—Past, Present, and Future—cont'd

Type of diet	Advantages	Disadvantages	Examples
Limited food choice diets	Reduce the number of food choices made by the users Limited opportunity to make mistakes Almost certainly low in Calories after the first few days	Deficient in many nutrients, depending on the foods allowed Monotonous—difficult to adhere to Eating out and eating socially are difficult Do not refrain dieters in acceptable eating habits Low long-term success rates No scientific basis for these diets	Banana and milk diet Grapefruit and cottage cheese diet Kempner rice diet Lecithin, vinegar, kelp, and vitamin B$_6$ diet Beverly Hills Diet Fit for Life
Restricted calorie, balanced food plans	Sufficiently low in Calories to permit steady weight loss Nutritionally balanced Palatable Include readily available foods Reasonable in cost Can be adapted from family meals Permit eating out and social eating Promote a new set of eating habits	Do not appeal to people who want a "unique" diet Do not produce immediate and large weight losses	Weight Watchers Diet Prudent Diet (American Heart Association) The I Love New York Diet UCLA Diet Time-Calorie Displacement (TCD) Fit or Fat Target Diet Take Off Pounds Sensibly (TOPS) Overeaters Anonymous
Fasting starvation diet	Rapid initial loss	Nutrient deficient Danger of ketosis >60% loss is muscle <40% loss is fat Low long-term success rate	ZIP Diet
High-carbohydrate diet	Emphasizes grains, fruits, and vegetables High in bulk Low in cholesterol	Limits milk, meat Nutritionally very inadequate for calcium, iron, and protein	Beverly Hills Diet Quick Weight Loss Diet Pritikin Diet Carbohydrate Cravers

less, although they do supply more empty calories for the body to deal with.

At the time of this writing, a large number of non-prescription appetite suppressants containing **phenylpropanolamine (PPA)** are being sold in supermarkets. Controversy concerning the safety of this active ingredient may alter its future availability. The drug is clearly dangerous for some people. People with high blood pressure, thyroid problems, diabetes, depression, and glaucoma should not use PPA. In addition, it can interact with other medications to produce potentially dangerous side effects. Like its prescription counterparts, the amphetamines, this drug has only short-term value in weight reduction programs.

NONAPPETITE SUPPRESSANT PHARMACEUTICAL AGENTS

Although far from being approved by the FDA for general use, three interesting new approaches for dealing with excessive weight and body fat have been identified. The first of these includes *orlistat,* a drug that reduces the percent of fat that can be absorbed from the digestive tract by slightly altering the action of enzymes needed to prepare dietary fat for movement into the blood stream.[18] The second pharmaceutical agent is a topically applied cream, *aminophyline,* that appears to stimulate fat cell metabolism in the area to which the cream has been applied.[19] Critics suggest that only localized dehydration has occurred. Regardless, the ability to "spot reduce" may be only

---

phenylpropanolamine (PPA) (fen ill pro pan **ol** ah meen) active chemical compound found in most over-the-counter diet products.

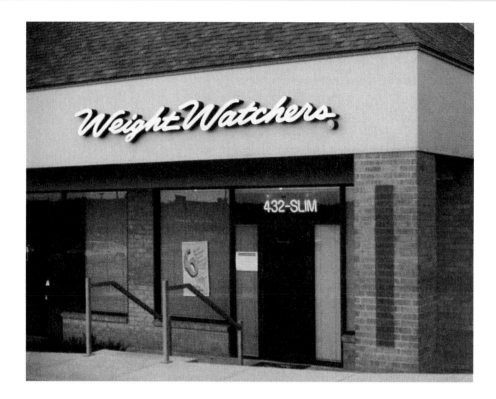

Health ACTION Guide

When Choosing A Diet Book

▼ Make sure the program incorporates a balanced diet, exercise program, and behavior modification.

▼ Beware of inflexible plans, such as those that require you to eat certain foods on certain days.

▼ Avoid plans that allow fewer than 1200 Calories a day, the minimum needed to get essential nutrients.

▼ Make sure the recommended rate of weight loss doesn't exceed 2 lb per week.

▼ Steer clear of books that promote vitamins, pills, shots, gimmicks, gadgets, or brand-name diet foods.

▼ Read reviews to see if the book got approval from a reputable nutrition expert, institution, or journal.

▼ Check the authors' credentials. They should be trained in nutrition from an accredited university, or they should use reliable sources for their information.

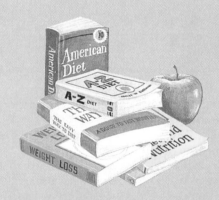

▼ Make sure the book is based on up-to-date scientific research.

▼ Beware of diets that promise fast, easy, or effortless weight loss, or "a new secret formula."

▼ Choose a plan that teaches how to keep the weight off once you've lost it.

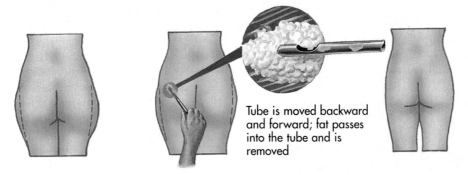

Tube is moved backward and forward; fat passes into the tube and is removed

Figure 6-7 Suction-assisted lipectomy. Liposuction is a controversial method for removing body fat.

slightly more realistic than is currently believed. The third approach to altering body composition is the use in men of testosterone patches. Initial research suggested that the testosterone absorbed through the skin was able to reduce some adipose tissue layered around the major abdominal organs.[20]

SURGICAL MEASURES

When weight loss is imperative and the initial level of obesity is great, surgical intervention may be considered. A *gastric resection* is a major operation in which a portion of the small intestine is bypassed in an attempt to decrease the body's ability to absorb nutrients. Although the procedure can produce major loss of body weight, it is associated with many unpleasant side effects (including diarrhea and liver damage) and various nutritional deficiencies. Not only will surgery be required for this approach, but lifetime medical management will also be necessary.

Gastroplasty (stomach stapling) is a surgical procedure that appears to be less dangerous than the intestinal bypass operation. During this operation about half of the stomach is sealed with surgical staples. Once the procedure is completed, the reduced capacity of the stomach decreases the amount of food that can be processed at any one time. As a result patients feel full more quickly after eating a small meal. This procedure is reversible but carries the risks associated with surgery and the costs of a major surgical procedure.

LIPOSUCTION (LIPOPLASTY)

Another form of surgical weight loss management is *liposuction* (Figure 6-7). During this expensive procedure, a physician inserts a small tube through the skin, and vacuum aspiration literally sucks away fat cells. This procedure is generally used for stubborn, localized pockets of fat and is usually appropriate for people under the age of 40.

Clearly, liposuction is more a cosmetic procedure than a general approach to weight loss. Along with unrealistic expectations, the risks of infection, pain and discomfort, bruising, swelling, discoloration, abscesses, and unattractive changes in body contours are

possible outcomes of liposuction. Therefore individuals seeking to undergo this procedure need to carefully investigate all aspects of the procedure, including the training and experience of the surgeon, to determine whether it is appropriate for them. An expanded version of liposuction, called liposuction fat transfer, has been performed on a limited basis. This procedure uses fat cells removed by liposuction to contour other areas of the body, including the breasts. Again, careful consideration is necessary before undergoing this procedure.

ACUPUNCTURE

Acupuncture is being used as a treatment for obesity, as well as for a variety of other health problems. The appearance of acupuncture rings and earrings in drugstores and novelty shops suggests that the procedure has moved into the nonprofessional domain. The majority of persons receiving acupuncture for the treatment of obesity are, fortunately, receiving treatment from skilled practitioners.

Behavior Change Strategies

In addition to dietary alterations, drugs, and surgical intervention, several approaches designed to change learned eating patterns have been tried by people desiring to lose weight. Because of the relatively small number of people involved in many of these approaches and the limited extent to which they have been scientifically studied, it is difficult to assess their long-term effectiveness. Nevertheless, they remain as alternatives to the approaches already described.

BEHAVIOR MODIFICATION

To the behaviorist, learned behavior can be "unlearned." If people have learned to eat in an appropriate manner and as a result have difficulty maintaining

---

acupuncture (**ack** you punc shur) insertion of fine needles into the body to alter electroenergy fields and cure disease.

their weight, then that pattern can be replaced by a more sensible pattern.[18] *Behavior modification* is an approach to accomplishing this more desirable pattern.

In the standard behavioral modification approach to weight loss, the individual would be taught to (1) recognize the environmental factors associated with the faulty eating pattern, (2) identify the reward system that accompanies that pattern, (3) establish a new environment in which to develop the new dietary pattern, and (4) institute a new reward system to support the newly adopted dietary pattern. Behavior modification programs can be undertaken in both group and individual formats. The following Health Action Guide box gives some approaches to behavior modification.

HYPNOSIS

Hypnosis appears to hold some promise as an effective weapon in the obesity battle. Studies involving hypnosis have appeared in the literature for at least 30 years. Many of these have reported excellent success rates, but most involve small numbers of patients and little has been reported on long-term success rates.

More recently, "private practitioners" of hypnosis are applying their skills in many nonprofessional settings such as motel rooms. Claims made for these programs have been extremely high. The cost of treatment is also high. On this basis, we would be cautious of using hypnosis.

PHYSICAL ACTIVITY

Most experts now believe that the most important component of a weight-loss program is regular physical activity. Physical activity contributes to weight loss and the maintenance of weight loss because activity burns Calories. It is important to remember that the need for Calories decreases with age and decreased activity.

At one time it was thought that physical activity could stimulate a 12- to 24-hour period of sustained elevation of the BMR. This elevated BMR was thought to result in more Calories being burned, even after moderate exercise was completed. It is now thought that a

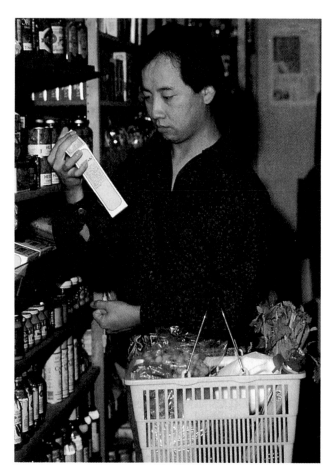

Has this person chosen to eat wisely?

Health ACTION Guide

To Change Your Eating Patterns

▼ Keep a log of the times, settings, reasons, and feelings associated with your eating.
▼ Set realistic long-term goals (for example, loss of a pound per week instead of 5 lb per week)
▼ Avoid the total deprivation of enjoyable foods (occasionally reward yourself with a small treat)
▼ Eat slowly and realize that the sacrifices you are making are what *you* feel are important for *your* health and happiness.

▼ Put more physical activity into your daily routine (taking stairs instead of elevators or parking in the distant part of a parking lot, for example)
▼ Reward yourself when you reach your goals (with new clothes, sporting equipment, a vacation trip)
▼ Share your commitment to weight loss with your family and friends (then they can support your efforts)
▼ Keep careful records of daily food consumption and weight change
▼ Be prepared to deal with occasional plateaus and setbacks in your quest for weight loss
▼ Remember that low-fat, low–saturated fat, and high-complex carbohydrate meals in combination with regular physical activity is the basis upon which these strategies are applied.

Health ACTION Guide

Weight Management Tips

TIPS FOR WEIGHT LOSS

▼ You probably didn't gain your excessive weight eating alone. Seek the encouragement and support of family and friends in your weight loss efforts.

▼ Eat only at the table. Leave the table immediately after finishing your meal. And by all means never take your meal with you into other rooms of the house.

▼ Stop eating after one serving. A second helping contributes more fat than your diet can afford.

▼ If you must snack between meals, choose small, nutritious, low-fat snacks.

▼ Stay away from the kitchen. An innocent look into the refrigerator will almost certainly lead to a taste, a snack, or even a meal.

TIPS FOR WEIGHT GAIN

▼ Make certain that there is no medical reason for your thinness.

▼ Have your current dietary practices evaluated so that appropriate modifications can be made.

▼ Begin a moderate exercise program to enhance your physical fitness.

▼ Incorporate the following recommendations into your dietary practice:
  • Substitute juice, soup, or hot chocolate for coffee.
  • Eat a healthy breakfast.
  • Learn appropriate portion sizes.
  • Replace junk foods with more healthy foods.

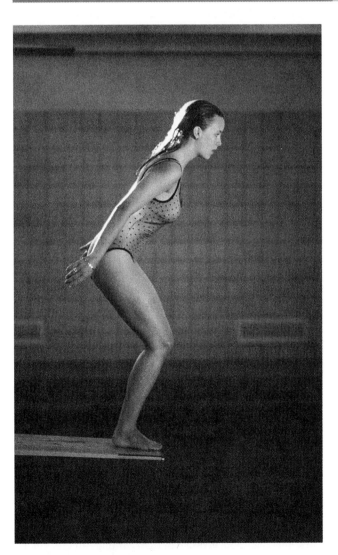

Exercise to expend calories.

more likely interval of BMR elevation (after moderate exercise) is 2 or 3 hours.[21]

An additional benefit derived from physical activity is that proportionately more fat is lost than is lost through dieting alone. Studies suggest that the weight loss achieved through physical activity is 95% fat and 5% lean tissue, such as muscle, in comparison with a loss of 75% fat and 25% lean tissue when dieting alone is used. Exercise also offers the additional benefits of increasing heart and lung endurance, muscular strength, and flexibility.

A Combination Approach

In a recent study on weight loss conducted for the FDA, nearly 50% of American adults are attempting to lose weight through dieting. The majority are able to lose weight, but very few are able to maintain their weight loss. Regardless of the weight loss method used, within 5 years all of the lost weight will be regained.[22] Further, in too many instances, the newly established weight is actually higher than the initial weight. This tendency for persons to lose weight only to end up *heavier* and then attempt to diet again is the **yo-yo syndrome.**

If we were to recommend a single approach to weight reduction that would, in theory, offer the maximum chance for success, we would suggest a program combining a well-planned diet and aerobic exercise. Specifically, the program would be as follows:

yo-yo syndrome the repeated weight loss, followed by weight gain, experienced by many dieters.

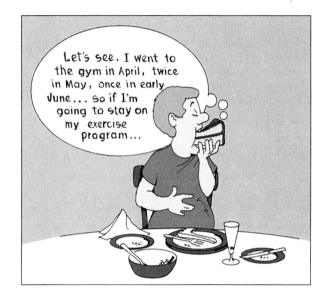

▼ A varied, balanced diet emphasizing portion control and low-fat, low–saturated fat, high-complex carbohydrate food items would be developed; with necessary modifications, the diet would be adopted by the entire family.

▼ Reasonable short-term weight-loss goals and weight loss maintenance goals would be established at the beginning of the program and assessed during and after the program.

▼ A professionally planned aerobic fitness component would be developed and implemented as a part of the total program format. A family-wide commitment to regular aerobic activity (walking, hiking, rollerblading, biking) would be even more helpful, particularly if it involved both younger and older family members.

▼ The family would participate and serve as a source of encouragement for the overweight person.

THE WEIGHT LOSS INDUSTRY

People generally tend to become fatter with age, but cultural norms emphasize thinness at almost any cost. As a consequence, millions of Americans are unhappy about their weight. So common is this feeling that nearly one half of adult women and one third of adult men consider themselves to be overweight.

In response to our near obsession with thinness, a thriving weight loss industry exists to assist us in our attempts to lose weight. In 1990 a House committee investigating questionable practices in the weight loss industry reported that Americans were spending $32 billion a year on various products and services in the quest for thinness.[23] A breakdown of this staggering sum indicated that $11.4 billion was spent on diet soft drinks alone. The weight loss industry, represented by

a wide variety of programs (see Table 6-6) and products, earned $9.9 billion, and health spas and exercise club memberships cost $8.5 billion. In addition to these expenditures, Americans spent $1.6 billion on luxury spas and $1.0 billion on artificial sweeteners.

Clearly, Americans are willing to spend money in the pursuit of thinness. In spite of the advice given by reputable health experts that we cannot prevent the gradual conversion of lean mass to fat and that weight loss is difficult to achieve, particularly when we do not increase caloric expenditure and modify behaviors, we remain willing to pay billions of dollars in an attempt to achieve our goal.

The financial success of the weight loss industry in this country has in part been due to its effective television advertising. Skillfully produced commercials featuring successful program members suggested likely success for the viewer willing to "sign" on. Before 1994, these were regular fare on daytime television. Today, however, commercials for diet programs such as Jenny Craig, Nutri/Systems, Weight Watchers, and others are considerably more restrained in their messages about success. Under directives issued by the FTC, today's advertisements cannot misrepresent program performance. They must disclose that most weight loss is temporary, and they now inform the viewer that their loss will most likely not approximate that of the successful subjects featured in their commercials.

EATING DISORDERS

Perhaps it is not surprising to find that some people have medically identifiable, potentially dangerous eating patterns. Two serious disorders that are sometimes seen among college students are anorexia and bulimia.

Anorexia Nervosa

A young woman, competitive and perfectionistic by nature, determines that her weight (and appearance) is unacceptable. She sets upon a course of disregarding hunger and appetite. Her food consumption virtually ceases.

The young woman in this description may be seen by her friends or roommates as active and intelligent and simply dieting and exercising with an unusual amount of commitment. Eventually, however, you would observe that her food consumption had virtually ceased. Her weight loss would continue beyond the point that is aesthetically pleasing—at least to you. Nevertheless, her activity level might remain high. When questioned about her weight loss, she would probably indicate that she still needed to lose more weight.

This person is suffering from a medical condition referred to as **anorexia nervosa.** This self-induced starvation is life threatening in 5% to 20% of cases. The stunning amount of weight that some anorexics lose—up to 50% of their body weight—eventually leads to kidney failure and cardiovascular collapse. Lowered blood potassium levels can produce irregular heartbeat patterns and sudden death.

Anorexia nervosa appears to be increasing among women, particularly from white middle- to upper-middle-class families. Some experts believe that the incidence of anorexia is on the rise because our society expects young women to be as glamorous, sexy, and thin as the women seen on television, in magazines, and on billboards. Indeed, anorexia patients typically come from families that place a heavy emphasis on high achievement, perfection, eating patterns, and physical appearances.

Fortunately for the anorexic, psychological intervention in combination with medical and dietary support can return the victim to a more life-sustaining pattern of eating. However, the anorexic first needs to seek professional help. Your obligation when you observe this condition in a friend is to secure immediate assistance for this person.

The prevalence of anorexia (and bulimia as well) has been very low in men as compared with women. Today, however, the incidence of both conditions is increasing in men as they begin to feel some of the same pressures that women feel to conform to the weight and body composition standards imposed by others. The "lean look" of young male models serves as a standard for more and more young men, whereas the requirements to "make weight" for various sports drives others. In the latter group, runners, wrestlers, jockies, and gymnasts frequently must lose weight quickly in order to meet particular standards for competition or the expectations of coaches and trainers. Life changes, such as the end of a relationship, the loss of employment, or the diagnosis of illness, also can stimulate the development of an eating disorder in men and women alike.

Researchers report that men are even less inclined than women to admit that they may have an eating disorder. Thus, they are even less likely to seek treatment. Also, physicians are still not as likely to suspect eating disorders in men as they are to suspect them in women. Hopefully, both of these aspects of eating disorders among men are beginning to change.

Bulimia Nervosa

Bulimia reflects a dietary practice pattern in which people gorge themselves with food. When people practice a pattern of massive eating followed by **purging,** they are said to suffer from *bulimarexia,* or bulimia nervosa. Most often, however, the term *bulimia* is used to describe this binge/purge pattern. This condition, like anorexia, can lead to weight loss, but it differs in terms of the victim's personality and specific behavioral patterns and the prospects for successful treatment. As with anorexics, most bulimics are young women, although the incidence in men is growing.

Bulimics lose weight or maintain weight not because they stop eating, but because they eat and then purge their digestive system by vomiting or using laxatives. Syrup of ipecac, a product used to help poisoning victims vomit, is so frequently abused by bulimics that efforts are underway to make this a prescription drug. Compared with anorexics, bulimics tend to be extroverted, socially active, and less perfectionistic. Your primary awareness of a bulimic's condition may be the paradox between high food intake and concurrent weight loss. In the mid-1980s, medical experts estimated that as many as 19% of 18- to 22-year-old women developed all the principal symptoms of bulimia. More recent estimates have dramatically lowered this to less than 2%.[23]

People with bulimia may gorge themselves with food (up to 10,000 Calories or more at a sitting) and then quietly disappear, only to return later seemingly unaffected by the foods they recently ate. In all likelihood, they have quickly and quietly regurgitated the food. Unlike anorexics, people with bulimia nervosa may demonstrate an extreme sensitivity to food. Thus they have many food likes and dislikes. This suggests that they have not managed to suppress their hunger. Bulimics feel hungry, overeat, and then resolve their guilt by vomiting or abusing laxatives.

anorexia nervosa (an oh **reck** see uh ner **vo** suh) disorder of emotional origin in which appetite and hunger are suppressed, and marked weight loss occurs.

bulimia (boo lee **me** uh) disorder of emotional origin in which binge eating patterns are established; usually accompanied by purging.

purging using vomiting or laxatives to remove undigested food from the body.

Treatment for Eating Disorders

The treatment of anorexia nervosa and bulimia nervosa is a complex and demanding undertaking. The components of therapy, drawn from medical and behavioral sciences, involve the cooperation of several health care providers. Each case of anorexia or bulimia must be approached from an individual perspective.

The initial physical care for anorexia most often begins with hospitalization of the individual to stabilize the physical deterioration associated with starvation. Nasogastric tubes and intravenous feedings are sometimes necessary, particularly when the patient will not (or cannot) eat. In addition, drug therapy to decrease hyperactivity and stimulate appetite is often used.

The psychological and familial components underlying anorexia require a variety of therapeutic approaches. Behavioral modification, including eating contracts, is employed, as is psychotherapy in both individual and group formats. Nutritional counseling and family therapy counseling complete the therapy.

Treatment for bulimia involves individual, family, and nutritional counseling. Unlike treatment for anorexia, however, bulimia treatment does not involve hospitalization as often. People with eating disorders need professional assistance. Unfortunately, the assistance available for treating bulimia appears to be less effective than that available to victims of anorexia nervosa. This may relate to the difficulty of dealing effectively with the lack of control experienced by the bulimic. The stress of binge eating followed by purging that is experienced by the bulimic is often coped with once again by the excessive consumption of food.

Resources for Anorexia and Bulimia Treatment

LOCAL RESOURCES

★ College/university health centers

★ College/university counseling centers

★ Comprehensive mental health centers

★ Crisis intervention centers

★ Mental health associations

TELEPHONE HOT LINES

★ ANAD (National Association of Anorexia Nervosa and Associated Disorders):
Highland Park, Ill
(708) 831-3438

★ Bulimia Anorexia Nervosa Association:
Windsor, Ont (Canada)
(519)253-7421 or 7545

UNDERNUTRITION

For some young adults, the absence of body weight is a concern of great importance. Particularly for individuals who have inherited an ectomorphic body build (tall, narrow shoulders/hips, tendency to thinness), attempts to gain weight are routinely undertaken, often

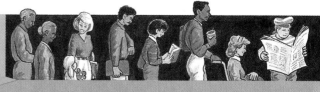

Learning FROM ALL Cultures

Eating Habits

All people satisfy hunger by eating, but because of cultural differences, when and how our appetites are satisfied vary. All people usually eat at least one meal in a 24-hour period. Some African tribes and other developing societies are accustomed to eating only one meal per day, the result of occasional or continual food shortages. Other substances are known to be used by some of these societies to suppress hunger such as coca leaves (which contain cocaine), peyote (a hallucinogen derived from a cactus), tobacco, coffee, and tea.[24] Appetite suppressants in the form of diet aids in the United States serve the same purpose but for different reasons.

Typically in North America, three meals a day is the custom, although skipping regular meals and snacking are common. The British usually eat four times a day, while continental European people may eat five or six times. Of course these practices vary according to changing lifestyles.[24]

For most, eating is a pleasurable experience but not just for the sake of nourishment. Business deals are made over lunch, agreements between countries are discussed over a meal, relationships are begun during a romantic dinner, and events are celebrated by the sharing of food.

Think about your own eating habits. Why and when do you eat? How do your eating habits reflect your culture and lifestyle?

Identification of Anorexia Nervosa and Bulimia

The American Psychological Association uses diagnostic criteria to identify anorexia nervosa and bulimia:

ANOREXIA

★ 15% or more below desirable weight

★ Fear of weight gain

★ Altered body image

★ Three or more missed menstrual periods

BULIMIA

★ Binge eating two or more times a week for 3 months

★ A lack of control over binging

★ Purging

★ Concern about body image

Characteristic symptoms that may be displayed include the following. However, it is unlikely that all the symptoms will appear in any one individual.

ANOREXIA

★ Looks thin and keeps getting thinner

★ Skips meals, cuts food into small pieces, moves food around plate to appear to have eaten

★ Loss of menstrual periods

★ Wears "layered look" in an attempt to disguise weight loss

★ Loss of hair from the head

★ Growth of fine hair on face, arms, and chest

★ Extreme sensitivity to cold

BULIMIA

★ Bathroom use immediately after eating

★ Inconspicuous eating

★ Excessive time (and money) spent food shopping

★ Shopping for food at several stores rather than one store

★ Menstrual irregularities

★ Excessive constipation

★ Swollen and/or infected salivary glands, sore throat

★ Bursting blood vessels in the eyes

★ Damaged teeth and gums

★ Dehydration and kidney disfunction

---

with limited success. If these persons are to be successful in gaining weight, they must discover an effective way to take in more Calories than they burn.

In the opinion of nutritionists, the healthiest way to gain weight is to increase the intake of Calorie-dense food. These foods are characterized by high fat density, resulting from high levels of vegetable fats (polyunsaturated fats). Particularly good foods in this regard are dried fruits, bananas, nuts, granola, and cheeses made from low-fat milk. It is important, however, to consume these foods later in a meal so that the onset of satiety that quickly follows eating fat-rich foods does not occur.

A second component of weight gain for those who are underweight is the curtailment of excessive physi-cal activity. By carefully reducing their activity level, they can prevent the "burning up" of calories and, thus, use them for development of body fat. Of course, activity should not be restricted to the point that cardiovascular conditioning declines or enjoyable activities are no longer available.

For those who cannot gain weight in spite of having tried the above approaches, a medical evaluation could possibly supply an explanation for being underweight. When it has been determined that no medical explanation can be found, the individual must then begin to accept the reality of his or her unique body type. Ironically, current fashion tends to emphasize thinness, and most people who are overweight would welcome a chance to experience thinness.

Summary

✔ Overweight and obesity are the most common forms of malnutrition in the United States and are associated with various health problems.

✔ Obesity results from an abnormal accumulation of fat.

✔ Obesity and overweight can be measured in a variety of ways.

✔ The principal methods for determining obesity are the body mass index and the waist-to-hip ratio.

✔ Body image may or may not align itself with actual scale weight and body composition.

✔ Maintaining a healthy body weight is desirable.

✔ Theories regarding the cause of obesity focus on factors from within the individual and from the environment.

✔ Theories that concern the role of inheritance, set point, feeding patterns, pregnancy, aging, inactivity, and family eating patterns are complex.

✔ Caloric balance influences weight gain, loss, and maintenance.

✔ The body's energy needs arise from three functions BMR, activity, and the thermic effect of food.

✔ Maintenance of weight and body composition is based on a lifetime commitment to a diet featuring low-fat and high-complex carbohydrate foods and regular aerobic activity.

✔ Weight loss can be attempted through dieting, which is the restricting of food intake.

✔ Drugs, behavior modification, and other techniques are used with limited success to achieve weight loss.

✔ Although most people can lose weight through dieting, very few who do are able to maintain that weight loss.

✔ The weight loss industry is facing increased pressure to be more honest with their customers about weight loss.

✔ Potentially serious eating disorders result, in part, from concerns about weight and body image.

✔ Calorie-dense foods and careful restriction of activity can aid underweight persons in gaining weight.

Review Questions

1. Why are obesity and overweight considered forms of malnutrition and potentially serious health problems?

2. How are obesity and overweight defined? Why is it possible to be overweight without being overfat? What is the role played by the set point?

3. In what ways can obesity be determined? What is body mass index?

4. Why is there concern among health experts about not only the amount of fat a person has but also the location of that fat on the body?

5. What is meant by the term *healthy body weight?* How does it differ from desirable body weight?

6. Describe the role that each of the following could play in causing obesity: heredity, set point, feeding patterns, pregnancy, aging, inactivity, and family eating patterns.

7. What is caloric balance? What are the body's three areas of energy needs? How does dieting influence caloric balance? How does exercise influence caloric balance?

8. What is the role of fad diets, fasting, drugs, surgery, behavior modification, and hypnosis in weight loss?

9. What are the two techniques that should be combined in order to maintain weight and body composition over the course of the adult years? When used as a weight-reduction approach, how do they compare in effectiveness to other techniques?

10. What are the two principal eating disorders seen within the college community? In what ways do they differ? How are eating disorders treated?

Think about This . . .

✔ What ways have you used to determine whether you are underweight, overweight, or obese?

✔ What are your attitudes toward people with weight control problems? Why do you feel this way?

✔ Do you believe that being underweight is as psychologically traumatic as being overweight?

✔ If you have ever attempted to lose weight, what methods have you used? Were any of your methods potentially dangerous?

✔ Regardless of your weight, what traits do you have that others find positive? How can you accentuate these attributes?

✔ If you are a person with a weight problem, do you agree or disagree that you have a responsibility to yourself and other people to adjust your weight?

REAL LIFE
REAL CHOICES

YOUR TURN

▼ Why do you think Kate isn't succeeding at getting weight off and keeping it off?

▼ What are some of the dangers of yo-yo dieting?

▼ What might be a realistic, workable approach for Kate to consider?

AND NOW, YOUR CHOICES . . .

▼ If you wanted to lose weight, what changes would you make in your diet and lifestyle? Would you see these changes as being temporary or permanent?

▼ Have you ever fasted or purged to lose weight, or have you ever considered doing so? Why or why not? ▼

References

1. Wardlaw GM, Insel PM: *Perspectives in nutrition,* St Louis, 1993, Mosby.
2. Crowley LV: *Introduction to human disease,* ed 3, Boston, 1992, Jones and Bartlett Publishers.
3. Interagency Board for Nutrition Monitoring and Related Research, Ervin B, Reed D, eds: Nutrition monitoring in the United States. In Chartbook I: *Selected findings from the National Nutrition Monitoring and Related Research Program,* Hyattsville, Maryland, 1993, *Public Health Service.*
4. *Nutrition and your health: dietary guidelines for Americans (1990),* Home and garden bulletin 232, United States Department of Agriculture/United States Department of Health and Human Services.
5. Bray GA: Obesity: a blueprint for progress, *Contemp Nutr* 12(7):1-2, 1987.
6. Prentice W: *Fitness for college and life,* ed 4, St Louis, 1994, Mosby.
7. Weighing the facts on obesity, **Worldview** 4(1):1-4, Spring 1992.
8. Mayer J: *Overweight,* Englewood Cliffs, NJ, 1968, Prentice Hall.
9. National Research Council: *Diet and health: implications for reducing chronic disease risk,* Washington, DC, 1989, National Academy Press.
10. Kemnitz J: Body weight set point theory, *Contemp Nutr* 10:1-2, 1985.
11. Walden TA, Foster GD, Letizia JL, Mullen JL: Long-term effects of dieting on resting metabolic rate in obese outpatients, *JAMA* 264(6):707-711, 1990.
12. Schauberger CW, Rooney BL, Brimer LM: Factors that influence weight loss in the puerperium, *Obstet Gynecol* 79(3):424-429, 1992.
13. Moffett D, Moffett S, Schauf C: *Human physiology: foundations and frontiers,* St Louis, 1993, Mosby.
14. Blair SW, et al: Body weight change, all-cause mortality, and cause-specific mortality in the Multiple Risk Factors Intervention Trial, *Ann Intern Med* 119(7):749-757, 1993.
15. Food and Nutrition Board: *Recommended dietary allowances,* Washington, DC, 1989, National Academy of Sciences, National Research Council.
16. Wardlaw GM, Insel PM, Seyler MF: *Contemporary nutrition: issues and insights,* St Louis, 1994, Mosby.
17. Losing weight: what works and doesn't work, *Consumer Reports* 58(6):347-352, June, 1993.
18. Elmer-Dewitt P: Cake eater's dream, *Time* 142(4):54, July 26, 1993.
19. Friend T: Cream may wipe fat from thighs, *USA Today* October 21, 1993, 1a.
20. Marin P, Krotkiewski M, Bjorntorp P: Androgen treatment of middle-aged, obese men—effects on metabolism, muscle and adipose tissue, European Journal of Medicine 1(6):329-336, 1992.
21. Kolata G: Metabolic catch-22 of exercise regimens, *Science* 236:146-147, 1987.
22. NIH Technology Assessment Conference Panel: Methods for voluntary weight loss and control, *Ann Intern Med* 116(11):942-949, 1992.
23. Burket RC, Hodgin JD: An eating disorders hotline: organization, implementation, and initial experience, *J Am Coll Health* 37(4):183-186, 1989.
24. Fieldhouse P: *Food and nutrition: customs and culture,* London, 1986, Cromm Helm.

Suggested Readings

Craig J, Wolfe BL: *Jenny Craig's what have you got to lose?* New York, 1992, Villard Books.

Designed to get dieters actively involved in their weight-loss program; emphasizes goal setting, record keeping, and self-monitoring; written in a workbook format.

Miller PM: *The Hilton Head diet for children and teenagers,* New York, 1993, Warner Books.

*An excellent book for parents of children 8 years and older; focuses on how to maintain weight and body composition within desirable ranges, or lose weight when necessary, for health reasons. Provides advice on ex-*ercise, eating behavior, food selection, convenience foods, and fast foods.

Spiller G: *The super pyramid eating program,* New York, 1993, Times Books.

A nutritionally-sound book that uses the newly approved USDA food grouping plan. Emphasis is on low-fat and high-carbohydrate foods.

Sutkamp JC, Mason T: *How to help your man lose weight: a guide for the concerned woman,* New York, 1992, Simon & Schuster.

If you believe that men can't or won't be responsible for their own health, particularly body weight, then this book is for you. For most readers, however, the title and premise are condescending.

It is our hope that the information you have mastered in Unit 2 will be helpful as you work on the five developmental tasks this book addresses. Of course, you must remember that all people work on these tasks in different ways and at varying speeds. However, it is through the completion of these developmental tasks that you will have a satisfying and productive life.

Forming an Initial Adult Identity

Developmentally speaking, traditional age students have as one of their major responsibilities the establishment of an initial adult identity. Even nontraditional students (and professors) find that they are often working on their adult identities. In forming these identities, we are expected to blend those traits we currently have with those that we desire. What are the roles for fitness, nutrition, and weight management in forming and re-forming our identities? Your enhanced fitness level, interest in nutrition, and body weight will be evident to you and transmitted to others as a sense of personal self-acceptance. In a sense, you are telling the world, "I like what I am and I hope you like it too."

Your interest in these areas is also a commitment to the future as you plan for your adult years and as others plan theirs with you in mind. You are likely to become a person who is more capable of living a productive and satisfying life.

Establishing Independence

Independence, a much-desired freedom for those nearing the end of their formal education, is achieved by the majority of adults regardless of whether they are interested in the health information presented in this unit. However, the quality of independence can be enhanced by a reasonable level of fitness and an interest in nutrition and weight management. Particularly in terms of your ability to cope with the new demands of independence, a well-developed state of fitness and a sound diet will help reduce stress and increase the level of alertness needed to master the demands of adulthood. For nontraditional students whose independence is already well-established, continued interest and involvement in physical activity, nutrition, and weight management can add a measure of renewal to your demanding life as an employee, single person, spouse, or parent.

Assuming Responsibility

As people move through adulthood, to whom should they be most responsible? As we mentioned earlier, people should probably be most responsible to themselves. But the responsibility to oneself does not limit the need to be responsible to others. The reasons that compel you to appreciate health and to promote it to the fullest extent reach beyond yourself to include others with whom you come into contact. For this reason, your fitness level, nutritional status, and weight management can affect your ability to perform optimally. Beyond this rather philosophical connection between high-level health and responsibility is another more concrete connection: Your motivation to maintain good cardiorespiratory fitness, nutrition, and weight management is an indicator of willingness and ability to assume responsibility. By being faithful to your fitness program and well-rounded diet, you assure yourself that you are a responsible person.

Developing Social Skills

As your social interaction increases with entry into or movement through the adult years, the relationship between this unit's content and your developing social skills becomes evident. Much social contact with other adults centers around food and physical activity. Exercise classes, parties, cycling groups, cafeteria meals, outdoor cookouts, evenings with friends, reunions, and athletic teams represent some social groups that cater to our fitness or food desires. Through your participation in these common social groupings, you will have a great opportunity to practice and improve social skills. Cherish these opportunities. Indeed, social interactions will form a principal basis for a kind of personal enjoyment that will last a lifetime.

Developing Intimacy

To enjoy all that accompanies intimate relationships, a dependable level of physical health is necessary. Limited physical conditioning can reduce the scope of activities in which you can interact. The enjoyment of food and a commitment to fitness can be areas of common interest within an intimate relationship.

UNIT THREE

There is little doubt in the minds of health professionals that the use, misuse, and abuse of many substances impair health. These substances not only alter the function of the body and the mind, but they also have an impact on the social, intellectual, and spiritual dimensions of health as well.

● Physical Dimension of Health

The relationship between substance use and the physical dimension of health is reasonably well understood, especially in relation to the long-term use of alcohol and tobacco. These substances clearly increase human illness and death.

The abuse of alcohol produces destructive changes in the structure and function of a variety of systems. Chronic alcohol use damages the heart, liver, brain, and tissues of the digestive system. Alcohol misuse and abuse can destroy families and innocent people.

Tobacco's damaging influence on physical health centers mainly on effects to the cardiovascular system and the tissues lining the air passages. Damage to the red blood cells, heart irregularities, and lung cancer are some serious effects of tobacco use.

Chronic misuse and abuse of most psychoactive drugs alter many central nervous system functions. Even the experimental use of psychoactive drugs presents the possibility of toxic overdose.

◆ Emotional Dimension of Health

Why do some people use alcohol, other drugs, and tobacco so extensively? Our understanding of these areas is far from complete. It is known, however, that psychoactive substances are capable of altering the normal function of the central nervous system. For individuals who seem predisposed to dependent relationships, chemical substances can become a readily available crutch. When growing emotional dependence combines with a physical dependence, major detrimental effects begin to surface.

■ Social Dimension of Health

The use of many psychoactive substances is associated with social interaction. In the minds of some people, the use of these substances seems to be a first step for enjoying the company of others. However, little social support exists for inappropriate substance use. In fact, the majority of society deplores the use of psychoactive drugs, misuse of beverage alcohol, and passive smoking.

Perhaps the most serious social consequence of these substances is the dulling effect they have on the learning of desirable social interaction skills. Successful social interaction demands discrimination and dissemination of a variety of cues and responses. The misuse of drugs, alcohol, and tobacco is likely to interfere with increased social growth.

▲ Intellectual Dimension of Health

Intellectual impairment is one part of the gradual decline of the body attributable to chemical abuse. People cannot perform well when they feel extremely high, extremely low, or are incapacitated by sensory impairment.

One important issue in the intellectual dimension centers on the disregard some people have for valid information related to the use, misuse, and abuse of chemical substances. This is an especially perplexing issue when it concerns college students—people whose education and intellectual abilities would suggest they can fully comprehend the dangers of drug use.

● Spiritual Dimension of Health

Although the use of chemical substances has a role in the religious practices of many people throughout the world, the nonceremonial misuse or abuse of chemical substances seems in conflict with the tenets of stewardship and service to others. The misuse of these substances seems an affront to the ideals of self-worth associated with many aspects of spiritual growth. It is unlikely that the development of one's spiritual life is improved by the use of chemical substances.

Products of Dependence

A Focus on Responsible Use

7

Psychoactive Drugs
Use, Misuse, and Abuse

The use of psychoactive drugs can be a tremendously disruptive factor in many people's lives. From tragic deaths and violence, to the loss of employment opportunities (63% of companies use drug testing to screen employees),[1] to the deterioration of personal relationships, drugs exert their negative influence on individuals. Realizing this, college students have generally moved away from the use of the most dangerous illegal drugs.[2]

Since the early 1980s, college students' illegal drug use has consistently dropped. However, a 1993 major survey of college students' drug use reported that this downward trend may have bottomed out.[3] For the first time in years, a slight increase was indicated in the percentage of students who reported using an illegal drug within the past year. (In 1991, 29.2% of college students used an illegal drug, but in 1992, 30.6% of college students used an illegal drug.) Overall, drug use remained steady or actually dropped in all drug categories except for hallucinogens and marijuana. (See Figure 7-1 for college students' drug use data.)

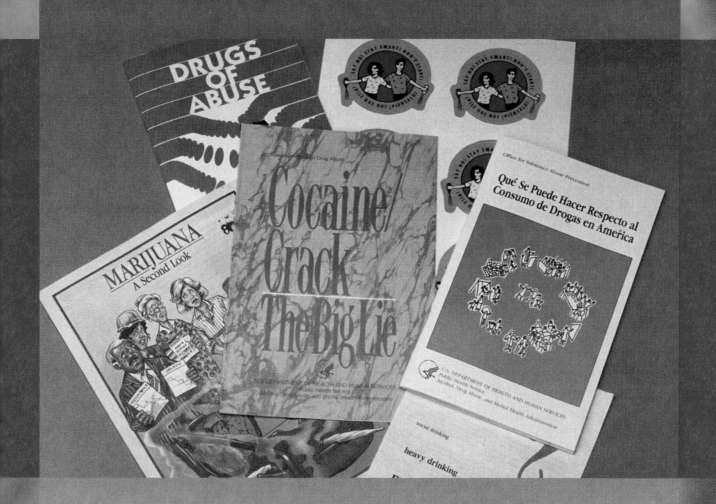

D R U G S

The following objectives are covered in this chapter:

▼ Reduce drug-related deaths to no more than 3 per 100,000 people. (Age-adjusted baseline: 3.8 per 100,000; p. 168.)

▼ Increase by at least 1 year the average age of first use of cigarettes, alcohol, and marijuana by adolescents aged 12 through 17. (Baseline: age 11.6 for cigarettes, age 13.1 for alcohol, and age 13.4 for marijuana in 1986; p. 169.)

▼ Reduce the proportion of young people who have used marijuana and cocaine in the past month to these year 2000 targets: marijuana/age 18 to 25 to 7.8% and cocaine/age 18 to 25 to 2.3%. (1988 Baselines: 15.5% for marijuana/age 18 to 25 and 4.5% for cocaine/age 18 to 25; p. 169.)

▼ Establish and monitor in 50 states comprehensive plans to ensure access to alcohol and drug-treatment programs for traditionally underserved people. (Baseline data unavailable; p. 172.)

▼ Extend adoption of alcohol and drug policies for the work environment to at least 60% of worksites with 50 or more employees. (Baseline data unavailable; p. 174.)

HEALTHY PEOPLE 2000 OBJECTIVES

REAL LIFE
REAL CHOICES

Drugs and Parenthood: Making Responsible Choices

▼ Name: Barry Wolf
▼ Age: 44
▼ Occupation: architect

Anyone who grew up in the sixties can tell you it was quite a trip. Protest marches, communes, beads, beards, tie-dyeing, peace, love, harmony, drugs ... and more drugs. In that tumultuous time, the door of a giant pharmaceutical cabinet swung open, and there it all was: acid (LSD), horse (heroin), speed (amphetamines), 'ludes (Quaaludes, a barbiturate)—and everything in between, from airplane glue to hashish brownies.

Barry Wolf remembers. Before he started college in 1969, he'd already checked out some popular potions. He tried LSD and had the classic bad trip; took a turn with downers and slept through classes; and finally settled on good old garden-variety marijuana. Like countless other students, Barry loved to light up, mellow out, see the inner essence of wallpaper patterns, divine the true meaning of the lyrics of "Jumping Jack Flash" . . . and go on those freaked-out 2:00 AM convenience store raids in search of the world's biggest package of Ring-Dings.

Barry's 5-year architecture program was demanding and tough—no way to learn this exacting discipline while sleeping or stoned. He applied himself to his studies, smoked dope only on weekends, and graduated with a 3.5 GPA.

Today, more than 20 years later, Barry is a prosperous, sought-after architect. He has a solid marriage, two great daughters, and plenty of friends. And he still smokes dope. Never at work or in front of the kids; never while driving or drinking—just at gatherings of college friends, where they do *The Big Chill*: light up, listen to Jefferson Airplane, and reminisce about old wild times.

Barry's wife, Linda, smoked dope in college and quit when she graduated. She's disturbed about Barry's marijuana use and wants him to quit, for his own good and also because their preteen daughters need guidance from their parents on drug use. Barry says an occasional hit is no big deal, he's not hooked, and he'll quit when the kids are "older."

As you study this chapter, think about Barry's behavior and reasoning, and prepare yourself to answer the questions in **Your Turn** at the end of the chapter. ▼

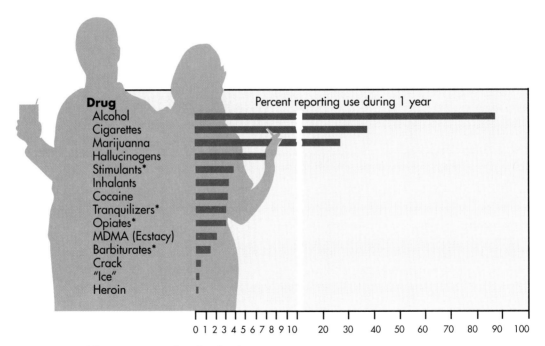

* Drug use was not under a doctor's orders.

Figure 7-1 Alcohol, cigarettes, marijuana, and hallucinogens are the four most common substances used by college students.

t is safe to say that in the mid 1990s drug use remains a significant problem for both college students and the general population. Alcohol is the major "problem drug" for most college students (see Chapter 8), but other drugs pose risks for certain students. (Some of these drugs are specified in the Healthy People 2000 Objectives.) Additionally, many nontraditional students see the impact of drug use in their neighborhoods and worry about their children being exploited by drugs and those who deal them.

ADDICTIVE BEHAVIOR

This chapter explores the health consequences of drug use, misuse, and abuse. Before talking about specific drugs, however, drug use should be put in the broader context of addictive behaviors. Experts in human behavior view drug use and abuse as just one of the many forms of addictive behaviors. Addictive behaviors include addictions to shopping, eating, gambling, sex, television, video games, and work, as well as addictions to alcohol, or other drugs.

The Process of Addiction

The process of developing an addiction has been a much studied topic. There seem to be three common aspects of addictive behaviors.

EXPOSURE

Initially, a person must be exposed to the drug or behavior. An addiction can begin after a person is exposed to a drug (such as alcohol) or a behavior (such as gambling) that he or she finds pleasurable. Perhaps this drug or behavior temporarily replaces an unpleasant feeling or sensation. The initial pleasure gradually (or in some cases quickly) becomes a focal point in the person's life.

COMPULSION

Increasingly more energy, time, and money are spent pursuing the drug or behavior. At this point in the addictive process, one can be said to have a compulsion for the drug or behavior. Frequently, repeated exposures to the drug or behavior continue despite negative consequences.

During the compulsion facet of the addictive behavior, a person's "normal" life is likely to degenerate while she or he searches for increased pleasures from the drug or the behavior. An addicted person's family life, circle of friends, work, or study patterns become less important than the search for increased "highs." The development of tolerance and withdrawal are distinct possibilities.

Why some persons seem to develop compulsions and others do not is difficult to pinpoint. Differences in genetic makeup, family dynamics, physiological processes, personality makeup, peer groups, and

Why People Use Drugs

★ Medication

★ To get high (a buzz)

★ To be cool

★ To get rid of pain

★ To experiment

★ Peer pressure

★ Family problems

★ To calm nerves

★ To get down

★ To escape

★ Because of friends

★ Because they like it

★ Because they are addicted

★ To work better

★ To be alert

★ Because they are bored

★ To hurt themselves

★ To hurt someone else

★ To get in a good mood

★ For a dare

★ Fear of stopping

★ To commit suicide

available resources for help may explain why some people become addicted and others do not.

LOSS OF CONTROL

Over time, the search for highs becomes an obsession with avoiding the effects of withdrawal from the drug or behavior. People lose their ability to control their behaviors. Despite overwhelming negative consequences (for example, loss of family and friends or loss of all financial resources), addicted people continue to behave in ways that make their lives worse. The person addicted to alcohol continues to drink heavily, the person addicted to shopping continues to run up heavy debts, and the person addicted to food continues to eat indiscriminately. These behaviors reflect a loss of control over one's life. Frequently, persons have addictions to more than one drug or behavior.

Intervention and Treatment

The good news for persons with addictive behaviors is that help is available. Within the last two decades, much attention has been focused on intervention and treatment for addictive behaviors. Many persons can be helped through programs such as those described at the end of this chapter. These programs often include inpatient or outpatient treatment, family counseling, and long-term aftercare counseling.

It is common for persons in aftercare treatment for addictive behaviors to belong to a self-help support group such as Alcoholics Anonymous, Gamblers Anonymous, or Sex Addicts Anonymous. These groups are often listed in the phonebook or the classified section of the newspaper.

DRUG TERMINOLOGY

Before discussing drug actions or drug behavior, you must first be familiar with some basic terminology. Much of this terminology has its origin in the field of *pharmacology,* or the study of the interaction of chemical agents with living material.

What does the term *drug* mean? Each of us may have different ideas about what a drug is. Although a number of definitions are available, we will consider a drug to be "any substance, natural or artificial, other than food, that by its chemical nature alters structure or function in the living organism."[4] Included in this broad definition are a variety of psychoactive drugs, medicines, and substances many people do not usually consider to be drugs.

Psychoactive (or *psychotropic*) **drugs** have the ability to alter the user's feelings, behaviors, perceptions, or moods. Psychoactive drugs include stimulants, depressants, hallucinogens, opiates, and inhalants. *Medicines* are drugs whose primary function is to heal unhealthy tissue. Medicines are also used to ease pain, prevent illness, and diagnose health conditions. Although some psychoactive drugs are consumed for medical reasons, as in the case of tranquilizers and some narcotics, the most commonly prescribed medicines are antibiotics, sulfa drugs, diuretics, oral contraceptives, and antihypertensive drugs. Substances not usually considered to be drugs (but which certainly are drugs) include caffeine, tobacco, alcohol, aspirin, and other over-the-counter (OTC) preparations. These common substances are used so frequently in our society that they are rarely perceived as true drugs.

For organizational reasons, this chapter primarily discusses psychoactive drugs. Alcohol, the most frequently used drug, is covered in Chapter 8. The effects of tobacco are discussed in Chapter 9. Prescription and OTC drugs and medicines are discussed at length in Chapter 17. Environmental pollutants are covered in Chapter 18.

Dependence

Psychoactive drugs have a strong potential for the development of **dependence.** When users take a psychoactive drug, the patterns of nervous system function are altered. If these altered functions provide perceived benefits for the user, drug use may continue, perhaps at increasingly larger dosages. If persistent use continues, the user can develop a dependence on the drug. Pharmacologists have identified two types of dependences—physical and psychological.

Persons can be said to have developed a *physical dependence* when their body cells have become reliant on a drug. Once this phenomenon has occurred, continued use of the drug is required, because body tissues have adapted to its presence.[5] Said in another way, the person's body needs the drug to maintain homeostasis, or dynamic balance. If the drug is not taken or is suddenly withdrawn, the user develops a characteristic **withdrawal illness** (abstinence syndrome). The symptoms of withdrawal reflect the attempt by the body's cells to regain normality without the drug. Withdrawal symptoms are always unpleasant (ranging from mild to severe irritability, depression, nervousness, digestive difficulties, and abdominal pain) and can be life threatening, as in the case of abrupt withdrawal from barbiturates or alcohol. The term *addiction* has been used interchangeably with physical dependence.

Continued use of most drugs can lead to the phenomenon of tolerance. **Tolerance** is an acquired reaction to a drug in which continued intake of the same dose has diminishing effects.[5] That is, the user needs more of a drug to receive the sensations felt previously at smaller doses. The continued use of depressants, including alcohol, and the opiates can cause users to quickly develop a tolerance to the drug.

College seniors who have engaged in 4 years of beer drinking can usually recognize tolerance occurring in their own bodies. Many such students can vividly recall their initial and subsequent sensations after drinking. For example, five beers consumed during a freshman social gathering might well have resulted in inebriation, but if the same students continued to drink beer regularly for 4 years, five beers would probably fail to produce the response they experienced as freshmen. Perhaps seven or eight beers would be needed to produce such a response. Clearly they would have developed a tolerance to alcohol.

Furthermore, tolerance developed for one drug may carry over to another drug within the same general category. This phenomenon is known as **cross-tolerance.** The heavy abuser of alcohol might require a larger dose of a preoperative sedative to become relaxed before surgery. The tolerance to alcohol "crosses over" to the other depressant drug.

Persons who possess strong desires to continue the use of a particular drug are said to have developed *psychological dependence.* People who are psychologically dependent on a drug think they need to consume the drug to maintain a sense of well-being. They crave the drug for emotional reasons, in spite of having persistent or recurrent physical, social, psychological, or occupational problems that are caused or worsened by the use of drugs. Abrupt withdrawal of a drug by these persons would not initiate the fully expressed withdrawal illness, although minor symptoms of withdrawal might be experienced. The term *habituation* is often used interchangeably with psychological dependence.

Drugs whose use can relatively quickly lead to both physical and psychological dependence are the depressants (barbiturates, tranquilizers, and alcohol), narcotics (the opiates: derivatives of the Oriental poppy—heroin, morphine, and codeine), and synthetic narcotics (Demerol and Methadone). Drugs whose use can lead only to various degrees of psychological dependence are the stimulants (amphetamines, caffeine, and, perhaps, cocaine), hallucinogens (LSD, peyote, mescaline, and marijuana), and inhalants (glues, gases, and petroleum products).

Drug Misuse and Abuse

So far in the chapter we have used the term *use (user)* in association with the taking of psychoactive drugs. At this point, however, it is important to both define use and to introduce the terms *misuse* and *abuse*.[5] By doing so we can more accurately describe the ways in which drugs are used.

The term *use* is an all-encompassing term that is used to describe drug taking in the most general way. For example, Americans use drugs of many types. The term *use* can also encompass the constructs of misuse and abuse. It is in this regard that we will most often employ the word.

The term **misuse** will be confined to the inappropriate use of legal drugs intended to be medications. Misuse may occur when a patient misunderstands the directions for use of a prescription or over-the-counter (OTC) drug or when a patient shares a prescription with a friend or family member for whom the drug was not prescribed. Misuse also occurs when a patient takes the prescription or OTC drug for a purpose or condition other than that for which it was intended or at a dosage other than that recommended.

The term **abuse** applies to any use of an illicit drug or any use of a legal drug when it is detrimental to health and well-being. The costs of drug abuse to the individual are extensive and include effects such as absenteeism and underachievement, loss of job, marital instability, loss of self-esteem, serious illnesses, and even death.

THE DYNAMICS OF THE ADDICTIVE PERSONALITY

Although the list that appears in the star box on p. 163 provides some insights as to why people use drugs, Figure 7-2 can further expand our understanding of this question. We must conclude from the appearance of Figure 7-2 that the answer is complicated.

There are many factors that influence drug-taking behavior, including individual factors, immediate environmental factors, and factors that are more global in origin. Specific aspects of each are discussed in this section.

Influence of Individual Factors

In the case of the individual, genetic predisposition, personality traits, attitudes and beliefs, interpersonal skills, and unmet developmental needs can form the basis of drug use.

GENETIC PREDISPOSITION

The importance of *genetic predisposition* (inherited vulnerability) to drug use has not been fully delineated. However, studies of alcoholics have demonstrated that genetic factors do play some role in the development of alcoholism.[6] Research on genetic predisposition to the abuse of other drugs is much further behind that for alcohol.

---

psychoactive (sye ko **act** ive) **drug** any substance capable of altering one's feelings, moods, or perceptions.

dependence general term that reflects the need to keep consuming a drug for psychological or physical reasons, or both.

withdrawal illness uncomfortable, perhaps toxic response of the body as it attempts to maintain homeostasis in the absence of a drug; also called abstinence syndrome.

---

tolerance an acquired reaction to a drug; continued intake of the same dose has diminishing effects.

cross-tolerance transfer of tolerance from one drug to another within the same general category.

misuse inappropriate use of legal drugs intended to be medications.

abuse any use of an illicit drug or the use of a legal drug when it is detrimental to health.

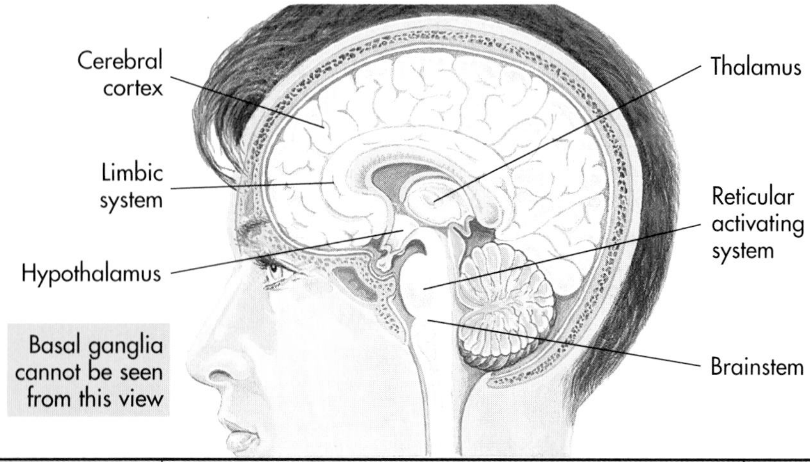

Neuro-anatomy	Function	Drug agents
Reticular activating system	Old sensory system—activates cortex in response to incoming stimuli	1+ 2- 3-
Hypothalmus	Control center for autonomic nervous system—interfaces CNS/ANS with endocrine system via pituitary gland	2- 3-
Brainstem	Control of vital funtions (respiration, cardiac, blood pressure)—houses reticular activating systems, sleep/wake center, coordination of motor functions	1+ 2- 3-
Cerebral cortex	Higher intellectual funtion, learning higher motor functions, elaboration (association) of sensory information	1+ 2- 4+
Basal ganglia	Execution of semiautonomic motor activity (body language)	3-
Thalamus	Two-gate controlling interchange among all CNS centers	2- 3- 4+
Limbic system	Connects cortex to thalamus—control of emotional states	3- 4-

Key: 1 Stimulates; 2 Depressants; 3 Opiates; 4 Halluciogens; 5 Inhalants*
+ Enhances normal level of function
- Decreased normal level of function
* Because of the variety of pharmacological agents delivered as inhalants (anesthetics, toxic solvents), no general influence can be assigned.

Figure 7-2 Psychoactive drugs alter the function of the brain and nervous system. (Refer to the key at the bottom of the chart for the corresponding drug agents.)

PERSONALITY TRAITS, ATTITUDES, AND BELIEFS

Although drug-taking behavior cannot always be predicted strictly on the basis of personality type, correlations have been noted with certain aspects of personality (or temperament). For example, children who are easily bored and need constant activity and challenge are more likely to engage in drug-taking behavior. A similar trend is seen in children who are driven to avoid negative consequences for their actions and who crave immediate external reward for their efforts. Clusters of traits (as measured by personality inventories) including rebelliousness, rejection of behavioral norms, resistance to authority, and a high tolerance for deviance are also reported in drug abusers.

The reader should be cautioned that a cause and effect relationship between personality and drug-taking behavior is difficult to prove. Perhaps, rather than a particular personality profile fostering drug abuse, the abuse of drugs (for other reasons) creates the personality traits described.

INTERPERSONAL SKILLS AND DEVELOPMENTAL TASK MASTERY

In addition to the personality traits and attitudinal stances described, drug abusers are usually deficient in interpersonal skills. They are very likely to score lower on tests that measure well-being, tolerance of others, and achievement. They also often demonstrate lower levels of self-esteem than those who do not abuse drugs. Again, the question of cause and effect must be raised.

The process of growth and development, at all stages of adult life, is supported by the successful accomplishment of daily undertakings.[7] When persons are lacking, for whatever reasons, in positive experiences in school, employment, parenting, and varied aspects of community involvement, they may attempt to compensate through chronic, heavy drug use. Of course, drug abuse removes them further from the involvement that is required for productive and satisfying growth and development, thus increasing compensatory use of drugs.

Influences of the Immediate Environment

Drug-taking behavior can be fostered by factors outside the individual, including the immediate environment. The immediate environment includes home and family, school, peers, and community.

HOME AND FAMILY

It has been suggested that when drug abuse begins in childhood, it is often associated with the home environment.[5] Children appear to be at greater risk when parents exhibit poor management skills, antisocial behavior, and even criminality. These families are often disorganized and have poorly defined roles for both parenting and being a productive member of society. In too many cases, adult family members abuse drugs themselves or tolerate others who do. As with tobacco use (see Chapter 9), parents can be the best (or worst) models that children can have.[8]

 Family Socialization and the Abuse of Drugs[5]

The family is one of the most important factors influencing drug-taking behavior. Adolescents who are likely to abuse drugs often come from families who foster the abuse of drugs. Listed below are contrasting patterns of child rearing.

"Traditional" or status-centered	"Modern" or person-centered
Each member's place in family is a function of age and sex status	Emphasis on selfhood and individuality of each member
Father is defined as boss and, more important, as agent of discipline. He receives "respect" and deference from mother and children	Father is more affectionate, less authoritative; mother becomes more important as agent of discipline
Emphasis on overt acts—what child does rather than why	Emphasis on motives and feelings—why child does what he does
Valued qualities of child are obedience and cleanliness	Values qualities of child are happiness, achievement, consideration, curiosity, self-control
Emphasis on "direct" discipline: physical punishment, scolding, threats	Discipline based in reasoning, isolation, guilt, threat of loss of love
Social consensus and solidarity in communication; emphasis on "we"	Communication used to express individual experience and perspectives; emphasis on "I"
Emphasis on communication from parent to child	Emphasis on two-way communication between parent and child; parent open to persuasion
Parent feels little need to justify demands to child; commands are followed with "because I say so"	Parent gives good reasons for demands: not "Shut up" but "Please keep quiet or go into the other room; I'm trying to talk on the telephone"
Emphasis on conforming to rules, respecting authority, maintaining conventional social order	Emphasis on reasons for rules; particular rules can be criticized in the name of "higher" rational or ethical principles
Child may attain a strong sense of social identity at the cost of loss of individuality and poor academic performance	Child may attain strong sense of selfhood but may have identity problems and feel guilt, alienation

Which pattern do you think would contribute most effectively to minimizing the abuse of drugs? Would a combination of patterns be even more effective? ★

SCHOOL

Children from disorganized or socially maladjusted families frequently have more difficulty adjusting to the organized environment of the school. The following chain of events has been suggested to explain the relationship of poor home environment and weak academic performance to drug abuse. An undesirable home environment contributes to poor school performance and poor social development. Failure at school leads to loss of self-esteem, aggressive behavior, and loss of interest in school. These factors, in turn, may foster truancy and drug experimentation during the later grades.

PEERS

A clear relationship exists between peer group drug-taking behavior and the drug-taking behavior of individual members.[5] It is unusual for a student to remain an active member of a peer group that is involved in drug-taking behavior and still abstain from using drugs. Certainly, to both abstain from and condone drug use would be highly unusual.

Conversely, when adolescent peer groups become involved in drug prevention activities (such as SADD), they are often successful in reducing the drug use in that school setting.

COMMUNITY

Each community varies in regard to drug availability, drug enforcement, drug education, and drug treatment and rehabilitation. As a consequence, drug abuse rates may differ from community to community on the basis of these factors. Nontraditional students who are parents may in particular be interested in assessing the degree to which their communities foster drug-taking behavior.

Influences within the Larger Society

Factors such as the existence of a youth subculture, modeling and advertising, and even technological advances influence drug-taking behavior.

YOUTH SUBCULTURE

For many reasons, there exists in this country (and in many other areas of the world) a distinct youth subculture (approximately ages 12-17). This subculture has its own expectations, roles, and standards, as well as its language, dress codes, and behaviors. Drug abuse was traditionally assumed to be higher in this group than in any other segment of American society.

Regardless of the recognition that the youth subculture receives, the perception that drug abuse is most severe in this group is not supported by research. A recent study indicates that higher levels of drug abuse occur in 18- to 34-year-olds.[9] Nevertheless, the abuse of drugs that does occur in the youth subculture is of concern, because patterns that are established at a

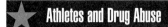

Athletes and Drug Abuse

Student athletes may be more susceptible to drug abuse than other students because of the stress they encounter. This stress arises from a unique combination of pressures from those outside, as well as stresses imposed by the student athletes themselves. In both college and high school, they may attempt to cope by turning to drugs. What specific components of these demands make drugs attractive as an initial coping strategy?

★ *High visibility* Continuous monitoring by fans, coaches, teammates, and other students allows little opportunity for student athletes to correct their mistakes. Thus they relentlessly strive toward flawless performances.

★ *Demands* Coaches, administrators, academic advisors, and fans are vigilant in noting academic performance. Simultaneously, parents, friends, and teachers expect student athletes to be unaffected by the pressure and behave like their nonathlete classmates.

★ *Improvements* Expectations to continuously improve as more stringently applied to student athletes. The stress of a plateau or poor performance may encourage them to abuse drugs.

★ *Limitations of time* The end of school, lessening eligibility, and serious injuries can limit the careers of student athletes to a few short years. When the curtain falls, the need to quickly fill the void is often forceful.

★ *Physical prowess* Initial gains mask the negative effects of drug abuse longer for student athletes than for nonathletes. Thus use may continue until dependence is firmly established.

★ *Separation* Student athletes spend much more time away from family and nonathlete friends, and drug use may compensate for this isolation.

★ *Media exposure* When drug abuse is established in student athletes, fear of media exposure may hinder movement into treatment. Failure to obtain effective early intervention may worsen the degree of dependence.

These combined factors, among others, enhance the possibility of drug abuse by today's student athletes. ★

young age carry into later life. In fact, during this period, experimentation with **gateway drugs** (nicotine, alcohol, and marijuana) begins, leading to the possible abuse of illicit drugs later. Specific Healthy People 2000 Objectives are targeted toward this age group.

MODELING AND ADVERTISING

The influence that others have on us by example of their own behavior is referred to as *modeling.* Modeling within the family and peer group regarding drug-taking behavior has already been presented. However, the modeling that occurs in conjunction with drug use by movie stars, musicians, and professional athletes exerts its own powerful influences on children and adolescents.

When models are employed by the media to sell products, advertising becomes an important factor in fostering drug-taking behavior. The marketing of tobacco and alcohol products is perhaps the best example of the influential use of modeling in advertising. "Beautiful people" are depicted enjoying a social drug (alcohol, coffee, tea, tobacco) in pleasant surroundings that some viewers can only hope to experience. Well-known celebrities participate in events sponsored by alcohol or tobacco companies. Company logos are seen on almost every item that appears on television, including the clothing and equipment of the participants, outfield walls, scoreboards, and race cars. Scenes of affluence and sexuality also abound.

TECHNOLOGICAL ADVANCES

The ability of people to engage in medical self-care makes drug-taking behavior easier and more socially acceptable than in the past. In a society conditioned by the effectiveness and availability of OTC and prescription medications, the use of other drugs, both legal and illicit, to "make ourselves feel better" seems more reasonable than ever before. It is in conjunction with this attitude that the self-care arena fosters drug misuse and, for some, drug abuse.

DRUG IMPACT ON THE CENTRAL NERVOUS SYSTEM

To better understand the disruption caused by the actions of psychoactive drugs, a general knowledge of the normal functioning of the nervous system's basic unit, the **neuron,** is required. Stimuli from the internal or external environment are received by the appropriate sensory receptor, perhaps an organ such as an eye or an ear.

Once sensed, these stimuli are converted into electrical impulses. These impulses are then directed along the neuron's **dendrite,** through the cell body, and along the **axon** toward the *synaptic junction* near an adjacent neuron. On arrival at the **synapse,** the electrical impulses stimulate the production and release of chemical messengers called *neurotransmitters.*[11] These neurotransmitters "transfer" the electrical impulses from one neuron to the dendrites of adjoining neurons. Thus neurons function in a coordinated fashion to send information to the brain for interpretation and to relay appropriate response commands outward to the tissues of the body.

The role of neurotransmitters is critically important to the transfer of information within the system. A substance that has the ability to alter some aspect of transmitter function holds the potential for causing a major disruption to the otherwise normally functioning system. Psychoactive drugs are capable of exerting these disruptive influences on the neurotransmitters. Drugs "work" by changing the way neurotransmitters work, often by blocking the production of a neurotransmitter or forcing the continued release of a neurotransmitter (see the box on p. 170).

DRUG CLASSIFICATIONS

Drugs can be categorized by the nature of the physiological effect they exert. Most drugs fall into one of six general categories: stimulants, depressants, hallucinogens, cannabis, narcotics, and inhalants (Table 7-1).

Stimulants

In general, **stimulants** excite or increase the activity of the central nervous system (CNS). Also called "uppers," stimulants alert the CNS by increasing heart rate, blood pressure, and brain function. Users feel uplifted and less fatigued. Examples of stimulant drugs include caffeine, amphetamines, and cocaine. Stimulants produce psychological dependence and tolerance relatively quickly, but they seem incapable of producing significant physical dependence when judged by life-threatening withdrawal symptoms.

---

gateway drugs easily obtained legal or illegal drugs (alcohol, tobacco, marijuana) whose use may precede the use of less common illegal drugs.

neuron (noor on) a nerve cell.

dendrite (den drite) portion of a neuron that receives electrical stimuli from adjacent neurons; neurons typically have several such branches or extensions.

axon (ax on) portion of a neuron that conducts electrical impulses to the dendrites of adjacent neurons; neurons typically have one axon.

synapse (sinn aps) location at which an electrical impulse from one neuron is transmitted to an adjacent neuron; also referred to as a synaptic junction.

stimulants (stim you lants) psychoactive drugs that stimulate the function of the central nervous system.

Drug Impact on the Central Nervous System

This illustration depicts the disruption caused by the actions of psychoactive drugs on the central nervous system.
(1) Neurotransmitters are chemical messengers that transfer electrical impulses across the synapse between nerve cells.
(2) Psychoactive drugs disrupt this process, thus interrupting the coordinated functioning of the nervous system.[10] ★

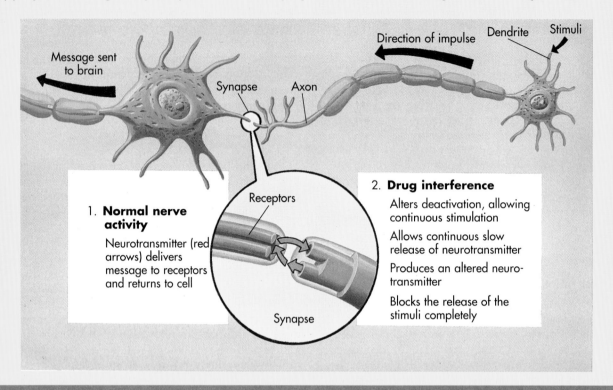

TABLE 7-1   **Psychoactive Drug Categories**

Drugs	Trade or common names	Medical uses	Possible effects
Stimulants			
Cocaine*	Coke, flake, snow, crack	Local anesthetic	Increased alertness, excitation, euphoria, increased pulse rate and blood pressure, insomnia, loss of appetite
Amphetamines	Biphetamine, Delcobese, Desoxyn, Dexedrine, mediatric, methamphetamine (ice)	Hyperactivity, narcolepsy, weight control	
Phendimetrazine	Prelu-2		
Methylphenidate	Ritalin, Methidate		
Other stimulants	Adipex, Bacarate, Cylert, Didrex, Ionamin, Plegine, PreSate, Sanorex, Tenuate, Tepanil, Voranil		
Depressants			
Chloral hydrate	Noctec, Somnos	Hypnotic	Slurred speech, disorientation, drunken behavior without odor of alcohol
Barbiturates	Amobarbital, Butisol, Phenobarbital, Phenoxbarbital, Secobarbital, Tuinal	Anesthetic, anticonvulsant, sedative, hypnotic	
Glutethimide	Doriden	Sedative, hypnotic	

*Designated a narcotic under the Controlled Substances Act.
†Not designated a narcotic under the Controlled Substances Act.

TABLE 7-1 Psychoactive Drug Categories—cont'd

Drugs	Trade or common names	Medical uses	Possible effects
Depressants—cont'd			
Methaqualone	Optimil, Parest, Quaalude, Somnafec, Sopor	Sedative, hypnotic	Slurred speech, disorientation, drunken behavior without odor of alcohol
Benzodiazepines	Ativan, Azene, Clonopin, Dalmane, Diazepam, Librium, Serax, Tranxene, Valium, Verstran	Anti-anxiety, anticonvulsant, sedative, hypnotic	
Other depressants	Equanil, Miltown, Noludar, Placidyl, Valmid	Anti-anxiety, sedative, hypnotic	
Hallucinogens			
LSD	Acid, microdot	None	Illusions and hallucinations, poor perception of time and distance
Mescaline and peyote	Mesc, buttons, cactus	None	
Amphetamine variants (designer drugs)	2,5-DMA, DOM, DOP, MDA, MDMA, PMA, STP, TMA	None	
Phencyclidine	Angel dust, Hog, PCP	Veterinary anesthetic	
Phencyclidine analogs	PCE, PCPy, TCP	None	
Other hallucinogens	Bufotenin, DMT, DET, Ibogaine, psilocybin, psilocyn	None	
Cannabis			
Marijuana	Acapulco gold, grass, pot, reefer, sinsemilla, Thai sticks	Under investigation	Euphoria, relaxed inhibitions, increased appetite, disoriented behavior
Tetrahydrocannabinol	THC	Under investigation	
Hashish	Hash	None	
Hashish oil	Hash oil	None	
Narcotics			
Opium	Dover's powder, Paregoric, Parapectolin	Analgesic, antidiarrheal	Euphoria, drowsiness, respiratory depression, constricted pupils, nausea
Morphine	Morphine, Pectoal syrup	Analgesic, antitussive	
Codeine	Codeine, Empirin compound with Codeine, Robitussin A-C	Analgesic, antitussive	
Heroin	Diacetylmorphine, horse, smack	Under investigation	
Hydromorphone	Dilaudid	Analgesic	
Meperidine (pethidine)	Demerol, Pethadol	Analgesic	
Methadone	Dolophine, Methadone, Methadose	Analgeisc, heroin substitute	
Other narcotics	Darvon,† Dromoran, Fentanyl, LAAM, Leitine, Levo-Dromoran, Percodan, Tussionex, Talwin,† Lomotil	Analgesic, antidiarrheal, antitussive	
Inhalants			
Anesthetic gases	Aerosols, petroleum products, solvents	Surgical anesthesia	Intoxication, excitation, disorientation, aggression, hallucination, variable effects
Vasodilators (amyl nitrite, butyl nitrite)	Aerosols, petroleum products, solvents	None	

*Designated a narcotic under the Controlled Substances Act.
†Not designated a narcotic under the Controlled Substances Act.

CAFFEINE

Caffeine, the tasteless drug found in chocolate, some soft drinks, coffee, tea, some aspirin products, and OTC "stay-awake" pills is a relatively harmless stimulant when consumed in moderate amounts (Table 7-2). Many coffee drinkers could not start the day successfully without the benefit of a cup or two of coffee in the morning.

Pregnant women are advised to consume caffeine sparingly.[12] For the average healthy adult, however, moderate consumption of caffeine is unlikely to pose any serious health effects. However, excessive consumption (equivalent to 10 or more cups of coffee daily) could lead to anxiety, diarrhea, restlessness, delayed onset of sleep or frequent awakening, headache, and heart palpitations.

AMPHETAMINES

Amphetamines produce an increase in activity and elevation in mood in almost all users. The amphetamines include several closely related compounds: amphetamine, dextroamphetamine, and methamphetamine. These compounds do not have any natural sources and are completely manufactured in the laboratory. Medical use of amphetamines is limited primarily to the treatment of obesity, **narcolepsy,** and **attention deficit disorder (ADD).**

Amphetamines are effectively ingested, injected, snorted, or inhaled. At low-to-moderate doses, amphetamines elevate mood and increase alertness and feelings of energy by stimulating receptor sites for two naturally occurring neurotransmitters. They also decrease activities of the stomach and intestine and decrease hunger. At high doses, amphetamines can increase heart rate and blood pressure to dangerous levels. As amphetamines are eliminated from the body, feelings of tiredness are experienced.

When used in a chronic abusive fashion, amphetamines produce rapid tolerance and strong psychological dependence. Other chronic effects include impotence and episodes of psychosis. Once chronic use is discontinued, periods of depression may develop.

Today the abuse of amphetamines is a more pressing concern than it has been in the recent past. Underlying this upturn in abuse is methamephetamine. Known by a variety of names, including "ice," "crystal," "meth," "speed," "crystal meth," and "Zip," methamphetamine is produced in illegal laboratories, primarily in the western states.

TABLE 7-2   Caffeine content of beverages, food, and drug preparations

Coffee (5 oz cup)	Caffeine (mg)	Soft drinks (12 oz)	Caffeine (mg)	Pain relievers	Caffeine (mg)
Drip method	110-150	Mountain Dew	54	Anacin	32
Percolated	64-124	Mello Yello	52	Excedrin	65
Instant	40-108	TAB	46	Midol	32
Decaffeinated	2-5	Coca-Cola	46	Plain aspirin	0
		Diet Coke	46	Vanquish	33
Tea (5 oz cup)		Shasta Cola	44		
1-min brew	9-33	Mr. Pibb	40	**Diuretics**	
3-min brew	20-46	Dr. Pepper	40	Aqua Ban	100
5-min brew	20-50	Sugar-free Dr. Pepper	40		
Instant tea	12-28	Pepsi Cola	38	**Cold remedies**	
Iced tea (12 oz)	22-36	Diet Pepsi	36	Coryban-D	30
		Pepsi Light	36	Dristan	0
Cocoa				Triaminicin	30
		Stimulants			
Made from mix	6			**Weight-control aids**	
Milk chocolate (1 oz)	6	NoDoz tablets	100	Dexatrim	200
Baking chocolate	35	Vivarin tablets	200	Prolamine	140
				Prescription pain relievers	
				Cafergot	100
				Darvon Compound	32
				Fiorinal	40
				Migralam	100

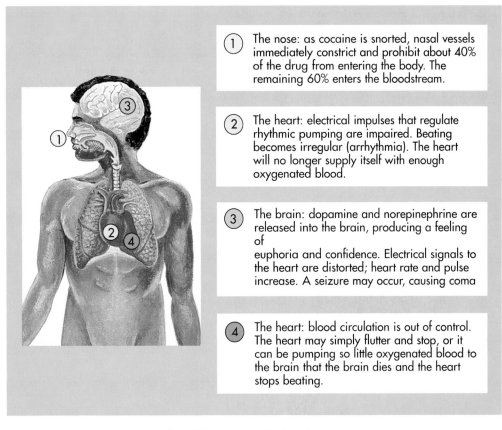

1. The nose: as cocaine is snorted, nasal vessels immediately constrict and prohibit about 40% of the drug from entering the body. The remaining 60% enters the bloodstream.

2. The heart: electrical impulses that regulate rhythmic pumping are impaired. Beating becomes irregular (arrhythmia). The heart will no longer supply itself with enough oxygenated blood.

3. The brain: dopamine and norepinephrine are released into the brain, producing a feeling of
euphoria and confidence. Electrical signals to the heart are distorted; heart rate and pulse increase. A seizure may occur, causing coma

4. The heart: blood circulation is out of control. The heart may simply flutter and stop, or it can be pumping so little oxygenated blood to the brain that the brain dies and the heart stops beating.

Figure 7-3 Cocaine's effect on the body.

Ice

"Crystal meth," or "ice," is among the most recent and potentially dangerous forms of methamphetamine. First appearing in Hawaii, ice is a very pure form of methamphetamine that looks like rock candy. When smoked, the effects of "ice" are felt in about 7 seconds as a wave of intense physical and psychological exhilaration. This effect lasts for several hours (much longer than the effects of crack) until the user becomes physically exhausted. Chronic use leads to nutritional difficulties, weight loss, reduced resistance to infection, and damage to the liver, lungs, and kidneys. Psychological dependence is quickly established. Withdrawal results in acute depression and fatigue but not physical discomfort.

COCAINE

Cocaine, perhaps the strongest of the stimulant drugs, has received much media attention. Cocaine is the primary psychoactive substance found in the leaves of the South American coca plant. The effects of cocaine are of short duration—from 5 to 30 minutes (Figure 7-3). Regardless of the form in which it is consumed, cocaine produces an immediate near-orgasmic "rush," or feeling of exhilaration. This euphoria is quickly followed by a period of marked depression. Used occa-

sionally as a topical anesthetic, today cocaine is generally inhaled (snorted), injected, or smoked (as freebase or crack). There is overwhelming scientific evidence to indicate that users quickly develop a strong psychological dependence to cocaine. There is considerable evidence that physical dependence is also quickly developed. However, cocaine's physical dependence is not a form that leads to death upon withdrawal.

The recent status of cocaine as a substitute for amphetamines (during the 1960s), as a recreational drug for the wealthy (during the 1970s), and as a widely abused drug by many segments of society (during the 1980s) is well documented. Most recently, cocaine use has decreased, although heavy use has increased. Today, freebasing and the use of crack cocaine have re-

narcolepsy (nar co lep see) sleep-related disorder in which a person has a recurrent, overwhelming, and uncontrollable desire to sleep.

attention deficit (def uh sit) **disorder (ADD)** above-normal physical movement; often accompanied by an inability to concentrate well on a specified task; also called hyperactivity.

placed the inhalation of "lines" of cocaine, which was the primary route of administration in the 1980s.

Freebasing

Freebasing and the use of *crack* cocaine represent the most recent techniques for maximizing the psychoactive effects of the drug. Freebasing first requires the common form of powdered cocaine (cocaine hydrochloride) to be chemically altered (alkalized). This altered form is then dissolved in a solvent, such as ether or benzene. This liquid solution is heated to evaporate the solvent. The heating process leaves the freebase cocaine in a powder form that can then be smoked, often through a waterpipe. Because of the large surface area of the lungs, smoking cocaine facilitates fast absorption into the bloodstream.

One danger in freebasing cocaine is the risk related to the solvents used. Ether is a highly volatile solvent capable of exploding and causing serious burns. Benzene is a known carcinogen associated with the development of leukemia. Clearly, neither solvent can be used without increasing the level of risk normally associated with cocaine use. This method of making smokeable cocaine led to a new epidemic of cocaine use, smoking crack.

Crack

In contrast to freebase cocaine, crack is obtained by combining cocaine hydrochloride with common baking soda. When this pastelike mixture is allowed to dry, a small rocklike crystalline material remains. This crack is heated in the bowl of a small pipe, and the va-

The Cocaine Pipeline

Colombia is the pipeline that supplies approximately 75% of the cocaine entering the United States and links the drug markets of North and South America. ★

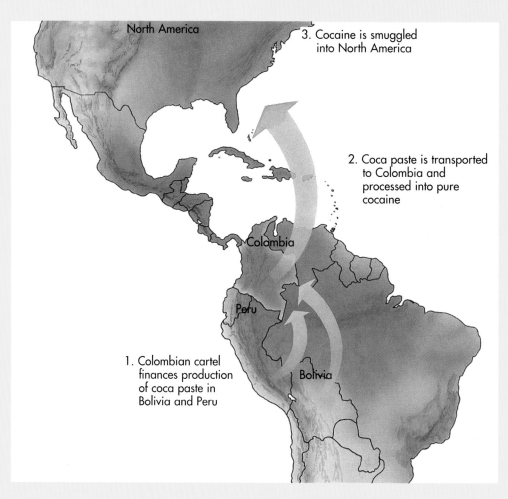

North America

3. Cocaine is smuggled into North America

2. Coca paste is transported to Colombia and processed into pure cocaine

Colombia

Peru

1. Colombian cartel finances production of coca paste in Bolivia and Peru

Bolivia

pors are inhaled into the lungs. Currently a single dose of crack sells for $10 to $20. Some crack users spend hundreds of dollars a day to maintain their habit.

The influence of crack is almost instantaneous. Within 10 seconds after inhalation, cocaine reaches the CNS and influences the action of several neurotransmitters at specific sites in the brain. As with use of other forms of cocaine, convulsions, seizures, respiratory distress, and cardiac failure have been reported with this sudden, extensive stimulation of the nervous system.

Within about 6 minutes, the stimulating effect of crack is completely expended, and users frequently enter into a state of depression. Dependence develops within a few weeks since users consume more crack in response to the short duration of stimulation and rapid onset of depression.

Intravenous administration has been the preferred route for cocaine abusers who are also regular abusers of heroin and other injectable drugs. Intravenous in-

jections result in an almost immediate high, or rush, which lasts about 10 minutes. A "smoother ride" is said to be obtained from a "speedball," the injectable mixture of heroin and cocaine (or methamphetamine).[5]

Cocaine and society

It is beyond the scope of this book to chronicle the way in which cocaine use has profoundly damaged our nation. However, we encourage students to watch or read the media reports that cover this topic on a daily basis. A few of the central reasons why civic and government leaders have declared war on the use of illicit drugs, especially cocaine, follow.

Although cocaine use hurts people from all walks of life, it most critically affects inner city minorities and the urban poor.[13] Cocaine use provides an instant, temporary escape from an unpromising future. For many inner-city youths, selling cocaine (crack) is the easiest way to escape poverty. However, drug dealing also brings with it an escalation in street gangs, crime, and

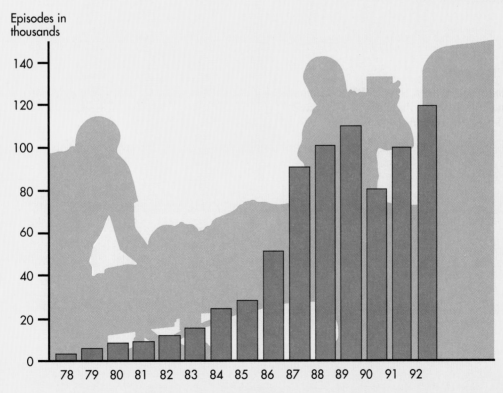

★ Cocaine-Related Hospital Emergency Room Episodes

Despite decreases in the overall number of cocaine users among Americans, heavy cocaine use remains a major drug problem. This is reflected in the continued increase in the number of hospital emergency room episodes related to cocaine use. In 1990 there were 80,400 episodes; in 1991 there were 101,200 episodes; and in 1992 there were 119,800 episodes. ★

Trends in cocaine-related emergency room episodes.

P E R S O N A L   A S S E S S M E N T

To assess whether you may be experiencing the symptoms of drug abuse, circle **Y** for yes and **N** for no.

1. A sudden increase or loss of appetite or sudden weight loss or gain.   Y   N
2. Moodiness, depression, irritability, or withdrawal.   Y   N
3. Disorientation, lack of concentration, or forgetfulness.   Y   N
4. Frequent use of eye drops or inappropriate wearing of sunglasses.   Y   N
5. Disruption or change in sleep patterns or a lack of energy.   Y   N
6. Borrowing money more and more, working excessive hours, selling personal items,
   or experiencing an incident of stealing or shoplifting.   Y   N
7. Persistent and frequent nosebleeds, sniffles, coughs, and other signs of upper
   respiratory infection.   Y   N
8. Change in speech patterns or vocabulary or a deterioration in academic performance.   Y   N
9. Feeling ill at ease with family members and other adults.   Y   N
10. Neglect of personal appearance.   Y   N

INTERPRETATION

A yes response to more than three questions indicates that there may be drug dependence, and professional help should be obtained.

TO CARRY THIS FURTHER . . .

See the box on p. 182 and the Health Reference Guide at the back of this text for information about national groups and hot lines for drug abuse. They will help you obtain additional information about drug dependence and how to combat it.

violence.[14] Crack houses are also notorious for the spread of HIV infection and other serious diseases. Tragically, a high percentage of babies born in large city hospitals are addicted to cocaine and have both physical and neurological difficulties. Some are born with HIV infection that soon leads to AIDS. Indeed the personal and social decay is enormous.

Depressants

Depressants (or sedatives) tend to sedate or slow down CNS function. Drugs included in this category are alcohol, barbiturates, and tranquilizers. Depressants produce tolerance in abusers, as well as strong psychological and physical dependence. (For a discussion of alcohol, see Chapter 8.)

BARBITURATES

Barbiturates are the so-called sleeping compounds that function by enhancing the effect of inhibitory neurotransmitters. They depress the CNS to the point where the user drops off to sleep or—as is the case with surgical anesthetics—the patient becomes anesthetized. Medically, barbiturates are used in widely varied dosages as anesthetics and for treatment of anxiety, insomnia, and epilepsy.[4] Regular use of a barbiturate quickly produces tolerance—even to the point where such a high dosage is required that the user finds that the drug effects linger through the next morning. Some abusers then begin to alternate barbiturates with stimulants, producing a vicious cycle of dependence. Other misusers combine alcohol and barbiturates or tranquilizers, inadvertently producing toxic, even lethal results—as was the fate of Marilyn Monroe. Abrupt withdrawal from barbiturate use frequently produces a withdrawal syndrome that can involve seizures, delusions, hallucinations, and even death.

Methaqualone (Quaalude, "ludes," Sopor) was developed as a sedative that would not have the dependence properties of other barbiturates.[4] Although this did not happen, Quaaludes were occasionally prescribed for anxious patients. Today compounds resembling Quaaludes are manufactured in home laboratories and illegally sold as products to combine with small amounts of alcohol for an inexpensive, drunklike effect.

TRANQUILIZERS

Tranquilizers are depressants that are intended to reduce anxiety and to relax persons who are having problems coping with the stressors of life. They are not specifically designed to produce sleep but rather to help people cope during their waking hours. Such tranquilizers are termed *minor tranquilizers,* of which diazepam (Valium) and chlordiazepoxide (Librium) may be the most commonly prescribed examples.

Some tranquilizers are further designed to control hospitalized psychotic patients who have suicidal tendencies or who are potential threats to others. These *major tranquilizers* subdue people physically but permit them to remain conscious. Their use is generally limited to institutional settings. All tranquilizers can produce physical and psychological dependence and tolerance.

Hallucinogens

As the name suggests, hallucinogenic drugs produce hallucinations—perceived distortions of reality. Also known as *psychedelic* drugs or *phantasticants,* **hallucinogens** reached their height of popularity during the 1960s. At that time young people were encouraged to use hallucinogenic drugs to "expand the mind," "reach an altered state," or "discover reality." Not all of the reality distortions, or "trips," were pleasant. Many users reported "bummers," or trips of negative, frightful distortions.

Hallucinogenic drugs include laboratory-produced lysergic acid diethylamide (LSD), mescaline (from the peyote cactus plant), and psilocybin (from a particular genus of mushroom). Consumption of hallucinogens seems to produce not physical dependence but rather mild levels of psychological dependence. The development of tolerance is questionable. *Synesthesia,* a process in which users report "hearing a color, smelling music, or touching a taste," is sometimes produced with hallucinogen use.

The long-term effects of hallucinogenic drug misuse and abuse are not fully understood. Questions about genetic abnormalities in offspring, *fecundity,* sex drive and performance, and the development of personality disorders have not been fully answered. One phenomenon that has been identified and documented is the development of *flashbacks*—the unpredictable return to a psychedelic trip that occurred months or even years earlier. Flashbacks are thought to result from the accumulation of a drug within body cells.

LSD

The most well-known hallucinogen is lysergic acid diethylamide (LSD). LSD is a drug that helped define the counterculture movement in the 1960s. In the 1970s and the 1980s, this drug lost considerable popularity. However, in the 1990s LSD is making a comeback, with some studies showing about one in ten high school students and one in twenty college students

hallucinogens (huh **loose** in oh jens) psychoactive drugs capable of producing hallucinations (distortions of reality).

have experimented with LSD. Fear of cocaine and other powerful drugs, boredom, low cost, and an attempt to revisit the culture of the '60s are thought to have increased LSD's attractiveness to today's young people.

LSD is manufactured in home laboratories and frequently distributed in blotter paper decorated with cartoon characters. Users place the paper on their tongue or chew the paper to ingest the drug. LSD can produce a psychedelic (mind-viewing) effect that includes altered perceptions of shapes, images, time, sound, and body form. Synesthesia is common to LSD users. Ingested in doses known as "hits," LSD produces a 6- to 9-hour experience (a "trip"). Hits range in price from $3 to $5.[15]

Although the hits today are about half as powerful as those in the 1960s, users still tend to develop high tolerance to LSD. Physical dependence does not occur. Not all LSD trips are pleasant. Hallucinations produced from LSD can be frightening and dangerous. Users can injure or kill themselves accidentally during a bad trip. Dangerous side effects include panic attacks, flashbacks, and occasional prolonged psychosis.

DESIGNER DRUGS

In recent years, chemists who produce many of the illicit drugs in home laboratories have managed to design versions of drugs listed on **FDA Schedule 1.** These *designer drugs* are similar to the controlled drugs on the FDA Schedule 1 but are sufficiently different so that they escape governmental control. They are either newly synthesized products that are similar to already outlawed drugs but for which no law yet exists, or they are reconstituted or renamed illicit substances. Designer drugs are said to produce effects similar to their controlled drug counterparts.

People who consume designer drugs do so at great risk, because the manufacturing of these drugs is unregulated. The neurophysiological impact of these home-made drugs can be quite dangerous. So far, a synthetic heroin product (MPPP) and several amphetamine derivatives with hallucinogenic properties have been designed for the unwary drug consumer.

STP (DOM), MDA ("love drug"), and MDMA (ecstasy) are examples of hallucinogenic designer drugs. These drugs produce mild LSD-like hallucinogenic experiences, positive feelings, and enhanced alertness. They also have a number of potentially dangerous effects. Experts are particularly concerned that MDMA can produce strong psychological dependence and can deplete serotonin, an important excitatory neurotransmitter associated with a state of alertness.[4]

PHENCYCLIDINE (PCP)

Phencyclidine (PCP, angel dust) has been classified variously as a hallucinogen, a stimulant, a depressant, and an anesthetic. PCP was studied for years during the 1950s and 1960s and was found to be an unsuitable animal and human anesthetic. PCP is an extremely unpredictable drug. Easily manufactured in home laboratories in tablet or powder form, PCP can be injected, inhaled, taken orally, or smoked. The effects vary. Some users report mild euphoria, although most users report bizarre perceptions, paranoid feelings, and ag-

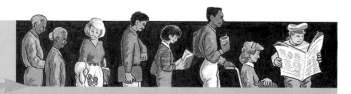

Learning FROM ALL Cultures

Hallucinogens and Religious Ceremonies

The use of hallucinogens became very popular in the United States in the 1960s, and they are still used today. Some of these substances are fairly recent discoveries, whereas others have been used for hundreds of years by certain societies. Some forms have and continue to be used by Native Americans as part of their religious ceremonies.[5]

Mescaline is a hallucinogen derived from the peyote cactus. Indian tribes in Mexico used peyote in religious ceremonies many years ago to enhance the spiritual experience. The practice then spread to Indian tribes in the United States. Today, the Native American Church of North America still uses peyote in religious ceremonies.[5]

Some Indian tribes have had to change their practices of peyote use because of state laws. The legality of using peyote for religious ceremonies is a state decision. A Supreme Court ruling in favor of the State of Oregon, prohibiting the use of peyote, stated that Indian tribes must comply with the state laws concerning the use of peyote in religious rituals. However, 23 other states allow ceremonial peyote use by the Native American Church.[16]

Other religious practices, such as the sacrifice of animals, have been questioned by some state governments. How far should government interfere in the practices of religious groups in their ceremonial rituals? ●

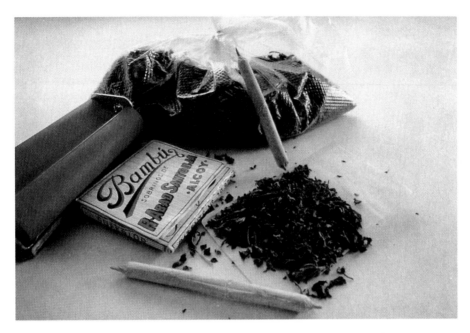

Marijuana.

gressive behavior. PCP overdose may cause convulsions, cardiovascular collapse, and damage to the brain's respiratory center.

In a number of cases, the aggressive behavior caused by PCP has led users to commit violent, brutal crimes against both friends and innocent strangers. PCP accumulates in cells and may stimulate bizarre behaviors months after initial use.

Cannabis

Cannabis (marijuana) has been labeled a mild hallucinogen for a number of years. However, most experts now consider it to be a drug category by itself. Marijuana produces mild effects like those of stimulants and depressants. The recent implications of marijuana in a large number of traffic fatalities make this drug one whose consumption should be carefully considered. Marijuana is actually a wild plant (*Cannabis sativa*) whose fibers were originally used in the manufacture of hemp rope. When the leafy material and small stems are crushed and dried, users can smoke the mixture in rolled cigarettes (joints) or pipes. The resins collected from scraping the flowering tops of the plant yield a marijuana product called *hashish*, or simply *hash*, commonly smoked in a pipe.

The potency of marijuana's hallucinogenic effect is determined by the percentage of the active ingredient THC, or tetrahydrocannabinol, present in the product. Based on the analysis of samples from drug seizures and street buys in the United States, the concentration of THC averages about 3.5% for marijuana, 7% to 9% for higher quality marijuana (sinsemilla), 8% to 14% for hashish, and as high as 50% for hash oil.[4,17]

THC is a fat-soluble substance and thus is absorbed and retained in fat tissues within the body. Before being excreted, THC can remain in the body for up to a month. With the sophistication of today's drug tests, trace amounts of THC can be detected in the bloodstream for months after consumption. It is possible that the THC that comes from passive inhalation (for example, during an indoor rock concert) can be detected.

Once marijuana is consumed, its effects vary from person to person. Being "high" or "stoned" or "wrecked" means different things to different people. Many persons report heightened sensitivity to music, cravings for particular foods, and a relaxed mood. Widespread consensus about marijuana's behavioral effects includes four probabilities: (1) users must learn to recognize what a marijuana high is like, (2) marijuana impairs short-term memory, (3) users overestimate the passage of time, and (4) users lose the ability to maintain focused attention on a task.[4]

The long-term effects of marijuana use are still being studied. Chronic abuse may lead to an *amotivational syndrome* in some people. The irritating effects of marijuana smoke on lung tissue are more pronounced than those of cigarette smoke, and some of the over 400 chemicals in marijuana are now linked to lung cancer development.

> **FDA Schedule 1** list comprising drugs that hold a high potential for abuse but that have no medical use.

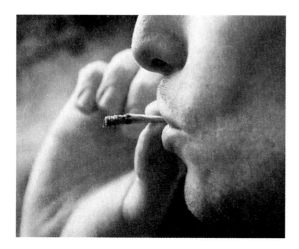

Smoking pot.

Long-term marijuana use is also associated with damage to the immune system, damage to male and female reproductive systems, and an increase in birth defects in babies born to parents who smoke marijuana.[4] The effect of long-term marijuana use on sexual behavior is not fully understood. Because the drug clearly can distort perceptions and thus perceptual ability (especially when combined with alcohol), its misuse or abuse by automobile drivers clearly jeopardizes the lives of many innocent persons.

In recent years, the only medical uses for marijuana have been to relieve the nausea from chemotherapy and to lower the buildup of pressure in the eyes of glaucoma patients. However, a variety of other drugs, many of which are nearly as effective, are also used for these purposes.

Narcotics

The **narcotics** are among the most dependence-producing drugs. Medically, the narcotics are used to relieve pain and induce sleep. Narcotics can be subgrouped on the basis of their origin into the natural, quasi-synthetic, and synthetic narcotics.

NATURAL NARCOTICS

Naturally occurring substances derived from the Oriental poppy plant include opium (the primary psychoactive substance extracted from the Oriental poppy), morphine (the primary active ingredient in opium) and thebaine (a compound not used as a drug). Morphine and related compounds have medical use as analgesics in the treatment of mild-to-severe pain.

QUASI-SYNTHETIC NARCOTICS

Quasi-synthetic narcotics are compounds created by chemically altering morphine. These laboratory-produced drugs are intended to be used as analgesics, but their benefits are largely compromised by a high de-

★ "Raves" and "Smart Drinks"

Since 1985, the designer drug MDMA (ecstasy) has been classified as a Schedule I compound by the Drug Enforcement Agency. This means that the drug has a high potential for abuse and no currently accepted medical use. MDMA is an amphetamine-like drug that reportedly produces both "warm feelings" (an enhanced mood, positive feelings, and increased feelings of sensuality) and mild hallucinations in users.

MDMA is also capable of producing some adverse side effects in users. Among these effects are muscle tightness and rigidity, jaw clenching, nausea, pulse and blood pressure changes, and neurotoxicity (as nerve cells become depleted of the neurotransmitter serotonin). MDMA is delivered in pill or capsule form.

Among counterculture youth in the early 1990s, MDMA has been a common drug used at all-night dancing parties called "raves." Raves originated in England and are fueled by "heavily mixed, electronically-generated sound, surrounded by computer-generated video and laser light shows."[21] It is common for rave participants to dance the entire night. Frequently, party goers buy "smart drinks" which are nontoxic, amino acid–laced beverages that users believe enhance alertness and energy.

Recently, the *Journal of the American Medical Association* reported that six youths had died at raves in England.[22] The cause of death was related to MDMA use, but apparently not solely associated with drug toxicity. Instead, the deaths were thought to be caused by heat stroke, from a combination of the drug and the prolonged vigorous dancing. At the time of this writing, no deaths had been reported in the United States from MDMA use at raves. ★

pendence rate and great risk of toxicity. The best known of the quasi-synthetic narcotics is heroin. Although heroin is a faster acting and more effective analgesic, it is extremely addictive. Once injected into a vein or "skin-popped" (injected beneath the skin surface), heroin produces dreamlike euphoria in users and, like all narcotics, produces strong physical and psychological dependence and tolerance.

As with use of all other injectable illicit drugs, the practice of sharing needles increases the likelihood of transmission of various communicable diseases, including HIV infection (see Chapter 12). Abrupt withdrawal from heroin use rarely produces death in abusers, but the discomfort during **cold turkey** withdrawal is reported to be overwhelming. The use of heroin has increased over the last decade. The purity of heroin is up, while the price is dropping. Cocaine abusers may use heroin to "come down" from the high associated with cocaine.

SYNTHETIC NARCOTICS

Meperidine (Demerol) and propoxyphene (Darvon), common postsurgical painkillers, and methadone, the drug prescribed during the rehabilitation of heroin addicts, are *synthetic narcotics*. These opiate-like drugs are manufactured in medical laboratories. They are not natural narcotics or quasi-synthetic narcotics because they do not originate from the Oriental poppy plant. Like true narcotics, however, these drugs can rapidly cause development of physical dependence. One major criticism of methadone rehabilitation programs is that they merely shift the addiction from heroin to methadone.

Inhalants

This drug classification includes a variety of volatile (quickly evaporating) compounds that generally produce unpredictable, drunklike effects in users. Users of **inhalants** may further experience some degree of delusionary and hallucinogenic effects. Some users may become quite aggressive. Drugs in this category include anesthetic gases (chloroform, laughing gas, and ether), vasodilators (amyl nitrite and butyl nitrite), petroleum products and commercial solvents (gasoline, kerosene, plastic cement, glue, typewriter correction fluid, paint, and paint thinner), and certain aerosols (found in some propelled spray products, fertilizers, and insecticides).

Most of the danger in using inhalants lies with the damaging, sometimes fatal, effects on the respiratory system. Furthermore, users may unknowingly place themselves in potentially dangerous situations because of the drunklike hallucinogenic effects. Aggressive behavior might also make users dangerous to themselves and others.

COMBINATION DRUG EFFECTS

Drugs taken in various combinations and dosages can alter and perhaps intensify the effects of the drugs.

A **synergistic drug effect** is a dangerous consequence that can occur when different drugs in the same general category are taken at the same time. The combined effect produces an exaggeration of each individual drug's effects. For example, the combined use of alcohol and tranquilizers will produce a synergistic effect greater than the total effect of each of the two drugs taken separately. In this instance a much-exaggerated, perhaps fatal, sedation will occur. In a simplistic sense, "one plus one equals four or five."

When two or more drugs are taken at or near the same time, these drug combinations can produce a variety of effects. Some drug combinations produce an additive effect, other combinations produce a potentiating effect, and still others produce an antagonistic effect. When two or more drugs are taken and the result is merely a combined total effect of each drug, the result is an **additive effect.** The sum of the effects is not

exaggerated. In a sense, "one plus one plus one equals three."

When one drug produces a intensified action of a second drug, the first drug is said to have a **potentiated effect** on the second drug. One popular drug-taking activity in the 1970s was the consumption of Quaaludes and beer. Quaaludes potentiated the inhibition-releasing, sedative effects of alcohol. This particular drug combination produced an inexpensive, but potentially fatal, drunklike euphoria in the user.

An **antagonistic effect** is an opposite effect one drug can have on another drug. One drug may be able to reduce another drug's influence on the body. Knowledge of this principle has been useful in the medical treatment of certain drug overdoses, as in the use of tranquilizers to relieve the effects of LSD or other hallucinogenic drugs.

SOCIETY'S RESPONSE TO DRUG USE

In the last 20 years, society's response to illegal drug use has been one of growing concern. For the vast majority of adults, drug abuse has been seen as a clear danger to society. This position has been supported by the development of community, school, state, and national organizations interested in the ultimate reduction of illegal drug use. These organizations have included such diverse groups as Parents Against Drugs, Parents for a Drug-Free Youth, Mothers Against Drunk Drivers (MADD), Narcotics Anonymous, and the federal Drug Enforcement Administration. Certain

narcotics (nar **cot** icks) opiates; psychoactive drugs derived from the Oriental poppy plant; they relieve pain and induce sleep.

cold turkey immediate, total discontinuation of use of a drug; associated with withdrawal discomfort.

inhalants (in **hay** lants) psychoactive drugs that enter the body through inhalation.

synergistic drug effect (sin er **jist** ick) heightened, exaggerated effect produced by the concurrent use of two or more drugs.

additive effect combined (but not exaggerated) effect produced by the concurrent use of two or more drugs.

potentiated effect (poe **ten** she ay ted) phenomenon whereby the use of one drug intensifies the effect of a second drug.

antagonistic effect (an tag oh **nist** ick) effect produced when one drug reduces or offsets the effects of a second drug.

National Groups and Hot Lines

NATIONAL GROUPS

★ PRIDE (Parent's Resource Institute for Drug Education): Atlanta (404) 577-4500; in Georgia (900) 998-7743

★ National Federation of State High School Associations Target Programs: Kansas City, Missouri (816) 464-5400

★ National Health Information Clearinghouse: (800) 336-4797

★ National Clearinghouse for Alcohol and Drug Information: Silver Spring, Maryland (800) 729-6686; (301) 468-2600

★ Narcotics Anonymous: Van Nuys, California (818) 780-3951

★ Toughlove: Doylestown, Pennsylvania (215) 348-7090

HOT LINES

★ National Institute on Alcohol and Drug Abuse Hot Line: (800) 662-HELP

★ National Cocaine Hot Line: (800) COCAINE

★ Alcohol Hot Line: (800) ALCOHOL

★ Cocaine Abuse Hot Line: (800) 888-9383; (800) 234-0420

COCAINE ANONYMOUS (CENTRAL OFFICES)

★ National Office: Culver City, California (213) 839-1141

★ California: Los Angeles (800) 347-8998
  Los Angeles area (818) 447-2887
  San Francisco (415) 821-6155
  Solana Beach (619) 268-9109

★ Connecticut: New Haven (203) 387-1664

★ Georgia: Atlanta (404) 255-7787

★ Illinois: Chicago (312) 202-8898

★ New Jersey: Summit (908) 273-4530

★ New York: Manhattan (212) 496-4266

★ Tennessee: Nashville (615) 747-5483

---

groups have concentrated their efforts on education, others on enforcement, and still others on the development of laws and public policy.

The personal and social issues related to drug use and abuse are very complex. Innovative solutions continue to be raised. Some believe that only through early childhood education will people learn alternatives to drug use. Starting drug education in the preschool years may have a more positive impact than waiting until the upper elementary or junior high school years. Some persons are advocating much harsher penalties for drug use and drug trafficking (including public executions).

Others support legalizing all drugs and having governmental agencies be responsible for drug regulation and control, as is the case with alcohol. Advocates for this position believe that drug-related crime and violence would virtually cease once the demand for illegal products is reduced. It is possible that sound arguments can be made on both sides of this issue. What are your opinions?

Unless significant changes in society's response to drug use take place soon, the disastrous effects of virtually uncontrolled drug abuse may continue. Families and communities will continue to be plagued by drug-related tragedies. Law enforcement officials will be pressed to the limit in their attempts to reduce drug flow. Our judicial system will be heavily burdened by

thousands of court cases. Health-care facilities could face over-whelming numbers of clients.

In comparison with other federally funded programs, the "war on drugs" is less expensive than farm support, NASA, food stamps, Medicare, and national defense. However, it remains to be seen whether any amount of money spent on enforcement, without adequate support for education, treatment, and poverty reduction, can reduce the illicit drug demand and supply. Currently, $12 billion are spent to fight the drug war in the United States: $8 billion are spent on law enforcement, and $4 billion are spent on education, prevention, and treatment.

Drug Testing

One clear response of society to concern over drug use is the development and growing use of drug tests. At present, the five largest drug-testing laboratories in the United States combined process over 1 million urine specimens per month.[18] The bulk of the specimens comes from corporations that screen employees for commonly abused drugs. Among these are amphetamines, barbiturates, benzodiazepines (the chemical bases for prescription tranquilizers such as Valium and Librium), cannabinoids (THC, hashish, and marijuana), methaqualone, opiates (heroin, codeine, and morphine), and PCP. With the exception of marijuana, most traces of these drugs are eliminated by the body

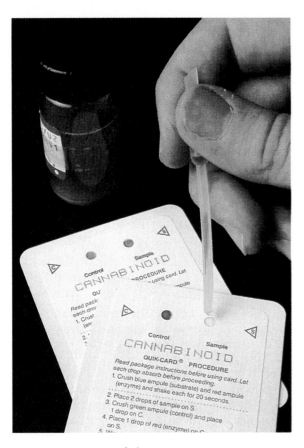

A drug test.

within a few days after use. Marijuana can remain detectable for weeks after use.[18]

How accurate are the results of drug testing? At typical cutoff standards, drug tests will likely identify 90% of recent drug users. This means that about 10% of recent users will pass undetected. (These 10% are considered false negatives). Nonusers whose drug tests indicate drug use (false positives) are quite rare. (Follow-up tests on these false positives would nearly always show negative results.) In the final analysis, human errors are probably more responsible than technical errors for inaccuracies in drug tests.[18]

Recently, scientists have been refining procedures that use hair samples to detect the presence of drugs.[19] These procedures seem to hold much promise, although certain technical obstacles remain. Watch for refinements in hair sample drug testing in the near future.

Most Fortune 500 companies, the armed forces, various government agencies, and nearly all athletic organizations have already implemented mandatory drug testing. Corporate substance abuse policies are being developed with careful attention being paid to legal and ethical issues (Figure 7-4).[20]

Do you think that the possibility of having to take such a drug test will have any impact on college students' use of drugs? Will the increased use of drug tests help the United States achieve its Healthy People 2000 Objectives?

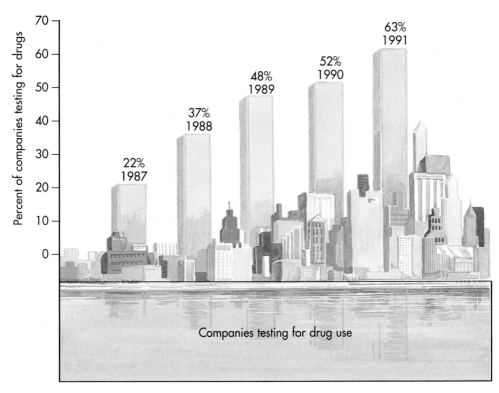

Companies testing for drug use

Figure 7-4 Drug testing is increasingly more likely to be a component of employment.

Health ACTION Guide

Reducing Drug Use

In whatever capacity you interact with others, particularly children and adolescents, you can play a part in reducing drug use. To accomplish this:

▼ *Be informed.* Be aware of possible drug use by learning to recognize early involvement.
▼ *Be firm.* Communicate firmly and clearly your position on drug use and your concerns about the be-

havior you are observing.
▼ *Be consistent.* Follow through with the rules and consequences that you have established about appropriate behavior.
▼ *Be a good listener.* Take time to listen to other views, even when you are in total disagreement with them.
▼ *Be available.* Make yourself available to help or console others who might be involved with drug use.
▼ *Be loving.* Demonstrate love and concern, but say "no" when you mean it.
▼ *Be an example.* Never do what you do not want others to do.
▼ *Be involved.* Give as much support as possible to those who are also concerned about drug use.

COLLEGE AND COMMUNITY SUPPORT SERVICES FOR DRUG DEPENDENCE

If students have drug problems and realize they need assistance, the assistance they might select could depend on the services available on campus or in the community near the university and the costs they are willing to pay for treatment services.

One recent approach to convince drug-dependent people to enter treatment programs is the use of *confrontation.* People who live or work with chemically dependent persons are being encouraged to confront them directly about their problems. Direct confrontation helps chemically dependent persons realize the impact their behaviors have on others. Once chemically dependent persons realize that others will no longer tolerate their behaviors, the likelihood of their entering treatment programs is increased significantly. Although effective, this approach is very stressful for family members and friends and may require the assistance of professionals in the field of chemical dependence. These professionals can be contacted at a drug treatment center in your area.

Treatment

Comprehensive drug treatment programs are found in very few college or university health centers. College settings for drug dependence programs are more commonly found in the university counseling center. At such a center the emphasis will probably be not on the medical management of dependence but on the behavioral dimensions of drug abuse. Trained counselors and psychologists who specialize in chemical dependence counseling will work with students to (1) analyze their particular concerns, (2) establish constructive ways to cope with stress, and (3) search for alternative ways to achieve new nonchemical "highs" (see p. 185).

Medical treatment for the management of drug problems may need to be obtained through the services of a community treatment facility administered by a local health department, community mental-health center, private clinic, or local hospital. Treatment may be on an inpatient or outpatient basis. Medical management might include detoxification, treatment of secondary health complications and nutritional deficiencies, and therapeutic counseling related to chemical dependence.

Some communities have voluntary health agencies that deliver services and treatment programs for drug-dependent persons. Check your telephone book for listings of drug-treatment facilities. Some communities have drug hot lines that offer advice for persons with questions about drugs.

Costs of Treatment for Dependence

Drug-treatment programs that are administered by colleges and universities for faculty and students generally require no fees. Local agencies may provide either free services or services based on a **sliding scale.** Private hospitals, physicians, and clinics are the most expensive forms of treatment. Inpatient treatment at a private facility may cost as much as $300 or more per day. Since the length of inpatient treatment averages about a month, a patient can quickly accumulate a very large bill. However, with many types of health insurance policies now providing coverage for alcohol and other drug dependencies, even these services may not require additional out-of-pocket expenses.

sliding scale method of payment by which patient fees are scaled according to income levels.

Nonchemical High Challenge

Experts agree that drug use provides only short-term, ineffective, and often destructive solutions to problems. We hope that you have found (or will find) innovative, invigorating, nondrug experiences that will make your life more exciting. Circle the number for each activity that reflects your intention to try that activity.

Use the following guide for indicating your responses:
1 No intention of trying this activity
2 Intend to try this within 2 years
3 Intend to try this within 6 months
4 Already tried this activity
5 Regularly do this activity

1. Learn to juggle	1 2 3 4 5	12. Go rockclimbing	1 2 3 4 5
2. Go backpacking	1 2 3 4 5	13. Take a role in a theater production	1 2 3 4 5
3. Complete a marathon race	1 2 3 4 5	14. Build a piece of furniture	1 2 3 4 5
4. Start a vegetable garden	1 2 3 4 5	15. Solicit funds for a worthy cause	1 2 3 4 5
5. Ride in a hot air balloon	1 2 3 4 5	16. Learn to swim	1 2 3 4 5
6. Snow ski or water ski	1 2 3 4 5	17. Overhaul your car engine	1 2 3 4 5
7. Donate blood	1 2 3 4 5	18. Compose a song	1 2 3 4 5
8. Go river rafting	1 2 3 4 5	19. Travel to a foreign country	1 2 3 4 5
9. Learn to play a musical instrument	1 2 3 4 5	20. Write the first chapter of a book	1 2 3 4 5
10. Cycle 100 miles	1 2 3 4 5		
11. Parachute from a plane	1 2 3 4 5	Your total points _____	

INTERPRETATION

61-100   You participate in many challenging experiences
41-60   You are willing to try some challenging experiences
20-40   You take few challenging risks described here

TO CARRY THIS FURTHER . . .

Looking at your point total, were you surprised at the degree to which you are aware of alternative activities? What are the top five activities, and can you understand their importance? What activities would you add to our list?

PERSONAL ASSESSMENT

Summary

✔ Drug use and abuse has a major impact on society.

✔ Exposure, compulsion, and loss of control are common aspects of addictive behaviors.

✔ Knowledge of the terms *misuse, abuse, tolerance,* and *dependence* as they relate to drugs is important for understanding the dynamics of drug use.

✔ A drug's impact on the CNS takes place through neurotransmitter activity on the neuron.

✔ Most drugs can be classified into six general categories: stimulants, depressants, hallucinogens, cannabis, narcotics, and inhalants.

✔ Combination drug effects include synergistic, additive, potentiated, and antagonistic effects.

✔ Society's response to drug abuse has been widely based and ranges from education, enforcement, treatment, and testing to searching for nondrug ways to achieve highs.

Review Questions

1. How is the term *drug* defined in this chapter? What are psychoactive drugs? How do medicines differ from drugs?

2. Explain what is meant by dependence. Identify and explain the two types of dependence.

3. Define the word *tolerance.* What is meant by cross-tolerance? Given an example of cross-tolerance.

4. Differentiate between drug misuse and drug abuse.

5. Identify some reasons commonly given for why people use psychoactive drugs.

6. Describe how neurotransmitters work.

7. Specify the six general categories of drugs. For each category, identify several examples of drugs, and explain the effects they would have on the user. What are designer drugs?

8. What is the active ingredient in marijuana? What are its common effects on the user? What is known about the long-term effects of marijuana use?

9. What is meant by synergistic effect, additive effect, potentiated effect, and antagonistic effect?

10. How accurate is drug testing?

Think about This . . .

✔ Can you identify any drugs on which you may have developed either a physical or psychological dependence?

✔ Do you find that you now require a larger dose of a particular drug to reach a high or low that you once felt with a smaller dose?

✔ Evaluate your own status as a user of drugs, including caffeine, tobacco, and aspirin. Do you consider your use of drugs to be a problem?

✔ Think about your own life experiences. What things have you done that have produced nondrug highs?

REAL LIFE REAL CHOICES

YOUR TURN

▼ Is marijuana addictive?

▼ What are the risks to Barry of continuing to smoke marijuana?

▼ Is Barry in a position to give his daughters good advice about drug use?

AND NOW, YOUR CHOICES...

▼ What would you do if you found out that one of your parents were using drugs, despite having told you repeatedly never to use drugs yourself?

▼ If you use drugs, what would you tell a younger brother or sister who asked you for guidance about drug use?

References

1. Percent of businesses using drug testing . . . , *USA Today*, March 29, 1991, p 1B.

2. Office of the National Drug Control Policy: *1992 National Drug Control Strategy: a nation responds to drug use*, Jan 1992, US Government Printing Office.

3. US Department of Health and Human Services: *Smoking, drinking and illicit drug use among American secondary school students, college students, and young adults, 1975-1992*, vol 2, NIH Pub No BKD-124, Washington DC, 1993, US Government Printing Office.

4. Ray O, Ksir C: *Drugs, society, and human behavior*, ed 6, St Louis, 1993, Mosby.

5. Pinger RR, Payne WA, Hahn DB, Hahn EJ: *Drugs: issues for today*, ed 2, St Louis, 1995, Mosby.

6. National Institute on Alcohol Abuse and Alcoholism: The genetics of alcoholism, *Alcohol Alert*, No 18 (PH 328), 1-3, October 1992.

7. Hahn DB, Payne WA: *Focus on health*, ed 2, St Louis, 1994, Mosby.

8. Manning TM: Perceived family environment as a predictor of drug and alcohol usage among offspring, *Journal of Health Education* 22(3):144-149 and 165, 1991.

9. US Department of Health and Human Services: *National household survey on drug abuse; population estimates 1992*, DHHS Pub No (SMA) 93-2053, Oct 1993, US Government Printing Office.

10. Moffett DF, Moffett SB, Schauf CL: *Human physiology: foundations and frontiers*, ed 2, St Louis, 1993, Mosby.

11. Thibodeau GA: *Structure and function of the body*, St Louis, 1992, Mosby.

12. Armstron BG, McDonald AD, Sloan M: Cigarette, alcohol and caffeine consumption and spontaneous abortion, *Am J Public Health* 82(1):85-87, 1991.

13. Cocaine: the first decade, 1992, *Rand Drug Policy Research Center Issue Paper* 1(1):1-4.

14. Moore J: Gangs, drugs, and violence, *National Institute of Drug Abuse Research Monograph*, 103, 1990, DHHS Publication No (ADM) 91-1721, pp 160-176.

15. Urban J: Thirty years later, LSD again becoming the drug of choice, *The Muncie Star*, March 21, 1993, p 6B.

16. Religion liberties, *Time*, April 30, 1990, p 85.

17. National Narcotics Intelligence Consumers Committee: *The NNICC report 1988*, Washington DC, April 1989, Drug Enforcement Agency.

18. Ackerman S: Drug testing: the state of the art, *Am Sci*, vol 77, 19-23, 1989.

19. Mieczkowski T: New approaches in drug testing: a review of hair analysis, *Ann Am Acad Pol Soc Sci* 521:132-150, 1992.

20. Comprehensive procedures for drug testing in the workplace, *National Institute on Drug Abuse*, 1991, DHHS Publication No (ADM) 91-1731.

21. Randall T: Ecstasy-fueled `rave' parties become dances of death for English youths, *Journal of the American Medical Association* 268(12):1505-1506, Sept 23/30, 1992.

22. Randall T: `Rave' scene, ecstacy use, leap Atlantic, *Journal of the American Medical Association* 268(12):1506, Sept 23/30, 1992.

Suggested Readings

Gold MS: *800-COCAINE*, ed 4, New York, 1990, Bantam Books.

A comprehensive manual for anyone needing information on any topic related to cocaine. It includes a self-test for addiction. The author founded the 24-hour cocaine hotline.

Pohl M, Kay DK: *Staying sane: when you care for someone with a chronic illness*. Deerfield Beach, Fla, 1993, Health Communications.

For caregivers of people with chronic illnesses. Provides exercises and ideas to lighten the burden of caring for ill persons. Appropriate for caregivers of addicted persons.

Twerski A: *Seek sobriety—find serenity*, New York, 1993, Pharos Books.

A rabbi, a physician, and an addiction specialist compiled this book of 365 daily meditations on a variety of topics related to healing from addiction. Topics range from self-esteem to sobriety to surviving.

Alcohol
Responsible Choices

The push for zero tolerance laws, the tightening of standards for determining legal intoxication, and the emergence of national groups concerned with alcohol misuse indicate that our society is more sensitive than ever to the growing misuse of alcohol. People are asking questions about the consequences of drunk driving, alcohol-related crime, and lowered job productivity. Recent national data indicate that per capita alcohol consumption has dropped in the United States[1] (Figure 8-1). Alcohol use remains the preferred form of drug use for the majority of adults, but as a society we are increasingly uncomfortable with the ease with which alcohol can be misused. Many Healthy People 2000 Objectives relate directly to alcohol use.

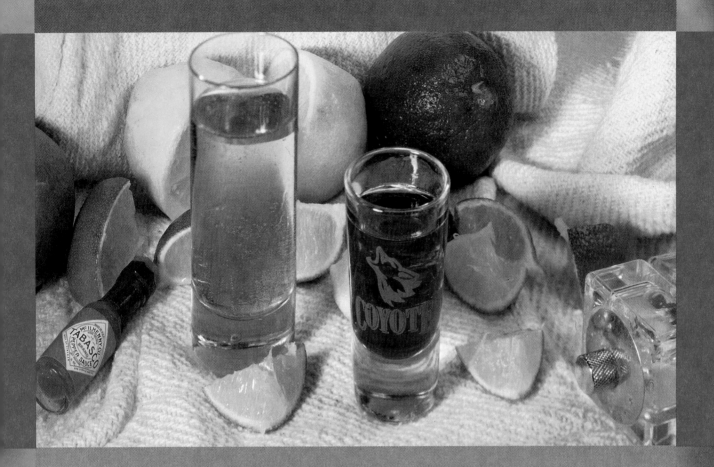

A L C O H O L

The following objectives are covered in this chapter:

▼ Reduce cirrhosis deaths to no more than 6 per 100,000 people. (Age adjusted baseline: 9.1 per 100,000 in 1987, p. 167.)

▼ Reduce deaths caused by alcohol-related motor vehicle crashes to no more than 8.5 per 100,000 people. (Age-adjusted baseline: 9.8 per 100,000 in 1987; p. 166.)

▼ Reduce the proportion of young people who have used alcohol in the past month to reach this year 2000 target: age 18-20 to 29%. (1988 baseline: 57.9% for age 18-20 in 1988; p. 169.)

▼ Reduce the proportion of high school seniors and college students engaging in recent occasions of heavy drinking of alcoholic beverages to no more than 28% of high school students and 32% of college students. (Baseline: 33% of high school seniors and 41.7% of college students in 1989; p. 170.)

▼ Extend to 50 states legal blood alcohol concentration tolerance levels of 0.04% for motor vehicle drivers age 21 and older and 0.00% for those younger than age 21. (Baseline: 0 states in 1990; p. 178.)

REAL LIFE
REAL CHOICES
Alcoholism: A Family Problem

▼ Name: Ricardo Diaz
▼ Age: 38
▼ Occupation: Vice squad detective

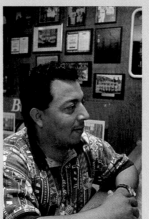

"I'll never be like that."

Those words—whispered, shouted, sobbed—were the anthem of Ricardo (Rick) Diaz's youth. The years that should have been carefree and adventuresome for Rick and his three younger brothers were instead an endlessly running horror movie. Rick tried to be a substitute dad to his siblings as their father, Geraldo, drank his way from life of the party to menacing bully, from successful machine-shop foreman to unemployed loafer, from proud family man to shameful secret. Geraldo died of cirrhosis of the liver in Rick's senior year in high school, and although he grieved his father's loss, he also secretly felt relief.

Now 38, Rick was recently promoted to detective lieutenant in a big-city police department. His wife,

Maria, is a successful accountant, and their two daughters and son are excellent students and all-around good kids. Rick and Maria don't drink, and he's proud that his life reflects his vow: "I'll never be like that."

Rick's not like that—but the same can't be said for his youngest brother, Rodrigo. Now 28, he seems to be headed into the same dark tunnel as his father, taking with him his frightened wife and 4-year-old twin daughters. Rick, ever the protective big brother, has tried everything to help Rodrigo, from "lending" him money and bringing him home from bars to "taking care of" his citations for drunk driving and making excuses for his behavior at family get-togethers.

As you study this chapter, think about Rick and Rod's situation and prepare yourself to answer the questions in **Your Turn** at the end of the chapter. ▼

The alcohol use patterns of many people are irresponsible. Frequent heavy drinking, drinking to purposely get drunk, drinking on the job, and drinking while driving are but a few of the irresponsible ways in which adults drink. The use patterns being formed today by young adults may tip the delicate balance that now exists between the use of alcohol as an agent for achieving satisfaction and social integration and use of alcohol as an agent for disruptive and life-threatening behavior.

CHOOSING TO DRINK

As plausible as all of the explanations in the box on p. 192 are in explaining why people might choose to drink an alcohol beverage, we believe that the last choice listed is ultimately the only reason most people drink alcohol: they drink to feel the effects of alcohol. Although most people will not admit it, they find alcohol an effective, affordable, and legal substance for altering the normal function of the central nervous system. As psychological restraints are removed by the influence of the alcohol, behaviors that are generally held in check by **inhibitions** are expressed. At least temporarily, drinkers become a different version

of themselves—more outgoing, relaxed, and adventuresome. If alcohol did not make these changes in people, little alcohol would be consumed. Do you agree or disagree?

ALCOHOL USE PATTERNS

From magazines to billboards to television, alcohol is one of the most heavily advertised consumer products in the country.[2] You cannot watch television, listen to a radio, or read a newspaper without being encouraged to buy a particular brand of beer, wine, or liquor. The advertisements create a warm aura about the nature of alcohol use. The implications are clear: alcohol use will bring you good times, handsome men or seductive women, exotic settings, and a chance to forget the hassles of hard work and study.

Perhaps as a consequence of the many pressures to drink, it is not surprising that most adults drink alcohol beverages. Two thirds of all American adults are classified as drinkers. Yet one in three adults does not drink. In the college environment, where surveys indicate that nearly 90% of all students drink,[3] it is difficult for many students to imagine that every third adult is an abstainer.

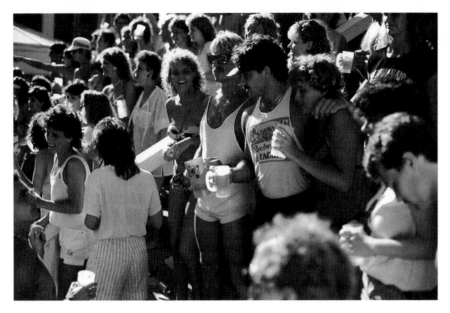

Do you see this behavior frequently on your campus?

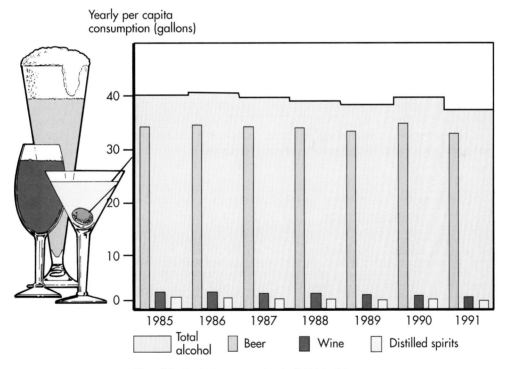

Figure 8-1 Alcohol consumption in the United States.

Alcohol consumption figures are reported in many different ways, depending on the researchers' criteria. Figures from various sources support the contention that one third of adults age 18 and older are abstainers, about one third are light drinkers, and one third are

inhibitions (in hib **ish** uns) inner controls that prevent a person's engaging in certain types of behavior.

Why Do I Choose an Alcohol Beverage?

★ Alcohol beverages are more thirst quenching than nonalcohol alternatives.

★ Alcohol beverages taste better—their flavor is unique and satisfying.

★ My friends always choose alcohol beverages—I've learned to do the same.

★ Alcohol drinks form an important part of the larger statement that I am making about myself. They reflect the fact that I am an adult.

★ Drinking alcohol beverages causes me to feel different—I like the changes that come about when I drink.

moderate to heavy drinkers. As a single category, heavy drinkers make up about 10% of the adult drinking population. Students who drink in college generally tend to classify themselves as light to moderate drinkers. It comes as a shock to our students though that many of them are considered to be heavy drinkers according to the criteria for each drinking classification. These classifications, based on the combination of quantity of alcohol consumed per occasion and the frequency of drinking, are shown in Table 8-1.

In a recent unpublished survey of our undergraduate health science classes, we found that 37% of the 200 students met the criteria for heavy drinking, 26% met the criteria for moderate drinking, 13% met the criteria

for light drinking, 11% were infrequent drinkers, and 13% were abstainers.[4] It is not surprising that many students, faculty, and administrators believe that alcohol abuse is a major problem on their campuses.

For large numbers of students who drink, the college years represent a time when they will drink more heavily than at other period during their lifetime. Some will suffer serious consequences as a result.[5] (Figure 8-2) These years will also be the entry years into a lifetime of problem drinking for some.

Binge Drinking

The abuse of alcohol by college students most frequently takes place through a drinking pattern called *binge drinking*. Binge drinking refers to the consumption of five drinks in a row, at least once in the previous 2-week period.[5] College students who fit the category of "heavy drinkers" rarely consume small amounts of alcohol each day, but instead, drink large amounts one or two nights each week. Some students in our classes openly admit that they plan to "get really drunk" on the weekend. They plan to binge drink.

By its very nature, binge drinking can be dangerous. Drunk driving, physical violence, property destruction, date rape, and police arrest are all highly associated with binge drinking. Reducing binge drinking is a goal of the Healthy People 2000 Objectives. The direct correlation between the amount of alcohol consumed and lowered academic performance remains crystal clear (see Figure 8-3). Frequently, the social costs of binge drinking can be very high, especially when intoxicated people demonstrate their level of immaturity. How common is binge drinking on your campus?

TABLE 8-1   Criteria for drinking classifications

Classification	Alcohol-related behavior
Abstainers	Do not drink or drink less often than once a year
Infrequent drinkers	Drink once a month at most and drink small amounts per typical drinking occasion
Light drinkers	Drink once a month at most and drink medium amounts per typical drinking occasion or drink no more than three to four times a month and drink small amounts per typical drinking occasion
Moderate drinkers	Drink at least once a week and small amounts per typical drinking occasion or three to four times a month and medium amounts per typical drinking occasion or no more than once a month and large amounts per typical drinking occasion
Moderate/heavy drinkers	Drink at least once a week and medium amounts per typical drinking occasion or three to four times a month and large amounts per typical drinking occasion
Heavy drinkers	Drink at least once a week and large amounts per typical drinking occasion

NOTE: Small amounts=One drink or less per drinking occasion.
Medium amounts=Two to four drinks per drinking occasion.
Large amounts=Five or more drinks per drinking occasion (binge drinking).
Drink=12 fluid oz of beer, 4 fluid oz of wine, or 1 fluid oz of distilled spirits.

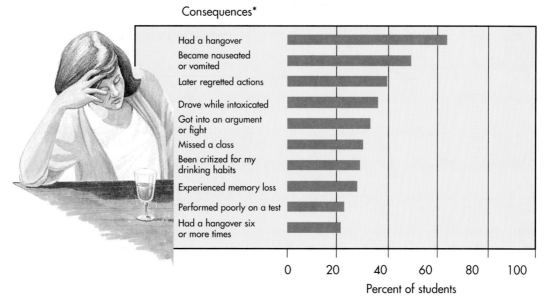

Figure 8-2 Negative consequences of alcohol and drug use as reported by college students. (* Occurred at least once in the past year.)

Uneven Distribution of Drinkers

One of the most interesting and frightening aspects of alcohol use patterns is the uneven distribution of drinkers in the United States. Figures that look at per capita alcohol consumption can be misleading because there are few drinkers who drink the "statistically average" amounts of alcohol. As you can see in Figure 8-4, approximately 70% of the drinking population consumes only 20% of all the alcohol sold. Thus 30% drink the other 80% of alcohol sold. Amazingly, one third of this group of heavy drinkers consumes 50% of all alcohol.[6] Figure 8-4 indicates how a group of 10 typical Americans would divide 10 drinks according to this uneven (but accurate) distribution of drinkers. It is clear that society's major alcohol health threat comes from the relatively small proportion of drinkers that drinks so heavily.

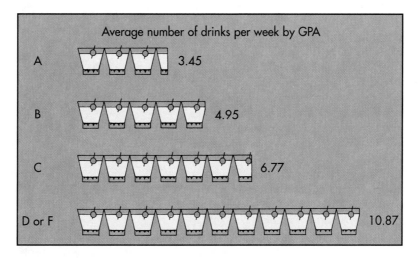

Figure 8-3 Average number of drinks per week by GPA.

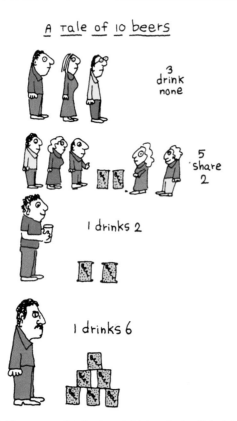

A Tale of 10 beers

3 drink none

5 share 2

1 drinks 2

1 drinks 6

Figure 8-4 The uneven distribution of drinkers in the United States and how they would divide 10 drinks.

THE NATURE OF ALCOHOL BEVERAGES

Alcohol (also known as ethyl alcohol or ethanol) is the principal product of **fermentation.** In this process *yeast* cells act on the sugar content of fruits and grains to produce alcohol and carbon dioxide. Alcohol was probably first discovered in prehistoric times when people consumed the juices of a berry mash that was exposed to airborne yeast cells. When this product produced more physical effects than the mere satisfaction of thirst, early man began the purposeful production of this crude wine. Alcohol became a celebrated elixir in a slowly developing world. Fermented juices have been consumed for at least 4000 years and have been used medically for hundreds of years as an analgesic and a sedative.

Until about 500 years ago, the principal beverages made with alcohol were wine (from fruit sources) and beer (from grain sources). These beverages were similar in their rather low percentage of alcohol concentration. At most, the early alcohol beverages contained 10% to 14% pure alcohol. Any greater concentration seemed to destroy the yeast cells. Not until the European development of the process of **distillation** in the fifteenth century did alcohol beverages contain a

higher percentage of alcohol.[7] By gathering the alcohol vapors from a fermented mixture that was heated in a device called a *still,* early distillers learned they could process a much more potent product. These vapors were then cooled and condensed to form distilled liquids, or spirits. Even after the addition of water and flavoring ingredients, the alcohol concentration of these new beverages exceeded 50%. Through the years, whiskey, rum, vodka, and gin were further developed to contain even higher concentrations of alcohol.

The alcohol concentration in distilled beverages today is expressed by the term *proof,* a number that is twice the percentage of alcohol by volume in a beverage. Thus 70% of the fluid in a bottle of 140 proof gin is pure alcohol. Most proofs in distilled beverages range from 80 to 160. The familiar, pure *grain alcohol* that is often added to fruit punches and similar beverages has a proof that approaches 200.

In its purest form, ethyl alcohol has little taste. This clear fluid, when consumed alone, usually produces an initial burning sensation of the oral cavity and esophagus. The various flavors that you notice in alcohol beverages are by-products of the sugar source (the type of fruit or grain) and any additional flavorings added to the fermenting mixture. Whereas wine and beer are generally not mixed with other nonalcohol liquids, distilled spirits are frequently combined with fruit juices, colas, and prepared mixes. (See Table 8-2 for the categories of alcohol beverages and the box on p. 196 for types of alcohol beverages.)

★ The Perfect Alternative?

Recently, many low-alcohol and nonalcohol malt beverages have entered the marketplace. Do you believe these products will have much influence on the beer industry? Would you consider using these beverages as an alternative to alcohol beverages at a party you would host? Why or why not? ★

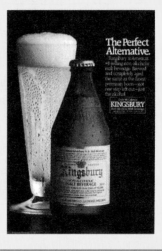

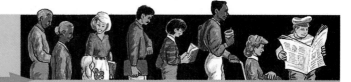

Learning FROM ALL Cultures

Alcohol Use

Whether or not individuals use alcohol often is a reflection of attitudes developed through the culture in which they live. How much they drink, what they drink, when they drink, and why they drink are all habits derived from their particular environments. Attitudes that a particular culture develops also influence rates of alcoholism. Times change, however, and countries are less isolated than they once were. Those cultural attitudes of a generation ago probably had more influence on behavior, such as drinking alcohol, than they do today. Still, culture does play a role in developing attitudes and behavior concerning the consumption of alcohol.

Italy is the second biggest wine-producing country in the world, and Italians have historically enjoyed drinking wine. And yet a generation ago, Italy's rates of alcoholism were low. Most Italians drank wine and approved of the practice. They typically would drink wine with the noon and evening meals. Excessive drinking and drunkeness, however, were unacceptable.[6]

Jews, like Italians, have had low rates of alcoholism. Their attitudes toward drinking and drinking habits have been very similar to those of Italians.[6]

Attitudes continue to change in various cultures, but there are a few factors that seem to affect the rate of alcoholism regardless. In societies where alcohol is introduced to children in small amounts on special occasions and within a sound family structure, the rates of alcoholism are low. This is also true when drinking is not the main focus of entertainment but accompanies another activity. Conversely, high rates of alcoholism among groups of people seem to occur when there are no standards on how to drink and how much to drink.[6]

Consider the attitudes toward drinking among your culture and family group. How do these attitudes and practices influence your own opinions toward alcohol use? ●

Recently, beer drinkers were given a new selection in their search for a favorite brew. Both American and Canadian breweries are now marketing "ice beer," a beverage designed to be more flavorful than most beers currently available. The term *ice* refers to the manner in which this beer is brewed and processed. After the beer is brewed and fermented, it is deep-chilled at 24 to 28 degrees Fahrenheit. This causes ice crystals to form in the mixture. Most brewers then remove the ice crystals and package the remaining liquid.

By removing the ice crystals (and thus, some water content) the beverage remaining has a greater concentration of alcohol. Regular beer and light beer typically contain less than 5% alcohol, whereas ice beers generally range from 5% to 6% alcohol content. Labatt's Maximum Ice (a Canadian ice beer) contains the highest concentration of alcohol at 7.1%.

With the advent of ice beer, beer drinkers have a greater selection of beers. Do you think many will choose this new alternative? If so, will their choice be made because of the reportedly "rich, zesty flavor" of ice beer or because of the greater amount of alcohol in ice beer? ★

The nutritional value of alcohol is extremely limited. Although the crude, early fermented mixtures of alcohol beverages did contain moderate amounts of vitamins and minerals, alcohol beverages produced today through modern processing methods contain only empty Calories—about 100 Calories per fluid ounce of 100 proof distilled spirits and about 150 Calories per each 12-ounce bottle or can of beer.[6] Alcohol contains few minerals and no vitamins, fats, or protein.

As a chemical compound, alcohol exists in many forms. Among the more familiar of these are methyl (wood alcohol), ethyl (grain alcohol), isopropyl (rubbing alcohol), and butyl. Only ethyl alcohol can be

---

fermentation (fur men **tay** shun) chemical process whereby plant products are converted into alcohol by the action of yeast cells on carbohydrate materials.

distillation (dis til **a** shun) production of alcohol beverages by the vaporization and condensation of the alcohol component of plant material; the process that produces liquor.

TABLE 8-2   Categories of alcohol beverages

Alcohol beverage	Alcohol content (%)	Normal measure
Beer		
Malt liquor	7	12-oz bottle
Ale	5	12-oz bottle
Ice beer	5.5	12-oz bottle
Lite beer	4	12-oz bottle
Regular beer	4	12-oz bottle
Low-alcohol beer	1.5	12-oz bottle
Nonalcohol beer	.5	12-oz bottle
Wine		
Fortified: port, muscatel, etc.	18	3-oz glass
Natural: red/white	12	4-oz glass
Champagne	12	4-oz glass
Wine cooler	6	12-oz bottle
Cider (hard)	10	6-oz glass
Liqueurs		
Strong: sweet, syrupy	40	1-oz glass
Medium: fruit brandies	25	2-oz glass
Distilled spirits		
Rum, gin scotch, vodka, whiskey	45	1-oz glass
Mixed drinks and cocktails		
Strong martini, manhattan	30	3 ½-oz glass
Medium: old-, fashioned, daiquiri, Alexander	15	4-oz glass
Light: highball, sweet and sour mixes, tonics	7	8-oz glass

★ Types of Alcohol Beverages

In all major alcohol beverages—beer, table wines, cocktail and dessert wines, liqueurs and cordials, and distilled spirits—the significant ingredient is identical: alcohol. Regardless of the type of alcohol beverage, the typical serving contains about half an ounce of pure alcohol. This amount of alcohol is found in:

★ A shot of spirits (1.5 oz of 40% alcohol—80 proof whiskey or vodka)

★ A glass of fortified wine (3 oz of 20% alcohol)

★ A larger glass of table wine (5 oz of 12% alcohol)

★ Beer (12 oz of 4.5% alcohol)

In addition, these beverages contain other chemical constituents. Some come from the original grains, grapes, or other fruits; others are produced during the chemical processes of fermentation, distillation, and storage. Some are added as flavoring or coloring.

These nonalcohol substances contribute to the effects of certain beverages either by directly affecting the body or by affecting the rates at which alcohol is absorbed into the blood. ★

The introduction of "lite" beer and low-Calorie wines has been in response to concerns over the number of Calories that alcohol beverages provide. Be certain to remember that these "lite" beverages are not low-alcohol beverages—merely low-Calorie beverages. Only beverages marked "low-alcohol" contain a lower concentration of alcohol than the usual beverages of that type.

THE PHYSIOLOGICAL EFFECTS OF ALCOHOL

First and foremost, alcohol is classified as a drug—a very strong *central nervous system depressant*. The primary depressant effect of alcohol is observed in the brain and spinal cord. Many people think of alcohol as a stimulant because of the way most users feel after consuming a serving or two of their favorite drink. Any temporary sensations of jubilation, boldness, or relief are attributed to alcohol's ability as a depressant drug to release personal inhibitions and provide temporary relief from tension.

Factors Related to the Absorption of Alcohol

The basic principle of *diffusion,* or the movement of a substance from an area of greater concentration to an area of lesser concentration, applies to the movement

consumed safely by humans. All other forms are toxic and thus unsafe for use in beverages. Consumption of alcohols other than ethyl has resulted in serious injury and death.

The addition of denaturing substances to nonethyl alcohols prevents many persons from ingesting a lethal dose. This is because a nauseating effect is produced once the denaturing chemicals are ingested. Be careful never to consume alcohol unless you are certain of its form. Too frequently, beverages purported to be "home brew" or "moonshine" have proven to be dangerously concocted from nonethyl alcohols.

of alcohol from the digestive tract into the bloodstream. This **absorption** of alcohol is influenced by several factors, most of which are capable of being controlled by the individual. These factors include:

▼ *Strength of the beverage.* The stronger the beverage, the greater the amount of alcohol that will accumulate within the digestive tract. Thus, 3 oz of gin will produce a greater concentration of alcohol in the bloodstream than 3 oz of beer.

▼ *Number of drinks consumed.* The greater the number of drinks that are consumed, the more alcohol that must be absorbed. If consumed in a relatively short time, a concentration gradient will develop that will foster the rapid movement of alcohol into the bloodstream.

▼ *Speed of consumption.* If consumed rapidly, even relatively few drinks will result in a large concentration gradient that will foster high blood alcohol concentrations.

▼ *Presence of food.* Food can compete with alcohol for absorption into the bloodstream, thus slowing the absorption of alcohol. By slowing alcohol absorption, removal of the alcohol already in the bloodstream can occur. Slow absorption favors better control of blood alcohol concentrations.

▼ *Presence of carbonation.* The presence of carbon dioxide in drinks such as sparkling wines and champagne speeds up the rate of alcohol absorption. Drinking alcohol with carbonated soft drinks (i.e., rum and cola) also speeds up alcohol absorption.

▼ *Body chemistry.* Each person has an individual pattern of physiological functioning that may affect the ability to process alcohol. Absorption time may be either slowed or quickened by anger, fear, stress, nausea, and the condition of the stomach tissues.

▼ *Sex.* Recently, a significant study in the *New England Journal of Medicine* reported that women produce much less alcohol dehydrogenase than men do.[8] This enzyme is responsible for breaking down alcohol in the stomach. With less alcohol dehydrogenase action, women absorb about 30% more alcohol into the bloodstream than men, despite identical number of drinks and equal body weight.

Three other reasons help explain why women tend to absorb alcohol more quickly than men of the same body weight: (1) Women have proportionately more body fat than men. Since alcohol is not very fat soluble, it enters the bloodstream relatively quickly. (2) Women's bodies have proportionately less water than men's of equal weight. Thus alcohol consumed by women does not become as diluted as it would in men. (3) Alcohol absorption is influenced by a woman's menstrual cycle. Alcohol is more quickly absorbed during the premenstrual phase of a woman's cycle. Also, there is evidence that women using birth control pills absorb alcohol faster than usual.[6]

With the exception of a person's body chemistry and sex, all other factors that influence absorption can be moderated by the user of alcohol.

Blood Alcohol Concentration

A person's **blood alcohol concentration (BAC)** level rises when alcohol is consumed at a rate faster than it can be oxidized by the liver (Figure 8-5). A fairly predictable sequence of effects takes place when a person drinks alcohol at a rate faster than one drink every hour. When the BAC reaches 0.05%, initial measurable changes in mood and behavior take place. Inhibitions and everyday tensions appear to be released, while at the same time judgment and critical thinking are somewhat impaired. This BAC level would be achieved by a 160-pound person taking about two drinks in an hour.

At a level of 0.10% (one part alcohol to 1,000 parts blood), the drinker typically loses significant motor coordination. Voluntary motor function becomes quite clumsy. At this BAC level most states consider a drinker legally intoxicated and thus incapable of operating a vehicle within the limits of safety. Although physiological changes associated with this BAC level are occurring, certain users may not feel intoxicated or outwardly appear to be impaired.

As a person continues to elevate the BAC from 0.20% to 0.50%, the health risk of acute alcohol intoxication increases rapidly. A BAC of 0.20% is characterized by the loud, boisterous, obnoxious drunk who staggers. A 0.30% BAC produces further depression and stuporous behavior, during which time the drinker becomes so confused that he or she may be fully incapable of understanding external stimuli. The 0.40% or 0.50% BAC produces unconsciousness. At this BAC a person can die, since brain centers that control body temperature, heartbeat, and respiration may be virtually shut down.

An important factor influencing the blood alcohol concentration that results from a given amount of alcohol is the individual's blood volume. The larger the person, the greater the amount of blood into which alcohol can be distributed. Conversely, the smaller individual has less blood into which alcohol can be distributed, and as a result a higher BAC will develop.

> **absorption** (ub **zorp** shun) passage of nutrients or alcohol through the walls of the stomach or intestinal tract into the bloodstream.
>
> **blood alcohol concentration (BAC)** percentage of alcohol in measured quantity of blood; BACs can be determined directly through the analysis of a blood sample or indirectly through the analysis of exhaled air.

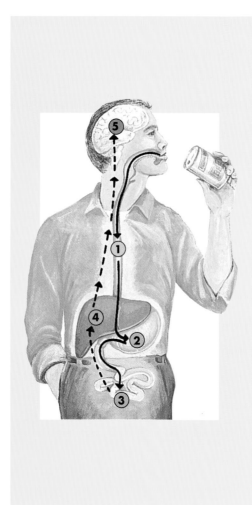

① When it is swallowed, alcohol travels through the esophagus to the stomach.

② Absorption of alcohol begins in the stomach. Approximately 20% passes directly into the venous drainage of the stomach wall. Food in the stomach will delay passage of the remaining alcohol into the small intestine.

③ The majority of alcohol (80%) is absorbed into the venous drainage of the small intestine. Absorption is proportional to the concentration of alcohol within the small intestine. Once in the venous drainage, alcohol is transported throughout the body and eventually reaches the liver for oxidation.

④ When it arrives in the liver, alcohol undergoes oxidation. The liver is capable of oxidizing approximately $\frac{1}{4}$ to $\frac{1}{3}$ ounce of pure alcohol per hour. Surplus alcohol is circulated throughout the body and BAC rises. Blood alcohol concentrations gradually fall as the liver oxidizes the remaining alcohol.

⑤ As BAC rises in the blood reaching the brain, predictable changes occur. At levels approximating 0.50%, central nervous system function can be so depressed that death can occur.

Figure 8-5 The body's absorption and oxidation of alcohol.

Sobering Up

Alcohol is removed from the bloodstream principally through the process of oxidation. **Oxidation** occurs at a constant rate (about $\frac{1}{4}$-$\frac{1}{3}$ oz of pure alcohol per hour) that cannot be appreciably altered. Since each typical serving of beer, wine, or distilled spirits contains about $\frac{1}{2}$ oz of pure alcohol, it takes about 2 hours for the body to fully oxidize one typical alcohol drink.[7]

Although people have attempted to sober up by drinking hot coffee, taking cold showers, or by exercising, the oxidation of alcohol remains unaffected. Thus far the U.S. Food and Drug Administration (FDA) has not approved any commercial product that can help people accomplish sobriety. Passage of time remains the only effective remedy for diminishing alcohol's effects.

First Aid for Acute Alcohol Intoxication

Not everyone who goes to sleep, passes out, or even becomes unconscious after drinking has a high BAC. People who are already sleepy, have not eaten well, are sick, or who are bored may drink a little alcohol and quickly fall asleep. However, people who drink heavily in a rather short time may be setting themselves up for an extremely unpleasant, toxic, potentially life-threatening experience. These people will have problems because of their high BAC.

As you watch people consuming alcohol at a social function, it can be important for you to carefully observe the drinking behavior and the resultant physical signs and symptoms exhibited by those drinking heavily. Although most cases of alcohol intoxication produce only uncomfortable hangovers and bruised egos, some social drinking episodes result in serious injury and death. A number of these deaths occur in college settings, often when inexperienced drinkers are encouraged to drink large amounts of alcohol in a relatively short time. Such behavior is not uncommon during days preceding or following the weekend's big

oxidation (ox ih **day** shun) the process that removes alcohol from the bloodstream.

How Do You Use Alcohol Beverages?

Answer the following questions in terms of your own alcohol use. Record your number of yes and no responses in the box at the end of the questionnaire.

Do you:

	Yes	No
1. Drink more frequently than you did a year ago?	____	____
2. Drink more heavily than you did a year ago?	____	____
3. Plan to drink, sometimes days in advance?	____	____
4. Gulp or "chug" your drinks, perhaps in a contest?	____	____
5. Set personal limits on the amount you plan to drink but then consistently disregard these limits?	____	____
6. Drink at a rate greater than two drinks per hour?	____	____
7. Encourage or even pressure others to drink with you?	____	____
8. Frequently want a nonalcohol beverage but then end up drinking an alcohol drink?	____	____
9. Drive your car while under the influence of alcohol or ride with another person who has been drinking?	____	____
10. Use alcohol beverages while taking prescription or OTC medications?	____	____
11. Forget what happened while you were drinking?	____	____
12. Have a tendency to disregard information about the effects of drinking?	____	____
13. Find your reputation fading because of alcohol use?	____	____
Total	____	____

INTERPRETATION

If you indicate a "yes" response on any of these questions, you may be demonstrating aspects of irresponsible alcohol use. Two or more "yes" responses indicates an unacceptable pattern of alcohol use and may reflect problem drinking behavior.

TO CARRY THIS FURTHER . . .

Ask your friends or roommates to take this assessment. Are they willing to take this assessment and then talk about their results with you? Be prepared to discuss any follow-up questions they might have about their (or your) alcohol consumption patterns. Your willingness to talk about drinking behaviors might help someone to realize that this topic can and should be discussed openly. Finally, be aware of how people in your area can get professional help with drinking problems or other drug concerns.

PERSONAL ASSESSMENT

Health ACTION Guide

Alcohol Intoxication

You should seek emergency help for acute alcohol intoxication when you find that a person drinking heavily:

▼ Cannot be aroused
▼ Has a weak, rapid pulse
▼ Has an unusual or irregular breathing pattern
▼ Has cool (possibly damp), pale or bluish skin

game, during social club gatherings, and during residence hall parties.

Although responsible drinking would prevent **acute alcohol intoxication** (poisoning), responsible drinking will never be a reality for everyone. As caring adults, what should we know about this health emergency that may help us save a life—perhaps even a friend's life?

The first real danger signs we need to recognize are the typical signs of **shock.** By the time these shock signs are evident, a drinker will already have advanced to an unconscious stage. He or she cannot be aroused from a deep stupor. The person will probably have a weak, rapid pulse (over 100 beats per minute). Skin will be cool and damp, and breathing will be increased to once every 3 or 4 seconds. These breaths may be shallow or deep but will certainly be irregular in pattern. Skin color will be pale or bluish. (In the case of a person with dark skin, these color changes will be more evident in the fingernail beds or the mucous membranes inside the mouth or under the eyelids.) Whenever any of these signs are present, seek emergency medical help immediately.

Involuntary regurgitation (vomiting) can be another potentially life-threatening emergency for a person who has consumed too much alcohol. When a drinker has consumed more alcohol than the liver can oxidize, the pyloric valve at the base of the stomach tends to close. Additional alcohol remains in the stomach. This alcohol irritates the lining of the stomach to the extent that involuntary muscle contractions force the stomach contents to flow back through the esophagus. By removing alcohol from the stomach, vomiting may be a lifesaving mechanism for conscious drinkers.

An unconscious victim who regurgitates may be lying in such a position that the airway becomes obstructed with the vomitus from the stomach. This victim can easily die from **asphyxiation.** As a first aid

measure, unconscious drinkers should always be rolled on their sides to minimize the chance of airway obstruction.[9] If vomiting occurs when you are with the victim, make certain that the head is positioned lower than the rest of the body. This position minimizes the chance that vomitus will obstruct the air passages.

It is also important to keep a close watch on anyone who "passes out" from heavy drinking. Unfortunately party goers sometimes make the mistake of carrying these persons to bed and then forgetting about them. By the next morning, these forgotten people may have died. We should do our best to monitor the physical condition of anyone who passes out from heavy drinking. If you really care about these unconscious people, you will observe them at regular intervals until they appear to be clearly out of danger. Although this may mean an evening of interrupted sleep for you, you may save a friend's life.

ALCOHOL-RELATED HEALTH PROBLEMS

The relationship of chronic alcohol use to the structure and function of the body is reasonably well understood. Heavy alcohol use causes a variety of changes to the body that lead to an increase in morbidity and mortality. Table 8-3 describes these changes. Some of these health problems are addressed specifically in the Healthy People 2000 Objectives.

In addition to the more specific changes listed in Table 8-3, recently reported research clearly shows that chronic alcohol use damages the immune system and the nervous system. These chronic users are at higher risk for a variety of infections and neurological complications.[1]

Fetal Alcohol Syndrome and Fetal Alcohol Effect

A growing body of scientific evidence indicates that alcohol use by pregnant women can result in a variety of birth defects in unborn children. When alcohol crosses the **placenta,** it enters the fetal bloodstream in a concentration equal to that in the mother's bloodstream. Because of the underdeveloped nature of the fetal liver, this alcohol is oxidized much more slowly than the alcohol in the mother. During this time of slow detoxification, the developing fetus is certain to be overexposed to the toxic effects of alcohol. Mental retardation frequently develops.

This exposure produces additional disastrous consequences for the developing fetus. Low birth weight, facial abnormalities (small head, widely spaced eyes), mental retardation, learning disability, joint problems, and heart problems are often seen in such infants (Figure 8-6). This combination of effects is called **fetal alcohol syndrome (FAS).** After Down syndrome, FAS

TABLE 8-3 Alcohol-Related Health Problems

Body system	Health problem
Digestive system	Malnutrition caused by faulty dietary practices (consumption of empty calories, resulting obesity); impaired food absorption; nausea; diarrhea; vomiting; prevalance of cancer of the mouth, larynx, esophagus, and liver
Oral cavity	When combined with smoking, alcohol use promotes cancer of the mouth, tongue, and throat
Esophagus	Irritation, impaired swallowing
Liver	Chemical imbalance: altered protein production, blood sugar imbalance, fat accumulation in the liver tissue
	Inflammation: impaired circulation, scar tissue formation, alcohol-related hepatitis
	Cirrhosis: impaired circulation, kidney failure, death
Stomach	Irritation, gastritis, ulceration
Pancreas	Inflammation (pancreatitis)
Circulatory system	Cardiomyopathy: shortness of breath, heart enlargement
	Arrhythmias: cardiac insufficiency
	Coronary artery disease: angina pectoris, myocardial infarction hemorrhagic stroke, hypertension
Reproductive system	
Women	Dysmenorrhea, infertility, miscarriage, fetal alcohol syndrome
Men	Impotence, low testosterone levels, low sperm count

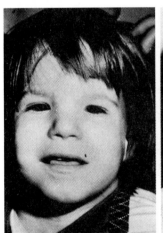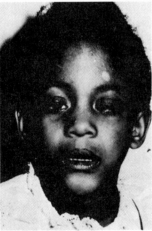

Figure 8-6 Widely spaced eyes are a facial characteristic of children with fetal alcohol syndrome.

remains the most common cause of mental retardation.[10] Recent estimates indicate that the full expression of this syndrome occurs at a rate of between one and three per thousand births. Partial expression, fetal alcohol effect (FAE), can be seen in three to nine per thousand live births.[1]

Is there a safe limit to the number of drinks one can consume during pregnancy? Since no one can accu-rately predict the impact of even small amounts of alcohol during pregnancy, the wisest plan would be to avoid alcohol altogether.

Because of the critical growth and development that occurs during the first months of fetal life, women who have any reason to think they are pregnant

acute alcohol intoxication potentially fatal elevation of the blood alcohol concentration, often resulting from heavy, rapid consumption of alcohol.

shock profound collapse of many vital body functions; evident during acute alcohol intoxication and other serious health emergencies.

asphyxiation (uhs fix ee **ay** shun) death resulting from lack of oxygen to the brain.

placenta (pluh **sent** uh) structure through which nutrients, metabolic wastes, and drugs (including alcohol) pass from the bloodstream of the mother into the bloodstream of the developing fetus.

fetal alcohol syndrome (FAS) characteristic birth defects noted in the children of some women who consume alcohol during their pregnancies.

"Moderate Drinking" Redefined

Alcohol Alert, a publication of the National Institute on Alcohol Abuse and Alcoholism, indicates that moderate drinking can be defined as no more than two drinks each day for most men and no more than one drink each day for women.[19] These levels of consumption are based on the amount of alcohol that can be consumed without causing problems, either for the drinker or society. (The gender difference is due primarily to the higher percentage of body fat in women and the lower level of an essential stomach enzyme in women.) Elderly persons are limited to no more than one drink each day, again due to the higher percentage of body fat in older persons.

These consumption levels are appropriate for most people. However, people who plan to drive, women who are pregnant, recovering alcoholics, people under age 21, people taking medications, and those with existing medical concerns should not consume alcohol. Additionally, although some studies have shown that low levels of alcohol may promote minor psychological and cardiovascular benefits, the NIAAA does not advise nondrinkers to start drinking. ★

should stop all alcohol consumption. Furthermore, women who are planning to become pregnant or women who are not practicing effective contraception must also consider keeping their alcohol use to a minimal level.

ALCOHOL-RELATED SOCIAL PROBLEMS

Beyond personal health problems, the misuse and abuse of alcohol is related to a variety of social problems. These problems effect the quality of interpersonal relationships, employment stability, and the financial security on which both the individual and family depend. Clearly, alcohol's negative social impact lowers our quality of life. In financial terms, the cost of alcohol abuse and dependence has been estimated at $136.3 billion for 1990 and $150 billion for 1995.[1]

The impact of alcohol consumption on several of these problems was summarized in the 1990 *7th Special Report to the U.S. Congress on Alcohol and Health*.[1] This major report documented reported findings in the area of accidents, crime and violence, and suicide.

Accidents

The four leading causes of accidental death (motor vehicle crashes, falls, drownings, and fires and burns) have significant statistical connections to alcohol use.

Approximately half of all fatal traffic crashes are alcohol related. Further, the likelihood of a fatal crash is about eight times higher for a drunk driver (0.10% BAC) than for a sober one.

Many are surprised to find that falls are the second leading cause of accidental death in the United States, with about 13,000 deaths per year. Alcohol use increases the risk of falls. Various studies suggest that alcohol is involved in between 17% and 53% of deadly falls, and between 21% and 77% of nonfatal falls.

Drownings represent the third leading cause of accidental death in the United States. Studies have shown that alcohol use is implicated in approximately 38% of these deaths. Over one third of boaters drink alcohol beverages while boating.

Fires and burns are responsible for an estimated 6000 deaths each year. This fourth leading cause of accidental death is also connected to alcohol use, with studies indicating that nearly half of burn victims have BACs above the legal limit.

Crime and Violence

You may have noticed at your college that most of the violent behavior and vandalism on university campuses is related to alcohol use. Indeed, the connection of alcohol to crime has a long history. Prison populations have large percentages of alcohol abusers and alcoholics. People who commit crimes are more likely to have alcohol problems than people in the general population. This is especially true for young criminals. Alcohol use has been reported in 67% of all homicides, with either the victim, the perpetrator, or both found to be drinking. In rape situations, rapists are intoxicated 50% of the time and victims 30% of the time.[6]

Because of research methodological problems, pinpointing alcohol's connection to family violence is difficult.[1] However, it seems clear that among a large number of families, alcohol is associated with violence and other negative interactions, including physical abuse, child abuse, psychological abuse, and abandonment.[6]

Suicide

The 1990 *7th Special Report to the U.S. Congress on Alcohol and Health* points to alcohol's relationship to suicide. Between 20% and 36% of suicide victims have a history of alcohol abuse or were drinking shortly before their suicides. Also, alcohol use is associated with impulsive suicides rather than with premeditated ones. Drinking is also connected with more violent and lethal forms of suicide, such as the use of firearms.[1]

For many of these social problems, alcohol use impairs critical judgment and allows a person's behavior to quickly become reckless, antisocial, and deadly. Because most of us wish to minimize problems associated with alcohol use, hosting a responsible party is a first step in this direction.

HOSTING A RESPONSIBLE PARTY

Some people might say that no party is totally safe when alcohol is served. These people are probably right when you consider the possibility of unexpected **drug synergism,** overconsumption, and the consequences of released inhibitions. Fortunately an increasing awareness of the value of responsible party hosting seems to be permeating college communities. The impetus for this awareness has come from various sources, including the respect for an individual's right to choose not to drink alcohol, the growing recognition of alcohol-related automobile accidents, and the legal threats related to **host negligence.**

For whatever reasons, hosting responsible parties at which alcohol is served is becoming a trend, especially among college-educated young adults. The Education Commission of the States' Task Force on Responsible Decisions about Alcohol has generated a list of guidelines for hosting a social event that includes the use of alcohol beverages. The list includes the following recommendations[11]:

▼ Provide other social activities as a primary focus when alcohol beverage is served.
▼ Respect an individual's decision about alcohol, if that decision is either to abstain or to drink responsibly.
▼ Recognize the decision not to drink and the respect it warrants by providing equally attractive and accessible nonalcohol drinks when alcohol is served.
▼ Recognize that drunkenness is neither healthful nor safe. One should not excuse otherwise unacceptable behavior either for that individual or for others solely because of "too much to drink."
▼ Provide food when alcohol is served.
▼ Serve diluted drinks and do not urge that glasses be constantly full.
▼ Keep the cocktail hour before dinner to a reasonable time and consumption limit.
▼ Recognize a responsibility for the health, safety, and pleasure of both the drinker and the nondrinker by avoiding intoxication and helping others to do the same.
▼ Make contingency plans for intoxication. If it occurs in spite of efforts to prevent it, assume responsibility for the health and safety of guests—transportation home, overnight accommodations, etc.
▼ Serve or use alcohol only in environments conducive to pleasant and relaxing behavior.

In addition to these suggestions, we would add that the use of a **designated driver** is an important component of responsible alcohol use. By planning to abstain or carefully limit their own alcohol consumption, designated drivers are able to safely transport friends who have been drinking. Have you noticed an increased use of designated drivers in your community? Would you be willing to be a designated driver?

ORGANIZATIONS SUPPORTING RESPONSIBLE DRINKING

The serious consequences of the irresponsible use of alcohol have led to the formation of a number of concerned-citizen groups. Although each organization has its specific approach, all attempt to deal objectively with two indisputable facts: alcohol use is part of our society, and irresponsible alcohol use can be deadly.

Mothers Against Drunk Drivers

Mothers Against Drunk Drivers (MADD) is a national network of over 400 local chapters in the United States and Canada. MADD attempts to educate people about alcohol's effects on driving and to influence legislation and enforcement of laws related to drunk drivers. This organization clearly had a major impact on the passage of a federal law requiring states to raise the drinking age to 21 or risk the loss of federal highway funds.

Students Against Driving Drunk

Students Against Driving Drunk (SADD) is an organization composed primarily of high school students whose goal is to reduce drinking-related deaths among teenagers. Founded in 1981, SADD now has approximately 15,000 chapters and about 4 million members. In this organization, students help to educate other students about the consequences of combining drinking and driving. One interesting feature of this organization's effort is the encouragement of a contract between students and their parents to provide transportation for each other if either is unable to drive safely after consuming alcohol. This pact also stipulates that no consequences are to be discussed until the following day.

Boost Alcohol Consciousness Concerning the Health of University Students

BACCHUS is an acronym for Boost Alcohol Consciousness Concerning the Health of University Students. Run by student volunteers, this college-

---

drug synergism (**sin** er jism) enhancement of a drug's effect as a result of the presence of additional drugs within the system.

host negligence (**neg** luh jence) a legal term that reflects the failure of a host to provide reasonable care and safety for persons visiting the host's residence or business.

designated driver a person who abstains or carefully limits alcohol consumption to be able to safely transport other people who have been drinking.

based organization promotes responsible drinking among university students who choose to drink. BACCHUS supports responsible party hosting, including providing quantities of food and nonalcohol beverages. The individual chapters of BACCHUS (now totaling well over 200) are encouraged to use a number of innovative educational approaches to promote alcohol awareness.

Other Approaches

Other responsible approaches to alcohol use are surfacing on a near daily basis. Even among college fraternity organizations, attitudes toward the indiscriminate use of alcohol are changing. Most fraternity rush functions are now conducted without the use of alcohol.

Another encouraging sign seen on college campuses is the increasing number of "alcohol use task forces." Although each of these study committees has its own focus and title, many of these groups are meeting to discuss alcohol-related concerns on their particular campus. These task forces often attempt to formulate detailed, comprehensive policies for alcohol use across the entire campus community. Membership on these committees often includes students (on-campus and off-campus, graduate and undergraduate), faculty and staff members, academic administrators, residence hall advisors, university police, health center personnel, alumni, and local citizens. Does your college have such an ongoing committee?

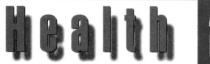

Tips to Help You Keep Drinking under Control

▼ Do not drink before a party.
▼ Avoid drinking when you are anxous, mad or depressed.
▼ Measure the liquor you put in mixed drinks (1-1½ oz).
▼ Eat ample amounts of food before and during your drinking.
▼ Avoid drinking games.
▼ Do not drive after drinking; use a "designated" nondrinking driver.
▼ Consume only a preplanned number of drinks.
▼ Stop alcohol consumption at a preplanned hour.

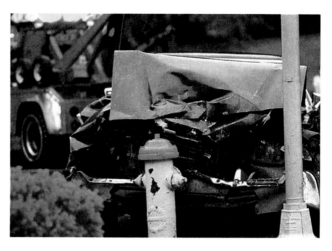

Drinking drivers frequently hurt themselves as well as others.

PROBLEM DRINKING AND ALCOHOLISM

Problem Drinking

At times, the line separating problem drinking from alcoholism is difficult to distinguish. There may be no true line with the exception that an alcoholic is unable to stop drinking. **Problem drinking** reflects a pattern of alcohol use in which a drinker's behavior creates personal difficulties or difficulties for other persons. What are some of these behaviors? Examples might be drinking to avoid life stressors, going to work intoxicated, drinking and driving, becoming injured or injuring others while drinking, solitary drinking, morning drinking, an occasional **blackout,** and being told by others that one drinks too much. For college students, two clear indications of problem drinking are missing classes and lowered academic performance as a result of alcohol involvement.

Problem drinkers are not always heavy drinkers. Problem drinkers might not be daily or even weekly drinkers. Unlike alcoholics, problem drinkers do not need to drink to maintain "normal" body functions. However, when they do drink, they (and others around them) experience problems—sometimes with tragic consequences. It is not surprising that problem drinkers are more likely than other drinkers to eventually develop alcoholism. Are there people around you that you believe may show signs of problem drinking?

Alcohol and Driving

Reports indicate that the percentage of traffic deaths resulting from alcohol use has dropped to below 50%. However, the 22,000 deaths attributed to drunk driving remain unacceptably high, and the additional serious injuries are great. Within the last few years, all states have raised the legal drinking age to 21 years.

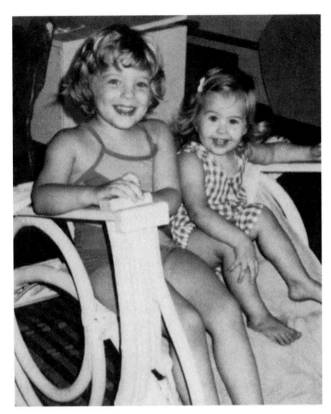

DRUNK DRIVING DOESN'T JUST KILL DRUNK DRIVERS.

Hannah and Sarah Fogleman, killed Dec. 12, 1988 at 2:22 pm on I-95 South, Brunswick, GA.

Next time your friend insists on driving drunk, do whatever it takes to stop him.

Because if he kills innocent people, how will you live with yourself?

FRIENDS DON'T LET FRIENDS DRIVE DRUNK.

Ad Council

U.S. Department of Transportation

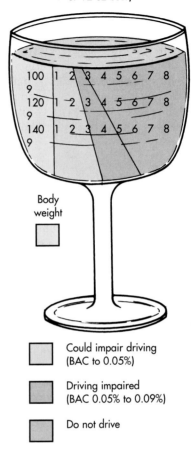

Number of drinks
in 2-hour period
(1½-oz 86-proof liquor
or 12-oz beer)

Body
weight

Could impair driving
(BAC to 0.05%)

Driving impaired
(BAC 0.05% to 0.09%)

Do not drive

Figure 8-7 For most states, a BAC of 0.10% represents legal intoxication. However, even a lower BAC can impair functioning enough to lead to a serious accident.

Most states have set 0.10% as the BAC level at which drivers are considered legally drunk (Figure 8-7). However, by January 1994, 10 states had lowered this standard to 0.08%, and legislative efforts were being made in many other states to follow this trend. Some states were enacting **zero tolerance laws** to help prevent underage drinking and driving. These laws may help the United States achieve one of its major health objectives for the year 2000.

Other programs and policies are being used that are designed to prevent intoxicated people from driving. Included among these are efforts to educate bartenders to recognize intoxicated customers, to establish designated drivers, to use off-duty police officers as observers in bars, to use police roadblocks, and to develop mechanical devices that prevent intoxicated drivers from starting their cars.

problem drinking alcohol use pattern in which a drinker's behavior creates personal difficulties or difficulties for other persons.

blackout temporary state of amnesia experienced by an alcoholic; an inability to remember events that occurred during a period of alcohol use.

zero tolerance laws as pertains to alcohol consumption, laws that severely restrict the right to operate motor vehicles for underage drinkers who have been convicted of driving under *any* influence.

Progressive Stages of Alcohol Dependence

Early	Middle	Late
Escape drinking	Loss of control	Prolonged binges
Binge drinking	Self-hate	Alcohol used to control
Guilt feelings	Impaired social relationships	withdrawal symptoms
Sneaking drinks	Changes in drinking patterns (more frequent	Alcohol psychosis
Difficulty stopping once drink-	binge drinking)	Nutritional disease
ing has begun	Temporary sobriety	
Increased tolerance	Morning drinking	
Preoccupation with drinking	Dietary neglect	
Blackouts		

Alcoholism

In 1992, a revised definition of **alcoholism** was established by a joint committee of experts in alcohol dependence.[12] This committee stated that alcoholism:

> . . . is a primary, chronic disease with genetic, psychosocial, and environmental factors influencing its development and manifestations. The disease is often progressive and fatal. It is characterized by impaired control over drinking, preoccupation with the drug alcohol, use of alcohol despite adverse consequences, and distortions in thinking, most notably denial. Each of these symptoms may be continuous or periodic.

This definition incorporates many of the recent concepts gained from addictions research in the last two decades. It is well recognized that alcoholics do not drink for the pleasurable effects of alcohol but to escape being sober. For alcoholics, being sober is a stressful experience.

Unlike problem drinking, alcoholism involves a physical addiction to alcohol.

For the true alcoholic, when the body is deprived of alcohol, physical and mental withdrawal symptoms become evident. These withdrawal symptoms can be life threatening. Uncontrollable shaking can progress into nausea, vomiting, hallucinations, shock, and ultimately to cardiac and pulmonary arrest. Uncontrollable shaking, combined with irrational hallucinations, represents *delirium tremens* (DTs), an occasional manifestation during an alcoholic's withdrawal.

The physical and emotional dependence encompassed by the term *alcoholism* has a complex and poorly understood cause. Why, when more than 100 million adults use alcohol without establishing a dependence relationship with it, do 10 million or more individuals lose their ability to control its use?

Could alcoholism be an inherited disease? Studies in humans and animals provide strong evidence that genetics play a role in some cases of alcoholism. Two forms of alcoholism are thought to be inherited: Type I

and Type II. Type I is thought to take years to develop and may not surface until the mid-life years. Type II is a more severe form and appears to be passed primarily from fathers to sons. This form of alcoholism frequently occurs earlier in a person's life and may start in adolescence.

Genetics also may account for some alcoholism seen in Asian people. In the case of these persons, low levels of aldehyde dehydrogenase (an enzyme necessary for the metabolism of alcohol) may account for an intolerance to alcohol. Genetic factors pertaining to the absorption rates of alcohol in the intestinal tract have been hypothesized to predispose American Indians to alcoholism. It is likely that more research will be undertaken concerning the role of genetic factors in all forms of chemical dependence.

The role of personality traits as conditioning factors in the development of alcoholism has received considerable attention. Factors ranging from unusually low levels of self-esteem to an antisocial personality have been described. Additional factors making persons susceptible to alcoholism may include excessive reliance on denial, hypervigilance, compulsiveness, and chronic levels of anxiety. Always complicating the study of personality traits is the uncertainty of whether the personality profile is a predisposing factor (perhaps from inheritance) or is caused by alcoholism.

Denial and Enabling

Problem drinkers and alcoholics frequently use the psychological defense mechanism of *denial* to maintain their drinking behavior. By convincing themselves that their lives are not affected by their drinking behavior, problem drinkers and alcoholics are able to maintain their drinking patterns. A person's denial is an unconscious process that is apparent only to rational observers.

Formerly, it was up to alcoholics to admit that their denial was no longer effective before they could be admitted to a treatment program. This is not the case today. Currently, family members, friends, or co-workers of alcohol-dependent persons are encouraged to intervene and force an alcohol-dependent person into treatment.

During treatment, it is important for chemically dependent persons to break through the security of denial and to admit that alcohol controls their lives. This process will be demanding and often time consuming, but no alternative exists if recovery is to be achieved.

For family and friends of chemically dependent people, denial can be evident in a process known as *enabling*. In this process, people close to the problem drinker or alcoholic inadvertently support drinking behaviors by denying that a problem really exists. Enablers unconsciously make excuses for the drinker, try to keep the drinker's work and family life intact, and in effect make the continued abuse of alcohol possible. Alcohol counselors contend that enablers are an alcoholic's worst enemy because they can significantly delay the onset of effective therapy. Do you know of a situation in which you or others have enabled a person with alcohol problems?

Codependence

Within the last decade, a new term has been used to describe the relationship betwen drug-dependent people and those around them—*codependence*. This term implies a kind of dual addiction. The alcoholic and the person close to the alcoholic are both addicted; one to alcohol and the other to a person. People who are codependents frequently find themselves denying and enabling the drug-dependent person.[6]

Unfortunately, this kind of behavior damages both the alcoholic and the codependent. The alcoholic's intervention and treatment may be delayed for a considerable time. Codependent people often pay a heavy price as well. Even if they do not become drug dependent themselves, they may suffer a variety of psychological consequences related to guilt, loss of self-esteem, depression, and anxiety. Codependents may place themselves at increased risk for both physical and sexual abuse.

Fortunately, research continues to explore this dimension of alcoholism. A number of students have found some of the resources listed in this chapter to be especially helpful.

Adult Children of Alcoholics

Just over 10 years ago, an additional dimension of alcoholism was recognized—the unusually high prevalence of alcoholism in the *adult children of alcoholics (ACOAs)*. Estimates are that these adult children are about four times more likely to develop alcoholism than children whose parents were not alcoholics. In the United States, there are an estimated 28 million

---

★ Common Traits of ACOAs

Adult children of alcoholics:

★ Guess what normal behavior is

★ Have difficulty following a project from beginning to end

★ Lie when it would be just as easy to tell the truth

★ Judge themselves without mercy

★ Have difficulty having fun

★ Take themselves very seriously

★ Have difficulty with intimate relationships

★ Overreact to changes over which they have no control

★ Constantly seek approval and affirmation

★ Feel that they are different from other people

★ Are super-responsible or super-irresponsible

★ Are extremely loyal, even in the face of evidence that the loyalty is undeserved

★ Tend to lock themselves into a course of action without giving consideration to consequences

---

ACOAs.[13] Clearly, large numbers of these ACOAs do not become alcoholics or even have major life crises, but even ACOAs who do not become alcoholics may have a difficult time adjusting to everyday living patterns. Janet Geringer Wotitz, author of the landmark book *Adult Children of Alcoholics*, describes 13 traits that, to some degree, most ACOAs exhibit (see the box above).[14]

The difficulties that ACOAs have can be traced to the years of living in an alcoholic family. When they were children, ACOAs had to learn survival behaviors to cope with the complexities of living in a dysfunctional family. A number of these behaviors were probably compulsive ones that permitted the child to adjust to the inconsistencies, embarrassment, shame, denial, secrecy, lying, and feelings of being trapped, isolated or different.[13] As these children grew up and moved into a more healthy environment, the behaviors they learned in the dysfunctional family may not have served them well.

> **alcoholism** a primary, chronic disease with genetic, psychosocial, and environmental factors influencing its development and manifestations.

Resources for Children of Alcoholics

Many experts agree that children of alcoholics who believe they have come to terms with their feelings sometimes face lingering problems. It can prove worthwhile to seek help if you experience the following:

★ Have difficulty in identifying your needs

★ Are always angry or sad

★ Cannot enjoy your successes

★ Tolerate inappropriate behavior

★ Are regularly afraid of losing control

Support groups to contact for more information include:

Al-Anon Adult Family Groups
1372 Broadway
New York, NY 10018-0862
(212) 302-7240

Children of Alcoholics Foundation, Inc.
P.O. Box 4185
Grand Central Station
New York, NY 10163
(212) 754-0656

National Council on Alcoholism and Drug Dependence
12 West 21st Street
New York, NY 10010
(212) 206-6770
(800) NCA-CALL (800-622-2255)

Many ACOAs have a difficult time discovering what "normal" behavior really is. For this reason, ACOAs have a tendency to marry alcoholics. In a sense, the ACOAs are familiar with the chaos of living with an alcoholic.

In response to the concern about ACOAs, support groups have been formed to assist adult sons and daughters in understanding their situations (see the box above). Through support groups, ACOAs can better learn about themselves. They must learn to be honest with themselves and others and to identify unhealthy patterns in their lives. They must learn that they did not cause their parents' drinking problems. They must learn that there are other ACOAs who have had similar struggles and that help is available, on both a professional and support group level. Finally, ACOAs must learn to take charge and seek help for themselves.[13]

Alcoholism and the Family

Because the alcoholic individual is afflicted and subsequently affects the entire family, there is considerable disruption in the families of alcoholics. Families are disrupted not only by the consequences of the drinking behavior (such as violence, illness, unemployment), but also by the uncertainty of their role in causing and prolonging the situation. Frequently, family members begin to adopt a variety of new roles that will allow them to cope with the presence of the alcoholic in the family. Among the more commonly seen roles are the family hero, the lost child, the family mascot, and the scapegoat.[6] Unless family members receive appropriate counseling, these roles may remain intact for a lifetime.

Once an alcoholic's therapy has begun, family members are encouraged to participate in many aspects of the recovery. This will also help them to better understand the ways in which they were affected by alcoholism. Should therapy and aftercare include participation in Alcoholics Anonymous, family members will be encouraged to affiliate with related support groups.

HELPING THE ALCOHOLIC: REHABILITATION AND RECOVERY

Once an alcoholic realizes that alcoholism is not a form of moral weakness but rather a clearly defined illness, the chances for recovery are remarkably good. It is estimated that as many as two thirds of the victims of alcoholism can recover. Recovery is especially enhanced when the victim has a good emotional support system, including concerned family members, friends, and employer. When this support system is not well established, the alcoholic's chances for recovery become considerably lessened.

Treatment methods for alcoholism will vary according to the specific needs of the individual. Following are three general steps in the treatment of alcoholism:

1. *Managing acute episodes of intoxication* to save a life and overcome the immediate effects of excess alcohol. This step usually includes inpatient medical care for the person suffering from severe intoxication or acute alcohol withdrawal. Depending on the severity of the acute medical problem, the alcoholic may spend up to 2 weeks receiving this medical care. Common procedures might include proper *hydration,* use of transquilizers to cope with withdrawal symptoms, and close supervision of food intake and **electrolyte balance.**

   Some therapists prescribe the deterrent drug disulfiram (Antabuse) in the initial weeks following detoxification. This drug is taken daily and produces an array of unpleasant symptoms if the patient should subsequently consume alcohol. These symptoms include nausea, vomiting, and pounding headaches. Used temporarily as an aid to other forms of supportive treatment, Antabuse can help the patient make the critical decision not to drink.

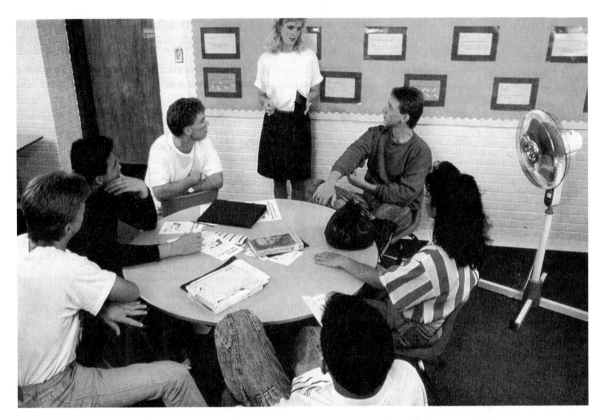

Problem drinkers and alcoholics need professional help.

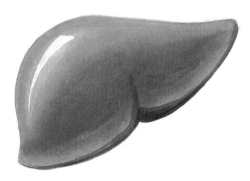

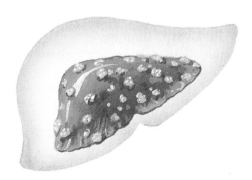

Figure 8-8 *Top*, normal liver; *bottom*, cirrhosis of the liver.

2. *Correcting chronic health problems* associated with alcoholism. During this stage of treatment, attempts are made to medically manage established diseases such as **cirrhosis (Figure 8-8),** *polyneuropathy,* and even psychiatric disorders that have an origin in alcoholism.
3. *Changing long-term behavior* of alcoholic individuals so that destructive drinking patterns are not continued. Through individual and group counseling, the alcoholic learns to focus on behaviors that can produce positive effects in a person's life. No one plan is effective for everyone. Attempts are often made to encourage the development of skills in assertiveness, stress management, problem solving, and relaxation.

electrolyte balance (ee **lek** tro lite) proper concentration of various minerals within the blood and body fluids.

cirrhosis (sir **oh** sis) pathological changes to the liver resulting from chronic, heavy alcohol consumption; a frequent cause of death among heavy alcohol users.

These three general steps to the treatment of alcoholism can be undertaken in various settings, including hospitals, clinics, and centers. Inpatient treatment usually lasts about 4 weeks and can cost between $10,000 and $20,000. Increasing evidence indicates that outpatient treatment can be as effective as inpatient treatment and costs less.

Twelve-Step Programs

People who seek recovery from alcohol addiction can become involved with "twelve-step programs." These programs may be run independently or jointly with traditional medical management procedures just described. Twelve-step programs are best represented by *Alcoholics Anonymous (AA).* AA is a voluntary fellowship of men and women whose primary purpose is to get sober, stay sober, and help others achieve sobriety. AA was started by two recovering alcoholics in 1934 in Akron, Ohio.[15]

Alcoholics Anonymous's only membership requirement is a person's desire to stop drinking. AA charges no dues for membership and is self-supported by personal contributions. AA is not organized around any sect or religious denomination. AA does not involve itself with politics or controversy and does not support or oppose any causes. Its only purpose is to help members retain sobriety.[16]

The term *twelve-step* comes from the 12 steps to recovery from alcoholism that AA members support. (See the box on the right.) Keys to accomplishing the twelve steps are a belief in personal humility coupled with a belief in a "higher power." The higher power is defined according to each AA member's personal interpretation. According to AA, to achieve sobriety, an alcoholic must admit that a power exists that is greater than himself or herself.[16] In this sense, there is a strong spiritual component to AA, although this spiritual component is defined solely by the alcoholic.

AA members do not attempt to scientifically understand their drinking behaviors. Rather, they attempt to rely on simple slogans or sayings to help them take being sober "one day at a time." The three most common slogans of AA are "first things first," "easy does it," and "live and let live." Most AA members have sponsors. These are sober men and women who have significant experience with AA and serve as confidants or mentors to newer AA members. Over 87,000 AA groups exist through the world. AA has members in 134 countries.

AL-ANON AND ALATEEN

Al-Anon and Alateen are parallel organizations to AA that give support to persons who live with alcoholics. Al-Anon is geared for spouses and other relatives, whereas Alateen focuses on children of alcoholics. Both organizations help members realize that they are not alone and that successful adjustments can be made

The Twelve Steps of Alcoholics Anonymous

1. We admitted we were powerless over alcohol—that our lives had become unmanageable.

2. Came to believe that a Power greater than ourselves could restore us to sanity.

3. Made a decision to turn our will and our lives over to the care of God *as we understood Him.*

4. Made a searching and fearless moral inventory of ourselves.

5. Admitted to God, to ourselves, and to another human being the exact nature of our wrongs.

6. Were entirely ready to have God remove all these defects of character.

7. Humbly asked Him to remove our shortcomings.

8. Made a list of all persons we had harmed, and became willing to make amends to them all.

9. Made direct amends to such people wherever possible, except when to do so would injure them or others.

10. Continued to take personal inventory and when we were wrong, promptly admitted it.

11. Sought through prayer and meditation to improve our conscious contact with God, *as we understood Him*, praying only for knowledge of His will for us and the power to carry that out.

12. Having had a spiritual awakening as the result of these steps, we tried to carry this message to alcoholics, and to practice these principles in all our affairs.[16]

to nearly every alcoholic-related situation. AA, Al-Anon, and Alateen chapter organizations are usually listed in the telephone book or in the classified sections of local newspapers.

Secular Recovery Programs

Despite the significant impact that AA and other twelve-step programs have had for many alcoholics, a growing body of people feel uncomfortable with the concept of having to admit that their lives are, ultimately, controlled by a higher power. They feel uncomfortable with notions of divine intervention and a spiritual guidance.

For these persons, *secular recovery programs* may be the answer for controlling their alcoholism. These programs maintain that sobriety comes from within the alcoholic. Secular programs place major emphasis on self-reliance and self-determination.[17] During their group meetings, they encourage rational thinking and attempt to identify the irrational thoughts some members might have concerning their alcoholic behavior.

Unlike most twelve-step programs, there are no sponsor systems in secular recovery programs. Personal independence is encouraged. Like twelve-step programs, secular recovery programs do not criticize any other recovery programs, do not have a political agenda, and are self-supporting through voluntary contributions from members.[18]

There are two especially notable secular recovery programs. Secular Organizations for Sobriety (SOS) was begun in 1985 by James Christopher, a recovering alcoholic. For additional information, SOS can be reached at SOS National Clearinghouse, P.O. Box 5, Buffalo, NY 14215-0015, phone: (716)-834-2922. A second well-known secular recovery program is called Rational Recovery Systems (RRS). Known simply as Rational Recovery, this program can be reached at: RRS, Box 800, Lotus, CA 95691. Since these programs are relatively new, you may have to search carefully to find out about local meetings.

WOMEN AND ALCOHOL

For decades, women have consumed less alcohol and had fewer alcohol-related problems than men have. As we move through the 1990s, evidence is mounting that a greater percentage of women are choosing to drink and some subgroups of women, especially young women, are drinking more heavily. Increased admissions of women to treatment centers may also reflect the fact that alcohol consumption among women is on the rise.[1]

Studies indicate that now there are almost as many female alcoholics as male alcoholics. However, there appear to be differences between men and women when it comes to alcohol abuse.[6] Some of the differences are as follows:

1. More women than men can point to a specific trigger or event (such as a divorce, death of a spouse, career change, or children leaving home) that started them drinking heavily.
2. Women's alcoholism often starts later and progresses more quickly than men's alcoholism.
3. Women tend to be prescribed more mood-altering drugs than men are. Thus women face the risks of drug interaction or cross-tolerance.
4. Nonalcoholic males tend to divorce their alcoholic spouses nine times more often than nonalcoholic females divorce their alcoholic spouses. Thus alcoholic women are not as likely to have a family support system to aid them in their recovery attempts.

5. Female alcoholics do not tend to receive as much social support as males in their treatment and recovery.
6. Unmarried, divorced, or single-parent women tend to have significant economic problems that may make entry into a treatment program especially difficult.[6]

In light of the generally recognized educational, occupational, and social gains made by women in the last 2 decades, it will be interesting to see whether these male/female differences in alcoholism continue to be found. What's your best guess?

ALCOHOL ADVERTISING

Every few years, careful observers can see subtle changes in the ways the alcohol beverage industry markets its products. Recently, the marketing push has been directed at minorities (through advertisements for malt liquor), women (through wine and wine cooler ads), and youth.

On the college campus, aggressive alcohol campaigns have used rock stars, beach party scenes, athletic event sponsorships, and colorful newspaper supplements as vehicles to encourage the purchase of alcohol. Critics of the alcohol beverage industry support a more visible role for the industry in the area of prevention. Critics claim that most of the collegiate advertising is directed at the "below age 21" crowd and that the prevention messages are not enough to offset the potential health damage to this population. As a college student, how do you feel about alcohol advertising on your campus? If you are a nontraditional student, do you find these advertising campaigns amusing or potentially dangerous?

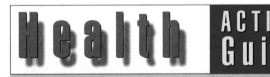

Advertising Ploys

The next time you watch television and see a beer commercial, you and your friends might analyze the commercial by considering the following points:

▼ How attractive are the actors in the commercial?
▼ What type of environment (or atmosphere) is presented?
▼ To what extent is responsibility encouraged?

Summary

✔ Alcohol is the drug of choice among college students and the rest of society.

✔ There are many factors that affect the rate of absorption of alcohol into the bloodstream.

✔ As the blood alcohol concentration (BAC) levels rise, predictable depressant effects take place.

✔ Persons in acute alcohol intoxication must receive first-aid care immediately.

✔ The health effects of chronic alcohol use are quite serious.

✔ Problem drinking reflects an alcohol use pattern in which a drinker's behavior creates personal difficulties or problems for others.

✔ Alcoholism is a primary, chronic disease with a variety of possible causes and characteristics.

✔ Denial, enabling, codependence, adult children of alcoholics, and alcohol advertising are current alcohol-related concerns.

✔ Through a variety of treatment programs, recovery from alcoholism is possible.

Review Questions

1. What percentage of American adults consume alcohol? Approximately what percentage of adults are classified as abstainers? What percentage of college students drink? What is binge drinking?

2. What is meant by the term *proof*? What is the nutritional value of alcohol? How do "lite" and low-alcohol beverages compare?

3. Identify and explain the various factors that influence the absorption of alcohol. Why is it important to be aware of these factors?

4. What is BAC? Describe the general sequence of physiological effects that takes place when a person drinks alcohol at a rate faster than the liver can oxidize it.

5. What are the signs and symptoms of acute alcohol intoxication? What are the first aid steps you should take to help a person with this problem?

6. Describe the characteristics of fetal alcohol syndrome and fetal alcohol effects.

7. Explain the differences between problem drinking and alcoholism.

8. What roles do denial and enabling play in alcoholism? What is codependence?

9. What are some common traits of ACOAs?

10. What special alcohol-related problems exist for women?

Think about This . . .

✔ How much is your decision to drink or not drink influenced by those around you?

✔ Did you know that drinking alcohol in cold weather actually causes heat loss? The feeling of warmth results from the loss of body heat related to the dilation of blood vessels under the skin. In effect you may feel warmer but are actually getting colder.

✔ This chapter refers to data indicating that about one third of college drinkers can be considered heavy drinkers. Do you think this is true at your college?

✔ What role should men play in the prevention of fetal alcohol syndrome?

✔ How can you tell whether you and your friends are drinking in a responsible manner?

✔ Do you believe it is your responsibility to make sure friends do not drink and drive?

✔ Do you think your drinking pattern will change when you are out of college?

REAL LIFE REAL CHOICES

YOUR TURN

▼ What role did Rick Diaz play as the oldest child in an alcoholic family?
▼ What is the term for the way Rick is behaving toward his alcoholic brother now?
▼ How could Rick be most helpful to his brother?

AND NOW, YOUR CHOICES. . .

▼ How do you think you would feel and behave if one of your parents were an alcoholic? If you have an alcoholic parent, how do you deal with the situation?
▼ How would you deal with a younger brother or sister you believed was drinking alcohol excessively? ▼

References

1. US Department of Health and Human Services: *Alcohol and health: seventh special report to the US Congress*, DHHS Pub No (ADM) 90-1656, Washington, DC, 1990, US Government Printing Office.

2. US Bureau of the Census: *Statistical abstracts of the United States, 1992*, ed 112, Washington, DC, 1992, US Government Printing Office.

3. US Department of Health and Human Services: *Smoking, drinking, and illicit drug use among American secondary school students, college students, and young adults, 1975-1992*, vol 2, NIH Pub No BKD-124, Washington, DC, 1993, US Government Printing Office.

4. Unpublished survey of students in HSC 160 class at Ball State University, 1994, Muncie, Indiana.

5. Presley CA, Meilman PW: *Alcohol and drugs on American college campuses: a report to college presidents, June 1992*, US Department of Education, Drug Prevention in Higher Education Program, (FIPSE Grant), Southern Illinois University Student Health Program Wellness Center.

6. Kinney J, Leaton G: *Loosening the grip: a handbook of alcohol information*, ed 5, St Louis, 1995, Mosby.

7. Ray O, Ksir C: *Drugs, society, and human behavior*, ed 6, St Louis, 1993, Mosby.

8. Frezza M, et al: High blood alcohol levels in women: the role of decreased gastric alcohol dehydrogenase activity and first-pass metabolism, *N Engl J Med* 322:(4)95-99, 1990.

9. American Red Cross: *Responding to emergencies*, St Louis, 1991, Mosby Lifeline Publishing.

10. Fetal alcohol syndrome, *The Harvard Mental Health Letter* 7:5, November 1990, pp 1-4.

11. Task Force on Responsible Decisions About Alcohol: Interim report No 2, Denver, Education Commission of the States.

12. Morse RM, et al: The definition of alcoholism, *JAMA* 268(8):1012-1014, 1992.

13. Maris M: *Adult children of alcoholics*, undated brochure, Muncie, Ind, Ball State University Alcohol Education Program, A.T. Wood Health Center.

14. Woititz JG: *Adult children of alcoholics*, Pompano Beach, Fla, 1983, Health Communications Inc.

15. Alcoholics Anonymous: *AA in treatment facilities*, Alcoholics Anonymous World Services, Inc, July 1991, pp 1-21.

16. Alcoholics Anonymous: *This is AA: an introduction to the AA recovery program*, Alcoholics Anonymous World Services, Inc, March 1992, pp 1-21.

17. Peterson KS: Rational Recovery's focus on self-reliance, *USA Today*, April 21, 1993, p 4-D.

18. Secular Organizations for Sobriety: *Save ourselves*, undated informational brochure, Council for Democractic and Secular Humanism (CODESH), Buffalo, NY, pp 1-5.

19. National Institute on Alcohol Abuse and Alcoholism: Moderate drinking, *Alcohol Alert*, #16, (PH 315), April, 1992, pp 1-4.

Suggested Readings

Beattie M: *The language of letting go*, San Francisco, 1990, Harper/Hazelden.
    The author of the best-selling Codependent No More *writes this meditation book for codependents. Presents daily readings (for January 1 through December 31) that encourage spiritual and emotional health. A calming book that focuses on self-esteem and acceptance.*

Rogers RL, McMillan CS: *Freeing someone you love from alcohol and other drugs*, New York, 1992, Perigee Books.

    A guide for people who have friends and loved ones who need treatment for their alcohol or other drug dependencies. Readers will learn the signs of addiction, treatment options, and how to get people into treatment.

ZP: *A skeptic's guide to the 12 steps*, Center City, Minn, 1991, Hazelden Educational Materials.
    Written by a psychologist who questions the value of a Higher Power in the twelve-step recovery programs, this book chronicles this skeptic's struggles with recognizing the value of a spiritual direction.

9

Tobacco Use

A Losing Choice

Today the evidence linking tobacco use to impaired health is beyond any serious challenge. The regular users of tobacco products, particularly cigarettes, and those who are exposed to their tobacco smoke, are more likely to experience serious health problems, and, perhaps, even die prematurely. In fact, in 1990, it was estimated that cigarette smoking cost 418,690 lives making it easily the single deadliest health behavior risk in the United States.[1] Consequently, any contention made by the tobacco industry suggesting that tobacco use is not dangerous is little more than a groundless statement that ignores the growing weight of scientific evidence.

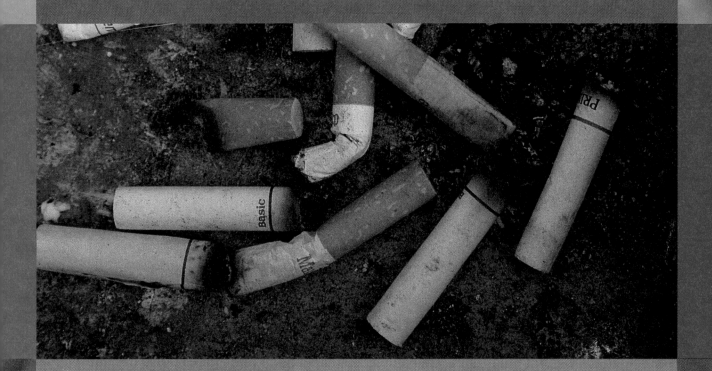

T O B A C C O

The following objectives are covered in this chapter:

▽ Slow the rise in lung cancer deaths to achieve a rate of no more than 42 per 100,000 people. (Age-adjusted baseline: 135 per 100,000 in 1987; p. 137.)

▽ Slow the rise in deaths from chronic obstructive lung disease (COLD) to achieve a rate of no more than 25 per 100,000 people. (Age-adjusted baseline: 18.7 per 100,000 in 1987; p. 138.)

▽ Reduce cigarette smoking to a prevalence of no more than 15% among people aged 20 and older. (Baseline: 29% in 1987; 32% for men and 27% for women; p. 140.)

▽ Reduce smokeless tobacco use by males aged 12 through 24 to a prevalence of no more than 4%. (Baseline: 6.6% among males aged 12 to 17 in 1988; 8.9% among males aged 18 to 24 in 1987; p. 147.)

▽ Reduce to no more than 20% the proportion of children aged 6 and younger who are regularly exposed to tobacco smoke at home. (Baseline: more than 39% in 1986, since 39% of households with one or more children aged 6 or younger had a cigarette smoker in the household; p. 146.)

REAL LIFE / REAL CHOICES — Smoking Can Be Hazardous to Your Health—and Relationships

▼ Names: Karen Heilmann and Steven Chu

▼ Ages: 24 and 23

▼ Occupation: Graduate students in molecular biology

Little more than a generation ago, smoking was considered sophisticated, sociable, and safe. Today there's ever-decreasing tolerance for smoking, and those who still cling to the habit may find it causes them heart problems—not only cardiovascular but also romantic.

That's the unhappy reality confronting Karen Heilmann and Steven Chu, who are both top students in their university's graduate program in molecular biology. They met as undergraduates and have been involved in a serious relationship for nearly 3 years. Although they don't plan to marry until they receive their doctorates, they intend to announce their engagement in the spring.

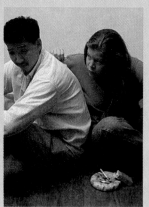

Karen and Steven seem to have everything going for them. But there's one big hang-up, at least in Steven's mind: Karen smokes. As a former smoker, Steven understands how easy it is to get "hooked" on nicotine and how difficult it can be to quit, but he's been putting increasing pressure on Karen to give it up. She smokes less than a pack a day, doesn't light up in Steven's apartment or car, and says she'll quit when she finishes her demanding graduate program. In the meantime, Steven and Karen have begun to spend more time arguing about smoking than enjoying each other's company, and last night Steven told Karen he wouldn't consider becoming engaged unless Karen agrees to quit smoking completely before they make the announcement.

As you study this chapter, think about steps Karen and Steven might take to resolve their conflict, and prepare yourself to answer the questions in **Your Turn** at the end of the chapter. ▼

TOBACCO USE IN AMERICAN SOCIETY

If you were to visit certain businesses, entertainment spots, or sporting events in your community, you might leave convinced that virtually every adult is a tobacco user. Certainly, for some segments of society, tobacco use is the rule rather than the exception. You may be quite surprised to find out that the great majority of adults do not use tobacco products.

On the basis of a variety of currently available statistics, less than 26% of all adults smoke cigarettes.[2] Further, data on smoking reveal that since 1964 the percentages of men and women who smoke cigarettes have declined steadily. For example, in 1965, 52.4% of adult males (age 20 and over) smoked compared with 28.1% in 1991. Among women (age 20 and over), 34.1% smoked in 1965 compared with 23.5% in 1991.[3]

Use Among Adolescents

As encouraging as it is that adults have moved away from smoking in recent decades, the most recent data about smoking by adolescents is discouraging. A recent report indicates that between 1992 and 1993 the daily use of cigarettes by high school seniors increased from 17% to 19%, whereas daily smoking by tenth graders and eight graders increased from 12% to 14% and from 7% to 8%, respectively.[3] The role of advertising targeted to adolescents in fostering this increase is discussed later in the chapter.

The Influence of Education

Regardless of other factors, the amount of formal education completed is associated with a lower rate of smoking. Among those with less than 12 years of formal education, 32% smoked during 1991, whereas among those with 16 or more years of education, only 13.6% were cigarette smokers.[2] Clearly, education appears to assist persons in understanding the risks of cigarette smoking. At this time, the group least likely to smoke cigarettes are African-American males enrolled in predominately black colleges.[4]

Alarmingly, however, studies since 1990 indicate a clear upturn in smoking among traditional-age college students. Are today's college students failing to understand the risks associated with smoking?

In contrast to the general population, where higher percentages of men than women smoke, college

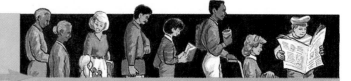

Learning FROM ALL Cultures

Tobacco Use

American cigarette companies are coping with the declining U.S. cigarette consumption by increasing their sales abroad, especially in developing nations. In the industrialized world, smoking is decreasing about 1% each year. However, in Asia and Latin America the incidence of smoking is growing 7% faster than the population. In Africa, it is growing 18% faster.[6]

Even with the availability of low and ultralow tar and nicotine cigarettes, given enough time, the health effects of cigarette smoking will begin to be seen in these countries. Who will take responsibility for the sickness and death that will occur?

Although the tobacco industry continues to advertise in developing countries, some governments of the Latin American countries are passing legislation restricting advertising and promotion of tobacco products. Fifteen Latin American countries have enacted legislation to discourage the use of cigarettes by adolescents and children, and thirteen of those fifteen countries have restricted the kind of advertising that targets young people. In six Latin American countries it is illegal to sell tobacco products to minors.[7]

Will legislation in these countries help reduce the use of tobacco? Is legislation that limits marketing and sales going to be enough? What else do these developing countries need to do to substantially reduce the use of tobacco products? ●

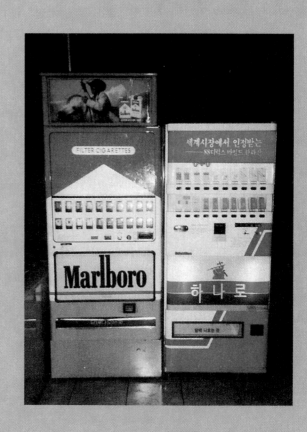

women are more likely to smoke than are college men. Approximately 16% of college women smoke, whereas only 12% of college men smoke.[5] When viewed in terms of daily smoking, 14.1% of all college students smoke. This rate has risen from 12.1% in 1990.[5] Very likely, the tendency for college students to be less likely to smoke than their noncollege peers is based on differences in cigarette use seen in high school.

Personal Preferences

Although the total percentage of the population using tobacco is lower now than it has been, the total number of persons using tobacco is at an all-time high. This finding reflects the continuing expansion of our population. Also, some evidence suggests that smokers are smoking more heavily than before. Regardless, cigarette sales are projected to begin a gradual decline as the number of young persons reaching "smoking age" declines and as more adult smokers stop.

In recent years the type of cigarettes preferred by smokers has changed. Today only a small percentage of all cigarette smokers prefer the small unfiltered cigarettes that were popular before and after World War II. Even the king-sized filtered cigarettes popular during the 1960s are losing popularity. High tar and high nicotine cigarettes have been replaced by low and ultralow tar and nicotine brands. Today *low tar and nicotine* brands (15 mg of tar or less) and *ultralow tar and nicotine* brands (less than 4 mg of tar) have the major share of the total cigarette market.

Advertising Approaches

The change in the American public's preference in cigarettes is a reflection of the strength of the tobacco industry in shaping demand for their products. Through continuous product development, skilled marketing, aggressive political lobbying, and diversification, the industry has managed to remain viable in the face of overwhelming evidence that their products are life-threatening. Several of their survival techniques are:

▼ Continued marketing of generic brands under the label of "value brands"
▼ Carefully targeted advertising, particularly to women, minorities, and less-educated young adults
▼ Youth-oriented advertisements (while simultaneously supporting public policy statements to control the access of cigarettes to minors)
▼ Increased marketing of tobacco products overseas where health restrictions are less forceful
▼ Acquiring nontobacco-related companies to minimize the loss of revenues from tobacco products
▼ Marshalling tobacco users into a "grass roots" effort to counter the growing political power of anti-smoking groups

Clearly, the tobacco industry remains healthy, while their products remain life-threatening to smokers and nonsmokers alike.

Pipe and Cigar Smoking

Many persons believe that pipe or cigar smoking is a safe alternative to cigarette smoking. Unfortunately, this is not the case. All forms of tobacco present users with a series of health threats.

When compared with cigarette smokers, pipe and cigar smokers have cancer of the mouth, throat, larynx (voice box), and esophagus at the same frequency. Cigarette smokers are more likely than pipe and cigar smokers to have lung cancer, chronic obstructive lung disease (COLD) and heart disease. However, the incidence of respiratory disease and heart disease in pipe and cigar smokers is greater than that among nonusers of tobacco.

★ Cigarette Advertising Approaches

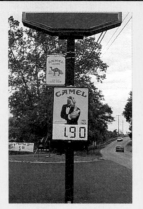

As the incidence of smoking declines within the general population, the tobacco industry has altered its advertising approaches to attract new markets and solidify their position in other markets. One tobacco company has attempted to target two groups: minorities from inner cities and undereducated "virile females." The R.J. Reynolds company unsuccessfully tried to test market a brand called Uptown. This cigarette was aimed principally at urban minorities. Test marketing was discontinued in 1990.

Reynolds also recently introduced a cigarette called Dakota. The group targeted for this cigarette is to be virile females—18- to 20-year-old females who have limited formal education and are holding entry-level factory jobs.

Philip Morris Tobacco Company targeted a different group with its super-thin, low-smoke cigarette Superslims. Apparently, marketing of Superslims has been aimed at a more sophisticated woman who is so concerned about her weight that she is willing to disregard the health risks of smoking in an attempt to remain thin.

"Misty" is a new value-brand (lower cost) cigarette being marketed to young women who are just beginning their professional careers. By producing this "fashionably inexpensive" cigarette, American Tobacco is offering a more affordable alternative to Virginia Slims and Slims. Of course, the model, Misty, appearing in the brand's initial advertisements, is thin. Although these brands are advertised to mature women, studies indicate that their appeal has been primarily to adolescent females.[8]

Macho males are not being spared the attention of tobacco companies either. New brands including Magna, Bucks, and a new version of Bull Durham, appeared in 1990. As more highly educated males continue to move away from tobacco use, these brands are designed to appeal to younger, less highly educated men.

Cartoon characters make seductive models. R.J. Reynolds' Old Joe Camel campaign has been so successful that Old Joe is a familiar face to American youngsters, rivaling that of Mickey Mouse.[9] Some health experts even suggest that Old Joe is largely responsible for adding 3000 new (adolescent age) smokers into the pipeline every day—the number needed by the tobacco industry to replace smokers who die or give up smoking. Regardless of whether they are new smokers or crossovers, preference for the Camel brand among younger smokers has increased from 2% to nearly 30%—five times the market share of the adult population. Few in the health field will be happy when Old Joe's soon to be introduced female friend joins in the promotion of Camels. Further, advertising experts suggest that the more Old Joe is criticized, the more attractive he will be to adolescents.

Reynolds, along with Philip Morris, the makers of Marlboro, use another marketing ploy to appeal to youth: the sale of promotional items such as magazines, calculators, T-shirts, caps, can holders, and posters. In the case of Camel cigarettes, these items can be bought with the "Camel Cash" coupons that accompany every package of Camel cigarettes purchased. ★

The Surgeon General's Warnings

Surgeon General's Warning:
Quitting smoking now greatly reduces serious risks to your health.

Surgeon General's Warning:
Cigarette smoke contains carbon monoxide.

Surgeon General's Warning:
Smoking by pregnant women may result in fetal injury, premature birth, and low birth weight.

Surgeon General's Warning:
Smoking causes lung cancer, heart disease, emphysema, and may complicate pregnancy.

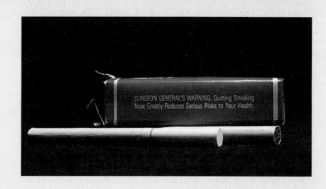

In addition to the health risks described, pipe and cigar smokers, like cigarette smokers, are not immune from the legal and social prohibitions against smoking. Whether pipe and cigar smoking even represents an "improvement" over cigarette smoking is open to debate. The use of smokeless tobacco, a third alternative to cigarette smoking, is discussed later in the chapter.

TOBACCO USE AND THE DEVELOPMENT OF DEPENDENCE

Dependence can imply both a physical and a psychological relationship. Particularly for the cigarette smoker, *physical dependence* or addiction, with its associated tolerance, withdrawal, and **titration;** and *psychological dependence* or habituation, with its accompanying psychological *compulsion* and *indulgence,* are frequently seen.

With dependence on tobacco, compulsion is a strong emotional desire to continue tobacco use despite restrictions and the awareness of health risks. Very likely, the user is "compelled" to engage in uninterrupted tobacco use in fear of the unpleasant physical, emotional, and social effects that result from discontinuing use. In comparison, indulgence is seen as "awarding" oneself for aligning with a particular behavior pattern (such as tobacco use). Indulgence is made possible by the existence of various reward systems built around the use of tobacco. From the peer group approval experienced by a beginning smoker to the sophisticated targeting of segments of the adult population by the tobacco industry, tobacco users are told that they "deserve" the benefits that are promised with tobacco use.

Much to the benefit of the tobacco industry, dependence (both addiction and habituation) on tobacco is easily established. Research indicates that 85% of all persons who experiment with cigarettes develop a dependent relationship. Typical cigarette smokers develop an addiction to nicotine, while at the same time they become emotionally dependent on its effect and the behaviors associated with obtaining it.

A small percentage of smokers, known as *"chippers,"* can smoke a few cigarettes on a daily basis without becoming dependent. Experts believe that they are less likely to use cigarettes to influence their mood and thus do not "require" cigarettes to feel a sense of pleasure.[10]

Physiological Factors Related to Dependence

Russell's bolus model[11] suggests that tobacco use is conditioned by the periods of neurohormonal arousal produced by each *bolus* (ball) of nicotine reaching the brain.

Nicotine activates receptors within the brain. Stimulation of the brain is seen as changes in electroencephalographic (EEG) patterns, reflecting an increase in the frequency of electrical activity. This is part of a general arousal pattern signaled by the release of the neurotransmitters norepinephrine, dopamine, acetylcholine, and serotonin.[11] It is likely that this increased activity within the central nervous system is perceived subjectively by the smoker as a feeling of well-being.

In a desire to maintain this feeling of arousal and well-being, the smoker inhales again and again. Several hundred puffs per day (approximately eight

titration (tie **tray** shun) particular level of a drug within the body; adjusting the level of nicotine by adjusting the rate of smoking.

per cigarette) quickly establish the schedule necessary to maintain the desired effect. Unique differences in smoking behavior (including the number of puffs per cigarette, the depth of inhalation, and the length of time the smoke is held in the lungs) and a variance in genetic predisposition to dependence account for the differing degrees of dependence noted among smokers. The speed at which dependence is established is also likely to be *dose related.*

A second theory of dependence suggests that nicotine stimulates the release of adrenocorticotropic hormone (ACTH) (see Chapter 3) from the pituitary gland, the "master gland" of the endocrine system. In response to the presence of ACTH, beta endorphins (naturally occurring opiate-like chemicals) are produced in specific areas of the brain, leading to mild feelings of euphoria. Nicotine has also been shown to have a stimulatory effect on the nervous system that, in itself, may be addictive for some individuals. It is probable that both of these factors play a part in the addictive process.

Yet another explanation called *self-medication* suggests that receptors for many mood-enhancing drugs, including nicotine, are located in the brain.[12] Smokers learn that they can physiologically "treat" periods of depression by using nicotine. Eventually they become physiologically and psychologically dependent on tobacco as a "medication" to make them feel better. Because tobacco is a legal drug, it becomes "preferred" over equally effective illicit drugs, such as cocaine and stimulants.

However, regardless of the mechanism involved, as tolerance to nicotine develops, smoking behavior is adjusted to maintain titration and prevent the occurrence of withdrawal symptoms. At some point the desire for constant arousal is probably negated by the smoker's desire not to experience withdrawal. Thus people smoke to protect themselves from the withdrawal effects rather than for the pleasure of being aroused.

As with any other psychoactive drug, cessation of nicotine can result in withdrawal symptoms. These symptoms are described in Chapter 7, p. 164.

THE ROLE OF NICOTINE

The importance of nicotine as the primary factor in establishing dependence on tobacco is supported by research that demonstrates that smokers will not select a nontobacco cigarette if a tobacco cigarette is available. Even tobacco cigarettes with a very low level of nicotine seem to be unacceptable to most smokers, as do cigarettes with very low nicotine but with high tar con-

How Much Do You Know About Smoking?

SMOKERS DIE YOUNGER

The death rate of cigarette smokers at all ages is higher than that of nonsmokers. It climbs in proportion to the number of cigarettes smoked, the number of years the smokers have smoked, and the age at which they started. According to the British Royal College of Physicians, "Cigarette smoking is now as important a cause of death as the great epidemics of typhoid, cholera, and tuberculosis in the past." The reason for the deadliness of cigarettes is the many different diseases they cause.

CIGARETTE-RELATED CANCERS IN MEN

Men who smoke less than half a pack a day have a death rate about 60% higher than that of nonsmokers; a pack to two packs a day, about 90% higher; and two or more packs a day, 120% above normal. Male cigarette smokers have about five times the normal risk of dying of mouth cancer as nonsmokers. Larynx cancer is six to nine times as frequent among cigarette smokers as among nonsmokers. Deaths from urinary bladder cancer are two to three times as numerous among cigarette smokers as among nonsmokers. Smokers are also more likely to develop pancreatic cancer.

CIGARETTE-RELATED CANCERS IN WOMEN

The lung cancer death rate of women has almost tripled in 15 years. Lung cancer is now the leading cause of cancer deaths in women. Pregnant women who smoke have a greater number of stillbirths than nonsmoking women, and their infants are more likely to die within the first month. Their babies more often weigh less than 5 ½ pounds (which is considered premature) and are exposed to more risk of disease and death.

SMOKING AND FIRES

In 1991, a total of 187,000 fires were specifically traced to being smoking related, resulting in 951 deaths, 3381 victims suffering from burns, and a total property loss of more than $443 million in the United States. About 9.2% of all U.S. fires are caused by smokers.[14]

FILTER CIGARETTES

Ninety-five percent of American smokers have switched to filter tips. Recent studies have shown that smokers who smoke filtered low-tar, low-nicotine cigarettes have a lower lung cancer death rate than those who smoke unfiltered high-tar, high nicotine cigarettes. But these rates are still far higher than for those who have never smoked. ★

Cigarette Vending Machines and Minors

Few things are as common as vending machines. Candy, soda, pastries, and, of course, cigarettes can be purchased by virtually anyone. Routinely, younger teens, and even children, can be observed purchasing cigarettes from these machines. In this country an estimated 1 billion cigarette packs are sold from these machines each year to persons under 18 years of age.[15] Equally as apparent is the direct sales of tobacco products to persons under 18 years of age.

Because cigarette use usually begins in the teen years, or even in the late preteen years, and dependence is established shortly thereafter, concern exists over young people's access to cigarettes through vending machines. Accordingly, 44 states and the District of Columbia have passed laws prohibiting the sale of cigarettes, including sales from vending machines, to persons under a particular age. The age for legal purchase of tobacco products varies (Figure 9-1). All of these states specify penalties for sales to minors, and 17 states require that signs be posted on vending machines. In addition, 23 states and the District of Columbia require that retailers and vending machine owners hold retail licenses for the sale of tobacco.

In spite of the attempts to prohibit sales of tobacco products to minors, only limited success has been achieved. A newly formulated amendment to the Public Health Service Act, the Synar Amendment, will require states to prohibit the sale and distribution of tobacco products to individuals under the age of 18, or risk forfeiture of Federal Substance Abuse Block Grant funds.[16] Perhaps the threat of losing these important funds will encourage the states to step up enforcement efforts to the higher levels needed to truly limit access of tobacco products to minors. ★

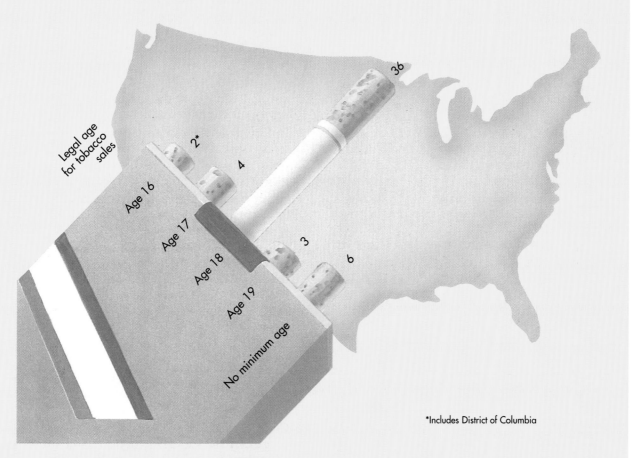

*Includes District of Columbia

Figure 9-1 Legal age for tobacco sales.

PERSONAL ASSESSMENT

ASSUMPTION

1. There are now safe cigarettes on the market.

2. A small number of cigarettes can be smoked without risk.

3. Most early changes in the body resulting from cigarette smoking are temporary.

4. Filters provide a measure of safety to cigarette smokers.

5. Low-tar, low-nicotine cigarettes are safer than high-tar, high-nicotine brands.

6. Mentholated cigarettes are better for the smoker than are nonmentholated brands.

7. It has been scientifically proven that cigarette smoking causes cancer.

8. No specific agent capable of causing cancer has ever been identified in the tobacco used in smokeless tobacco.

9. The cure rate for lung cancer is so good that no one should fear developing this form of cancer.

10. Smoking is not harmful as long as the smoke is not inhaled.

11. The "smoker's cough" reflects underlying damage to the tissue of the airways.

12. Cigarette smoking does not appear to be associated with damage of the heart and blood vessels.

13. Because of the design of the placenta, smoking does not present a major risk to the developing fetus.

DISCUSSION

F Depending on the brand, some cigarettes contain less tar and nicotine; none are safe, however.

F Even a low level of smoking exposes the body to harmful substances in tobacco smoke.

T Some, however, cannot be reversed—particularly changes associated with emphysema.

T However, the protection is far from adequate.

T Many persons, however, smoke low-tar, low-nicotine cigarettes in a manner that makes them just as dangerous as stronger cigarettes.

F Menthol simply makes cigarette smoke feel cooler. The smoke contains all of the harmful agents found in the smoke from regular cigarettes.

T In particular, cigarette smoking causes lung cancer and cancers of the larynx, esophagus, oral cavity, and urinary bladder.

F Unfortunately, smokeless tobacco is no safer than tobacco that is burned. The user of smokeless tobacco swallows much of what the smoker inhales.

F Approximately 13% of those persons having lung cancer will live the 5 years required to meet the medical definition of "cured."

F Because of the toxic material in smoke, even its contact with the tissue of the oral cavity introduces a measure of risk in this form of cigarette use.

T The cough occurs in response to an inability to clear the airway of mucus as a result of changes in the cells that normally keep the air passages clear.

F Cigarette smoking is, in fact, the single most important risk factor in the development of cardiovascular disease.

F Children born to women who smoked during pregnancy show a variety of health impairments, including smaller birth size, premature birth, and more illnesses during the first year of life. Women who are smokers also have more stillbirths. Even second-hand smoke is now known to effect fetal development.

14. Women who smoke cigarettes and use an oral contraceptive should decide which they wish to continue, because there is a risk in using both.

T Women over 35 years of age, in particular, are at risk of experiencing serious heart disease if they continue using both cigarettes and an oral contraceptive.

15. Air pollution is a greater risk to our respiratory health than is cigarette smoking.

F Although air pollution does expose the body to potentially serious problems, the risk is considerably less than that associated with smoking.

16. Addiction, in the sense of physical addiction, is found in conjunction with cigarette smoking.

T Dependence, including true physical addiction, is widely recognized in cigarette smokers.

17. The best "teachers" a young smoker has are his or her parents.

T There is a positive correlation between cigarette smoking of parents and the subsequent smoking of their children. Parents who do not want their children to smoke should not smoke.

18. Nonsmoking and higher levels of education are directly related.

T The higher one's level of education, the less likely one is to smoke.

19. About as many women smoke cigarettes as do men.

T Although in the past more men smoked than did women, the trend is changing. In the future cigarette smoking could become a woman's pasttime.

20. Fortunately, for those who now smoke, stopping is relatively easy.

F Unfortunately, relatively few smokers can quit. The best advice is never to begin smoking.

TO CARRY THIS FURTHER . . .

Were you surprised at the number of items that you answered correctly? In what areas did you hold misconceptions regarding cigarette smoking? Do you think that most university students are as knowledgeable as you? Where do you see the general public in terms of their understanding of cigarette smoking? How can the health care community do a better job in educating the public about tobacco use?

PERSONAL ASSESSMENT

tent. Interestingly, users of low nicotine cigarettes tend to inhale more frequently and deeply to obtain as much nicotine as possible.

Attempts to market cigarettes with extremely low levels of nicotine have occurred in the past, including test marketing of Next by Philip Morris. The acceptance of this brand could be difficult because the low level of nicotine may not meet the physiological needs of addicted smokers. Further, a focus on nicotine levels may prove to be unappreciated by a public conditioned to be concerned about "tar."

Snuff and chewing tobacco

Although not burned, snuff and chewing tobacco deliver nicotine effectively through the mucous membranes of the mouth and nose. Cigar and pipe smoke, when not inhaled, manage to transmit some nicotine to the smoker, but in amounts considerably below those associated with cigarettes.

Psychosocial Factors Related to Dependence

In the view of behavioral scientists, dependence on tobacco can also be explained on the basis of psychosocial factors. Both research and general observation support many of the powerful influences these factors have on the beginning smoker.

MODELING

Because tobacco use is a learned behavior, it is reasonable to accept that *modeling* acts as a stimulus to experimental smoking. Modeling suggests that susceptible persons smoke to emulate smokers whom they admire or with whom they share other types of social or emotional bonds. Particularly for adolescents, smoking behavior correlates with the smoking behavior of peers, older siblings, and to some degree, parents.

This is particularly true when smoking is a central factor in peer group formation and peer group associ-

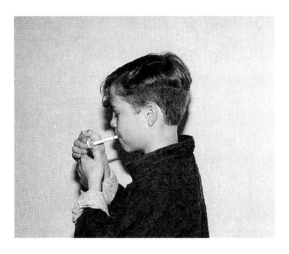

Does smoking make young people appear older?

ation, and can lead to a shared behavioral pattern, which differentiates the group from others, as well as from adults. Further, when risk-taking behavior and disregard for authority are common to the group, smoking becomes the behavioral pattern that most consistently identifies and bonds the group. Particularly for those young persons who lack self-efficacy, or the ability to resist the opportunity, initial membership in a tobacco-using peer group may become unescapable.

Further, when adolescents have lower levels of self-esteem and are searching for an avenue to improve self-image, a role model who smokes is often seen as tough, sociable, and sexually attractive.[13] The latter two traits have been played up by the tobacco industry in their carefully crafted advertisements.

MANIPULATION

In addition to modeling as a psychosocial link with tobacco use, tobacco use may meet the beginning smoker's need to manipulate something and at the same time provide the manipulative "tool" necessary to offset boredom, feelings of depression, or social immaturity. Clearly the availability of affordable smoking paraphernalia provides smokers with ways to reward themselves. A new cigarette lighter, a status brand of tobacco, or a beach towel with a cigarette's logo are all reinforcements to some smokers. For others, the ability to take out a cigarette or fill a pipe adds a measure of structure and control to situations in which they might otherwise feel somewhat ill at ease. The cigarette becomes a readily available and dependable "friend" to turn to during stressful moments.

SUSCEPTIBILITY TO ADVERTISING

The images of the smoker's world portrayed by the media can be particularly attractive. For adolescents, women, minorities, and other carefully targeted groups of adults, the tobacco industry has paired suggestions of a "better world" with the use of their products. To these users and potential users, the self-reward of power, liberation, affluence, sophistication, or adult status is achieved by using the products that they are told are associated with these desired states. Thus the self-rewarding use of tobacco products become an almost instantaneous means of achievement.

With this multiplicity of forces at work, it is possible to understand why so many who experiment with tobacco use find that they quickly become tobacco dependent. Human needs, both physiological and psychosocial, are many and complex. Tobacco use meets the needs on a short-term basis, whereas dependence, once established, replaces these needs with a different, more immediate set of needs.

In spite of the needs that are met through continuing to use tobacco, approximately 90% of adult smokers have, on at least one occasion, expressed a desire to quit, and 80% have actually attempted to become non-smokers. It therefore seems apparent that tobacco use is a source of **dissonance**. This dissonance stems from the need to deal emotionally with a behavior that is both enjoyable and dangerous. The degree to which this dissonance exists and the extent to which it negates the effectiveness of tobacco use as a coping technique probably varies greatly from user to user.

TOBACCO: THE SOURCE OF PHYSIOLOGICALLY ACTIVE COMPOUNDS

When burned, the tobacco in cigarettes, cigars, and pipe mixtures is a source of an array of physiologically active chemicals, many of which are closely linked to significant changes in normal body structure and function. At the burning tip of the cigarette, the 900° C (1,652° F) heat oxidizes tobacco (as well as paper, wrapper, filler, and additives). With each puff of smoke, the body is exposed to over 4000 chemical compounds, hundreds of which are known to be physiologically active, toxic, and carcinogenic. An annual 50,000 puffs taken in by the one-pack-a-day cigarette smoker result in a regularly occurring environment that makes the most polluted urban environment seem mild by comparison.

Cigarette, cigar, and pipe smoke can be described on the basis of two phases or components. These phases include a particulate phase and a gaseous phase. The **particulate phase** includes nicotine, water, and a variety of powerful chemical compounds known collectively as "tar." Tar includes phenol, cresol, pyrene, DDT, and a benzene-ring group of compounds that includes benzo [*a*] pyrene. The majority of the carcinogenic compounds are found within the tar.

The **gaseous phase** of tobacco smoke, like the particulate phase, is composed of a variety of physiologically active compounds, including carbon monoxide, carbon dioxide, ammonia, hydrogen cyanide, isoprene, acetaldehyde, and acetone. *Carbon monoxide* is the most damaging compound found in this component of tobacco smoke. Its impact is discussed shortly.

Nicotine

Nicotine is a powerful psychotropic (psychoactive) chemical agent found in the particulate phase of tobacco smoke. When drawn into the lungs, about one fourth of the nicotine in the inhaled smoke passes into the **systemic** circulation, through the brain barrier, and into the brain within 10 seconds of inhalation. *Nicotine receptors* within the brain are activated and produce a variety of responses, the majority of which are stimulating. The effects of low to moderate levels of nicotine include altered **EEG patterns** and behavior arousal as

a result of the increased production of neurotransmitters, including norepinephrine, dopamine, acetylcholine, and serotonin. High levels of nicotine, however, depress the central nervous system and result in the relaxation associated with heavy smoking. These phenomena suggest that nicotine is a neurotransmitter blocking agent, as well as a neurotransmitter stimulant.[17] (Refer to Chapter 7 for a more detailed discussion of neurotransmitter function.)

The remaining nicotine absorbed into the blood travels throughout the body to nicotinic receptors located in a variety of tissues. Among the presently understood additional effects of nicotine are the reduction of intestinal activity, the release of epinephrine from the adrenal glands, the release of **norepinephrine** from peripheral nerves, increase in heart rate, the constriction of peripheral blood vessels, and the dilation of airways within the respiratory system.

Nicotine that enters the body by routes other than inhalation produces similar effects, but at a much slower rate. Smokeless tobacco, for example, reaches its fullest physiological effect by the end of 20 minutes, nicotine patches within 30 minutes, and transdermal patches within several hours.[18]

Carbon Monoxide

Like every inefficient engine, a cigarette, cigar, or pipe burns (oxidizes) its fuel with less than complete conversion into carbon dioxide, water, and heat. As a result of this incomplete oxidation, burning tobacco forms carbon monoxide gas. Carbon monoxide is one of the most harmful components of tobacco smoke.

---

dissonance (**dis** son ince) feeling of uncertainty that occurs when a person believes two equally attractive but opposite ideas.

particulate phase (par **tick** you lut) portion of the tobacco smoke composed of small suspended particles.

gaseous phase (**gas** ee us) portion of the tobacco smoke containing carbon monoxide and many other physiologically active gaseous compounds.

nicotine (**nick** oh teen) physiologically active, dependence-producing drug found in tobacco.

systemic (sis **tem** ick) throughout the body.

EEG patterns patterns reflecting the type and extent of electrical activity occurring in the cerebral cortex of the brain.

norepinephrine (nor epp in **eff** rin) adrenalin-like chemical produced within the nervous system.

Carbon monoxide is a colorless, odorless, tasteless gas that possesses a very strong physiological attraction for hemoglobin, the oxygen-carrying pigment on each red blood cell. When carbon monoxide is inhaled, it quickly bonds with hemoglobin and forms a new compound, *carboxyhemoglobin.* In this form, hemoglobin is unable to transport oxygen to the tissues and cells where it is needed. In comparison with nonsmokers who normally have 0.5% to 1% of the total hemoglobin in the form of carboxyhemoglobin, smokers may have levels from 5% to 10%.[12]

The presence of excessive levels of carboxyhemoglobin in the blood of smokers leads to shortness of breath and lowered endurance. Because adequate oxygen supply to all body tissues is critical for normal functioning, any oxygen reduction can have a serious impact on health. Brain function may be reduced, reactions and judgment are dulled, and of course, cardiovascular function is impaired. Fetuses are especially at risk for this oxygen deprivation, because fetal development is so critically dependent on a sufficient oxygen supply from the mother.

ILLNESS, PREMATURE DEATH, AND TOBACCO USE

For persons who begin tobacco use as adolescents or younger adults, smoke heavily, and continue to smoke, the likelihood of premature death is virtually ensured. Two-pack-a-day cigarette smokers can expect to die 7 to 8 years earlier than their nonsmoking counterparts. (Only nonsmoking-related deaths that can afflict both smokers and nonsmokers alike keep the difference at this level rather than much higher.) Not only will these persons die sooner, but they also will probably be plagued with painful, debilitating illnesses for an extended time. Smoking is responsible for over 434,000 premature deaths each year.[3]

CARDIOVASCULAR DISEASE AND TOBACCO USE

Cardiovascular disease is the leading cause of death among all adults, accounting for 923,000 deaths in the United States in 1991.[19] Tobacco use, and cigarette smoking in particular, is clearly one of the major factors contributing to this cause of death. While overall progress is being made in reducing the incidence of cardiovascular-related deaths, tobacco use affects these efforts. So important is tobacco use as a contributing factor in deaths from cardiovascular disease that the cigarette smoker doubles the risk of experiencing a **myocardial infarction,** the leading cause of death from cardiovascular disease (Figure 9-2). Smokers also increase their risk of **sudden cardiac death** by two to four times.[19] Fully one third of all cardiovascu-

lar disease can be traced to cigarette smoking.

The relationship between tobacco use and cardiovascular disease is centered on two major components of tobacco smoke: nicotine and carbon monoxide.

Nicotine and Cardiovascular Disease

The influence of nicotine on the cardiovascular system occurs when it stimulates the nervous system to release norepinephrine. This powerful stimulant increases the rate at which the heart contracts. In turn an elevated heart rate increases cardiac output, thus increasing blood pressure. The extent to which an elevated heart rate is dangerous depends in part on the coronary circulation's ability to supply blood to the rapidly contracting heart muscle. The development of **angina pectoris** and the possibility of sudden heart attack are heightened by this sustained elevation of heart rate, particularly in those individuals with existing coronary artery disease (see Chapter 10).

In addition to its influence on heart rate, nicotine is also a powerful vasoconstrictor of the peripheral blood vessels. As these vessels are constricted by the influence of nicotine, the pressure against their walls increases. The resultant hypertensive change elevates blood pressure, thus compounding any existing hypertension.

Nicotine also increases blood **platelet adhesiveness.**[20] As the platelets become more and more likely to "clump," an individual will be more likely to develop a blood clot. In persons already prone to cardiovascular disease, more rapidly clotting blood is an unwelcome liability. Heart attacks occur when clots form within the coronary arteries or are transported to the heart from other areas of the body.

In addition to other influences on the cardiovascular system, nicotine possesses the ability to decrease the proportion of high-density lipoproteins (HDLs) and to increase the proportion of low-density lipoproteins (LDLs) and very-low-density lipoproteins that constitute the body's serum cholesterol. Low-density lipoproteins appear to support the development of atherosclerosis and are clearly increased in the bloodstreams of smokers. (See Chapter 10 for further information about cholesterol's role in cardiovascular disease.)

Carbon Monoxide and Cardiovascular Disease

A second substance contributed by tobacco influences the type and extent of cardiovascular disease found among tobacco users. Carbon monoxide interferes with oxygen transport within the circulatory system.

As described earlier in the chapter, carbon monoxide is a component of the gaseous phase of tobacco smoke and readily joins with the hemoglobin of the red blood cells. Carbon monoxide has an affinity for hemoglobin 200 times that of oxygen. Once the hemoglobin of a red cell has accepted carbon monoxide molecules, the hemoglobin is transformed into *carboxyhe-*

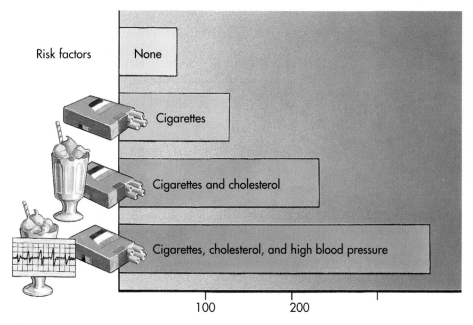

Risk factors

None

Cigarettes

Cigarettes and cholesterol

Cigarettes, cholesterol, and high blood pressure

100   200

Figure 9-2 The danger of heart attack increases with the number of risk factors present. Smoking is the most significant of the three risk factors listed.

moglobin. Thereafter the carboxyhemoglobin makes the red blood cell permanently weaker in its ability to transport oxygen. These red blood cells remain relatively useless during the remainder of their 120-day life. Levels of carboxyhemoglobin in heavy smokers are associated with significant increases in the incidence of myocardial infarction.

When a person has impaired oxygen-transporting abilities, physical exertion becomes increasingly demanding on both the heart and the lungs. The cardiovascular system will attempt to respond to the body's demand for oxygen, but these responses are themselves impaired as a result of the influence of nicotine on the cardiovascular system. If tobacco does create the good life, as advertisers claim, it also unfortunately lowers the ability to participate actively in that life.

CANCER DEVELOPMENT AND TOBACCO USE

Over the past 40 years, research from the most reputable institutions in this country and abroad has consistently concluded that tobacco use is a significant factor in the development of virtually all forms of cancer and the most significant factor in cancers involving the respiratory system.

In describing cancer development, the currently used reference is *20 pack-years,* or an amount of smoking equal to smoking one pack of cigarettes a day for 20 years. Thus the two-pack-a-day smoker can anticipate cancer development in as early as 10 years, while the half-pack-a-day smoker may have 40 years to wait.

Regardless, the opportunity is there for all people to confirm these data. We hope that most people will think twice before disregarding this evidence.

Data supplied by the American Cancer Society (ACS) indicate that during 1993 an estimated 1,170,000 Americans developed cancer.* These cases were nearly equally divided between the sexes and resulted in approximately 526,000 deaths. In the opinion of the ACS, 30% of all cancer cases are heavily influenced by tobacco use. Lung cancer alone accounted for about

*Excluding about 700,000 cases of nonmelanoma skin cancer.

---

carbon monoxide (CO) (kar bun mon **ox** ide) chemical compound that can "inactivate" red blood cells.

myocardial infarction (mye oh **car** dee uhl in **farc** shun) heart attack; the death of heart muscle as a result of a blockage in one of the coronary arteries.

sudden cardiac death immediate death resulting from a sudden change in the rhythm of the heart.

angina pectoris (an **jie** nuh peck **tor** is) chest pain that results from impaired blood supply to the heart muscle.

platelet adhesiveness (**plate** let ad **he** sive ness) tendency of platelets to clump together, thus enhancing speed at which the blood clots.

170,000 of the new cancer cases and 149,000 deaths in 1993. Fully 85% of male lung cancer victims were cigarette smokers. Cancer of the respiratory system, including lung cancer and cancers of the mouth and throat, accounted for about 185,000 new cases of cancer and 151,000 deaths.[21] Despite these high figures, not all smokers develop cancer. Perhaps a "smoking gene" makes some smokers at greater risk for tobacco-related cancer than others.

Recall that tobacco smoke produces both a gaseous and a particulate phase. The particulate phase contains the tar fragment of tobacco smoke. This rich chemical environment contains over 4000 known chemical compounds, hundreds of which are known as possible carcinogens.

In the normally functioning respiratory system, particulate matter suspended in the inhaled air settles on the tissues lining the airways and is trapped in **mucus** produced by specialized *goblet cells.* This mucus with its trapped impurities is continuously swept upward by the beating action of hairlike **cilia** of the ciliated columnar epithelial cells lining the air passages (Figure 9-3). On reaching the throat, this mucus is swallowed and eventually removed through the digestive system.

When tobacco smoke is drawn into the respiratory system, however, its rapidly dropping temperature allows the particulate matter to accumulate. This brown, sticky tar contains compounds known to harm the ciliated cells, goblet cells, and the *basal cells* of the respiratory lining. As the damage from smoking increases, the cilia become less effective in sweeping mucus upward to the throat. When cilia can no longer clean the airway, tar accumulates on the surfaces and brings carcinogenic compounds into direct contact with the tissues of the airway.

At the same time that the sweeping action of the lining cells is being slowed, substances in the tar are stimulating the goblet cells to increase the amount of mucus they normally produce. The "smoker's cough" is an attempt to remove this excess mucus.

With prolonged exposure to the carcinogenic materials in tar, predictable changes will begin to occur within the respiratory system's *basal cell layer* (Figure 9-3). The basal cells begin to display changes characteristic of all cancer cells. In addition, an abnormal accumulation of cells occurs. Collectively these changes in the basal cell layer signal the beginning of lung cancer.

By the time lung cancer is usually diagnosed, its development is so advanced that the chance for recovery is very poor. Only 13% of all lung cancer victims survive for 5 years or more after diagnosis.[21] Most die in a very agonizing, painful way (Figure 9-4).

Cancerous activity in other areas of the respiratory system, including the *larynx,* and within the oral cavity (mouth) follows a similar course. In the case of oral cavity cancer, carcinogens found within the smoke and within the saliva are involved in the cancerous changes. Tobacco users, such as pipe smokers, cigar smokers, and the users of smokeless tobacco, have a very high rate of cancer of the mouth, tongue, and voice box.

In addition to drawing smoke into the lungs, tobacco users swallow saliva that contains an array of

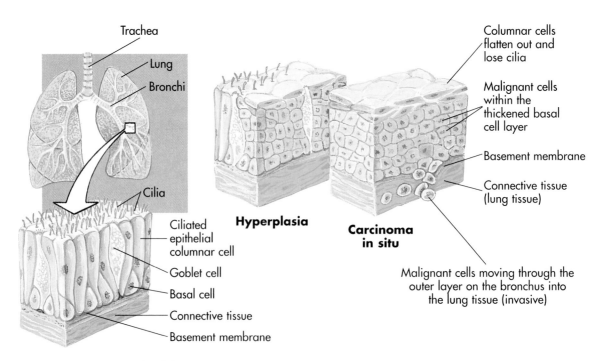

Figure 9-3 Histological changes associated with bronchogenic carcinoma

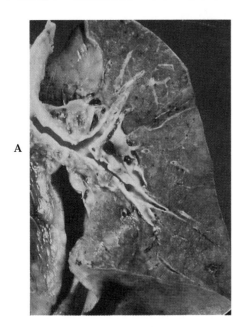 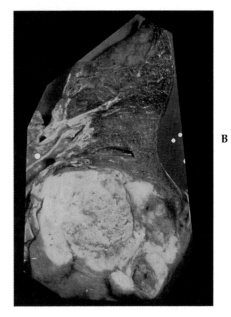

Figure 9-4 A, Normal lung; **B,** cancerous lung.

chemical compounds from tobacco. As this saliva is swallowed, carcinogens are absorbed into the circulatory system and transported to all areas of the body. The filtering of the blood by the liver, kidneys, and bladder may account for the higher than normal levels of cancer in these organs among smokers.

Although the tobacco industry may take some comfort in the difficulty that the scientific community has in proving that tobacco products "cause" many of these cancers, the degree of association between tobacco use and the incidence of many cancers is too great to be dismissed.

CHRONIC OBSTRUCTIVE LUNG DISEASE AND TOBACCO USE

Chronic obstructive lung disease (COLD) is a chronic disorder in which air flows in and out of the lungs becomes progressively limited. COLD is a disease state that is made up of two separate but related diseases: **chronic bronchitis** and **pulmonary emphysema.**

With chronic bronchitis, excess mucus is produced in response to the effects of smoking on airway tissue, and the walls of the bronchi become inflamed and infected. This produces a characteristic narrowing of the air passages. Breathing becomes difficult, and activity can be severely restricted. With cessation of smoking, chronic bronchitis is reversible.[22]

Emphysema causes irreversible damage to the tiny air sacs of the lungs, the **alveoli.** Chest pressure builds when air becomes trapped by narrowed air passages (chronic bronchitis) and the thin-walled sacs rupture.

Emphysema patients develop the characteristic "barrel chest" as they lose the ability to exhale fully. They feel as though they are suffocating.

More than 10 million Americans suffer from COLD. It is responsible for a greater limitation of physical activity than any other disease, including heart disease.[22] COLD patients tend to die a very unpleasant, prolonged death, often from a general collapse of normal cardiorespiratory function that results in *congestive heart failure* (see Chapter 10).

mucus (myoo cus) clear, sticky material produced by specialized cells within the mucous membranes of the body; mucus traps much of the suspended particulate matter within tobacco smoke.

cilia (sill ee uh) small, hairlike structures that extend from cells that line the air passages.

chronic bronchitis (kron ick bron **kie** tis) persistent inflammation and infection of the smaller airways within the lung.

pulmonary emphysema (pul mon air ee em fiz **ee** muh) irreversible disease process in which the alveoli are destroyed.

alveoli (al **vee** oh lie) thin, saclike terminal ends of the airways; the site at which gases are exchanged between the blood and inhaled air.

Persons with COLD are almost always older people who have smoked for many years. In fact, COLD is rarely seen in nonsmokers.

ADDITIONAL HEALTH CONCERNS

In addition to the serious health problems stemming from tobacco use already described, other health-related changes are routinely seen. These include a generally poor state of nutrition, the gradual loss of the sense of smell, and premature wrinkling of the skin. Tobacco users are also more likely to experience strokes (a potentially fatal condition), lose bone mass leading to osteoporosis, experience more back pain and muscle injury, and find that fractures heal more slowly. Further, smokers who have surgery spend more time in the recovery room. Although not perceived as a "health-problem" by persons who continue smoking in order to control weight, smoking does appear to minimize weight gain. In studies using identical twins, twins who smoked were 6 to 8 pounds lighter than their nonsmoking siblings.[23]

TOBACCO AND CAFFEINE USE

As discussed in Chapter 7, caffeine is the psychotropic drug in coffee, tea, cocoa, many soft drinks, and several OTC drugs, and it produces a stimulatory effect on the central nervous system. Because of caffeine's presence in such widely used and legal products, it may be the most used (and potentially misused) drug in this country. Coffee consumption has, however, fallen from 3.12 cups per day in 1962 to 1.75 cups today.[24] Refer back to Table 7-2, which depicts the amount of caffeine in various soft drinks, the major sources of caffeine for children and for many adults.

Think about how often you see someone light up a cigarette while enjoying a cup of coffee. Perhaps you have done this yourself. Did you know that when caffeine is consumed, it is rapidly absorbed into the blood stream and its effects are observable within 30 minutes? The exact action of the drug on the body is not fully understood, but its stimulatory effects are widespread. In low doses, consumption results in increased mental awareness, alertness, and a quickening of thought processes. At higher doses, restlessness, agitation, tremors, and cardiac dysrhythmia occur. Dependence on caffeine, including addiction and habituation, develop rapidly (some studies suggest within a matter of a few days). Unpleasant withdrawal symptoms develop within several hours following the end of consumption. Those experiencing caffeine withdrawal report fatigue, runny nose, persistent yawning, tension, and anxiety. For those who smoke, this becomes a second dependence added to their nicotine addiction.

Chronic heavy consumption of caffeine is called *caffeinism,* and is associated with a number of physiological indicators including nervousness, irritability, tremors, insomnia, heart palpitation, and gastrointestinal disturbances.[25] Efforts have been made to link caffeine consumption to coronary heart disease, pancreatic cancer, fibrocystic breast disease, and most recently, bone loss. To date, there has been little conclusive evidence relating serious health problems and caffeine consumption. However, caffeine does appear to be associated with a risk for miscarriage during pregnancy and should not, therefore, be consumed by women during pregnancy.[26] Regardless, for other adults, caffeine should most likely be consumed in moderation, particularly in light of its widespread presence in foods and products.

SMOKING AND REPRODUCTION

In all of its dimensions, the reproduction process is impaired by the use of tobacco, particularly cigarette smoking. Problems can be found in association with infertility, problem pregnancy, breastfeeding, and the health of the newborn.

Infertility

Recent research indicates that cigarette smoking by both males and females can reduce levels of fertility. Among men, smoking adversely affects sperm motility and sperm shape and can inhibit sperm production. Among women, lower levels of estrogen (a hormone necessary for uterine wall development), a reduced ability to conceive, and a somewhat earlier onset of menopause appear to be related to cigarette smoking.

Problem Pregnancy

The harmful effects of tobacco smoke on the course of pregnancy are principally the result of the carbon monoxide and nicotine to which the mother and her fetus are exposed. Carbon monoxide from the incomplete oxidation of tobacco is carried in the maternal blood to the placenta, where it diffuses across the placental barrier and enters the fetal circulation. Once in the fetal blood, the carbon monoxide bonds with the *fetal hemoglobin* to form *fetal carboxyhemoglobin.* As a result of this exposure to carbon monoxide, the fetus is deprived of normal oxygen transport and literally suffocates.

Nicotine also exerts its influence on the developing fetus. Thermographs of the placenta and fetus show signs of marked vasoconstriction within a few seconds after inhalation by the mother. This constriction further reduces oxygen supplies. In addition, nicotine stimulates the mother's stress response, placing the mother and fetus under the potentially harmful influence of elevated epinephrine and corticoid levels (see Chapter 3). Any fetus exposed to all of these agents is more likely to be *miscarried* or be *stillborn*. Children born to mothers who smoked during pregnancy have lower birth weights and may show other signs of a stressful intrauterine life.

Breastfeeding

For women who decide to breastfeed their infants, smoking during this period will continue to expose their children to the harmful effects of tobacco smoke. It is well recognized that nicotine appears in breast milk and thus is capable of exerting its vasoconstricting and stress-response influences on nursing infants. Mothers who stop smoking during pregnancy should be encouraged to continue to refrain from smoking while they are breastfeeding.

Neonatal Health Problems

Babies born to women who smoked during pregnancy will, on average, be shorter and have a lower birth weight than children born to nonsmoking mothers. During the earliest months of life, babies born to mothers who smoke experience an elevated rate of death caused by sudden infant death syndrome.[27] Statistics also show that infants are more likely to develop chronic respiratory problems, be hospitalized, and have poorer overall health during their early years of life. These problems are compounded when the children are exposed to involuntary smoking (see p. 232) in the household environment. Recent studies, in fact, suggest that the harmful effect of passive smoke exposure may approach that seen when the biological mother smoked during pregnancy.[28]

Parenting, in the sense of assuming responsibility for the well-being of children, does not begin at birth. In the case of smoking, this is especially true. Pregnant women who continue smoking are disregarding the well-being of the children they are carrying. Other

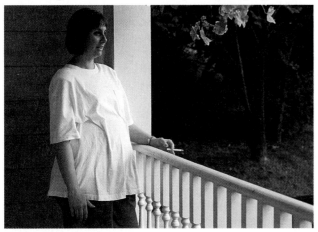

Tobacco use during pregnancy is dangerous.

family members, friends, and co-workers who subject pregnant women to cigarette, pipe, or cigar smoke are, in a sense, contributing a measure of their own disregard for the health of the next generation.

ORAL CONTRACEPTIVES AND TOBACCO USE

Women who smoke and use oral contraceptives are placing themselves at a much greater risk of experiencing a fatal cardiovascular accident (heart attack, stroke, **embolism**) than oral contraceptive users who do not smoke. This risk of cardiovascular complications is further increased for oral contraceptives users 25 years of age or older. Women who both smoke and use oral contraceptives are four times more likely to die from myocardial infarction (heart attack) than women who only smoke.[29] Because of this adverse relationship, *it is strongly recommended that women who smoke should not use oral contraceptives.*

SMOKELESS TOBACCO USE

Chewing Tobacco and Snuff

What do "Red Man," "Skoal," and "Copenhagen" have in common? They have all served to introduce 22 million Americans to a bit of the past—the use of smokeless tobacco.

Thanks to the resurgence of smokeless tobacco use, no longer are professional baseball players the only Americans to know the value of an empty coffee can or soft drink cup. These discarded containers are becoming standard equipment for people who dip and chew smokeless tobacco.

As the term implies, smokeless tobacco is not burned; rather, it is placed into the mouth. Once in place, the physiologically active nicotine and other soluble compounds are absorbed through the mucous membranes and into the blood. Within a few minutes, chewing tobacco and snuff generate blood levels of nicotine in amounts equivalent to those seen in cigarette smokers. The user of smokeless tobacco experiences the effects of nicotine without being exposed to the carbon monoxide and tar generated by burning tobacco.

Chewing tobacco is taken from its foil pouch, formed into a small ball (called a "wad," "chaw," or "chew"), and placed into the mouth. Once in place, the bolus of

> **embolism** (**em** boe liz um) potentially fatal condition in which a circulating blood clot lodges itself in a smaller vessel.

Health ACTION Guide

Smokeless Tobacco Use

If you use smokeless tobacco, you are at risk for serious health problems. If you have any of the following signs, see your dentist or physician immediately.

▼ Lumps in the jaw or neck area
▼ Color changes or lumps inside the lips
▼ White, smooth, or scaly patches in the mouth or on the neck, lips, or tongue
▼ A red spot or sore on the lips or gums or inside the mouth that does not heal in 2 weeks
▼ Repeated bleeding in the mouth
▼ Difficulty or abnormality in speaking or swallowing

tobacco is sucked and occasionally chewed, but not swallowed. Some users develop great skill at spitting the copious dark brown liquid residue into an empty coffee can, out a car window, or onto the sidewalk.

Snuff, a more finely shredded smokeless tobacco product, is marketed in small round cans. Snuff is formed into a small mass (or "quid") for dipping. The quid is placed between the jaw and the cheek; the user sucks the quid, then spits out the brown liquid—in cans, on the street, or next to urinals. Snuff, as once used, was actually a powdered form of tobacco that was inhaled through the nose.

Although smokeless tobacco would seem to free the tobacco user from many of the risks associated with smoking, chewing and dipping are not without their own substantial risks. The presence of leukoplakia (white spots) and erythroplakia (red spots) on the tissues of the mouth indicate precancerous changes.[30] In addition, an increase in **periodontal disease** (with the pulling away of the gum from the teeth and later tooth loss), the abrasive damage to the enamel of the teeth, and the high concentration of sugar in processed tobacco all contribute to health problems seen among users of smokeless tobacco. In those individuals who develop oral cancer, the risk is dramatically heightened if the cancer metastasizes from the site of origin in the mouth to the brain. Clearly, it is important that users be aware of any signs of damage being done by their use of smokeless tobacco.

In addition to the damage done to the tissues of the mouth, the need to process the inadvertently swallowed saliva that contains dissolved carcinogens places both the digestive and urinary system at risk of cancer.

In the opinion of health experts, the use of smokeless tobacco and its potential for life-threatening disease is presently at the place cigarette smoking was 40 years ago. Consequently, television advertisement has been banned, and the following warnings have been placed in rotation on all smokeless tobacco products:

WARNING: THIS PRODUCT MAY CAUSE MOUTH CANCER.

WARNING: THIS PRODUCT MAY CAUSE GUM DISEASE AND TOOTH LOSS.
WARNING: THIS PRODUCT IS NOT A SAFE ALTERNATIVE TO CIGARETTE SMOKING.

Clearly, smokeless tobacco is a dangerous product. There is little doubt that continued use of tobacco in this form is a serious problem to health in all of its dimensions.

INVOLUNTARY (PASSIVE) SMOKING

The smoke generated by the burning of tobacco can be classified as either **mainstream smoke** (the smoke inhaled and then exhaled by the smoker) or **sidestream smoke** (the smoke that comes from the burning end of the cigarette, pipe, or cigar). When either form of tobacco smoke is diluted and stays within a common source of air, it is referred to as **environmental tobacco smoke.** All three forms of tobacco smoke lead to involuntary smoking and can present health problems for both nonsmokers and smokers.

Surprisingly, mainstream smoke makes up only 15% of our exposure to involuntary smoking. This is because much of the nicotine, carbon monoxide, and particulate matter are retained within the active smokers.

Sidestream smoke is responsible for 85% of our involuntary smoke exposure. Because it is not filtered by the tobacco, the filter, or the smoker's lungs, sidestream smoke contains more free nicotine and produces higher yields of both carbon dioxide and carbon monoxide. Much to the detriment of nonsmokers, sidestream smoke has 20 to 100 times the quantity of highly carcinogenic N-nitrosamines that mainstream smoke has.[31]

Current scientific opinion suggests that smokers and nonsmokers are exposed to very much the same smoke when tobacco is used within a common airspace. The important difference is the quantity of smoke inhaled by smokers and nonsmokers. It is likely that for each pack of cigarettes smoked by a smoker, nonsmokers who must share a common air supply with the smokers will involuntarily smoke the equivalent of three to five cigarettes per day. Because of the

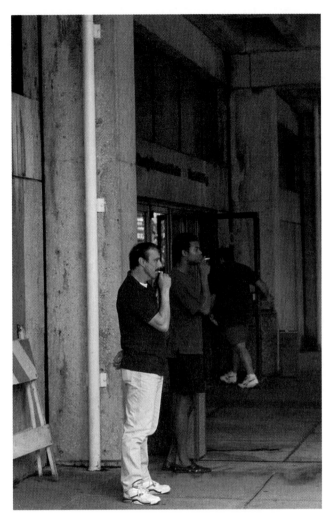

A designated smoking area outside the workplace.

★ Restrictions on Smoking

Texas restricts smoking in elevators, health facilities, libraries, museums, schools, and theaters, whereas Kansas restricts it in schools, and South Carolina bans smoking in school buses and on forms of public transit. In fact all but eight states ban smoking in certain public settings, and 14 states restrict smoking in private work settings. There are no statewide restrictions in Alabama, Illinois, Louisiana, Missouri, North Carolina, Tennessee, Virginia, and Wyoming, although local restrictions may apply.

The bans on smoking described above are the result of concerns about the health effects of "involuntary" smoke, including sidestream smoke. Accordingly, nonsmokers are applying pressure on legislatures to respond to a health threat that the U.S. Environmental Protection Agency calls "the leading cause of toxic exposure."

In opposition to these bans, smokers and representatives of the tobacco industry contend that restricting smoking is of questionable legality since the sale and use of tobacco are legal. Further, they contend that restrictions are largely unenforceable and that smokers are reasonable people who know how and when to control their own behavior. They also suggest that in the private sector the power of the nonsmokers as consumers can force restaurants and threatens to eliminate smoking from their business establishments.

In light of this information, what is your position on this topic? If you were a legislator, would you support legislation to ban smoking even more extensively? ★

small size of the particles produced by burning tobacco, environmental tobacco smoke cannot be completely removed from the worksite by even the most effective ventilation system.[31]

On the basis of recently reported research, involuntary smoke exposure may be responsible for between 10,000 and 20,000 premature deaths per year among nonsmokers in the United States (other estimates range upward to 53,000 premature deaths).[32] In addition, large numbers of persons exposed to involuntary smoke develop eye irritation, nasal symptoms, headaches, and a cough. Furthermore, most nonsmokers dislike the odor of tobacco smoke.

For these reasons, state, local, and private-sector initiatives to restrict smoking have been introduced. Most buildings in which people work, study, play, reside, eat, or shop now have some smoking restrictions. Some have complete smoking bans. The most highly visible of these bans occurred in 1994 when McDonald's announced that all 1400 company-owned restaurants were smoke-free. Franchised-owned stores

began the movement to smoke-free in the belief that such an environment is in the best interest of children and is preferred by adults.[33] Arby's and Wendy's have banned smoking in some stores as well. Nowhere is smoking more noticeably prohibited than in the U.S. airline industry. Currently, smoking is banned on all domestic plane flights of less than 6 hours. American

periodontal disease (pare ee oh **don** tal) destruction to soft tissue and bone that surround the teeth.

mainstream smoke smoke inhaled and then exhaled by a smoker.

sidestream smoke smoke that comes from the burning end of a cigarette, pipe, or cigar.

environmental tobacco smoke tobacco smoke that is diluted and stays within a common source of air.

Airlines has extended the band on smoking to selected international flights as well.

Involuntary smoking poses major threats to nonsmokers within residential settings.[34] Spouses and children of smokers are at greatest risk for involuntary smoking. Scientific studies suggest that nonsmokers married to smokers are three times more likely to experience heart attacks than nonsmoking spouses of nonsmokers, and they have a 30% greater risk of lung cancer than nonsmoking spouses of nonsmokers.

The children of parents who smoke are twice as likely as children of nonsmoking parents to experience bronchitis or pneumonia during the first year of life. In addition, throughout childhood, these children will experience more wheezing, coughing, and sputum production than children whose parents do not smoke.[34] Of course the impact on children who have two parents who smoke is greater than on children who have only one parent who smokes.

STOPPING WHAT YOU STARTED

As in the case of weight reduction, there are several ways to attempt to stop smoking. Among these are the *cold turkey* approach, a gradual reduction in cigarette use, organized smoking cessation programs, and the use of medically prescribed drug treatment.

Although it is far from easy to stop smoking, the majority of the 1.3 million persons who quit smoking each year do so by throwing their cigarettes away and going cold turkey.[35] After days, weeks, and even months of discomfort, the body will eventually begin functioning normally without nicotine. Respiratory capacity will return, the ability to taste will return, and if undertaken soon enough, tissues of the airways will begin returning to a more normal appearance. For most, some weight will be gained (about 6 to 8 pounds), but this represents a minimal health risk in comparison to the benefits of not smoking. On a less pleasant note, it may take years before the mental pictures of "smoking pleasures" have faded.

For those who fear the discomfort of going cold turkey, a more gradual approach can be attempted. The Health Action Guide on p. 235 provides several suggestions for cutting down on tobacco consumption until such time that stopping totally is possible. In the absence of being able to quit completely, these techniques may provide some hope for being able to smoke more safely.

As mentioned above, a wide variety of group-based smoking abatement programs exists in most communities. These programs are generally operated by hospitals, universities, health departments, voluntary health agencies, private physicians, and even local churches. Perhaps the best that can be said is that the better programs will have limited success—a 20% to 50% success rate as measured over 1 year—whereas

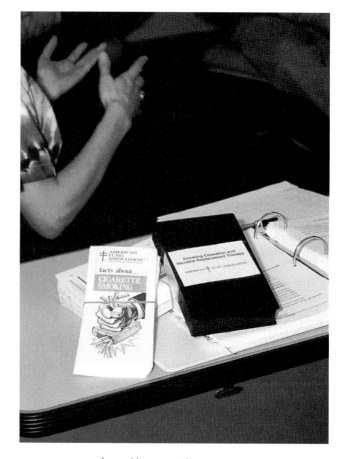

A smoking cessation program.

the remainder will have even poorer levels of success. In fact, persons entering these programs should recognize the high likelihood of failure and predetermine the number of attempts they will make before seeking another approach to cessation.

Two medically supervised approaches for weaning smokers from cigarettes to a nontobacco source of nicotine dependency are nicotine-impregnated chewing gum (Nicorette) and the transdermal nicotine patches (Nicoderm, Habitrol, Prostep) that allow nicotine to slowly diffuse through the skin surface into the body. The chewing gum has been on the market for a number of years and, when used correctly along with other smoking cessation therapies, has demonstrated a success rate of 40% or more. The more recently developed transdermal nicotine patches appear to be somewhat less effective than the chewing gum but easier to use. Concern about fatal heart attacks in persons who use the nicotine patches and continue to smoke has been recently reviewed by the FDA. At the present time, the transdermal nicotine patches remain on the market as prescription items intended to be used under close medical supervision and with other smoking cessation approaches.

Health ACTION Guide

To Reduce Your Smoking

Instead of reaching for a cigarette, reach out for life and health. Start with the following steps suggested by the American Cancer Society:

▼ Pick a quit day, sometime within the next 2 weeks. Plan either to stop cold turkey or to cut down gradually.

▼ Plan ahead for how you will handle tough times in your first few days off cigarettes.

▼ Think of one sentence that expresses your personal reason for wanting to quit smoking. Repeat the sentence to yourself often.

▼ Stock up on low- or no-Calorie snacks.

▼ On your quit day, drink a lot of water, and keep busy.

▼ Call the American Cancer Society for more information about quitting: self-help, how-to's, and group sessions in your community.

An alternative to total cessation is, of course, to reduce exposure to tobacco. This reduction can be accomplished through one or more of the following approaches:

▼ Reduce the consumption of your present high-tar and nicotine brand by smoking fewer cigarettes, inhaling less often and less deeply, and by smoking the cigarette only halfway down.

▼ Switch to a low-tar and nicotine brand of cigarette. Your smoking behavior, other than the brand change, must remain the same, however, do not compensate by inhaling more deeply and frequently.

▼ Switch to a low-tar and nicotine brand of cigarette and in addition, reduce the number smoked, the depth and number of inhalations, and smoke only a limited portion of the cigarette.

▼ Switch to a smokeless form of tobacco, but be prepared for potential problems (discussed earlier in this chapter).

A third medical approach to substituting nicotine dependence from cigarettes to a nontobacco source is through nicotine inhalation. Although still being clinically tested, this system, which uses the same extensive absorptive surface of the lungs, is seen as a promising tool in weaning smokers from their cigarettes.

TOBACCO USE: A QUESTION OF RIGHTS

Let us offer two simple questions concerning the issues of smokers' versus nonsmokers' rights:

▼ To what extent should smokers be allowed to pollute the air and endanger the health of nonsmokers?

▼ To what extent should nonsmokers be allowed to restrict the personal freedom of smokers, particularly since tobacco products are sold legally?

At this time answers to these questions are only partially available, but one trend is developing: the tobacco user is being forced to give ground to the nonsmoker. Today, in fact, it is becoming more a matter of when the smoker will be allowed to smoke, rather than a matter of when smoking will be restricted. Increasingly, smoking is tolerated less and less. The health concerns of the majority are prevailing over the dependence needs of the minority.

 Tobacco Industry Liability

For years, ill and dying smokers (and their survivors) have been suing, without success, tobacco companies for damages resulting from tobacco-induced illnesses. The success for the industry in countering these suits has been built around the contention that before 1964 they were unaware of any suspected dangers, and since 1966 they have warned smokers of the dangers they faced when using cigarettes. Accordingly, smokers were found to be responsible for their own poor judgment and the tobacco companies free of liability because of their compliance with mandates to warn smokers.

For the first time, in a Supreme Court ruling on June 24th, 1992, the door was opened for smokers (or their families) to attempt to prove that the smoking-induced illness resulted because smokers were enticed into smoking by the tobacco industry in spite of its compliance with governmental mandates to warn smokers of the risk of cigarette smoking. In other words, the Court is allowing plaintiffs to attempt to prove that the tobacco companies said one thing (our products are potentially dangerous) and did another (made smoking appear safe and attractive). Only time will tell whether plaintiffs will be successful. Expert opinion is clearly divided on the issue of their success.

A recent discovery that the tobacco industry manipulates nicotine levels in cigarettes and uses high nicotine tobacco (Y-1) has led the FDA to consider whether cigarettes are a drug delivery system. ★

Health ACTION Guide

Tips to Help You Quit Smoking

As powerful as a dependence on cigarettes can be, many people have been able to quit smoking. We hope that suggestions appearing below will assist you in making a concerted effort to stop. Are you ready to try?

▼ Get mad at yourself for having become less fully self-directed than you could be. Few smokers can contend that they are fully self-directed when they can barely function in the absence of their cigarettes.

▼ Observe nonsmokers. Note that nonsmokers are not missing out on anything as the result of not smoking. Recognize that the price you will pay for no longer smoking is not as high as it might have first appeared.

▼ Limit your contact with other cigarette smokers. Keep in mind that once you quit, smokers won't go out of their way to assist you in your efforts.

▼ Stay clear, as much as possible, of the locations and activities that are now associated with your smoking. Old habits will be hard to break, but at least you do not have to be constantly reminded by their presence.

▼ Establish a series of rewards that you will give yourself as you progress through your smoking cessation program.

Having done the above, you will be ready to make an attempt at quitting. Good luck. ▼

ENHANCING COMMUNICATION BETWEEN SMOKERS AND NONSMOKERS

Exchanges between smokers and nonsmokers are sometimes strained and, in many cases, friendships are damaged beyond the point of repair. As you have more than likely observed, roommates are changed, dates are refused, and memberships in groups are withheld or rejected because of the opposing rights of these two groups.

Recognizing that social skill development is an important task for young adults, the following simple considerations or approaches can reduce some conflict presently associated with smoking:

▼ Ask whether smoking would bother others in close proximity to you.

▼ When in a neutral setting, seek physical space in which you will be able to smoke and in a reasonable way not interfere with nonsmokers' comfort.

▼ Accept the validity of the nonsmoker's statement that your smoke "smells up everything and everyone."

▼ Respect stated prohibitions against smoking.

▼ If a nonsmoker requests that you refrain from smoking, respond with courtesy, regardless of whether you intend to comply.

▼ Practice "civil smoking" by applying a measure of restraint when you recognize that smoking is offensive to others. Particularly, respect the aesthetics that should accompany any act of smoking—ashes on dinner plates and cigarette butts in flower pots are hardly popular with others.

The suggestions above can become skills for the social dimension of your health that can be applied to other social conflicts. Remember that as a smoker you are part of a statistical minority living in a society that often makes decisions and resolves conflict based on majority rule.

For those of you who are nonsmokers, we would suggest several approaches we believe will make you more sensitive and skilled in dealing with smoking behavior:

▼ Attempt to develop a feeling for or a sensitivity to the power of the dependence that smokers have on their cigarettes.

▼ Accept the reality of the smoker's sensory insensitivity—an insensitivity that is so profound that the odors you complain about are not even recognized.

▼ When in a neutral setting, allow smokers their fair share of physical space in which to smoke. So long as the host does not object to smoking, you, as a guest, do not have the right to infringe on a person's right to smoke.

▼ When asking a person not to smoke, use a manner that reflects social consideration and skill. State your request clearly, and accept a refusal gracefully.

▼ Respond with honesty to inquiries from the smoker as to whether the smoke is bothering you.

For those who are contemplating smoking, we ask you to explore closely whether the social isolation that appears to be more and more common for smokers will be offset by the benefits you might receive from cigarettes. The ability to find satisfaction through social contact may be one of the most important dimensions in a productive and satisfying adult life.

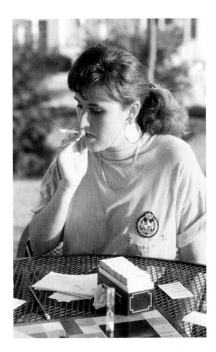

Unfortunately, more and more young women are smoking. Do you recognize yourself here?

Summary

✔ The percentage of American adults who smoke is continuing to decline.

✔ Increasingly, the American tobacco industry is diversifying into nontobacco product lines.

✔ As domestic tobacco sales decline, the tobacco industry is expanding its international sales of cigarettes and other tobacco products.

✔ Dependency, including addiction and habituation, is established quickly through tobacco use. Modeling, self-reward, and self-medication play important roles in the development of tobacco dependency.

✔ Most states have laws limiting the sales of tobacco to minors, whereas the majority have laws restricting the sales of cigarettes through vending machines.

✔ The tobacco industry is constantly targeting new markets, such as women, minorities, and adolescents.

✔ Tobacco smoke can be divided into gaseous and particulate phases. Each phase has its unique chemical composition.

✔ Nicotine, carbon monoxide, and phenol have damaging effects on various body tissues.

✔ Nicotine has predictable effects on the function of the cardiovascular system when used at relatively low doses. Several hundred carcinogenic agents are found in tobacco smoke.

✔ The majority of forms of cancer are worsened by tobacco use. Lung cancer progresses in a predictable fashion.

✔ Caffeine consumption and smoking produces predictable changes in nervous system function, but its long term effect on health is uncertain.

✔ Several areas of reproductive health are negatively influenced by tobacco use. Cigarette smoking and long-term use of oral contraceptives are not compatible.

✔ Smoking alters normal structure and function of the body, as seen in premature wrinkling, diminished ability to smell, and bone loss leading to osteoporosis.

✔ Smokeless tobacco carries its own health risks, including oral cancer.

✔ Stopping smoking can be undertaken in any one of several ways, including going "cold turkey."

✔ Nicotine gum, patches, and inhalants can be effective in a smoking cessation program.

✔ Involuntary smoke carries with it a wide variety of threats to the spouse, children, and co-workers of the smoker.

✔ Both smokers and nonsmokers have certain rights regarding the use of tobacco. Effective communication can be established between smokers and nonsmokers.

Review Questions

1. What percentage of the American adult population smokes? In what direction has change been occurring?

2. In what way do modeling and advertising explain the development of emotional dependency on tobacco? How do self-esteem, self-image, and self-efficacy relate to tobacco use?

3. What are the principal components of the gaseous and particulate phases of tobacco smoke?

4. What are the specific influences of nicotine, carbon monoxide, and phenol on the normal function of the body?

5. In what ways does cigarette smoking contribute to cardiovascular disease? What effect does nicotine have on the cardiovascular system?

6. To what extent is tobacco use a factor in cancer? What specific airway tissues are involved in lung cancer?

7. What is the traditional progression of chronic obstructive lung disease? In what ways does tobacco use decrease reproductive health?

8. In what ways is smokeless tobacco the equal of smoking in the development of serious health concerns?

9. What is our current understanding about chronic caffeine consumption and smoking as a health problem?

10. What is the most effective way to stop smoking? What is the average weight gain after stopping smoking? How effective are other approaches to stopping smoking? What are the principal nicotine replacements systems in use today?

11. What is involuntary smoking? Why is there growing concern about the effects of involuntary smoke on spouses and children?

12. What rights do smokers and nonsmokers have in public places? How can communication be enhanced between smokers and nonsmokers?

Think about This . . .

✔ Why do proportionally more highly educated women than highly educated men smoke cigarettes?

✔ What impact does smoking have on the general appearance of people you know who smoke? Would you be willing to discuss this with them?

✔ If you saw a minor being sold cigarettes, would you feel comfortable mentioning your concern to the merchant?

✔ If you are a smoker, do you understand why you are more "winded" than nonsmokers whom you try to compete with athletically?

✔ Should the nonsmoking majority continue to pay the health costs accrued by smokers?

✔ If you are a consumer of caffeine (coffee, colas, tea), have you thought of alternative beverages? How difficult would it be for you to stop drinking coffee or caffeinated soft drinks?

✔ Do you believe that a pregnant woman who smokes is being a responsible parent? Might this be considered a form of child abuse?

✔ Considering the large amount of information available on the risks associated with smoking, if you smoke, why do you continue to smoke?

✔ If you are a smoker, have you ever been asked to extinguish your cigarette? How did you react? How did you feel about this?

REAL LIFE
REAL CHOICES

YOUR TURN

▼ Do you identify more strongly with Karen or with Steven in this situation? Give reasons for your answer.

▼ If you smoke, how do friends, classmates, and others treat you, and how do you feel about their behavior?

▼ If you don't smoke, what is your attitude toward smoking and smokers? Why do you think and feel the way you do?

AND NOW, YOUR CHOICES . . .

▼ If you were a smoker and your partner didn't smoke, would you be willing to quit to save the relationship?

▼ If you didn't smoke and were involved with someone who did, would you consider ending the relationship if your partner refused to quit?

References

1. Public Health Services: *Healthy people 2000: national health promotion and disease prevention objectives*—full report, with commentary, Washington, DC, 1991, US Department of Health and Human Services, Public Health Service, DHHS Publication (PHS)41-91-50212.

2. Current Trends: Cigarette smoking among adults—United States, 1991, *MMWR* 42(12):230-233, 1993.

3. US Department of Health and Human Services: *Preventing tobacco use among young people: a report of the Surgeon General*, Atlanta, Ga, 1994, US Department of Health and Human Services, Public Health Service, Centers for Disease Control and Prevention, National Center for Chronic Disease Prevention and Health Promotion, Office on Smoking and Health.

4. Austin A: *The American freshman: national norms for 1989*, Los Angeles, 1990, UCLA Higher Education Research Institute.

5. National survey results on drug use. From *The monitoring the future study, 1875-1992*, vol 11, Washington, DC, 1993, National Institute on Drug Abuse, NIH Publication No. 93-3598.

6. Chapman S, Richardson J: Tobacco exercise and declining tobacco consumption: the case of Papua New Guinea, *Am J Public Health* 80(5):537-540, 1990.

7. US Department of Health and Human Services: *Smoking and health in the Americas*, Atlanta, 1992, US Department of Health and Human Services, Public Health Service, Centers for Disease Control, National Center for Chronic Disease Prevention and Health Promotion, Office of Smoking and Health.

8. Pierce JP, Lee L, Gilpin MS: Smoking initiation by adolescent girls, 1944 through 1988: an association with targeted advertising, *JAMA* 271(8):608-611, 1994.

9. Fishcher PM, et al: Brand logo recognition by children aged 3 to 6 years: Mickey Mouse and Old Joe the camel, *JAMA* 266:3145-3148, 1991.

10. Shiffman S: Chippers—individual differences in tobacco dependence, *Psychopharmacology* 97(4):539-547, 1989.

11. Russell M: Cigarette smoking: natural history of a dependency disorder, *Br J Med Psych* 44:1-16, 1971.

12. Pinger RE, Payne WA, Hahn DB: *Drugs: issues for today*, ed 2, St Louis, 1994, Mosby.

13. Glass RM: Blue mood, blackened lungs: depression and smoking, *JAMA* 264(12):1583-1585, 1990.

14. Allison Miller, National Fire Protection Association, Fire Analysis and Research Division, Quincy, Mass, telephone interview, March 9, 1994.

15. State laws restricting minors' access to tobacco, *MMWR* 39(21):351, 1990.

16. American Public Health Association: The Synar amendment: youth access to tobacco, *1993 Section News Letter*, June 1993, pp 7-8.

17. Ray O, Ksir C: *Drugs, society, and human behavior*, ed 6, St Louis, 1993, Mosby.

18. Palmer KJ, Bucklet MM, Faulds D: Transdermal nicotine: a review of its pharmacodynamics and pharmacokinetic properties, and therapeutic efficacy as an aid to smoking cessation, *Drugs* 44(3):498-529, 1992.

19. *America Heart Association, 1993 heart and stroke facts*, Dallas, 1992, The Association.

20. Nowak J, et al: Biochemical evidence of a chronic abnormality in platelet and vascular function in healthy individuals who smoke cigarettes, *Circulation* 76(1):6-14, 1987.

21. American Cancer Society: *Cancer facts & figures—1993*, Atlanta, Ga, 1993, The Society.

22. Crowley LV: *Introduction to human disease*, ed 3, Boston, 1992, Jones and Bartlett.

23. Eisen S, Lyon M, Goldberg J, True W: The impact of cigarette and alcohol consumption on weight and obesity: an analysis of 1911 monozygotic male twin pairs, *Arch Intern Med* 153(21):2457-2463, 1993.

24. Coffee cup doesn't Runneth over. *USA Today*, February 10, 1994, 1d.

25. Gilbert RJ: *Caffeine: The most popular stimulant*. Encyclopedia of psychoactive drugs, New York, 1986, Chelsea House Publishers.

26. Caffeine during pregnancy: grounds for concern? *JAMA* 270(24):2973, 1993 (editorial).

27. Kahn A, Groswasser J, Sottiaux M, et al: Parental exposure to cigarettes in infants with obstructive sleep apneas, *Pediatrics* 93(5):778-783, 1994.

28. Eliopoulos C, Klein J, My Khanh P, et al: Hair concentrations of nicotine in women and their newborn infants, *JAMA* 271(8)621-623, 1994.

29. Hatcher RA, et al: *Contraceptive technology, 1992-93,* ed 17, New York, 1992, Irvington Publishers.

30. Oral snuff, a preventable carcinogenic hazard, *Lancet II* (8500):198-200, 1986.

31. U.S. Department of Health and Human Services, *The health consequences of involuntary smoking: a report of the Surgeon General,* Centers for Disease Control Pub No 87-8938, Washington, DC, 1986, U.S. Government Printing Office.

32. Glantz SA, Parmely WW: Passive smoking and heart disease: epidemiology, physiology, and biochemistry, *Circulation* 83(1):1-12, 1991.

33. Moore MT: McDonald's says hold the smoke, *USA Today.* February 24, 1994, 2b.

34. Overpeck MD, Moss AJ: Children's exposure to environmental cigarette smoke before and after birth: United States, 1988. Advanced data from vital and health statistics; no 202, Hyattsville, Maryland, 1991, National Center for Health Statistics.

35. Fiore MC, et al: Methods used to quit smoking in the United States, *JAMA* 263(20):2760-2765, 1990.

Suggested Readings

Delaney S: *Women smokers can quit—a different approach,* Evanston, IL, 1990, Women's Healthcare Press.

Authored by a former heavy smoker, this book details information about the special concerns women have when they try to stop smoking. Emphasis is on quitting smoking without gaining weight and on learning new ways of coping with stress.

Douville JA: *Active and passive smoking in the workplace,* New York, 1990, Von Nostrand Reinhold.

A chemist and information scientist clearly explains the health effects of environmental tobacco smoke. This is an excellent guide for employers who must provide a healthful workplace. The author examines programs that have worked in different companies.

Farquhar JW, Spiller GA: *The last puff,* New York, 1990, WW Norton.

Shares the stories of 30 former smokers and their battles to quit smoking. The reader will learn that there are many motivations to quit and many ways to reach success. Provides inspiration to those who are thinking about quitting.

King S: *Nightmares and dreamscape,* New York, 1993, Viking Penguin.

A futuristic account of smokers as a sub-tribe of persons whose habit limits their involvement with society.

Understandably, relationships could exist between your decisions concerning substance use and all five of the developmental tasks of growth and development. Look within the chapters of this unit for specific information to support our beliefs about drugs, alcohol, and tobacco use and their effects on developmental task mastery.

Forming an Initial Adult Identity

For most of you, this period of life is a time when you will discover more about yourself—about who you really are. All of life's experiences will help you find out who you are. With these experiences, you begin to take on an identity that probably differs somewhat from the one you had a few years ago when you were younger and less independent. The relative freedom you now have allows you to develop a unique identity that might carry you through all of your adult life.

Decisions to use or avoid drugs, alcohol, and tobacco will reflect your uniqueness and how you view yourself. Some people will judge you either positively or negatively solely on use or misuse of these substances. Will your current drug use patterns support or hinder self-identity as you wish it to be 15 years in the future?

Establishing Independence

Living where you want, pursuing a career for which you have prepared, and marrying the person of your choice are among the more obvious dimensions of the independence enjoyed by adults. There are, however, less obvious dimensions of independence that can also be important. Substance use, such as that seen in conjunction with smoking, can influence independence in these less obvious dimensions.

You may have seen a substance abuser experience a partial loss of independence—not the absence of independence to reside, work, or marry as you choose—but rather the independence to make decisions free from substance addiction. While none of us is totally independent, the user of dependence-producing substances is relatively less independent.

Developing Social Skills

Not only is the use or misuse of substances such as alcohol, psychoactive drugs, and tobacco damaging to the user, but it also injures the health and sense of well-being of others with whom the user has contact. Alcohol abusers and drug users frequently find themselves unable (physically and psychologically) to interact socially with a wide range of people. As a result, the user may cease social communication. With tobacco use in particular, we see substance abuse having a negative impact on others' health.

For those who are contemplating using dependence-producing substances, explore closely whether the social isolation that appears to be more and more common for users will be offset by the benefits you might receive from the substance. The importance of social acceptance cannot be taken lightly.

Assuming Responsibility

College requires students to accept increasing levels of academic responsibility. Adult life in general demands additional responsibilities—everything from paying taxes to managing a growing family. Job requirements force us to assign priorities to schedules and personal activities. Clearly, adulthood is marked by our assumption of more and more responsibility.

Will you be able to accept these complex responsibilities if you find yourself incapable of functioning because of substance abuse? If you recognize now that your preferred method of coping with stress is to rely on alcohol or drugs, then you need to explore alternatives in light of the level of responsibility that lies ahead of you.

Developing Intimacy

As suggested in the social dimension of health, the misuse or abuse of drugs, alcohol, and tobacco can easily diminish social resourcefulness. Consider the role that social interaction skills play in all forms of intimacy; reducing the effectiveness of these skills through substance misuse and abuse eventually limits intimacy. The search for illicit drugs and the loss of control resulting from chronic heavy alcohol use can diminish the quality of an intimate relationship very quickly. Also, smoking can have a powerful influence in reducing the opportunity to be a friend, mentor, and even a dating partner.

UNIT FOUR

Unit 4 consists of three chapters that focus on disease processes. Throughout your lifetime, each illness you contract or develop has the potential to influence your overall health status and each of its five dimensions.

● Physical Dimensions of Health

We usually associate illness with pain, fear, discomfort, and limitations. While many of these factors do go hand in hand with illness, it is also possible that health problems can contribute positively to the physical dimension of health. Exposure to certain infectious diseases may allow your body to develop immunity. This is a very beneficial effect. Illness can also force you to rest, reduce your work load, reconsider your health behaviors, and take better care of yourself. Weight loss, smoking cessation, improved dietary practices, genetic counseling, or a renewed commitment to physical fitness may follow your recovery from an illness.

◆ Emotional Dimension of Health

Emotionally healthy people feel good about themselves and other people and are generally able to cope with most of the demands of life. Being diagnosed with some form of illness or disease can seriously jeopardize emotional resources. Until the disease is under control, we can feel frightened, depressed, anxious, isolated, and vulnerable. Fortunately, as you will discover in this unit, medical science has enhanced the prospects of recovery from many diseases.

■ Social Dimension of Health

Rarely do people face an illness or chronic health condition alone. Friends, family members, physicians, nurses, and therapists often interact with you when you have health problems. In fact, it is possible that health problems may lead you to meet many new people who might challenge and reward your social skills and insights. People who have heart disease, cancer, diabetes, or AIDS often establish relationships with others who have the same condition or with members of support groups. Illnesses can test your ability to be a friend. When friends are ill, you have an opportunity to practice the friendship skills you have sharpened over the years. Occasionally, however, social interactions with friends who are ill might expose you to unnecessary risks of disease. It may be in your best interest to temporarily avoid close contacts with these persons until they are no longer infectious.

▲ Intellectual Dimension of Health

Our ability to use the various intellectual processes of reasoning, analysis, interpretation, synthesis, creativity, and memory is best accomplished when we are free from health problems. When we are ill, we may not even want to exercise our higher reasoning powers. In some cases, diseases or medications affect our bodies in ways that make some intellectual processes impossible.

For some people, however, illnesses and other health problems can prove to be important learning experiences. Ill people can learn much about their bodies, their personalities, and health care technology. In fact, most physicians encourage their patients to learn as much as possible about managing their conditions. Although health problems frequently cause short-term decreases in intellectual function, they can also help people grow intellectually. Do you agree?

● Spiritual Dimension of Health

What relationships exist between the spiritual dimension of health and illness? Certainly, our ability to serve others can be damaged by a major health problem. A person can easily feel victimized after being diagnosed with a serious illness. This feeling may be the first testing that one experiences about the nature of life and the purpose of living. Some persons who believe in the existence of a loving God may begin to question that belief.

Diseases

Obstacles to a Healthy Lifestyle

10

Cardiovascular Disease

Turning the Corner

The title of this chapter implies that medical science is making steady advances in its efforts to reduce the deaths and disabilities that result from heart and blood vessel disorders. According to The American Heart Association, between 1981 and 1991, death rates from *cardiovascular* diseases declined by 25.7%.[1] With combined efforts in medicine, technology, research, and education, we are finally turning the corner on these dreaded diseases. The incidence of death from heart disorders should continue to decline into the twenty-first century. Surely we will all eventually succumb to some health condition, but it may be possible that persons who study the current literature in this area and then apply suggested preventive measures will be least likely to develop cardiovascular disease.

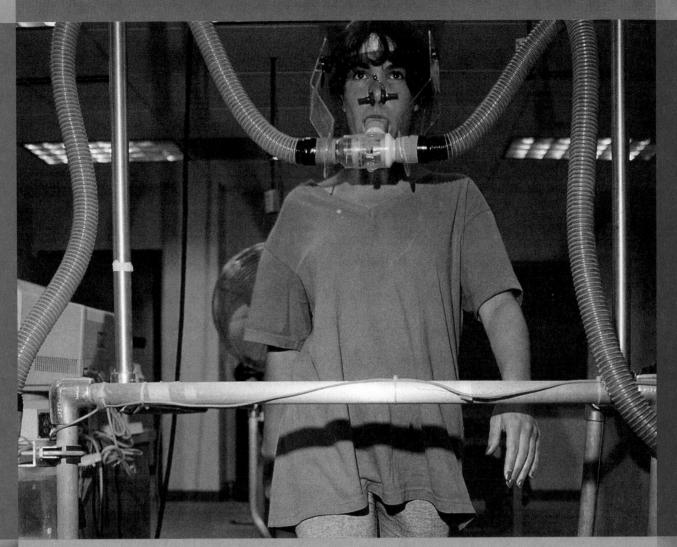

CARDIOVASCULAR DISEASE

The following objectives are covered in this chapter:

▼ Reduce coronary heart disease deaths to no more than 100 per 100,000 people. (Age-adjusted baseline: 135 per 100,000 in 1987; p. 394.)

▼ Reduce stroke deaths to no more than 20 per 100,000 people. (Age-adjusted baseline: 30.3 per 100,000 in 1987; p. 396.)

▼ Increase to at least 50% the proportion of people with high blood pressure whose blood pressure is under control. (Baseline: an estimated 24% controlled high blood pressure in 1982-84; p. 398.)

▼ Reduce the mean serum cholesterol level among adults to no more than 200 mg/dl. (Baseline: among people aged 20-74 in 1976-80: 211 mg/dl for men and 215 mg/dL for women, p. 400.)

▼ Increase to at least 50% the proportion of worksites with 50 or more employees that offer high blood pressure or cholesterol education and control activities to their employees. (Baseline: 16.5% offered high blood pressure education activities and 16.8% offered nutrition education activities in 1985, p. 406.)

REAL LIFE
REAL CHOICES
Straight From the Heart: One Kid's Story

▼ Name: Greg Chulick
▼ Age: 12
▼ Occupation: Student, Boy Scout, Little Leaguer

"Enjoy being a kid—you'll be a grown-up soon enough!"

If Greg Chulick had a nickel for every time he's heard those words from an older relative, he'd be a lot closer to affording that Duke Snider card at the Baseball Bonanza store downtown. He knows there are a lot of great things about being his age: like lazy afternoons fishing for carp in the Criders' pond, playing first base on the Little League team, and going on overnights with his scout troop.

As much as he has going for him, though, right now Greg is terrified. Why? Because for the last 3 days he's had a sore throat, and this morning it isn't any better. Like most kids, Greg ordinarily tells one of his parents when he isn't feeling well. But not this time.

If Greg were somebody else, a sore throat would be no bigger deal than a scrape, a bruise, or a belly-flop in the Y pool. But Greg isn't somebody else: he's the for-

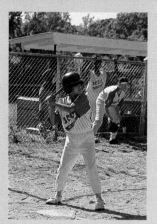

mer big brother of Joey, a chunky, spunky 5-year-old who 3 years ago woke up one morning with a sore throat and a month later was buried in All Saints Cemetery. Joey's sore throat turned out to have been caused by an infection that wasn't treated in time to prevent him from developing the disease that killed him—rheumatic fever.

Greg never talks about his little brother, because who would understand the hole in his life Joey left when he died? Who but Greg shared a room with him, traded secrets and jokes and kid crimes, helped him climb out on the roof one August night so they could watch a meteor shower while the rest of the family slept?

And now it's Greg's turn. He's got the sore throat that won't go away, the sore throat that isn't just *any* sore throat, except that's what everyone thought Joey had . . .

As you study this chapter, think about what Greg is experiencing and prepare yourself to answer the questions in **Your Turn** at the end of the chapter. ▼

PERVASIVENESS OF CARDIOVASCULAR DISEASE

Cardiovascular diseases are directly related to over 40% of deaths in the United States and indirectly related to a large percentage of additional deaths. Heart disease, stroke, and related blood vessel disorders combined to kill nearly 1 million Americans in 1991 (Figure 10-1). This figure represents more deaths than were caused by cancer, accidents, pneumonia, lung disease, diabetes, and AIDS combined. Indeed, cardiovascular disease is our nation's number one "killer."

However, recent advances in medical science, including early detection and innovative treatment methods, have helped reduce the numbers of premature deaths and disabilities. It is highly likely that the United States will reach its Healthy People 2000 goal of fewer than 100 coronary heart disease deaths per 100,000 people. The outlook is brighter than it has ever been, yet many people remain vulnerable to heart disease.

Who are the Potential Victims of Cardiovascular Diseases?

Each of us is a potential victim. Currently, one in five Americans has some form of cardiovascular disease.[1] Every 34 seconds, someone dies from cardiovascular disease. That's more than 2500 deaths each day! Young, middle-aged, and older persons are all vulnerable to various forms of cardiovascular disease.

For years, the general public has considered heart disease to be primarily a men's health issue. Indeed, heart disease strikes men more frequently than women during the years of middle age. One in six men aged 45 to 64 has some form of heart disease compared to one in seven women aged 45 to 64. However, by age 65, women catch up to men in heart disease prevalence. One in three *men and women* aged 65 and older has heart disease. The increase in heart disease in older women is due primarily to the severe reduction in estrogen experienced by women as they move through menopause. Until menopause, this female hormone protects women from heart disease.

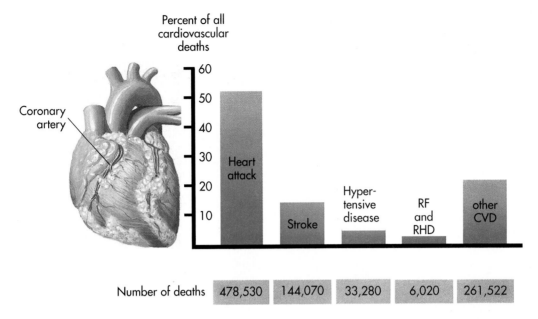

Figure 10-1 Of the 923,422 deaths in the United States in 1991 resulting from cardiovascular diseases, over half were attributable to heart attack.

Additional statistics also do not favor women. High blood pressure is more prevalent among older women than older men. In 1990, more women (87,391) died from stroke than men (56,697).[1] Cholesterol levels in women aged 50 and older are actually higher than men's levels. However, some young women are also at risk for heart problems. For example, women who use oral contraceptives and smoke are 39 times more likely to have a heart attack and 22 times more likely to have a stroke than women who neither use oral contraceptives nor smoke. Also, a small percentage of pregnant women experience complications because of high blood pressure during the last trimester of pregnancy. When you consider the fact that heart disease kills ten times more women each year than breast cancer, it becomes clear how important this health concern must be for women.

The Costs

Beyond the personal tragedies of heart disease, the economic costs are profound. The American Heart Association's estimate of the cost of cardiovascular disease in 1994 was $128 billion.[1] Included in this total are costs for lost productivity from disability, medications, hospital and nursing home services, physician services, and nursing services.

An academic understanding of cardiovascular diseases must begin with basic anatomical and physiological considerations. This information is presented next; then the various forms of cardiovascular disease are specifically discussed. The risk factors that predispose people to cardiovascular disease follow. Finally,

we discuss specific ways that people might reduce the impact of certain risk factors in their lives.

NORMAL CARDIOVASCULAR FUNCTION

The cardiovascular or circulatory system is a transportation system that uses a muscular pump to send a complex fluid on a continuous trip through a closed system of tubes. The pump is, of course, the heart, the fluid is blood, and the closed system of tubes is the network of blood vessels.

The Vascular System

The vascular system refers to the body's blood vessels. Although we might be familiar with the arteries (vessels that carry blood away from the heart) and the veins (vessels that carry blood toward the heart), arterioles, capillaries, and venules are also included in the vascular system. Arterioles are the farther, smaller diameter extensions of arteries. These arterioles lead eventually to capillaries, the smallest extensions of the vascular system. At the capillary level, exchanges of oxygen, food, and waste occur between cells and the blood.

cardiovascular (kar dee oh **vas** kyoo lar) pertaining to the heart (cardio) and blood vessels (vascular).

Learning FROM ALL Cultures

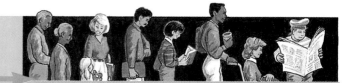

Coronary Heart Disease

Lifestyle and culture will affect your risk for coronary heart disease. For example, Japanese people who live in the United States have a greater risk of developing heart disease than Japanese people who live in Japan. Diet seems to be the factor. People who eat a low-fat diet experience less incidence of heart disease, regardless of where they live. Conversely, individuals who maintain a diet high in saturated fats, wherever they live, have a higher incidence of coronary heart disease.[16]

Developed Western countries seem to have a fairly high incidence of coronary heart disease, some of which can be attributed to lifestyle and diet. Early evidence of this was reported in a 5-year study of middle-aged men in the late 1950s and early 1960s. The Seven Countries Study reported that the death rate from heart attacks was three to ten times greater for men from Finland, the United States, and the Netherlands than for men from Greece, Yugoslavia, Italy, and Japan. Some of the difference was explained by determining blood cholesterol levels; they were much higher for men in the United States, Finland, and the Netherlands than for men from the other four countries. Men from the three high-risk countries consumed greater amounts of saturated fats in their diets than those from Japan and the Mediterranean countries.[16]

Consider your risk factors that can be changed. Then consider your lifestyle. Are your eating habits typical of those of a number of Americans, too high in saturated fats? What kinds of changes have you made or could you make to lower your risk factor of lifestyle and culture? ●

Once the blood leaves the capillaries and begins its return to the heart, it drains into small veins, or venules. The blood in the venules flows into increasingly larger vessels called veins. Blood pressure is highest in arteries and lowest in veins, especially the largest veins, which empty into the right atrium.

Generally arteries carry blood that has been oxygenated in the lungs. Veins usually carry deoxygenated blood and cellular waste products. Exceptions are the pulmonary arteries and pulmonary veins. The pulmonary arteries carry deoxygenated blood from the heart to the lungs for oxygenation, whereas the pulmonary veins transport oxygenated blood from the lungs back to the left atrium.

The Heart

The heart is a four-chambered pump designed to create the pressure required to circulate blood throughout the body. Usually considered to be about the size of a person's clenched fish, this organ lies slightly tilted between the lungs in the central portion of the **thorax.** The heart does not lie exactly in the center of the chest. Rather, approximately two thirds of the heart is to the left of the body midline and one third to the right.[2]

Two upper chambers called *atria* and two lower chambers called *ventricles* form the heart. The thin-walled atrial chambers are considered collecting chambers, whereas the thick-walled muscular ventricles are considered pressure chambers, or pumping

chambers. The right and left sides of the heart are divided by a partition called the *septum* (Figure 10-2).

Blood is circulated through the heart in a continuous, predictable fashion. Deoxygenated blood enters the right atrium from the **superior vena cava** and the **inferior vena cava.** On contraction of the right atrium, blood is forced through the **tricuspid valve** into the right ventricle. When the right ventricle contracts, the blood is forced through the **pulmonary valve** into the pulmonary arteries for distribution to the right and left lungs. In the smallest branches of the lungs, the alveoli, the blood is reoxygenated and its carbon dioxide exchanged.

The oxygen-rich blood returns to the heart by means of four pulmonary veins that empty into the left atrium. When the left atrium contracts, blood is forced through the **mitral (bicuspid) valve** into the left ventricle. When the left ventricle contracts, blood is pushed or forced under great pressure through the **aortic valve** into the *aorta,* the largest artery of the body. The aorta quickly branches into smaller arteries, which supply blood to heart muscle, the brain, and the rest of the body.

For the heart muscle to function well, it must be supplied with adequate amounts of oxygen. The two main **coronary arteries** (and their numerous branches) accomplish this. These arteries are located outside of the heart (see Figure 10-1). If the coronary arteries are diseased and not functioning well, a heart attack is possible.

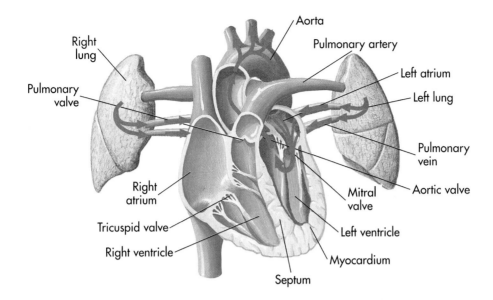

Figure 10-2 The heart functions like a complex double pump. The right side of the heart pumps deoxygenated blood to the lungs. The left side of the heart pumps oxygenated blood through the aorta to all parts of the body. Note the thickness of the walls of the ventricles. These are the primary pumping chambers.

Heart Stimulation

The heart contracts and relaxes through the delicate interplay of **cardiac muscle** tissue and cardiac electical centers called *nodes*. Nodal tissue generates the electrical impulses necessary to contract heart muscle. The *pacemaker*, also called the *sinoatrial* or *SA node*, provides the depolarization necessary for establishing the electrical current required first to contract the two atria simultaneously, and then to simultaneously contract the two ventricles.[3] The heart's electrical activity can be measured by an electrocardiograph (ECG or EKG). This instrument provides a printout (electrocardiogram) that can be evaluated to determine cardiac electrical functioning.

Blood

The average-sized adult has approximately 6 quarts of blood in the circulatory system. From the time we are small children with cuts and scrapes, we are conditioned to realize that blood is a critical body fluid. Indeed, the functions of blood are many. They are quite similar to the overall functions of the circulatory system. These functions include the following:

▼ Transportation of nutrients, oxygen, wastes, hormones, and enzymes
▼ Regulation of water content of body cells and fluids
▼ Buffering to help maintain appropriate pH balance of body fluids
▼ Regulation of body temperature; the water component in the blood absorbs heat and transfers it

thorax (thor ax) the chest; portion of the torso above the diaphragm and within the rib cage.

superior vena cava (vee na **Kay** va) body's largest vein; the vessel that brings blood from the upper body regions back to the right atrium of the heart.

inferior vena cava large vein that returns blood from lower body regions back to the right atrium of the heart.

tricuspid valve (try kus pid) three-cusp (leaf) valve that regulates blood flow between the right atrium and the right ventricle of the heart.

pulmonary valve (pull mon air ee) valve that controls the flow of blood into the pulmonary arteries from the right ventricle of the heart.

mitral (bicuspid) valve (my tral) two-cusp valve that regulates blood flow between the left atrium and the left ventricle of the heart.

aortic valve (a or tik) valve that controls the blood flow into the aorta from the left ventricle of the heart.

coronary arteries (kore oh nare ee) vessels that supply oxygenated blood to heart muscle tissues.

cardiac muscle (kar dee ack) specialized smooth muscle tissue that forms the middle (muscular) layer of the heart wall.

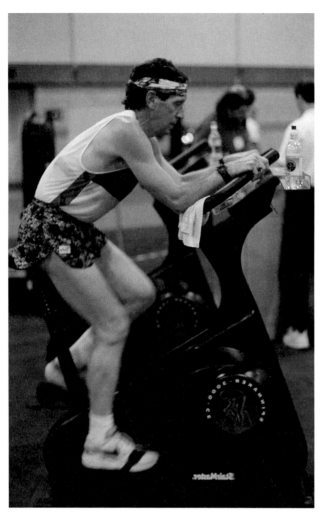

Exercise helps to maintain cardiovascular health.

These four requirements are:

▼ The heart muscle must be adequately nourished and oxygenated. This is accomplished by healthy coronary arteries.
▼ The heart must beat in an appropriate rhythm or pattern. This is coordinated by the heart's electrical system.
▼ The body's blood vessels must be able to dilate (widen) and constrict (narrow) in order to adjust to changes in cardiac output. Healthy, flexible blood vessels can do this when we exercise and when we relax.
▼ The blood vessels must carry adequate amounts of oxygen. Our red blood cells can do this well, unless they are damaged through disease or are exposed to dangerous substances (carbon monoxide, for example).

FORMS OF CARDIOVASCULAR DISEASE

The American Heart Association[4] describes the five major forms of cardiovascular disease (CVD) as coronary heart disease, hypertension, stroke, congenital heart disease, and rheumatic heart disease. A person may have just one of these five diseases or a combination of forms at the same time. Each form exists in varying degrees of severity. All forms are capable of causing secondary damage to other body organs and body systems. Table 10-1 shows current estimates of prevalence.

▼ Prevention of blood loss; by coagulating or clotting, the blood can alter its form to prevent blood loss through injured vessels
▼ Protection against toxins and microorganisms, accomplished by chemical substances (antibodies) and specialized cellular elements circulating in the bloodstream.

Your blood does all of these functions on a daily, full-time basis.

REQUIREMENTS FOR OVERALL CARDIOVASCULAR HEALTH

To promote overall good health, the cardiovascular system must be maintained in its own state of optimal health. Four primary functions can be used as indicators of the system's own health status. If these functions are impaired, then the system itself is no longer a dependable transportation system.

TABLE 10-1	Estimated Prevalence of Major Cardiovascular Diseases (CVDs)
CVD	**Number of Persons**
Coronary heart disease	6,300,000
Hypertension	50,000,000
Stroke	3,060,000
Congenital heart disease	940,000
Rheumatic heart disease	1,340,000
TOTAL CVDs*	56,450,000

* The sum of the individual estimates exceeds 56,450,00, because many persons have more than one cardiovascular disorder.

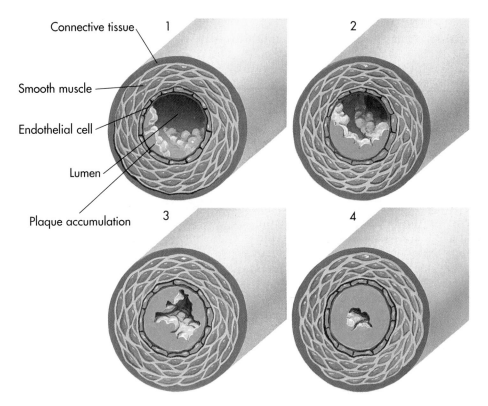

Connective tissue
Smooth muscle
Endothelial cell
Lumen
Plaque accumulation

Figure 10-3 Progression of artherosclerosis. This diagram shows how plaque deposits gradually accumulate to reduce the amount of lumen (space) within an artery. Although enlarged here, coronary arteries are only as wide as a pencil lead.

Coronary Heart Disease

This form of CVD, also known as coronary artery disease, involves damage to the vessels that supply blood to the heart muscle. The bulk of this blood is supplied by the coronary arteries. Any damage to these important vessels can cause a reduction of blood (and its vital oxygen and nutrients) to specific areas of heart muscle. The ultimate result of inadequate blood supply is a heart attack.

ATHEROSCLEROSIS

The principal culprit in the development of coronary heart disease is a condition known as atherosclerosis (Figure 10-3). **Atherosclerosis** is a condition that produces a narrowing of the coronary arteries. This narrowing stems from the long-term buildup of fatty deposits (plaque) on the inner walls of the arteries. This buildup reduces the blood supply to specific portions of the heart. Some arteries of the heart can become so blocked (occluded) that all blood supply is stopped. Heart muscle tissue begins to die when it is deprived of oxygen and nutrients. This damage is known as **myocardial infarction.** In lay terms, this event is called *heart attack.* The box on p. 254 discusses the signals and action of a heart attack. (Arteriosclerosis, a dangerous condition of the arteries that is distinctly different from atherosclerosis, is discussed on p. 258.)

A myocardial infarction can also result from a blood clot or a fatty clot that blocks a coronary artery. These clots might be circulating clots *(emboli)* that form in a distant artery, travel, and eventually lodge themselves in a narrowed coronary artery. Clots may also form directly within the coronary artery. Such stationary clots are called *thrombi.* Heart crises produced by clots are appropriately labeled coronary embolism, coronary thrombosis, or coronary occlusion, depending on the nature of the origin of the blockage.

Cholesterol and lipoproteins

For many years, scientists have known atherosclerosis as a complicated disease that has many causes. Some of these causes are not well understood, but others are clearly understood. *Cholesterol,* a fatty substance in al-

atherosclerosis (ath er oh scler **oh** sis) buildup of plaque on the inner walls of arteries.

myocardial infarction (in **fark** shun) heart attack; the death of heart muscle as a result of a blockage in one of the coronary arteries.

cohol form, is manufactured in the liver and small intestine and is a necessary element in the formation of sex hormones, bile salts, and nerve fibers. Elevated levels of serum cholesterol (above 200 milligrams per deciliter) are known to be associated with an increased risk for developing atherosclerosis. Slightly over half of American adults exceed the 200 mg/dl cholesterol level. With the average adult's cholesterol level now dropping to 205 mg/dl,[5] the Healthy People 2000 objective of 200 mg/dl seems within reach. However, about one out of five adults has a "high" blood cholesterol level, that is, 240 mg/dl or greater.[1]

Initially, most people can help lower their serum cholesterol by adopting three dietary changes. These include lowering the intake of saturated fats, lowering the intake of dietary cholesterol, and lowering caloric intake to a level that does not exceed body requirements. The aim is to reduce excesses in our diet (fats, cholesterol, excess Calories) while promoting sound nutrition. By carefully following such a diet plan, persons with elevated serum cholesterol levels typically are able to reduce their cholesterol levels 30 to 55 mg/dl.[6] However, dietary changes do not affect persons equally; some will experience greater reductions than others. Some will not respond at all to dietary changes.

Another factor related to the development of atherosclerosis concerns structures called lipoproteins. Lipoproteins are particles that circulate in the blood and transport lipids (including cholesterol and triglycerides) and proteins.[7] Three major classes of lipoproteins exist: *very low-density lipoproteins (VLDL)*, *low-density lipoproteins (LDL)*, and *high-density lipoproteins (HDL)*. The VLDLs contain 10% to 15% of the serum cholesterol; the LDLs contain 60% to 70%; and the HDLs contain 20% to 30% of the serum cholesterol.[6]

After much scientific study, it has been determined that high levels of LDL are a major cause of atherosclerosis.[3] This makes sense, because LDLs carry the greatest percentage of cholesterol. High LDL levels are determined partially by inheritance, but they are also clearly associated with smoking, poor dietary patterns, obesity, and lack of exercise. High levels of HDLs are associated with a decreased risk of heart disease. Lifestyle alterations that increase this type of lipoprotein (quitting smoking, reducing obesity, and exercising) are recommended for everyone.

Reducing total serum cholesterol (including LDL levels) is a significant step in reducing the risk of death from coronary heart disease. For persons with elevated cholesterol, a 1% reduction in serum cholesterol yields about a 2% reduction in the risk of death from heart disease. Thus a 10% to 15% cholesterol reduction can reduce risk by 20% to 30%.[6] Study Table 10-2 for cholesterol classifications and current recommended follow-up.

Angina pectoris

When coronary arteries become narrowed, chest pain or *angina pectoris* is often felt. This pain results from a diminished supply of oxygen to heart muscle tissue. Usually angina is felt when the patient becomes stressed or exercises too strenuously. Angina reportedly can range from a feeling of mild indigestion to a severe viselike pressure in the chest. The pain may radiate from the center of the chest to the arms and even up to the jaw. Generally the more severe the blockage, the more pain is felt.

Some cardiac patients relieve angina with the drug *nitroglycerin*, a powerful vasodilator. This prescription drug, available in slow-release skin pads or small pills that are placed under a person's tongue, causes the

Health ACTION Guide

To Help Lower Your Cholesterol

▼ Reduce saturated fats
▼ Reduce intake of excess calories
▼ Exercise regularly
▼ Quit smoking

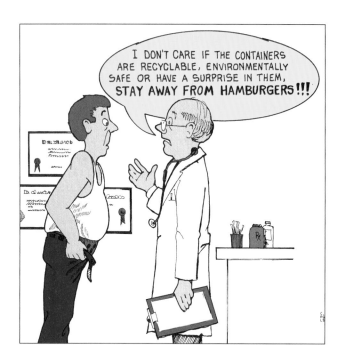

TABLE 10-2   Initial Classification and Recommended Follow-up Based on Total Cholesterol

Total cholesterol	Classification	Recommended follow-up
< 200 mg/dl	Desirable blood cholesterol	Repeat test within 5 years
200-239 mg/dl	Borderline-high blood cholesterol	*Without* definite CHD or two other CHD risk factors (one of which may be male sex): Dietary modification and annual retesting *With* definite CHD or two other CHD risk factors: Lipoprotein analysis; further action based on LDL-cholesterol level
≥ 240 mg/dl	High blood cholesterol	Lipoprotein analysis; further action based on LDL-cholesterol level

Health ACTION Guide

Your Cholesterol Levels

The next time you get your blood cholesterol levels checked, try to find out more than just your total cholesterol level. Ask for the following three measurements and compare them with the desirable measurements for adults, listed in the right column.

Readings	Mine	Desirable
HDL level: mg/dl	_____	Above 45
LDL level: mg/dl	_____	Below 130
Total level: mg/dl	_____	Below 200

Having compared your readings with the desirable measurements, how do your levels measure up? If they are not satisfactory, refer to Table 10-2 and the accompanying Health Action Guide. ▼

coronary arteries to dilate and allow more blood to flow into heart muscle tissue. Other cardiac patients may be prescribed drugs such as **calcium channel blockers** or **beta blockers.**

EMERGENCY RESPONSE TO HEART CRISES

Heart attacks are not always fatal. The consequences of any heart attack depend on the location of the damage, the extent to which heart muscle is damaged, and the speed with which adequate circulation is restored. Injury to the primary pumping chambers (ventricles) may very well prove fatal unless medical countermeasures are immediately undertaken. The recognition of heart attack is critically important.[8] See the box on p. 254.

Cardiopulmonary resuscitation (CPR) has been demonstrated to be one of the most important immediate countermeasures that trained people can use when confronted with a victim of heart attack. Public education programs sponsored by the American Red Cross and the American Heart Association teach people how to recognize, evaluate, and manage heart attack emergencies. CPR trainees are taught how to restore breathing (through mouth-to-mouth resuscitation) and circulation (through external chest compressions) in victims who require such emergency countermeasures. Frequently colleges offer CPR classes through health science or physical education departments. We encourage every student to enroll in a CPR course.

In the event of a coronary crisis, medical therapies available to aid the victim include both drug- and non-drug-centered approaches. Drugs can be used to enlarge coronary arteries (thus improving blood flow), to lower blood pressure (reducing the heart's work load), and to regulate the heart rate (reducing **arrhythmias).** Anticoagulant drugs may also be administered to help dissolve clots and prevent the formation of new clots.

Although not a drug therapy, electric shock pads can also be used in emergency situations to stimulate the return of a normal heart rate, especially in victims of *ventricular fibrillation*, a condition in which the ventricles are merely fluttering in a weak, nonproductive manner.

calcium channel blockers drugs that prevent arterial spasms; used in the long-term management of angina pectoris.

beta blockers (**bay** tah) drugs that prevent overactivity of the heart, which results in angina pectoris.

arrhythmias (uh **rith** mee uhs) irregularities of the heart's normal rhythm or beating pattern.

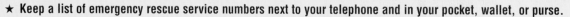

★ Heart Attack—Signals and Action

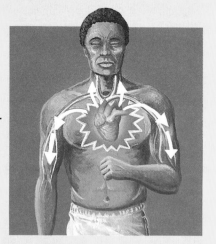

Know the Warning Signals of a Heart Attack

★ Uncomfortable pressure, fullness, squeezing, or pain in the center of your chest lasting 2 minutes or longer.

★ Pain spreading to your shoulders, neck, or arms.

★ Severe pain, dizziness, fainting, sweating, nausea, or shortness of breath.

Not all of these warning signs occur with every heart attack. If some start to occur, however, don't wait. Get help immediately!

Know What to Do in an Emergency

★ Find out which hospitals in your area have 24-hour emergency cardiac care.

★ Determine (in advance) the hospital or medical facility that is nearest your home and office, and tell your family and friends to call this facility in an emergency.

★ Keep a list of emergency rescue service numbers next to your telephone and in your pocket, wallet, or purse.

★ If you have chest discomfort that lasts for 2 minutes or more, call the emergency rescue service.

★ If you can get to a hospital faster by going yourself and not waiting for an ambulance, have someone drive you there.

Be a Heart Saver

★ If you are with someone experiencing the signs of a heart attack—and the warning signs last for 2 minutes or longer—act immediately.

★ Expect a "denial." It is normal for someone with chest discomfort to deny the possibility of something as serious as a heart attack. Don't take "no" for an answer. Insist on taking prompt action.

★ Call the rescue service (dial "911") *or* get to the nearest hospital emergency room that offers 24-hour emergency cardiac care.

★ Give CPR (mouth-to-mouth breathing and chest compressions) if it is necessary and if you are properly trained.

DIAGNOSIS AND CORONARY REPAIR

Once a victim's vital signs have stabilized, further diagnostic examinations can reveal the type and extent of damage to heart muscle. Initially a victim might have an electrocardiogram (ECG or EKG) taken. This test analyzes the electrical activity of the heart. *Heart catheterization,* also called coronary arteriography, is a minor surgical procedure that starts with the introduction of a thin plastic tube in an arm or leg artery. This tube, or catheter, is guided through the artery until it reaches coronary circulation, where a *radiopaque dye* is then released. X-ray pictures called angiograms then record the progress of the dye through the coronary arteries. Areas of occlusion are relatively easily identified. **Radionuclide imaging** (including thallium tests or scans) and **magnetic resonance imaging (MRI scan)** represent more recent innovative diagnostic procedures.[4]

Once the extent of damage is identified, a physician or team of physicians can decide on a medical course of action. Currently popular is an extensive form of surgery called **coronary artery bypass surgery.** An estimated 407,000 bypass surgeries were performed in 1991.[1] The purpose of such surgery is to detour (bypass) areas of coronary artery obstruction. This is achieved by using a section of a vein from the patient's leg (often the saphenous vein) or an artery from the patient's chest (the internal mammary artery) and grafting it from the aorta to a location just beyond the area of obstruction. Multiple areas of obstruction result in double, triple, or quadruple bypasses. Each operation costs between $40,000 and $50,000.

Coronary bypass surgery requires a highly specialized team of surgeons, anesthesiologists, and nurses. Doctors perform delicate procedures that include a major incision directly through the sternum (breastbone), procedures to connect the patient's heart to the **heart-lung machine,** microsurgery to complete the vessel grafting procedures, and techniques to restimulate the normal heartbeat. Within a few months after

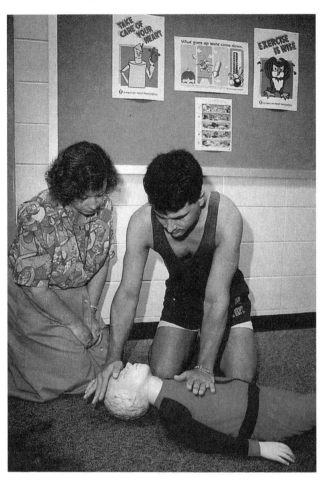

Could you provide help during a cardiac emergency?

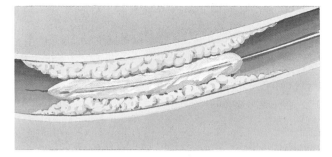

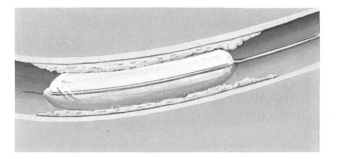

Figure 10-4 Angioplasty.

In 1990, a new FDA-approved device for clearing heart and leg arteries was introduced. This device is called a motorized scraper.[9] Inserted through a leg artery and held in place by a tiny inflated balloon, this motor-driven cutter shaves off plaque deposits from inside the artery. A nose cone in the scraper unit stores the plaque until the device is removed.

The use of laser beams to dissolve artery blockage has been slowly evolving. Presently, the FDA has approved three laser devices for use in clogged leg arteries. In 1992, the FDA approved the use of an "excimer" laser for use in coronary arteries.[10]

surgery, patients often report reduced chest pain, increased physical activity, and the feeling of a "new lease on life."

However, there is increasing evidence that coronary bypass surgery does not prolong survival in most cardiac patients. Thus there is some concern among health professionals that too many bypass operations are being performed.

Angioplasty

Angioplasty, an alternative to bypass surgery, involves the surgical insertion of a doughnut-shaped "balloon" directly into the narrowed coronary artery (Figure 10-4). When this balloon is inflated, plaque and fatty deposits are compressed against the artery walls. This enlarges the inner diameter of the artery, so that blood can flow more easily. These balloons usually remain within the artery for less than 1 hour. It has been found that renarrowing of the artery will occur in about one fourth of angioplasty patients. About 331,000 angioplasty procedures were performed in 1991.[1] Balloon angioplasty can be used for blockages in the heart, kidneys, arms, and legs.

radionuclide imaging (ray dee oh **new** klide) a diagnostic test in which small amounts of radioactive substances (radionuclides) are injected into the bloodstream; computer-generated pictures are then able to see how well the heart muscle is functioning

magnetic resonance (rez oh nence) **imaging (MRI scan)** a diagnostic test in which a powerful magnet is used to generate an image of body tissue

coronary artery bypass surgery surgical procedure designed to improve blood flow to the heart by providing alternate routes for blood to take around points of blockage.

heart-lung machine device that oxygenates and circulates blood during bypass surgery.

Aspirin

Studies released in the late 1980s highlighted the role of aspirin in reducing the risk of heart attack in men who had no history of previous attacks. Specifically, the studies concluded that for men with hypertension, elevated cholesterol, or both, taking one aspirin per day was a significant factor in reducing their risk of heart attack. Aspirin works by making the blood less able to clot. This reduces the likelihood of blockage in the blood vessels. Presently there is differing opinion regarding the age at which this preventive action should begin. Some researchers have suggested that men with known risk factors should begin taking one baby aspirin per day by age 35. Others disagree and indicate that aspirin therapy can cause potentially serious side effects including excessive bleeding, stomach ulcers, and gastrointestinal upset. The safest advice is to check with your physician before starting aspirin therapy.

Alcohol

For years, scientists have been uncertain about the extent to which alcohol consumption is related to a reduced risk for heart disease. The current thinking is that moderate drinking (defined as no more than two drinks per day for men and one drink per day for women) is related to a lower heart disease risk.[11,12] However, the benefit is much smaller than proven risk reduction behaviors such as stopping smoking, reducing cholesterol, lowering blood pressure, and increasing physical activity. Experts caution that heavy drinking increases cardiovascular risks and that non-drinkers should not start to drink just to reduce heart disease risk.

Heart transplants and artificial hearts

For approximately 30 years, surgeons have been able to surgically replace a person's damaged heart with that of another human being (Figure 10-5). Although very risky, these transplant operations have added years to the lives of a number of patients who otherwise would have lived only a short time. In 1992, nearly 2000 heart transplants were performed in the United States.[1] (See Figure 10-5.) Aside from the seriousness of this surgery, two major difficulties must be overcome in the process of heart transplantation: (1) finding a suitable donor heart and (2) coping with the recipient's possible rejection of the newly transplanted heart.

With an increased national awareness of the importance of organ donations, it is hoped that more hearts will become available for transplantation. Donor hearts must be removed immediately from the bodies of deceased donors and transported to the recipient's hospital as quickly as possible. This can be a complicated process. Once transplant surgery is completed, tissue rejection by the recipient is possible. However, with the use of a combination of antirejection drugs, it is estimated that more than 70% of heart transplant recipients will be able to live at least 5 years.[1]

Artificial hearts have also been developed and implanted in humans. These mechanical devices have extended the lives of patients. Artificial hearts have also served as temporary hearts while patients are waiting for a suitable donor heart. One of the major difficulties with artificial heart implantation has been the control of blood clots that may form, especially around the artificial valves.

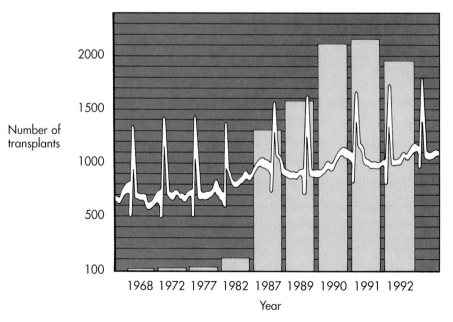

Figure 10-5 The increase in heart transplants.

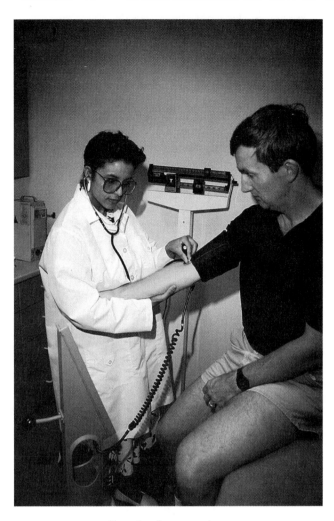

Hypertension screening.

Hypertension

Just as your car's water pump recirculates water and maintains water pressure, your heart recirculates blood and maintains blood pressure. When the heart contracts, blood is forced through your arteries and veins. Your blood pressure is a measure of the force that your circulating blood exerts against the interior walls of your arteries and veins.

Blood pressure is measured with a *sphygmomanometer*. A sphygmomanometer is attached to an arm-cuff device that can be inflated to stop the flow of blood temporarily in the brachial artery. This artery is a major supplier of blood to the lower arm. It is located on the inside of the upper arm, between the biceps and triceps muscles.

A physician, nurse, or technician using a stethoscope will listen for blood flow as the pressure in the cuff is released. Two pressure measurements will be recorded. The **systolic pressure** is the blood pressure against the vessel walls when the heart contracts. The

diastolic pressure is the blood pressure against the vessel walls when the heart relaxes (between heartbeats). Expressed in millimeters of mercury displaced on the sphygmomanometer, blood pressure is recorded in the form of a fraction, 115/82, for example. Because blood pressure drops when the heart relaxes, the systolic pressure is always higher than the diastolic pressure.

Although many persons still consider 120/80 as a "normal" or safe blood pressure for a young adult, variances from this figure do not necessarily indicate a medical problem. In fact, many young college women of average weight will indicate blood pressures that seem to be relatively low (105/65 for example), yet these lowered blood pressures are quite "normal" for them. Any major deviation from 120/80 in your blood pressure should be discussed with a physician.

Hypertension refers to a consistently elevated blood pressure. Generally, concern about a young adult's high blood pressure begins when he or she has a systolic reading of 140 or above or a diastolic reading of 90 or above. Fifty million American adults and children have hypertension. According to the American Heart Association, African Americans, Puerto Ricans, Cuban Americans, and Mexican Americans are more likely to suffer from hypertension than are Anglo Americans. Asian Americans and Pacific Islanders have significantly lower rates of hypertension, however.[1]

It is estimated that in 90% to 95% of the cases of hypertension, the cause is not clearly known. This form of hypertension is called *essential hypertension*.[4] Essential hypertension does appear to be statistically related to age, heredity, and diet, since epidemiological studies have indicated that this disease tends to strike older persons, to run in families, and to afflict persons who eat a diet high in saturated fat and salt. Unresolved stress may be a factor in essential hypertension, but the relationship has not been clearly established. (Two important points are worth remembering. First, persons under a lot of stress do not necessarily have hypertension. Second, hypertension and hyperactivity are two completely different conditions.)

A second form of hypertension is called *secondary hypertension*. This form of hypertension appears to be

systolic pressure (sis **tol** ick) blood pressure against blood vessel walls when the heart contracts.

diastolic pressure (die uh **stol** ick) blood pressure against blood vessel walls when the heart relaxes.

triggered by a specific cause. **Arteriosclerosis,** endocrine gland disorders, and kidney diseases may all be causes of secondary hypertension. Scientific research also implicates unresolved stress as another possible contributor to secondary hypertension.

The cardiovascular health risks produced by uncontrolled hypertension are many. Hypertension accelerates atherosclerosis (see p. 251). Thus the heart is required to work much more forcefully to pump blood through narrowed vessels. This requirement places too much demand on the coronary arteries and the ventricles, which must carry the brunt of the work load. Heart attack and heart failure may result.

Throughout the body, hypertension also accelerates arteriosclerosis. This process makes arteries and arterioles become less elastic and thus incapable of dilating under a heavy work load. Brittle, calcified blood vessels can burst unexpectedly and produce serious strokes (brain accidents), kidney failure (renal accidents), or eye damage **(retinal hemorrhage).** Furthermore, it appears that blood and fat clots are more easily formed and dislodged in a vascular system influenced by hypertension. Clearly hypertension is a potential killer.

Ironically, despite its deadly nature, hypertension is referred to as "the silent killer," because victims of hypertension rarely, if ever, are aware that they have the condition. Victims cannot feel the sensation of high blood pressure. Hypertension does not produce dizziness, headaches, or memory loss, unless one is experiencing a medical crisis. Because it is a silent killer, estimates are that 35% of the people who have hypertension do not realize they have it. Many who are aware of their hypertension do little to control it. Only a small percentage of people (21%) who have hypertension control it adequately, generally through dietary control, supervised fitness, relaxation training, and drug therapy.[1] Thus reaching the Healthy People 2000 objective (50%) may be difficult. Essential hypertension is not thought of as a curable disease; rather, it is a controllable disease. Once therapy is stopped, the condition returns.

PREVENTION AND TREATMENT

Weight reduction, physical exercise, moderation in alcohol use, and sodium restriction are often used to reduce hypertension. For heavy or obese persons, a reduction in body weight may produce a significant drop in blood pressure. Physical activity helps lower blood pressure by expending Calories (which leads to weight loss) and improving overall circulation. Reducing alcohol consumption to less than 2 ounces daily helps reduce blood pressure in some people.[4]

The restriction of sodium (salt) in the diet also helps some people to reduce hypertension. Interestingly, this strategy is effective only for those who are **salt sensitive**—estimated to be about 25% of the population.

Reducing salt intake would have little effect on the blood pressure of the rest of the population. Nevertheless, since our daily intake of salt vastly exceeds our need for salt, the general recommendation to curb salt intake still makes good sense.

Many of the stress reduction activities discussed in Chapter 3 are receiving increased attention in the struggle to reduce hypertension. In recent years behavioral scientists have reported the success of meditation, biofeedback, controlled breathing, and muscle relaxation exercises in reducing hypertension. Look for further research in these areas in the years to come.

Drugs used to lower high blood pressure are called *antihypertensives.*[13] *Diuretic drugs* work by forcing fluid from the bloodstream, thereby reducing blood volume. *Vasodilators* relax the muscles in the walls of blood vessels (especially the arterioles), allowing the vessels to dilate (widen). Also used are calcium channel blockers, beta blockers (p. 253), and other drugs that work in various ways to relax blood vessels. The most disturbing aspect of drug therapy for hypertension is that many patients refuse to take their medication on a consistent basis, probably because of the mistaken notion that "you must feel sick to be sick."

A number of people taking these medications report uncomfortable side effects, including depression, reduced libido (sex drive), muscle weakness, impotence, dizziness, and fainting. Thus the treatment's side effects may seem worse than the disease. Because of the poor record of patient compliance with hypertension drug therapy, numerous television and radio announcements are geared to the hypertensive patient. Nutritional supplements, such as calcium, magnesium, potassium and fish oil are not effective in lowering blood pressure.[14]

As a responsible adult, you might push yourself to use every opportunity you can find to measure your blood pressure. Ask to have your blood pressure checked when you are in a physician's office or in the student health center. (You may have to pry these measurements from the nurse or technician; you do have a right to this information!) You could also check with nursing majors to see whether they might check your blood pressure. Use the free machines that measure blood pressure in shopping malls or drug stores. (Do not count on completely accurate measurements from these machines, however.) Become familiar with your own potential silent killer.

Stroke

Stroke is a general term for a wide variety of crises (sometimes called *cerebrovascular accidents* or CVAs) that result from blood vessel damage in the brain. African Americans have a 60% greater risk of stroke than white Americans do, probably because African Americans have a greater likelihood of having hypertension than whites do. Data for 1991 indicate that

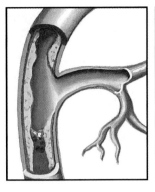
Thrombus

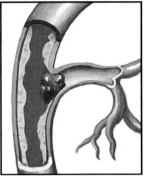
Embolus

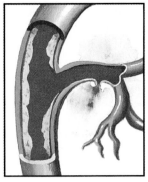
Hemorrhage

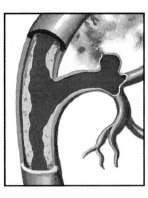
Aneurysm (ruptured)

Figure 10-6 Causes of stroke.

over 144,000 deaths and half a million new cases of stroke occurred.[1] Just as heart muscle needs adequate blood supply, so does the brain. Any disturbance in the proper supply of oxygen and nutrients can pose a hazardous situation.

Perhaps the most common form of stroke results from the blockage in a cerebral (brain) artery. Similar to coronary occlusions, **cerebrovascular occlusions** can be initiated by a clot (thrombus) that forms within an artery or by a clot (embolus) that travels from another part of the body to the brain (Figure 10-6, *A* and *B*). The resultant accidents (cerebral thrombosis or cerebral embolism) cause between 70% and 80% of all strokes. The portion of the brain deprived of oxygen and nutrients can literally die.

The extent of damage depends on the location of the occlusion and the degree of blockage. Thus an occlusion in a portion of brain tissue that serves as a speech center can result in a person's inability to speak. Occlusion in motor coordination areas can result in paralysis. Memory, behavior, and thought patterns can also be affected by stroke. Obviously a massive occlusion or an occlusion in a critical area (such as a center that controls respiration, temperature, or coronary function) can initiate a life-threatening situation.

Strokes can also result from an artery that bursts to produce a crisis called *cerebral hemorrhage* (Figure 10-6, *C*). Damaged, brittle arteries can be especially susceptible to bursting when a person has hypertension. Brittle arteries may result from arteriosclerosis. Arteriosclerosis tends to increase as we age or as a consequence of other disease processes, such as diabetes or hypertension. Cerebral hemorrhage produces two key problems: (1) the brain tissue supplied by the damaged artery is deprived of oxygen and nutrients and (2) the accumulation of blood places added pressure on surrounding brain tissue. Because the skull (cranium) will not expand, this pressure buildup can be life threatening in itself.

A fourth form of stroke is a *cerebral aneurysm.* An aneurysm is a ballooning or outpouching on a weakened area of an artery (Figure 10-6, *D*). Aneurysms may occur in various locations of the body and are not always life threatening. The development of aneurysms is not fully understood, although there seems to be a relationship between aneurysms and hypertension. It is quite possible that many aneurysms are congenital defects. In any case, when a cerebral aneurysm bursts, a stroke results. See the box on p. 260 for warning signs of stroke.

TREATMENT

A person who reports any warning signs of stroke or any little stroke **(transient ischemic attack [TIA])** will undergo a battery of diagnostic tests, which could in-

arteriosclerosis (are **teer** ee oh scler **oh** sis) calcification within the artery's wall that makes the vessel less elastic, more brittle, and more susceptible to bursting; hardening of the arteries.

retinal hemorrhage (**ret** in al **hem** or edge) uncontrolled bleeding from arteries within the eye's retina.

salt sensitive description of people who overreact to the presence of sodium by retaining fluid, and thus experience an increase in blood pressure.

cerebrovascular occlusions (ser **ee** bro **vas** kyou lar oh **klu** shun) blockages to arteries supplying blood to the cerebral cortex of the brain; strokes.

transient ischemic attack (TIA) (**tran** see ent iss **key** mick) strokelike symptoms caused by temporary spasm of cerebral blood vessels.

clude a physical examination, a search for possible brain tumors, tests to identify areas of the brain affected, use of the electroencephalogram, cerebral arteriography, and the use of the **CAT** (computerized axial tomography) **scan** or MRI (magnetic resonance imaging) scan. Many additional tests are also available.

Treatment of stroke patients depends on the nature and extent of the damage. Some patients require surgery (to repair vessels and relieve pressure) and acute care in the hospital. Others undergo drug treatment, especially the use of anticoagulant drugs, including aspirin.

The advancements made in the rehabilitation of stroke victims are amazing. It is true that some severely damaged patients have little hope of improvement. However, increasing advancements in the application of computer technology to such disciplines as speech therapy and physical therapy do offer encouraging signs for stroke patients and their families.

Congenital Heart Disease

A congenital defect is one that is present at birth. It is estimated that each year 25,000 babies are born with a congenital heart defect. In 1991, 5800 children (mostly infants) died of congenital heart disease.[1]

A variety of abnormalities may be produced by congenital heart disease, including valve damage, holes in the walls of the septum, blood vessel transposition, and an underdevelopment of the left side of the heart.[4] All of these problems ultimately prevent a newborn baby from adequately oxygenating tissues throughout the body. A bluish skin color (cyanosis) is seen in some infants with such congenital heart defects. These infants are sometimes referred to as "blue babies."

The cause of congenital heart defects is not clearly understood, although one cause, *rubella,* has been identified. Mothers who contract the rubella virus during the first 3 months of pregnancy place their child at great risk of developing *congenital rubella syndrome* (*CRS*), a catchall term for a wide variety of congenital defects, including heart defects, deafness, cataracts, and mental retardation. Other hypotheses about the development of congenital heart disease implicate environmetal pollutants, use of drugs including alcohol, and unknown genetic factors.

TREATMENT

Treatment of congenital defects centers on surgery, although some conditions may respond well to drug therapy. Defective blood vessels and certain malformations of the heart can be surgically repaired. So successful is this surgery that many children respond quite quickly to the increased circulation and oxygenation. Many are able to lead normal active lives.

Rheumatic Heart Disease

Rheumatic heart disease is the final stage in a series of complications started by a streptococcal infection of

Warning Signs of Stroke

Although many stroke victims have little advance warning of an impending crisis, there are some warning signals of stroke that should be recognized. The American Heart Association encourages everyone to be aware of the following signs:

★ Sudden, temporary weakness or numbness of the face, arm, and leg on one side of the body

★ Temporary loss of speech or trouble in speaking or understanding speech

★ Temporary dimness or loss of vision, particularly in one eye

★ Unexplained dizziness, unsteadiness, or sudden falls

★ Many major strokes are preceded by "little strokes," warning signals like the above, experienced days, weeks, or months before the more severe event

Prompt medical or surgical attention to these symptoms may prevent a fatal or disabling stroke from occurring. ★

the throat (strep throat). This bacterial infection, if untreated, can result in an inflammatory disease called *rheumatic fever* (and a related condition, scarlet fever). Rheumatic fever is a whole-body (systemic) reaction that can produce fever, joint pain, skin rashes, and possible brain and heart damage. Once having had rheumatic fever, a person is more susceptible to subsequent attacks. Rheumatic fever tends to run in families. Approximately 6000 Americans died from rheumatic fever and rheumatic heart disease in 1991.[1]

Damage from rheumatic fever centers on the heart's valves. For some reason, the bacteria prefer to proliferate in the region of the heart valves.

Defective heart valves may fail either to open fully (*stenosis*) or to close fully (*insufficiency*). Diagnosis of valve damage might initially come when a physician hears a backwashing or back flow of blood (a **murmur**). Further tests—including chest x-rays, cardiac catheterization, and echocardiography—can reveal the extent of valve damage.[4] Once identified, a faulty valve can be replaced surgically with a metal and plastic artificial valve or a valve taken from an animal's heart. The success rate of such surgery is quite high. Patients with only moderate valve damage might forego surgery, instead receiving regular, periodic reexaminations, possible long-term antibiotic treatment, and careful monitoring of physical exercise. Those with mild damage, as evidenced by only a slight murmur, may have no physical restrictions imposed on them. In fact, to the relief of most parents, most murmurs initially identified by physicians are labeled "innocent murmurs," because they are not related to streptococcal damage and will never impair a child's normal development.

PREVENTION AND TREATMENT

Rheumatic heart disease is best prevented by recognizing that *any* sore throat might be strep throat. Although most sore throats are not caused by streptococcal bacteria, any unusually sore throat of sudden onset, especially in children ages 5 to 15, should be examined by a physician.[4] A throat culture and possibly a strep antibody test would determine the causative agent or at least rule out strep as a probable cause. If strep throat is diagnosed, antibiotic treatment would likely follow.

RELATED CARDIOVASCULAR CONDITIONS

Besides the cardiovascular diseases already discussed, the heart and blood vessels are also subject to other pathological conditions. Tumors of the heart, although rare, are known to occur. Infectious conditions involving the pericardial sac that surrounds the heart (*pericarditis*) and the innermost layer of the heart (*endocarditis*) are more commonly seen. In addition, inflammation of the veins (*phlebitis*) is troublesome to some people, and *peripheral artery disease (PAD)* and *congestive heart failure* are serious conditions.

Peripheral Artery Disease

Peripheral artery disease (PAD), also called peripheral vascular disease (PVD), is a blood vessel disease characterized by serious changes to the arteries and arterioles in the extremities (primarily the legs and feet, but sometimes in the hands). These changes result from years of atherosclerotic and arteriosclerotic damage to the blood vessels. The result of PAD is severely restricted blood flow to the extremities. The reduction in blood flow is responsible for leg pain or cramping during exercise, numbness, tingling, coldness, and loss of hair in the affected limb. The most serious consequence of PAD is the increased likelihood of developing ulcerations and tissue death. These conditions can lead to gangrene and may eventually necessitate amputation.

The management of PAD consists of multiple approaches and may include efforts to improve lipid profiles (through diet, exercise, or drug therapy), reduce hypertension, reduce body weight, and eliminate smoking. Blood vessel surgery may be a possibility, but only after other approaches (including the use of drugs that dilate the affected blood vessels) are first explored.

Congestive Heart Failure

Congestive heart failure is a condition in which the heart lacks the strength to continue to circulate blood normally throughout the body. During congestive heart failure, the heart continues to work, but it cannot function well enough to maintain appropriate circulation. Venous blood flow starts to "back up." Swelling occurs, especially in the legs and ankles. Fluid can collect in the lungs and cause breathing difficulties and shortness of breath, and kidney function may be damaged. Without medical care, congestive heart failure can be fatal.[4]

Congestive heart failure can result from heart damage caused by congenital heart defects, lung disease, rheumatic fever, heart attack, atherosclerosis, or high blood pressure. Generally, congestive heart failure is treatable through a combined program of rest, proper diet, modified daily activities, and the use of appropriate drugs. Without medical care, congestive heart failure can be fatal.

CARDIOVASCULAR RISK FACTORS

A *cardiovascular risk factor* is an attribute that a person has or is exposed to that increases the likelihood that he or she will develop some form of cardiovascular disease. However, merely having one or even a few risk factors does not always mean that a person will develop a disease. You may even know some at-risk people who never seem to develop clinical symptoms of heart disease.

CAT scan computerized axial tomography; x-ray procedure designed to visualize structures within the body that would not normally be seen through conventional x-ray procedures.

rheumatic heart disease (roo **mat** ick) chronic damage to the heart (especially heart valves) resulting from a streptococcal infection within the heart; a complication associated with rheumatic fever.

murmur atypical heart sound that suggests a backwashing of blood into a chamber of the heart from which it just left.

peripheral artery disease (PAD) (per **if** er all) damage resulting from restricted blood flow to the extremities, especially the legs and feet.

congestive heart failure (con **jest** ive) inability of the heart to pump out all the blood that returns to it; can lead to dangerous fluid accumulations in veins, lungs, and kidneys.

"Big Four" Risk Factors for Cardiovascular Disease

★ Cigarette smoking   ★ High cholesterol level

★ Hypertension   ★ Physical inactivity

Factors that Cannot Be Changed

★ Heredity

★ Sex

★ Race

★ Age

Factors that Can Be Changed

★ Cigarette smoking

★ High blood pressure

★ Blood cholesterol levels

★ Physical inactivity

Contributing Factors

★ Diabetes

★ Obesity

★ Stress

Other Heart Disease Risk Factors

RISK FACTORS FOR CONGENITAL HEART DISEASE

★ Fetal exposure to rubella, other viral infections, pollutants, alcohol or tobacco smoke during pregnancy

RISK FACTORS FOR RHEUMATIC HEART DISEASE

★ Streptococcal infection

Common Symptoms of Strep Throat

★ Sudden onset of sore throat, particularly with pain when swallowing

★ Fever

★ Swollen, tender glands under the angle of the jaw

★ Headache

★ Nausea and vomiting

★ Tonsils covered with a yellow or white exudate (discharge or pus)

Risk Factors for Coronary Artery Disease, Hypertension, and Stroke

Medical science can only predict that our chances of developing heart disease are increased if we have multiple risk factors. (See the Star box above for lists of the factors that can and cannot be changed, as well as a list of contributing factors.) Interestingly, some scientists believe that we really understand only about half of the risk factors that may cause heart disease.

However, most health professionals are convinced that *now* is the best time for people to take a close look at the risk factors they can control. They are convinced that cardiovascular diseases are lifestyle diseases—diseases that closely parallel the way people choose to live their lives.

While you may think that "everything is bad for your heart" and that heart disease will occur "regardless of what I do," this just is not the case. Virtually every person can benefit from living a heart-healthy lifestyle.

Many chapters in this textbook will help you in your quest to reduce your heart disease risk. For ways to improve your physical activity and physical fitness, refer to Chapter 4. Chapters 5 and 6 discuss nutrition and weight management. Ways to stop cigarette smoking are discussed in Chapter 9.

Through lifestyle changes in fitness, nutrition, and smoking, you can have a profound impact on your cardiorespiratory system, your dietary intake, your weight, and your cholesterol level. Efforts to improve your mental health (Chapter 2) and stress management (Chapter 3) and to avoid diabetes (Chapter 11) will also be beneficial for your heart.

Although no one can promise you freedom from heart and blood vessel diseases, conscious efforts to control the "big four" risk factors (cigarette smoking, hypertension, high cholesterol level, and physical inactivity) can pay healthful benefits throughout your lifetime.[15] In addition to the disease prevention benefits of controlling the "big four" risks, you will probably find personal satisfaction with this lifestyle. In our health science classes, our nontraditional students who have restructured their lifestyle behaviors frequently report overwhelming personal benefits. They report having much more energy, self-esteem, and satisfaction with the course of their lives. The time to start these changes is *now*.

Risk Factors for Congenital Heart Disease and Rheumatic Heart Disease

It may already be apparent to you that the risk factors for stroke, coronary artery disease, and high blood pressure differ considerably from the factors that appear to be correlated with the development of congenital heart disease and rheumatic heart disease. Most of the causal factors of congenital heart disease are not

Health ACTION Guide

Can a Good Diet Include Fries?

In earlier chapters of this book, you learned that the recommended level of daily fat intake was 25% to 30% of the overall Calories. Knowing this, you can closely approximate how that "regular order of french fries" fits into your dietary plan.

▼ For example, you are allowed about 2800 Calories each day in your diet (a ballpark estimate for college males). By multiplying 2800 by .25, you find that you can consume about 700 Calories from fat each day.

▼ You know that each gram of fat is equal to 9 calories. Thus you can consume about 80 grams of fat each day and still be in the suggested healthful range.

▼ At your favorite fast food place, ask for the nutrition information guide. You will discover that the regular size fries have 12 to 15 grams of fat.

▼ You will not abandon your nutritious eating plan by eating french fries. You still have up to 65 more grams of fat to eat on that day.

▼ Plan to do this regularly with healthful selections from the five main food groups.

---

well understood. A mother's contraction of rubella during pregnancy has been specifically linked to congenital heart abnormalities, and other maternal insults during pregnancy (alcohol or drug abuse, exposure to other disease processes or environmental pollutants) are thought to contribute to heart defects in newborn children.

These risk factors can be minimized by a woman's careful control of her body before conception and during pregnancy, including being immunized before becoming pregnant, reducing exposure to environmental pollutants and tobacco smoke, and limiting drug and alcohol use during pregnancy. Appropriate obstetrical supervision and proper nutrition are other factors that might enhance the chances of giving birth to a healthy baby—one who is free of congenital heart problems.

The greatest risk factor related to rheumatic heart disease is the failure to control the streptococcal (bacterial) infection commonly called strep throat. Administration of appropriate antibiotic drugs (primarily penicillin) before bacteria spread to the heart valves is the best way to check the spread of this potentially serious disease.

Since this disease most commonly strikes children ages 5 to 15, it is important for parents to be reasonably concerned about children's sore throats.[4] For people of all ages, high-level health can reduce susceptibility to a wide variety of infections, including strep infection. Adequate sleep, regular exercise, and proper diet (factors that are sometimes difficult for college students to control) can all contribute to your high level of physical health.

Health ACTION Guide

Reduce Your Risk of Heart Attack

The American lifestyle—high-fat diets, lack of regular exercise, being overweight, and cigarette smoking—is a major contributor to heart attacks. To reduce your risks of suffering a heart attack you should:

▼ Have your blood pressure checked regularly. If it is high, cooperate with your doctor to keep it under control.

▼ Do not smoke cigarettes.

▼ Eat foods that are low in saturated (animal) fats and cholesterol.

▼ Maintain proper weight. If you are overweight, follow the Heart Association's suggestions to reduce weight while maintaining a balanced and nutritious diet.

▼ Exercise regularly to maintain cardiovascular fitness. Check with your doctor before beginning an exercise program.

▼ Have regular medical checkups and follow your doctor's advice about reducing your risks of heart attack.

PERSONAL ASSESSMENT

CHOLESTEROL

**Your serum cholesterol
 level is:**
   0 190 or below
 + 2 191 to 230
 + 6 231 to 289
 +12 290 to 319
 +16 Over 320

**Your HDL
 cholesterol is:**
 −2 Over 60
   0 45 to 60
 + 2 35 to 44
 + 6 29 to 34
 +12 23 to 28
 +16 Below 23

SMOKING

You smoke now or have in the past:
   0 Never smoked, or quit more than 5 years ago
 +1 Quit 2 to 4 years ago
 +3 Quit about 1 year ago
 +6 Quit during the past year

You now smoke:
 + 9 ½ to 1 pack a day
 +12 1 to 2 packs a day
 +15 More than 2 packs a day

The quality of the air you breathe is:
   0 Unpolluted by smoke, exhaust **or** industry at
      home **and** at work
 +2 Live **or** work with smokers in unpolluted area
 +4 Live **and** work with smokers in unpolluted area
 +6 Live **or** work with smokers and live or work in
      air-polluted area
 +8 Live **and** work with smokers and live and work
      in air-polluted area

BLOOD PRESSURE

Your blood pressure is:
   0 120/75 or below
 + 2 120/75 to 140/85
 + 6 140/85 to 150/90
 + 8 150/90 to 175/100
 +10 175/100 to 190/110
 +12 190/110 or above

EXERCISE

Your exercise habits are:
   0 Exercise vigorously 4 or 5 times a week
 +2 Exercise moderately 4 or 5 times a week
 +4 Exercise only on weekends
 +6 Exercise occasionally
 +8 Little or no exercise

WEIGHT

Your weight history is:
   0 Always at or near ideal weight
 +1 Now 10 percent overweight
 +2 Now 20 percent overweight
 +3 Now 30 percent or more overweight
 +4 Now 20 percent or more overweight and have
      been since before age 30

STRESS

You feel overstressed:
   0 Rarely at work or at home
 + 3 Somewhat at home but not at work
 + 5 Somewhat at work but not at home
 + 7 Somewhat at work **and** at home
 + 9 Usually, at work **or** at home
 +12 Usually, at work **and** at home

ALCOHOL

You drink alcoholic beverages:

  0 Never or only socially, about once or twice a month, or only one 5-ounce glass of wine or 12-ounce glass of beer or 1 ½ ounces of hard liquor about 5 times a week

+2 Two to three 5-ounce glasses of wine or 12-ounce glasses of beer of 1 ½-ounce cocktails about 5 times a week

+4 More than three 1 ½-ounce cocktails or more than three 5-ounce glasses of wine or 12-ounce glasses of beer almost every day

DIABETES

Your diabetic history is:

  0 Blood sugar always normal

+2 Blood glucose slightly high (prediabetic) or slightly low (hypoglycemic)

+4 Diabetic beginning after age 40 requiring strict dietary or insulin control

+5 Diabetic beginning before age 30 requiring strict dietary or insulin control

INTERPRETATION

Add all scores and check below.

0 to 20:   Low risk. Excellent family history and lifestyle habits.

21 to 50:   Moderate risk. Family history or lifestyle habits put you at some risk. You might lower your risks and minimize your genetic predisposition if you change any poor habits.

51 to 74:   High risk. Habits and family history indicate high risk of heart disease. Change your habits now.

Above 75:   Very high risk. Family history and a lifetime of poor habits put you at very high risk of heart disease. Eliminate as many of the risk factors as you can.

TO CARRY THIS FURTHER . . .

Were you surprised with your score on this assessment? What were your most significant risk factors? Do you plan to make any changes in your lifestyle to reduce your cardiovascular risks? Why or why not?

PERSONAL ASSESSMENT

Summary

✔ Cardiovascular diseases are responsible for more disabilities and deaths than any other disease.

✔ The cardiovascular system consists of the heart, blood, and blood vessels. This system performs many functions.

✔ Our overall health depends on the health of the cardiovascular system.

✔ The major forms of cardiovascular diseases include coronary heart disease, high blood pressure, stroke, congenital heart disease, and rheumatic heart disease. Each disease develops in a specific way and may require a highly specialized form of treatment.

✔ A cardiovascular risk factor is an attribute that a person has or is exposed to which increases the likelihood of disease.

✔ The "big four" risk factors are cigarette smoking, hypertension, high cholesterol, and physical inactivity. These are controllable risk factors.

✔ Heredity, sex, race, and age are risk factors that cannot be controlled.

✔ Contributing risk factors are diabetes, obesity, and stress.

Review Questions

1. What are some of the factors that are helping to reduce the deaths from cardiovascular diseases?
2. Describe a potential victim of cardiovascular disease.
3. Identify the principal components of the cardiovascular system. Trace the path of blood through the heart and cardiovascular system.
4. How much blood does the average adult have? What are some of the major functions of blood?
5. What four important requirements reflect a healthy cardiovascular system?
6. What are the major forms of cardiovascular disease? For each of these diseases, describe what the disease is, its cause (if known), and its treatment. What role does atherosclerosis play in each of these diseases? How does arteriosclerosis differ from atherosclerosis?
7. Why is hypertension referred to as "the silent killer"?
8. What are the warning signals of stroke?
9. Define cardiovascular risk factor. What relationship do risk factors have to cardiovascular disease? Describe the role of cholesterol and lipoproteins as risk factors in cardiovascular disease.
10. Identify those risk factors for cardiovascular disease that cannot be changed. Identify those risk factors that can be changed. Identify those risk factors that are contributing factors.

Think about This . . .

✔ Have you ever thought of yourself as a potential victim of heart disease?

✔ In the last week, what have you done to improve your cardiovascular system?

✔ To get an accurate measure of your blood pressure, it is a good idea to take several readings and average them. When was the last time you had your blood pressure checked? What were the readings?

✔ What role should men play in reducing the threats of congenital heart disease?

✔ Are you comfortable talking with your relatives about their possible risk factors?

REAL LIFE
REAL CHOICES

YOUR TURN

▼ What specific kind of throat infection might Greg Chulick be dealing with?

▼ What can happen to someone who has this kind of throat infection and doesn't get medical treatment?

▼ What is your reaction to Greg's fear of telling his parents about his sore throat?

AND NOW, YOUR CHOICES . . .

▼ If you were one of Greg's parents, how could you encourage Greg to tell you when he got a sore throat without adding to his fears arising from his brother's death?

▼ If you were Greg's older brother or sister and he told you about his sore throat, how would you try to help him? ▼

References

1. American Heart Association: *Heart and stroke facts: 1994 statistical supplement*, Dallas, 1993, The Association.
2. Thibodeau GA: *Structure and function of the body*, ed 9, St Louis, 1992, Mosby.
3. Thibodeau GA, Patton KT: *The human body in health and disease*, St Louis, 1992, Mosby.
4. American Heart Association: *Heart and stroke facts*, Dallas, 1993, The Association.
5. Dietary measures and cholesterol: an update, *The Harvard Heart Letter* 4(5):1-3, 1994.
6. *High blood cholesterol: what it means*, The Search for Health, A Report from the National Institutes of Health, 1989, Bethesda, Md, US Department of Health and Human Services.
7. Wardlaw GM, Insel PM, Seyler MF: *Contemporary nutrition: issues and insights*, St Louis, 1994, Mosby.
8. Papazian R: Heart attack: the golden hour, *Harvard Health Letter* 17(10):6-8, 1992.
9. Farley D: Help for hearts and blood vessels: balloons, lasers, and scrapers, *FDA Consumer* 25(3):22-27, 1991.
10. Friend T: Laser OK'd to unclog heart arteries, *USA Today*, Feb 7, 1992, 1D.
11. Moderate drinking, *Alcohol Alert*, National Institute on Alcohol Abuse and Alcoholism, US Department of Health and Human Services, PHS Pub No 16(PH315), April 1992.
12. Is alcohol good for the heart?, *The Johns Hopkins Medical Letter—Health After 50* 4(8):3, 1992.
13. Which drug for hypertension? *The Harvard Heart Letter* 3(1):1-6, 1992.
14. Trials of Hypertension Prevention Collaborative Research Group: The effects of nonpharmacologic interventions on blood pressure of persons with high normal levels: results of the trials of hypertension prevention, Phase 1, *JAMA* 267(9):1213-1220, 1992.
15. *University of California at Berkeley Wellness Letter* 8(11):1, 1992, pg. 1.
16. Kleiman C, Osborn K: *If it runs in your family: heart disease: reducing your risk*, New York, 1991, Bantam Books.

Suggested Readings

Diethrich EB, Cohan C: *Women and heart disease*, New York, 1992, Times Books.

Co-authored by renowned heart expert, E.B. Diethrich. Women are encouraged to assess their risk for heart disease. Since diagnosis is particularly problematic for women, the reader is guided through a step-by-step process.

Kwiterovich PO, Jr: *The Johns Hopkins complete guide for preventing and recovering from heart disease*, Rocklin, Calif, 1993, Prima Publishing.

Written by the Chief of the Lipid Research and Atherosclerosis Unit of the Johns Hopkins University School of Medicine, all aspects of heart disease prevention, treatment, and recovery are included. Topics include cholesterol, genetic factors, treatment drugs, menus, children and heart disease, and an action diet plan. An American Heart Association Award of Excellence winner.

11

Cancer and Chronic Conditions

Most of you can attest to the disruptive influence an illness can have on your ability to participate in day-to-day activities. When feeling ill, your school, employment, and leisure activities are replaced by periods of reduced activity, and may even require periods of bed rest or hospitalization. When your illness is chronic, the impact of being ill may extend over a period of time. Ultimately, you, like virtually all people with chronic illness, must eventually find a balance between day-to-day function and the continuous presence of your illness. Unlike the diagnosis, treatment and recovery pattern associated with most *acute* (develops abruptly and subsides after a short time) conditions, *chronic* (develops slowly and persists for a long time) illness requires a management approach that may remain part of your daily activity for the remainder of your life.

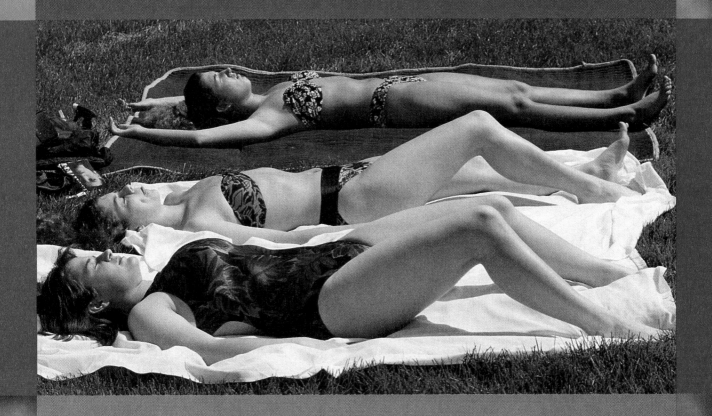

CANCER AND CHRONIC CONDITIONS

The following objectives will be covered in this chapter:

▼ Reverse the rise in cancer deaths to achieve a rate of no more than 130 per 100,000 people. (Age-adjusted baseline: 133 per 100,000 people; p. 418.)

▼ Reduce breast cancer deaths to no more than 20.6 per 100,000 women. (Age-adjusted baseline: 22.9% in 1987; p. 420.)

▼ Reduce colorectal cancer deaths to no more than 13.2 per 100,000 people. (Age-adjusted baseline: 14.4 people in 1987; p. 422.)

▼ Slow the rise in lung cancer deaths to achieve a rate of no more than 42 per 100,000 people. (Age-adjusted baseline: 37.9 per 100,000 in 1987; p. 420.)

▼ Reduce diabetes-related deaths to no more than 34 per 100,000 people. (Age-adjusted baseline: 38 per 100,000 in 1986; p. 456.)

▼ Reduce to no more than 8% the proportion of people who experience a limitation in major activity caused by chronic conditions. (Baseline: 9.4% in 1988; p. 446.)

REAL LIFE REAL CHOICES

Sunny Side Up: Are You Dying for a Tan?

▼ Name: Tina Mavrakos
▼ Age: 19
▼ Occupation: College student/camp counselor

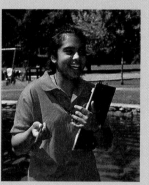

"Let's hit the beach!"

If Tina Mavrakos has a signature phrase, it's those four words. She's lived all her life in a small seaside town in southern New Jersey where her father and older brothers operate a small fishing boat, and she's loved the ocean and the shore ever since she picked up her first shell. When it came time to choose a college, Tina went straight for the "Sunshine State;" she's now a marketing major at a large university in southeastern Florida, where the palm-lined beach is her second home. During the summer she returns to New Jersey and works as a counselor at—what else?—a sailing camp for kids.

Tina loves the whole ocean experience, and she's got the tan to prove it. Her naturally olive-toned skin, a gift of her Greek heritage, is always the deep bronze of people in high-fashion magazines. Unlike her fair-haired friends, who apply the maximum-SPF sunscreen before even walking to the beach, Tina never uses sun protection and laughs when someone advises her to be careful. Whatever she'd put on would just wash off, she says breezily, because she's always getting wet while swimming, sailing, or helping her father and brothers unload a day's catch from their boat.

Anyway, she's never gotten sunburned—well, *almost* never. A few times—or maybe it's more than that—Tina has felt her unprotected skin begin to tighten and tingle after a couple of hours in the sun. She never wears more than a swimsuit or cutoffs and a tank top, and she can't understand why her father and brothers always go out on their boat clad in long pants, T-shirts or jerseys, and long-billed caps.

As you study this chapter, think about the risks of Tina's sun-worshipping life, and prepare yourself to answer the questions in **Your Turn** at the end of the chapter. ▼

CHRONIC HEALTH CONCERNS

Now that you have completed the study of cardiovascular disease in Chapter 10, we turn to selected chronic conditions. Cancer, the second leading cause of death for adults, will be studied in detail.[1] Additionally, three other chronic conditions, diabetes mellitus, multiple sclerosis, and asthma will be presented. These three chronic conditions were chosen as representative of the hundreds of chronic conditions that can influence our health. In most chronic conditions, many factors can contribute to the development and the extent to which they influence overall health and lifestyle. These factors include genetic predisposition, behavioral patterns, and environmental factors. Watch for indications of these factors in your own life in each of the conditions presented.

Information about other chronic conditions is given throughout this text. Low back pain is presented in Chapter 4 with physical fitness. Rheumatoid arthritis and allergic disorders are discussed as part of the immune system function in Chapter 12, whereas PMS (premenstrual syndrome) and fibrocystic breast condition are found with the discussion of menstruation in

Chapter 13. Sickle cell disease and trait accompany the discussion of reproduction in Chapter 16. Last, osteoarthritis and osteoporosis are presented in Chapter 20 with aging, and epilepsy appears in Appendix 2 on first aid.

Cancer: A Problem of Cell Regulation

In much the same manner that a corporation depends on competent individuals to staff its various departments, the body depends on its basic units of function—the cells. Cells band together as tissues to perform a prescribed function. Tissues, in turn, join to form organs, and organs are assembled into the body's several organ systems. Such is the "corporate structure" of the body.

If individuals and cells are the basic units of function for their respective organizations, the failure of either to perform in a prescribed, dependable manner can erode the overall organization to the extent that it might not be able to continue. Cancer, the second leading cause of death among adults, is a condition reflecting cell dysfunction in its most extreme form. In cancer the prescribed behavior of normal cells ceases.

CELL REGULATION

The tissues of the body lose cells over time. With the exception of a few types of tissues, this ongoing loss of cells requires that replacement cells be brought forward on a regular basis from areas of young and initially less specialized cells. The process of *differentiation* required to turn the less specialized cells into a mature form is carefully controlled by genes within the cells. Upon achieving specialization appropriate to the tissues they are joining, these newest cells replicate or copy themselves through a process of cellular division called mitosis. This **doubling** process is carefully monitored by the cells' **regulatory genes.** However, if the replication process becomes faulty because of failure of the regulatory genes to function, or because damage to genetic material by outside forces is beyond the cells' ability to repair, abnormal cells will be recognized and removed by the immune system (see Chapter 12).

In addition to their normal role of controlling cell replacement, the regulatory genes also can become cancer-causing genes, or **oncogenes** (regulatory genes that are not yet oncogenes can be called **protooncogenes**).[2]

How protooncogenes become oncogenes is a question that cannot be completely answered at this time. Although a detailed explanation lies outside the scope of this textbook, a simplified explanation follows.

ONCOGENE FORMATION

Recognizing that all cells have protooncogenes, what events alter otherwise normal regulatory genes so that they become cancer-causing genes? Three mechanisms, genetic mutations, viral infections, and carcinogens, have received much attention.

Genetic mutations develop when dividing cells miscopy genetic information. If the gene that is miscopied is a protooncogene, the oncogene that results will stimulate the formation of cancerous cells. A variety of factors, including aging, radiation, and an array of carcinogens are associated with genetic mutations that result in the faulty cell regulation that we call cancer.

In both animals and humans, cancer-producing *viral* infections have been identified. The cancer-producing virus seeks out cells of a particular type and alters their genetic material to convert these cells into virus-producing cells. In so doing, however, they change the makeup of the cells' protooncogenes, making them oncogenes. Once converted into oncogenes, the altered regulatory genes are passed on through cell division.

A third possible explanation for the conversion of protooncogenes into oncogenes involves the presence of environmental agents known as **carcinogenes.** Over an extended period, carcinogenes, such as chemicals found in tobacco smoke, polluted air and water, toxic wastes, and even foods, may convert protooncogenes into oncogenes. These carcinogens may work alone or in combination (*cocarcinogens*). Thus persons might de-

velop lung cancer only if they are exposed to the right combination of carcinogens over an extended period.

At the time of this writing our understanding of the role of genes in the development of cancer is expanding rapidly. In conjunction with the *Human Genome Project,* the scientific community now has identified over 100 faulty genes that function as oncogenes in a variety of human cancers, including most recently colon cancer.[3,4] In addition, a recently recognized role for a second form of cancer genes, the **suppressor genes,** has been established. Intended to hold faulty regulatory genes activity in check, suppressor genes themselves may be altered by carcinogenic activity or faulty replication and, as a consequence, may no longer be able to check abnormal regulation of cell activity. Some experts believe that a combination of oncogenes, including those of regulatory and suppressor origin, may be necessary for a malignancy to develop. Perhaps even a third form of genes, **repair genes,** may be necessary in cancer development.[5] When these genes are faulty too, they may be unable to repair the damage done to regulatory genes, thereby allowing cancer to become established.

Clearly, speculation remains about the number of oncogenes and even about their origin and role in both normal and abnormal cellular activity.

acute (a **kute**) begins abruptly and subsides after a short period.

chronic (**kron** ick) develops slowly and persists for a long period.

doubling (**dub** ling) mitotic reproductive division undertaken by cells of a particular tissue.

regulatory genes (reg **you** luh tory) genes within the cell that control cellular replication or doubling.

oncogenes (**on** ko genes) genes that are believed to activate the development of cancer.

protooncogene (**pro** toe **on** ko gene) normal regulatory gene that may be altered by mutation or recombination with a viral gene to become an oncogene.

carcinogens (**kar** sin oh jens) chemical compounds found in the environment that stimulate the formation of malignant or cancerous cells.

suppressor gene (sa **press** er) gene intended to monitor cell regulatory activity and stop faulty regulatory activity.

repair gene (gene intended to repair DNA), the cell's genetic blueprint, following mutational change.

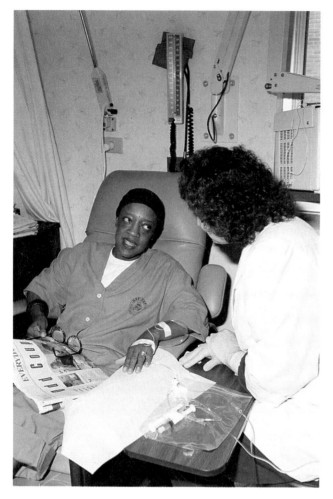

The effects of chemotherapy are carefully monitored.

THE MALIGNANT CELL

Contrary to general belief, cancer cells do not necessarily divide more quickly than do normal cells; in fact, they can divide at the same rate or even more slowly. Cancer cells' ability to overrun normal cells, however, results from their inability to respond to the negative feedback process that occurs in normal tissue maintenance. Because malignant (cancerous) cells do not possess the **contact inhibition** of normal cells, they accumulate and eventually alter the structure of a body organ. A decrease in **cellular cohesiveness** allows cancer cells to invade surrounding tissues or spread through the circulatory or lymphatic system to distant points *(metastasis)*.[2] A malignancy that has metastasized has been present in the body longer than a tumor of the same origin that has not yet spread. Metastasis (Figure 11-1) increases the difficulty of diagnosis and treatment because cancerous cells are no longer localized in a single area of the body.

Because of the growth rate of cancer cells, an extended time may be required for a **tumor** mass to reach a size in which normal function of the tissue or organ is impaired. Clinical identification of a malignant mass may not be possible until approximately 30 *doublings* (generations of cells) have taken place. Thus if a single doubling in a cancer cell requires 2 or more months, 5 or more years may pass before a tumor is recognized.[2]

Like a normal cell, a malignant cell requires metabolic material to sustain itself. An **angiogenesis factor** is believed to give some malignant cells an advantage over normal cells in establishing a rich blood supply.[2] Cancer cells, however, are not endowed with an infinite life expectancy, and *necrosis,* or cell death, is observed within tumors. Furthermore, uniqueness in the cell division process increases the length of time that a cancer cell's genetic material is susceptible to the destructive effects of radiation and chemotherapy drugs.

BENIGN TUMORS

Noncancerous, or **benign,** tumors can also form in the body. These tumors are usually encapsulated by a fiberous membrane and do not spread from their point of origin as cancerous tumors can. Benign tumors are dangerous, however, when they crowd out normal tissue within a confined space.

TYPES OF CANCER AND THEIR LOCATIONS

Malignancies can be categorized by the tissues in which they occur and by the varying rates to which specific organs are subjected to the development of malignancies. Although oncologists and pathologists use a far more extensive nomenclature, the classifications below are examples of those used in medicine to describe the origins of malignancy.

▼ **Carcinoma** Found most frequently in the skin, nose, mouth, throat, stomach, intestinal tract, glands, nerves, breasts, urinary and genital structures, lungs, kidneys, and liver; approximately 85% of all malignant tumors are classified as carcinomas.

▼ **Sarcoma** Formed in the connective tissues of the body; bone, cartilage, and tendons are the sites of sarcoma development; only 2% of all malignancies are of this type.

▼ **Melanoma** Arises from the melanin-containing cells of skin; found most often in individuals who have sustained extensive sun exposure, particularly a deep, penetrating sunburn; although it is rare, its prevalence has increased markedly in recent years. It remains among the most deadly forms of cancer.

▼ **Neuroblastoma** Originates in the immature cells found within the central nervous system; neuroblastomas are rare; usually found in children.

▼ **Adenocarcinoma** Derived from cells of the endocrine glands.

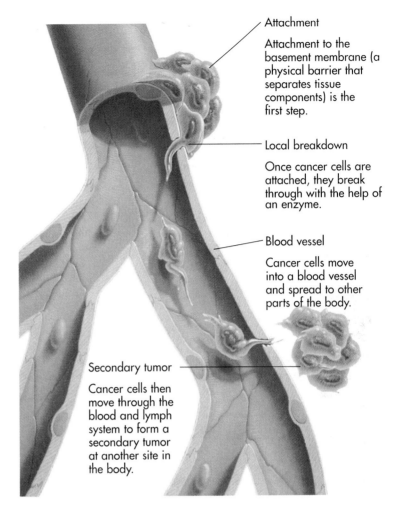

Attachment

Attachment to the basement membrane (a physical barrier that separates tissue components) is the first step.

Local breakdown

Once cancer cells are attached, they break through with the help of an enzyme.

Blood vessel

Cancer cells move into a blood vessel and spread to other parts of the body.

Secondary tumor

Cancer cells then move through the blood and lymph system to form a secondary tumor at another site in the body.

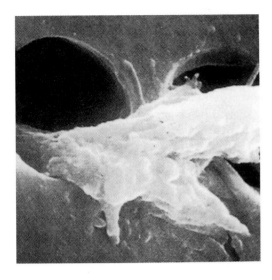

Figure 11-1 How cancer spreads: locomotion is integral to the entire process of metastasis. Scientists have identified a protein, named autocrine motility factor, that causes cancer cells to grow arms, or pseudopodia, enabling them to begin to move to other parts of the body.

▼ **Hepatoma** Originates in the cells of the liver; although not thought to be directly caused by alcohol use, hepatomas are more frequently seen in individuals who have experienced **sclerotic changes** in the liver.

▼ **Leukemia** Found in cells of the blood and blood-forming tissues; characterized by abnormal, immature white blood cell formation; multiple forms found in children and adults.

▼ **Lymphoma** Arises in cells of the lymphatic tissues or other immune system tissues; includes lymphosarcomas and Hodgkin's disease, characterized by abnormal white cell production and decreased resistance.

Figure 11-2 presents data on the incidence and deaths from cancer in various sites for both men and women.

contact inhibition (**in** hi **bish** shun) ability of a tissue, on reaching its mature size, to suppress additional growth.

cellular cohesiveness (**sell** you lar koe hee **siv** ness) tendency of normal cells to "stick together" rather than to move independently throughout the body.

tumor (**too** mer) mass of cells; may be cancerous (malignant) or noncancerous (benign).

angiogenesis factor (**an** gee oh **jen** a sis) chemical messenger that stimulates the development of additional capillaries into the tumor.

benign (be **nine**) noncancerous; tumors that do not spread.

sclerotic changes (skluh **rot** ick) thickening or hardening of tissues.

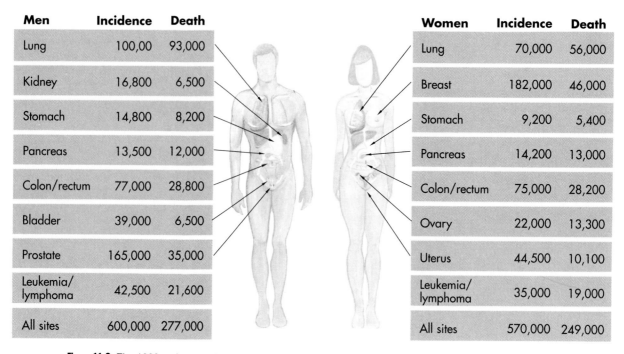

Men	Incidence	Death
Lung	100,00	93,000
Kidney	16,800	6,500
Stomach	14,800	8,200
Pancreas	13,500	12,000
Colon/rectum	77,000	28,800
Bladder	39,000	6,500
Prostate	165,000	35,000
Leukemia/ lymphoma	42,500	21,600
All sites	600,000	277,000

Women	Incidence	Death
Lung	70,000	56,000
Breast	182,000	46,000
Stomach	9,200	5,400
Pancreas	14,200	13,000
Colon/rectum	75,000	28,200
Ovary	22,000	13,300
Uterus	44,500	10,100
Leukemia/ lymphoma	35,000	19,000
All sites	570,000	249,000

Figure 11-2 The 1993 estimates of cancer incidence and cancer deaths reveal some significant similarities between men and women. Note that lung cancer is the leading cause of cancer deaths for *both* sexes.

CANCER AT SELECTED SITES IN THE BODY

A second and more familiar way to describe cancer is on the basis of the organ (or tissue) site at which it occurs. The American Cancer Society annually reports the incidence and deaths associated with cancer in some 12 sites, comprising nearly 40 organs or tissues.[6] The following discussion relates to some of these more familiar sites. Therefore, regular examination of these sites (see the box on pp. 276-277) can lead to early identification.

Lung

Lung cancer is one of the most lethal forms of cancer that is frequently diagnosed. Primarily because of the advanced stage at the time symptoms first appear, only 13% of all lung cancer victims survive 5 years beyond diagnosis.[6] By the time victims are sufficiently concerned about their persistent cough, blood-streaked sputum, and chest pain, their fate has often been sealed.

Today it is thought that a genetic predisposition could be important in the development of lung cancer. Perhaps as many as 70% of the persons who develop this form of cancer have an inherited "headstart."[7] When persons who are genetically at risk also smoke, their level of risk for developing lung cancer is hundreds of times greater than it is for nonsmokers. About 30% of lung cancer cases appear in persons who smoke but are not genetically predisposed. Environmental agents, such as radon, asbestos, and air pollutants, contribute to a lesser degree to the development of lung cancer.

According to the World Health Organization, the incidence of lung cancer has risen 200% for women, paralleling their increased smoking. Currently, lung cancer exceeds breast cancer as the leading cause of cancer death in women. The incidence of lung cancer has shown an encouraging decline in men as their use of tobacco dropped.

Breast

Surpassed only by lung cancer, breast cancer is the second leading cause of death from cancer in women. Now, nearly one in eight women will develop breast cancer.[6] As they age, women are increasingly at risk for developing breast cancer. The following rates reflect the role of age in breast cancer development:

Age	Incidence	Age	Incidence
25	1 in 19,608	60	1 in 24
30	1 in 2,525	65	1 in 17
35	1 in 622	70	1 in 14
40	1 in 217	75	1 in 11
45	1 in 93	80	1 in 10
50	1 in 50	85	1 in 9
55	1 in 33	Ever	1 in 8

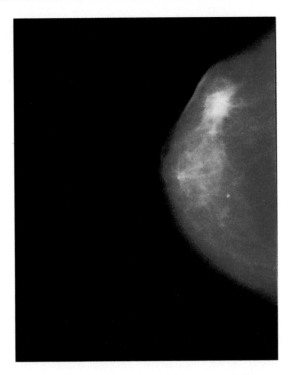

Cancerous tissue can be seen in the dense area of this mammogram.

For tens of thousands of other women, waiting to learn whether a suspicious lump is benign or is a fluid-filled cyst will be stressful. Early detection is the key to complete recovery.

Although all women (and men) are at some risk for developing breast cancer, women whose menstrual periods began when they were young and for whom menopause was late, women who had no children or had their first child later in life, and women with a family history of breast cancer are at greater risk.[8] Also, women whose diets are high in saturated fats and who have excessive fat in the waist/hip area are more likely to develop breast cancer,[9] although the role of dietary fats is currently being reassessed since a 1992 study discounted the role of dietary fat in breast cancer.[10] Alcohol consumption, use of an oral contraceptive, and use of estrogen replacement therapy (ERT) (which is thought by some to be a causative factor) still foster controversy regarding their roles in women's risk for developing breast cancer.

Breast self-examination is recommended for women 20 years of age and older (see box on p. 276). Mammograms are recommended every year for women 50 years of age and older if they have had no earlier symptoms. Many physicians, however, recommend beginning mammograms as early as 35 years of age, particularly for women with earlier symptoms or a family history of breast cancer.

At the time of this writing, however, there is some dispute about the effectiveness of mammography in detecting breast cancer in young women when compared with the same effectiveness that it has for women older than 50 years of age. Because of this finding, health care plans currently under consideration in Washington could exclude coverage for mammograms for younger women. Medicare does pay for routine mammography for older women. Regardless of age, each woman is unique in terms of her risk profile and, therefore, the recommendation of her individual physician should be given careful consideration.

In addition to breast self-examination (see the Health Action Guide on p. 278 and Figure 11-3) and mammography, new techniques for detection are being considered. Among these are magnetic resonance imaging (MRI). Although much more expensive than mammography, the MRI can see through dense tissue areas and collected breast fluid more effectively than X-rays for analysis of possible cancer cells.

Regardless of the method of detection, if a lump is found, a breast biopsy can determine what the lump is. If the lump is cancerous, treatment is highly effective if the cancer is found in an early stage. Since many choices exist about the type of surgery required to remove the cancer, women should seek a second opinion. The least extensive surgery possible is the most desirable. Today, breast reconstruction is often possible even after radical surgery.

Although breast cancer is far less common in young women than in women over 50 years of age, the rate at which it occurs is rising in younger women. Particularly troubling about breast cancer in young women is the more lethal nature of the cancer, possibly

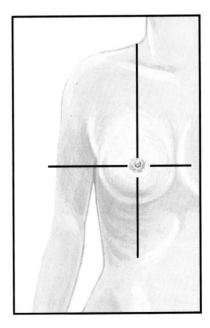

Figure 11-3 Breast cancer most often develops in the upper outer quadrant.

Cancer-Related Checkups

Following are guidelines for the early detection of cancer in people without symptoms. Talk with your doctor—ask how these guidelines relate to you. Remember, these guidelines are not rules and apply only to people without symptoms. If you have any of the seven warning signals of cancer, see your doctor or go to your clinic without delay.

AGE 20 TO 40: CANCER-RELATED CHECKUP EVERY 3 YEARS

Should include the procedures listed below plus health counseling (such as tips on quitting smoking) and examinations for cancers of the thyroid, testes, prostate, mouth, ovaries, skin, and lymph nodes. *Some people are at higher risk for certain cancers and may need to have tests more frequently.*

Breast

★ Examination by doctor every 3 years

★ Self-examination every month

★ One baseline mammogram between ages 35 and 40

Higher risk for breast cancer: personal or family history of breast cancer, never had children, first child after 30.

Uterus

★ Pelvic exam every 3 years

Cervix

★ Pap test—after three initial negative tests 1 year apart—at least every 3 years; includes women under 20 if sexually active

Higher risk for cervical cancer: early age at first intercourse, multiple sex partners

AGE 40 AND OVER: CANCER-RELATED CHECKUP EVERY YEAR

Should include the procedures listed below plus health counseling (such as tips on quitting smoking) and examinations for cancers of the thyroid, testes, prostate, mouth, ovaries, skin, and lymph nodes. *Some people are at higher risk for certain cancers and may need to have tests more frequently.*

Breast

★ Examination by doctor every year

★ Self-examination every month

★ Mammogram every year after age 50 (between ages 40 and 50, ask your doctor)

Higher risk for breast cancer: personal or family history of breast cancer, never had children, first child after 30

Uterus

★ Pelvic examination every year

Cervix

★ Pap test—after three initial negative tests 1 year apart—at least every 3 years

Higher risk for cervical cancer: early age at first intercourse, multiple sex partners

---

reflecting its tendency to be more estrogen-sensitive than are the forms seen in older women. Younger women are more inclined to select a "lumpectomy" over more extensive surgery, which increases the possibility of recurrence. Additionally, chemotherapy drugs used in support of the less extensive surgical approach can lead to the early onset of menopause.

With these factors in mind, the need for early routine medical care for younger women is important, as well as the routine use of self–breast examination. Early diagnosis and appropriate treatment of breast cancer is, regardless of age, the first step toward recovery and cure.

Uterus

In 1993, approximately 44,500 new cases of cancer of the uterus were anticipated in the United States.[6] Included in this figure were 31,000 cases of cancer of the uterus lining (endometrial) and 13,500 cases of cancer of the uterine neck (cervical) cancer. Fortunately, the death rate from uterine cancer has dropped greatly

since 1950, largely because of the use of the **Pap test**. This test looks for precancerous changes in the cells taken from the cervix.

The importance of women having a Pap test for cervical cancer done on a routine basis cannot be overemphasized. Without screening, a 20-year-old of average risk has a 250 in 10,000 chance of getting cervical cancer and a 118 in 10,000 chance of dying from it. With screening, a 20-year-old of average risk has a 35 in 10,000 chance of getting this form of cancer and only a 11 in 10,000 chance of dying from it.[11] The Pap test is not perfect however. About 5% to 15% of the tests will miss finding abnormal changes. Additionally, the National Cancer Institute is reassessing the extent to which abnormal tissue (as determined by Pap test) requires aggressive treatment such as removal by laser or whether observation alone is sufficient in anticipa-

Pap test cancer screening procedure in which cells from the cervix are examined.

★ Cancer-Related Checkups—cont'd

AGE 20 TO 40: CANCER-RELATED CHECKUP EVERY 3 YEARS

Testes

★ Self-examination every month

★ Consult doctor when an abnormality is present

Higher risk for testicular cancer: personal or family history of testicular cancer, undescended testicles not corrected during early childhood; more prevalent in whites and in men under 35 years of age.

AGE 40 AND OVER: CANCER-RELATED CHECKUP EVERY YEAR

Endometrium

★ Endometrial tissue sample at menopause if at risk

Higher risk for endometrial cancer: infertility, obesity, failure of ovulation, abnormal uterine bleeding, estrogen therapy

Testes

★ Self-examination every month

★ Consult doctor when an abnormality is present

Higher risk for testicular cancer: personal or family history of testicular cancer, undescended testicles not corrected during early childhood; more prevalent in whites; risk declines with increasing age

Colon and Rectum

★ Digital rectal examination every year

★ Guaiac slide test every year after age 50

★ Proctoscopic exam—after two initial negative tests 1 year apart—every 3 to 5 years after age 50

Higher risk for colorectal cancer: personal or family history of colon or rectal cancer, personal or family history of polyps in the colon or rectum, ulcerative colitis

Prostate

★ Digital rectal and PSA test examination every year

Higher risk for prostate cancer: a history of previous urinary tract infections and in men over 50 years of age ★

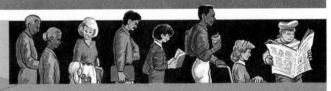

Learning FROM ALL Cultures

Breast Cancer

Research on breast cancer has identified a number of risk factors, which are identified in this text. Some of these factors can be changed or controlled, whereas others cannot. The following is additional information about the incidence of breast cancer. In demographic terms, breast cancer is likely to occur in the following:

• Women much more often than in men; it is 100 times more common in women.
• Whites more often than blacks; however, one factor may be greater awareness and better access to medical resources by the white population.

• Women over 50 more frequently than in younger women.
• Women who are obese rather than thin.
• Smokers rather than nonsmokers.
• Women of Western cultures; Japanese women living in Japan seem to have a low rate of incidence. However, for those Japanese women who move to Western cultures, the rate of incidence increases. Women in the Netherlands are reported as having the highest rates of all countries.[12]

Consider this last risk factor. What can you hypothesize about the Western culture and the increased incidence of breast cancer? ●

Health ACTION Guide

The Breast Self-Examination

The following explains how to do a breast self-examination:

▼ *In the shower:* Examine your breasts during a bath or shower; hands glide more easily over wet skin. With your fingers flat, move gently over every part of each breast. Use right hand to examine left breast, left hand for right breast. Check for any lump, hard knot, or thickening. This self-examination should be done monthly, preferably a day or two after the end of the menstrual period.

▼ *Before a mirror:* Inspect your breasts with arms at your sides. Next, raise your arms high overhead. Look for any changes in contour of each breast, a swelling, dimpling of skin, changes in the nipple, rest palms on hips, and press down firmly to flex your chest muscles. Left and right breast will not exactly match—few women's breasts do.

▼ *Lying down:* To examine your right breast, put a pillow or folded towel under your right shoulder. Place right hand behind your head—this distributes breast tissue more evenly on the chest. With left hand, fingers flat, press gently in small circular motions around an imaginary clock face. Begin at outermost top of your right breast for 12 o'clock, then move to 1 o'clock, and so on around the circle back to 12 o'clock. A ridge of firm tissue in the lower curve of each breast is normal. Then move in an inch toward the nipple; keep circling to examine *every part of your breast,* including the nipple. This requires at least three more circles. Now slowly repeat the procedure on your left breast with a pillow under your left shoulder and left hand behind head. Notice how your breast structure feels. Finally, squeeze the nipple of each breast gently between thumb and index finger. Any discharge, clear or bloody, should be reported to your doctor immediately.

Breast cancer can occur in men too. Therefore this examination should be performed monthly by men. Regular inspection shows what is normal for you and will give you confidence in your examination. ▼

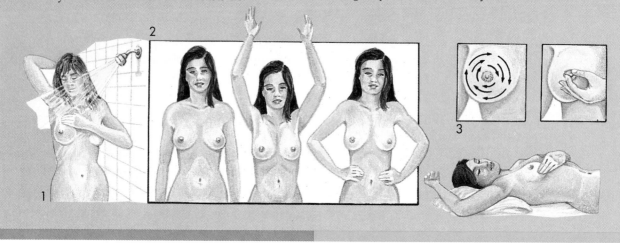

tion that tissue will return to normal. New Pap tests—including Virapap, to identify HPV, ThinPrep, and My-pap, a home Pap test—could add to the current level of effectiveness.

In addition to changes discovered by a Pap test, symptoms suggesting cancer of the uterus include abnormal bleeding between periods. Risk factors associated with developing this form of cancer include early age of first intercourse, number of sexual partners, history of infertility, HPV (human papilloma virus) infections, and excessive fat tissue around the waist. A lower level of risk for uterine cancer is seen in women who have used barrier contraceptives (condoms, diaphragms, and spermicides), suggesting that this form of cancer may have a sexually transmitted (viral) component.

A higher incidence of endometrial cancer in women who were given estrogen following the onset of menopause is also reported. This, however, must be balanced against the risk of osteoporosis, which is discussed further in Chapter 20.

Vagina

Although rare, cancer of the vagina (the passage leading to the uterus) is of concern to a particular group of younger women. These women are the daughters of over 3 million mothers who, when 30 to 35 years of age, were given the drug DES to prevent miscarriages. Because of the effect of DES on the developing reproductive system, these daughters now face the risk of developing a form of vaginal (and cervical) cancer

Breast Implants

For a woman who must undergo *mastectomy*, the option of having breast reconstruction surgery exists. Various techniques can be used in rebuilding the breast. One is to insert packets containing silicone or saline (implants) within the chest wall to fashion a breast while also using tissue taken from the abdominal wall. The decision to have reconstructive surgery can be made before removal of the breast. When this is done, it is often possible for the surgeon to retain tissue that will allow reconstruction to be done immediately after removal of the breast. Surgical reconstruction can also be done later if the patient decides to wait.

A woman who undergoes mastectomy but chooses not to have reconstructive surgery has nonsurgical options available. A breast prosthesis can be worn to recreate her former appearance. A self-adhering or bra-inserted prosthesis can be purchased in stores specializing in medical supplies. Depending on the type of prosthesis being used, virtually all types of activities and styles of clothing can be accommodated. Of course, if a woman chooses, there is no need to return to the presurgical image of the chest. Once

healing has occurred, normal activity can resume.

Implants have also become popular for women who wish to enlarge their breasts for cosmetic purposes *(breast augmentation)*. Today, however, women must be aware of the concerns about the safety of breast implants. A major concern is the safety of the silicone-filled implants and the possibility that they might leak at any time, rupture, become infected, stimulate an autoimmune response, or harden and obscure the tissues underlying the implants. The FDA has greatly reduced their use, allowing only a limited number to be implanted.

In March of 1994, a settlement was reached between the manufacturers of silicone implants and women able to demonstrate adverse health effects following implantation. Each victim should receive around 2 million dollars.

An alternative to the silicone implant, the saline-filled implant, has also come under closer watch. Physicians who favor saline to silicone implants believe that saline implants are less likely to harden, wrinkle, or interfere with detection of underlying breast cancer. ★

 Ovarian Cancer—The Silent Killer

Since the death of Gilda Radner in 1989, public awareness of ovarian cancer has increased in this country. In 1993, it was estimated that 22,000 new cases would be identified and 13,300 women would die. Most cases develop in women who are older than 40 years of age and who have not had children or began menstruation at an early age. Earlier breast cancer also appears to heighten the risk of developing ovarian cancer. The highest rate is in women over the age of 60. Today ovarian cancer causes more deaths than any form of female reproductive system cancer.

Because of its vague symptoms, ovarian cancer has been referred to as a *silent* cancer. Digestive disturbances, gas, and stomach distention are often its only symptoms. Today, diagnosis of this highly lethal cancer is made using transvaginal ultrasound and surgery. Wide scale screenings for all women does not, however, seem practical at this time. Because of the likelihood that cancer could spread before the development of symptoms, exploratory surgery should also be given serious consideration.[13]

A newly discovered and approved drug, Taxol, obtained from the bark and needles of the Pacific yew tree is now available for use as a treatment. The extent of its effectiveness remains under investigation. ★

called *clear cell cancer*. Since the risk was identified 25 years ago, the medical community has been following large groups of daughters to better assess their level of risk. To date, about 1 in every 1000 exposed daughters has developed this rare form of cancer, some as early as 15 years of age.

Prostate

Cancer of the prostate is the third most common form of cancer in men and a leading cause of death from cancer in older men. On the basis of current statistics, approximately one out of eleven men will develop this form of cancer.[6] Men with a family history of prostate cancer are at greater risk of developing this form of cancer.[14] Additionally, a link between prostate cancer and dietary patterns, such as red meat consumption, has been suggested.[15] Prostate cancer is found more frequently in African-American men than in white men.

The symptoms of prostate disease, including prostate cancer, are shown in the Health Action Guide on p. 280. If these symptoms appear, particularly in men 50 years of age and older, a physician should be consulted. Screening for prostate cancer should begin by age 40 and involves an annual rectal examination

mastectomy (mas **teck** toe me) removal of breast tissue.

★ Symptoms of Prostate Disease

★ **Difficulty in urinating**

★ **Frequent urination, particularly at night**

★ **Continued wetness for a short time after urination**

★ **Blood in urine**

★ **Low back pain**

★ **Achiness in upper thighs**

and the newly developed PSA (prostatic specific antigen) blood test.[16] An ultrasound rectal examination is used in men whose PSA scores are too high.

Traditionally, prostate cancer has been treated through surgery or use of radiation and chemotherapy, with a survival rate of 50% to 76%. Today, reevaluation of early treatment is occurring.

Testicle

Cancer of the testicles is among the least common forms of cancer; however, it represents the most common solid tumor in men between the ages of 20 and 34 years. Cancer of the testicles shows a tendency to run in families and is more common in men whose testicles were undescended during childhood. The incidence of this cancer has been increasing in recent years. In 1993, 6,600 new cases were diagnosed and 350 deaths occurred.[6]

Symptoms of cancer of the testicles include a small, painless lump on the side of the testicle, a swollen or enlarged testicle, or heaviness or a dragging sensation in the groin or scrotum. Risk factors include confirmed injury, mumps, and hormonal treatments given to the mother before the child's birth.

The importance of testicle self-examination and early diagnosis and prompt treatment cannot be overemphasized for men in the at risk age-group of 20 to 34 years (see the box on p. 277).

Colon and Rectum

Cancer of the colon and rectum has a combined incidence and death rate second only to that of lung cancer. Two types of tumors, carcinoma and lymphoma, can be found in both the colon and rectum. Fortunately, when diagnosed in a localized state, cancer of both the colon and rectum has relatively high survival rates (91% for colon and 85% for rectal).[6] As discussed earlier, two genes, including a suppressor gene, have been discovered that are believed to be responsible for the tendency for colon and rectal cancer to run in families. These forms of cancer are also seen in persons whose diets are high in saturated fats from red meat and low in fiber. Most recently, an association between colorectal cancer and smoking has been identified, suggesting that carcinogens may be ingested or pass into the digestive system from the blood stream.[17]

Symptoms associated with colon and rectal cancers include bleeding from the rectum, blood in the stool, or a change in bowel habits. Also a family history of inflammatory bowel disease, polyp formation, or cancer of the colon or rectum should make one more alert

Health ACTION Guide

The Testicular Self-Exam

Your best hope for early detection of testicular cancer is a simple 3-minute monthly self-examination. The following explains how to do a testicular self-examination. The best time is after a warm bath or shower, when the scrotal skin is most relaxed.

▼ Roll each testicle gently between the thumb and fingers of both hands.

▼ If you find any hard lumps or nodules, you should see your doctor promptly. They may not be malignant, but only your doctor can make the diagnosis.

After a thorough physical examination, your doctor may perform certain x-ray studies to make the most accurate diagnosis possible.

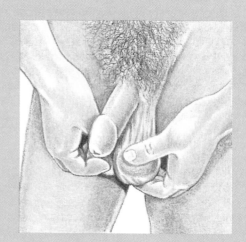

Testicular self-examinations are as important for men as breast self-examinations are for women. ▼

to symptoms. In persons over 50 years of age, any sudden change in bowel habits that lasts 10 days or longer should be evaluated by a physician. Preventive health care that includes digital rectal examination after age 40, a stool blood test after age 50, and proctosigmoidoscopic examination every 3 to 5 years after age 50 is recommended by the American Cancer Society. Prompt removal of polyps has recently been shown to be effective in lowering the risk of developing colorectal cancer.[18] Further, there is evidence that the development of colon and rectal cancer may be prevented or slowed through regular exercise and through the regular use of aspirin.[19]

Today, the treatment of colon and rectal cancer involves surgery, the possible use of chemotherapy drugs, and immunological agents. A **colostomy** is required in 15% of the cases of colon and rectal cancer.

Pancreas

Pancreatic cancer is one of the most lethal forms of cancer to develop, with a survival rate of only 3% at 5 years after diagnosis. In light of that organ's important roles in both digestion and metabolic processes (see diabetes mellitus), its destruction leaves the body in a state incompatible with living.

In 1993, 27,700 new cases of pancreatic cancer were identified. The disease is more common in men than women and occurs most frequently in African-American men.[6] Early detection of pancreatic cancer is difficult because of the absence of symptoms until late in its course. Risk of developing this form of cancer increases with age; with diabetes mellitus, pancreatitis, and cirrhosis; and with diets high in fat. To date, little in the way of effective treatment has been found.

Skin

Thanks in large part to our desire for a fashionable tan, we are spending more time in the sun (and in tanning booths) than our skin can tolerate. As a result, skin cancer, once common only among those people who had to work in the sun, is occurring with alarming frequency. In 1992, nearly 700,000 Americans developed basal or squamous cell skin cancer, and 32,000 cases of highly dangerous malignant melanoma were diagnosed.[6] Severe sunburning during childhood and chronic sun exposure during adolescence and younger adulthood are responsible for these increases in skin cancer.

Although many doctors may not emphasize this point enough, the key to successful treatment of skin cancer lies in early detection. In the case of basal cell or squamous cell cancer, the development of a pale, waxlike, pearly nodule or red, scaly patch may be the first symptom (Figure 11-4). For others, skin cancer may be noticed as a gradual change in the appearance of an already existing skin mole. If such a change is noted, a physician should be contacted. Melanomas usually be-

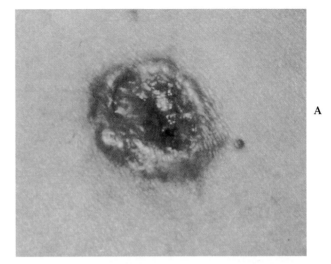

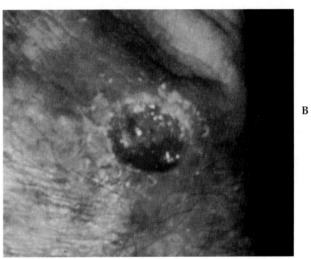

Figure 11-4 **A**, Basal cell carcinoma. **B**, Squamous cell carcinoma.

gin as a small, molelike growth that increases progressively in size, changes color, ulcerates, and bleeds easily. For use in detecting these melanomas, the American Cancer Society recommends the guidelines (Figure 11-5) shown on p. 282.

A is for asymmetry
B is for border irregularity
C is for color (change)
D is for a diameter greater than 6 mm

When nonmelanoma skin cancers are found, an almost 100% cure rate can be expected. Treatment of these skin cancers will be based on surgical removal, destruction through burning or freezing, or the use of

colostomy (koe **las** ta mee) surgically created opening on the abdominal wall for the elimination of body wastes.

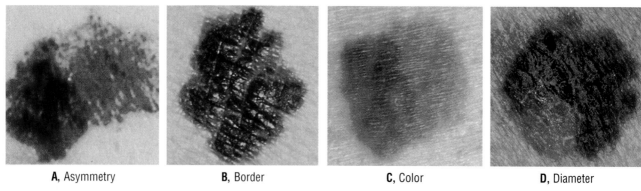

A, Asymmetry   **B,** Border   **C,** Color   **D,** Diameter

Figure 11-5 Guidelines for detecting melanomas.

X-ray therapy. When the more serious melanomas are found in an early stage, a high cure rate is accomplished by using the same techniques. However, when malignant melanomas are more advanced, extensive surgery and chemotherapy is necessary, and unfortunately, recovery will be very difficult. At the time of this writing, a vaccine developed for use in treating this form of skin cancer has shown initial promise. More studies are underway.[20]

Prevention of skin cancers should be a high priority for persons who enjoy the sun or must work outdoors. The use of sunscreens is of great importance. Table 11-1 provides guidance in selecting the sunscreen that is appropriate for your skin. In addition, parents can help their children prevent skin cancer later in life by restricting their outdoor play during the 11:00 AM-to-2:00 PM period, requiring them to wear hats that shade their faces, and applying a sunscreen with SPF 15 on their children regardless of skin tone. Recent studies suggest that regular use of sunscreens is effective in preventing the cellular changes that are associated with the development of basal cell carcinoma. However, the ability to prevent the development of melanoma is questionable.[21]

THE DIAGNOSIS OF CANCER

Is cancer survivable? The answer is, of course, yes. The chances for survival (living 5 years after diagnosis) depend greatly on the promptness of identification, diagnosis, and treatment.

In addition to the three factors affecting survival from cancer mentioned above, survival is also dependent on the type of cancer and the stage of its development. Without exception, a person's chances for surviving cancer are highest when treatment is undertaken while the disease is localized, and lowest when the disease is more generalized (spread).

Thus the chances for recovery from cancer are best when cancer is detected early. The familiar "cancer's

TABLE 11-1	**Sunscreen Guide**		
Skin type	**Pigmentation**	**Sunburn/tanning history**	**Sun protection factor (SPF)**
I	Very fair skin; freckling; blond, red, or brown hair	Always burns easily; never tans	15-30
II	Fair skin; blond, red, or brown hair	Always burns easily, tans minimally	15-20
III	Brown hair and eyes, darker skin (light brown)	Burns moderately, tans gradually and uniformly	8-15
IV	Light brown skin; dark hair and eyes (moderate brown)	Burns minimally; always tans well	8-15
V	Brown skin; dark hair and eyes	Rarely burns, tans profusely (dark brown)	Recommend same as skin type IV
VI	Brown-black skin; dark hair and eyes	Never burns, deeply pigmented (black)	Recommend same as skin type IV

NOTE: Although formulas as high as 60 are available, an SPF of 30 is usually appropriate for use, perhaps requiring more frequent applications *As deterioration of the ozone layer continues, it may be necessary to use an even more protective sunscreen.*

Cancer's Seven Warning Signals

1. **Change in bowel or bladder habits**

2. **A sore that does not heal**

3. **Unusual bleeding or discharge**

4. **Thickening or lump in breast or elsewhere**

5. **Indigestion or difficulty in swallowing**

6. **Obvious change in wart or mole**

7. **Nagging cough or hoarseness**

If you have a warning signal that persists for more than 5 days, see your doctor! ★

NOTE: While weight loss can be an indicator of cancer, weight loss is not always caused by cancer. Therefore, weight loss is a less reliable indicator.

seven warning signals" can serve as a basis for early detection (see the box above). As widely discussed and familiar as these signals are, they are frequently disregarded. Many people may recognize a cancer warning sign but prefer to attribute it to other (noncancer) causes. An awareness of these seven warning signals, nevertheless, remains the first line in the process of early cancer identification. Also, unexplained weight loss can be a signal for the presence of a malignancy. *Weight loss*, however, is not usually an early indicator of cancer. Persistent headaches and vision changes should be evaluated by a physician.

In addition to the recognition of danger signals, undergoing regularly scheduled *screening* for malignancy-related changes is important. Note that breast self-examination for all women over the age of 20 is recommended. Further, we would strongly recommend testicular self-examination for men. Step-by-step procedures for both of these self-examinations are provided in the boxes on pp. 278 and 280. The remaining screening procedures require the service of a medical practitioner.

In spite of the availability and effectiveness of various screening and diagnostic tests and procedures, a significant percent of the adult population fails to participate on a regular basis. Most experts attribute this to the anxiety and fear associated with the possibility that cancer might be found. In a sense, people believe that "no news is good news," at least in terms of cancer.

Because of the relationship between fear and nonparticipation in screening and diagnostic procedures for the detection of cancer, many hospitals are offering short courses (of 6 weeks) to assist people in mastering their fear and anxiety. To date, these programs have been very helpful, raising the rate of breast self-examination to 70% and mammography from 74% to 100% participation.[22]

Treatment

In today's approach to cancer treatment, proven therapies and promising new experimental approaches are often combined. The traditional therapies are surgery, radiation, and chemotherapy. Used independently or in combination, they form the backbone of our increasingly successful efforts in treating cancer. Newer, more experimental therapies are also being employed on a limited basis. One or more of these experimental approaches may combine surgery, radiation, and chemotherapy as a basis for treatment.

Beyond the technical aspects of cancer treatment that will be described, the treatment of cancer also involves a variety of factors that are understandable on the basis of human emotions. These include pain, discomfort, fear, confidence, trust, and a willingness to be compliant. Treatment for cancer, regardless of the particular therapy used, is demanding. Patients must accept the need for therapy as being in their best interest. They must participate fully in their own treatment. And, for some, eventual death must be faced. (See Chapter 20 for a discussion of a hospice program.)

In the section that follows, a brief description of each treatment scheme is described.

SURGERY

Surgical removal of tissue suspected to contain cancerous cells is the oldest approach to cancer therapy. When undertaken early in the course of the disease, surgery is particularly suited for cancers of the skin, gastrointestinal tract, breast, uterus, cervix, prostate, and testicles. Minimal procedures are undertaken whenever possible, and radiation or chemotherapy is often used with surgery to ensure maximum effectiveness.

RADIATION

The treatment of malignancies through the use of radiation or high-energy particles is both an old and a new approach. The implantation of radioactive materials and the use of supervoltage x-ray and cobalt are well-established therapies. More recent use of radiation and high-energy sources include the injection of tumor-specific sources of radioactive material, linear accelerators for the production of photons and electrons, and cyclotrons capable of producing high-energy particles.

Regardless of the procedure employed, the intent is to destroy cancer cells through disruption of their reproductive process. In doing so the therapist must balance loss of healthy tissue against the radiation's destructive influence on malignant cells. Radiation may be used in an attempt to achieve a cure or as a **palliative** measure against pain and suffering. For some tu-

palliative (**pal** ee ah tive) measure taken to reduce pain and discomfort but not to cure a disease.

PERSONAL ASSESSMENT

Are You at Risk for Skin, Breast, and Cervical Cancer?

Some people may have more than an average risk of developing particular cancers. These people can be identified by certain risk factors.

This simple self-testing method is designed by the American Cancer Society to help you assess your risk factors for three common types of cancer. These are the major risk factors but by no means represent the only ones that might be involved.

Check your response to each risk factor. Add the numbers in the parentheses to arrive at a total score for each cancer type. Find out what your score means by reading the information in the right column. You are advised to discuss the information with your physician if you are at a higher risk.

SKIN CANCER

1. Frequent work or play in the sun
   a. Yes (10)   **b.** No (1)
2. Work in mines, around coal tars, or around radioactivity
   a. Yes (10)   **b.** No (1)
3. Complexion—fair skin or light skin
   a. Yes (10)   **b.** No (1)

Your total points _____

EXPLANATION

Excessive ultraviolet light causes skin cancer. Protect yourself with a sunscreen.
These materials can cause skin cancer.

Light complexions need more protection than others.

INTERPRETATION

Numerical risks for skin cancer are difficult to state. For instance, a person with a dark complexion can work longer in the sun and be less likely to develop cancer than a light-complected person. Furthermore, a person wearing a long-sleeved shirt and a wide-brimmed hat may work in the sun and be less at risk than a person who wears a bathing suit for only a short period. The risk increases greatly with age.

The key here is if you answered "yes" to any question, you need to realize that you have above-average risk.

BREAST CANCER

1. Age group
   a. 20-34 (10)   **b.** 35-49 (40)   **c.** 50 and over (90)
2. Race/nationality
   a. Oriental (5) **c.** White (25)
   b. Black (20)   **d.** Mexican American (10)
3. Family history of breast cancer
   a. Mother, sister, or grandmother (30)
   b. None (10)

4. Your history
   a. No breast disease (10)
   b. Previous noncancerous lumps or cysts (25)
   c. Previous breast cancer (100)
5. Maternity
   a. First pregnancy before age 25 (10)
   b. First pregnancy after age 25 (15)
   c. No pregnancies (2)

Your total points _____

INTERPRETATION

Under 100   Low-risk women should practice monthly breast self-examination (BSE) and have their breasts examined by a doctor as part of a cancer-related checkup.

100-199   Moderate-risk women should practice monthly BSE and have their breasts examined by a doctor as part of a cancer-related checkup. Periodic mammograms should be included as your doctor may advise.

200 or more   High-risk women should practice monthly BSE and have the examinations and mammograms described earlier.

CERVICAL CANCER*

1. Age group
   a. Less than 25 (10)   **c.** 40-54 (30)
   b. 25-39 (20)   **d.** 55 and over (30)

2. Race/nationality
   a. Oriental (10)   **d.** White (10)
   b. Puerto Rican (20)   **e.** Mexican American (20)
   c. Black (20)

3. Number of pregnancies
   a. 0 (10)   **c.** 4 and over (30)
   b. 1 to 3 (20)

4. Viral infections
   a. Herpes and other viral infections or ulcer formations on the vagina (10)
   b. Never (1)

5. Age at first intercourse
   a. Before 15 (40)   **c.** 20-24 (20)
   b. 15-19 (30)   **d.** 25 and over (10)

6. Bleeding between periods or after intercourse
   a. Yes (40)   **b.** No (1)

Your total points _____

EXPLANATION

The highest occurrence is in the 40-and-over age group. The numbers represent the relative rates of cancer for different age groups. A 45-year-old woman has a risk three times higher than a 20-year-old.

Puerto Ricans, Blacks, and Mexican Americans have higher rates of cervical cancer.

Women who have delivered more children have a higher occurrence.

Viral infections of the cervix and vagina are associated with cervical cancer.

Women with earlier intercourse and with more sexual partners are at a higher risk.

Irregular bleeding may be a sign of uterine cancer.

INTERPRETATION/TO CARRY THIS FURTHER . . .

40-69   This is a low-risk group. Ask your doctor for a Pap test. You will be advised how often you should be tested after your first test.

70-99   In this moderate-risk group, more frequent Pap tests may be required.

100 or higher   You are in a high-risk group and should have a Pap test (and pelvic exam) as advised by your doctor.

* Lower portion of uterus. These questions would not apply to a woman who has had a complete hysterectomy.

PERSONAL ASSESSMENT

mors, such as cancer of the larynx, skin, cervix, uterus, and lymphoid tissue, radiation will be the primary therapy, whereas treatment for others combine radiation and surgery.

CHEMOTHERAPY

The major advances in successful treatment of cancer can be attributed to advances in chemotherapy, both in terms of new drugs and the more effective combination of familiar chemotherapeutic agents. Most often, these drugs work by destroying cancer cells' ability to use important materials within cellular processes or carry out cell division in a normal manner. Because chemotherapy influences cell division, it will influence noncancerous cells that divide frequently. Among the most susceptible to this influence are the cells that make up bone marrow, the lining of the intestinal tract, and the hair follicles. People who are undergoing chemotherapy often experience side effects directly related to these changes—immune system suppression, diarrhea, and hair loss.

IMMUNOTHERAPY

Immunotherapy refers to the use of a variety of substances to trigger a person's own immune system to attack cancer cells or prevent cancer cells from becoming activated. Among these new forms of immunotherapy are the use of interferon, monoclonal antibodies, interleukin-2, tumor necrosis factor (TNF), and certain bone marrow growth regulators. Some of these products are being produced by genetic engineering technology.

HYPERTHERMIA

Through the use of *ultrasound* or microwaves, the internal temperatures of cancer cells can be raised, thus subjecting critical protein-synthesizing processes to the destructive effects of heat.

HYPERBARIC THERAPY

For radiation therapy to have its maximal effect, the tissue being treated must possess an adequate level of oxygen. Because the central portions of solid tumors have little oxygen, radiation is less than maximally effective in these areas. Treatment delivered in a hyperbaric chamber, allowing greater oxygenation, increases the effectiveness of the radiation therapy.

As cancer research progresses, the prognosis for survival will certainly increase. The box on the right lists resources offering support for cancer victims.

ALTERNATIVE CANCER THERAPIES

In spite of advances made in the diagnosis and treatment of cancer during this century, cancer rates are climbing as we move toward the next century. In response to climbing rates and to requests made by cancer victims and many clinicians to expand the range of

Resources Offering Support for Cancer

For cancer victims and their families, many telephone lines have been set up offering information and referrals:

★ **American Cancer Society National Hot Line:** (800) ACS-2345. Also, ACS recommends calling local ACS chapters for support group information.

★ **National Cancer Institute Cancer Information Service:** (800) 4-CANCER.

★ **National Coalition for Cancer Survivorship** (umbrella group for cancer survivor units nationwide): (301) 650-8868.

★ **Candlelighters Childhood Cancer Foundation:** Information on support groups for children with cancer and their families: (301) 657-8401 and (800) 366-2223.

★ **Surviving:** Support group. Publishes newsletter for Hodgkin's survivors.
Stanford University Medical Center
Radiology Dept, Room C050
300 Pasteur Dr
Stanford, CA 94305

★ **Vital Options:** Support group for young adults, 17 to 40, who are cancer survivors: (818) 508-5657.

★ **The Resource Center**
American College of Obstetricians and Gynecologists
409 12th St. S.W.
Washington, DC 20224-2188
Send a self-addressed, business-size envelope for *Detecting and Treating Breast Problems.*

★ **American College of Radiology,** for accredited mammography centers.
(800) ACR-LINE (members only) or (703) 648-8900; ask for mammography.

treatments, the National Institutes of Health have begun an in-depth, $2 million study of alternative or nonconventional cancer treatments.[23] Through the use of new and carefully controlled studies and the reassessment of research and records already available, an attempt will be made to expand treatment options for patients to improve their chances of recovery.

Among the treatments to be given closer and more careful consideration are chiropractic (the manipulation of the spine), acupressure (finger and thumb pressure to relieve pain), and acupuncture (needles inserted to relieve pain and promote the flow of energy within the body). Additional areas of investigation will include ayurveda (traditional Indian use of herbs, diet, and lifestyle), biofeedback (monitoring of body functions to control body processes), homeopathy (use of minuscule doses of toxic substances), and naturopathy (use of natural remedies including sunshine and vitamins). Further focus will be directed toward oxidizing agents (substances believed to kill viruses), reflexology (the massaging of points on the feet), therapeutic touch (redirecting of "life forces" through touching areas of the body), and visualization (learning to "see" cure occurring).

Time and study will answer many questions about the effectivness of these methods of treating cancer. If these areas prove to be more effective than traditional medical science now believes, their incorporation will probably be very gradual.

ENVIRONMENTAL RISK FOR DEVELOPING CANCER AND RISK REDUCTION

How important is the environment in determining whether a person will develop cancer? Some experts suggest that 85% of all cancers are influenced to varying degrees by the environmental choices that people make: what we eat, drink, wear, expose ourselves to, and even where we choose to live and work. In the list appearing below, several specific risk factors are identified. Take the time to ask yourself, "Am I healthy enough for the cancer risk that I have assumed?" If the answer is "no," you may wish to consider modification in your life-style. In regard to the first stated risk, think carefully about how being someone's daughter or son can be a cancer-related risk factor.

▼ *Select your parents carefully.* This statement seems absurd, but is intent is constructive: you are the recipient of the genetic strengths and weaknesses of your biological parents. If cancer is prevalent in your family medical history, you cannot afford to disregard this fact. Individuals with a familial predisposition to breast cancer, for instance, must faithfully carry out monthly self-examinations, which are already recommended, of course, for all women.

▼ *Select your occupation carefully.* Because of recently discovered relationships between cancer and occupations that bring employees into contact with carcinogenic agents, you must be aware of risks with certain job selections and assignments. Gainful employment is an important facet of modern life, but to risk that life in a carcinogenic work environment is hardly wise.

▼ *Do not use tobacco products.* You may want to review the discussion on the overwhelming evidence linking all forms of tobacco use (including smokeless) to

Health ACTION Guide

Reducing Cancer Risk

The American Cancer Society recommends the following dietary precautions to help reduce the risk of getting cancer:

▼ Avoid obesity
▼ Reduce total fat intake
▼ Eat more high-fiber foods
▼ Include foods rich in vitamins A and C in your daily diet
▼ Include cruciferous vegetables in your diet
▼ Avoid smoked, salt-cured, and nitrate-cured foods
▼ Moderate alcohol consumption

the development of cancer. Smoking cigarettes will increase your risk of developing lung cancer by a factor of nine or ten. So detrimental is smoking to health that it is considered the number one preventable cause of death.

▼ *Follow a prudent diet.* Return to Chapter 5 and review the relationships that exist between certain dietary practices and the incidence of various diseases, including cancer. Current preliminary research is focusing on the role of nutrients in preventing cancer. Vitamin A family compounds, calcium, vitamins B_6, B_{12}, and E, folic acid, and selenium are currently being studied. Should research demonstrate a clear role for these nutrients, "chemoprevention" may become an even more widely practiced component of cancer prevention. In planning meals and preparing food, increase consumption of foods high in fiber and low in saturated fats, avoid burning or overgrilling meat, and limit food that is high in nitrates. Certainly by reducing saturated fats in your diet and increasing the fiber, you may be able to decrease your risk of developing certain cancers.

▼ *Control your body weight.* Particularly for women, obesity is related to a higher incidence of cancer of the uterus, ovary, and breast. Maintaining a desirable body weight could improve overall health and lead to more successful management of cancer should it develop.

▼ *Limit your exposure to sun.* It is important to heed this message, even if you enjoy many outdoor activities. Particularly for people with light complexions, the radiation received through chronic exposure to the sun may foster the development of skin cancers.

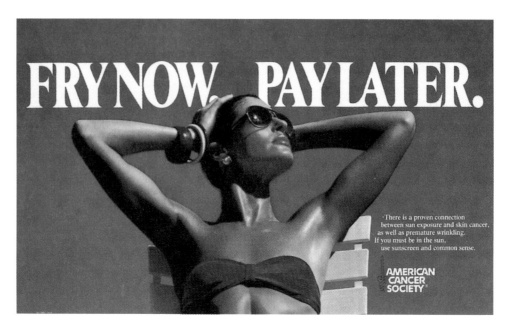

How much sun is enough?

Although most skin cancers are readily treatable, one form, malignant melanoma, can be life threatening.

▼ *Consume alcohol in moderation.* Although the evidence linking alcohol use and an increased rate of cancer is at best circumstantial, heavier users of alcohol do experience an increased prevalence of cancer of the oral cavity, larynx, and esophagus. Whether this results directly from the presence of carcinogens in alcohol or is more closely related to the alcohol user's tendency to smoke is not yet established. It is known, however, that people who have developed alcohol-related changes in the liver are more likely to develop a malignancy at that site.

All risk factor reduction is, in the final analysis, relative in nature. Our observation and experiences lead us to believe that life cannot be totally structured around the desire to achieve maximum longevity or reduce morbidity at all costs. Most people need a balance between life that is emotionally, socially, and spiritually satisfying and life that is structured solely for the purpose of living a long time and minimizing exposure to illness.

OTHER HEALTH CONDITIONS

Diabetes Mellitus

Diabetes mellitus is not a single condition but rather two conditions with important similarities and differences.

NONINSULIN-DEPENDENT DIABETES MELLITUS (TYPE II)

In persons who do not have diabetes mellitus, the body's need for energy is met through the "burning" of glucose (blood sugar) within the cells. Glucose is absorbed from the digestive tract and carried to the cells by the blood system. Passage of glucose into the cell is achieved through a transport system that moves the glucose molecule across the cell's membrane. Activation of this glucose transport mechanism requires the presence of the hormone insulin. Specific receptor sites for **insulin** can be found on the cell membrane.[24] In addition to its role in the transport of glucose into sensitive cells, insulin is also required for the conversion of glucose into glycogen in liver cells, the formation of fatty acids in adipose cells, and the movement of amino acids into cells for the synthesis of protein.

Insulin is produced in the cells of the islets of Langerhans within the pancreas. The release of insulin from the pancreas corresponds to the changing levels of glucose within the blood.

In adults with a **genetic predisposition** for developing noninsulin-dependent diabetes mellitus (NIDDM), a trigger mechanism (most likely obesity) begins a process through which the body cells become increasingly less sensitive to the presence of insulin, although a normal amount of insulin, and possibly even an excessive amount, is being produced by the pancreas. The growing ineffectiveness of insulin in getting glucose into cells results in the buildup of glucose in the blood. Elevated levels of glucose give rise to *hyperglycemia,* a hallmark symptom of noninsulin-dependent diabetes mellitus.

How Forms of Diabetes Mellitus Differ

INSULIN-DEPENDENT (TYPE I)
The following usually develop rapidly.

★ Extreme hunger

★ Extreme thirst

★ Frequent urination

★ Extreme weight loss

★ Irritability

★ Weakness and fatigue

★ Nausea and vomiting

NONINSULIN-DEPENDENT (TYPE II)
The following symptoms usually develop gradually.

★ Any of the symptoms for insulin-dependent diabetes

★ Blurred vision or a change in sight

★ Itchy skin

★ Tingling or numbness in the limbs

   If you notice these symptoms occurring, bring them to the attention of your physician. ★

In response to the build up of glucose in the blood, the kidneys begin the process of filtering glucose from the blood. Excess glucose then spills over into the urine. This removal of glucose in the urine demands large amounts of water. *Diuresis,* a second important symptom of adult onset diabetes, is experienced as fluid is drawn from the body to accommodate the need for urination. Although uncommon, a type of coma can develop as fluid is withdrawn from cells, including nerve cells, in an attempt to dilute the high levels of glucose in the blood.[24]

The current treatment of noninsulin-dependent diabetes mellitus is undergoing constant refinement as more is learned about insulin insensitivity. For many adults with diabetes, dietary restriction is the only treatment required to maintain an acceptable level of glucose use. Weight loss will improve the condition by "releasing" more insulin receptors, and as a consequence, the person can return to a more normal state of functioning.[24]

For people whose condition is more advanced, dietary restriction and weight loss alone will not accomplish the level of management required, and oral drugs or even insulin may be necessary. For those who

require insulin, management of the condition becomes much more demanding.

In addition to genetic predisposition and obesity as important factors in noninsulin-dependent diabetes mellitus, unresolved stress appears to play a role in the development of hyperglycemic states. Although stress alone probably cannot produce a diabetic condition, it is likely that stress, through the presence of epinephrine (see Chapter 3), can create a series of endocrine changes that can lead to a state of hyperglycemia.

Diabetes can cause serious damage to several important structures within the body. The rate and extent to which persons with diabetes develop these changes can be markedly influenced by the nature of their particular condition and the type of management to which they comply. For those who already have diabetes, understanding of the condition and a commitment to management are important elements in living with diabetes mellitus.

INSULIN-DEPENDENT DIABETES MELLITUS (TYPE I)

A second type of diabetes mellitus is insulin-dependent diabetes mellitus (IDDM), or Type I diabetes. The onset of this type of diabetes generally occurs before the age of 35, most often during childhood. In fact, it is still called by its old name, juvenile diabetes mellitus, by some. In contrast to NIDDM, in which insulin is produced but is ineffective because of insensitivity, with IDDM the body does not produce insulin. Destruction of the insulin-producing cells of the pancreas by the person's immune system accounts for this sudden and irreversible loss of insulin production.[24]

In most ways the two forms of diabetes are similar, with the important exception that IDDM requires the use of insulin from an outside source. Today this insulin is obtained either from animals or through genetically engineered bacteria and is taken by injection (one to four times per day) or through the use of an insulin pump that provides a constant supply of insulin to the body. Inhalation of insulin via a nasal spray may soon be available as well. Development of the glucometer, a highly accurate device for measuring the amount of glucose in the blood, allows for sound management of this condition and a life expectancy that is essentially normal. Today, people with diabetes mellitus check their blood several times a day, inject several

insulin (in suh lin) pancreatic hormone required by the body for the effective metabolism of glucose (blood sugar).

genetic predisposition inherited tendency to develop a disease process if necessary environmental factors exist.

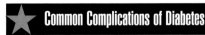

Common Complications of Diabetes

★ **Cataract formation**

★ **Glaucoma**

★ **Blindness**

★ **Dental caries**

★ **Stillbirths/miscarriages**

★ **Neonatal deaths**

★ **Congenital defects**

★ **Cardiovascular disease**

★ **Kidney disease**

★ **Gangrene**

★ **Impotence**

times a day, and appear to be experiencing much improved management compared with the practice of injecting only once or twice a day.

Of course, with both forms of diabetes mellitus, sound dietary practice, planned activity, and control of stress are important for keeping blood glucose levels within normal ranges. In the absence of good management of diabetes mellitus, several serious problems can result, including blindness, gangrene of the extremities, kidney disease, and heart attack. People who cannot establish good control are likely to live a shorter life than those who can establish better control.

Multiple Sclerosis

For proper nerve conduction to occur within portions of the brain and spinal cord, an insulating sheath of *myelin* must surround *neurons.* In the progressive disease multiple sclerosis (MS) the cells that produce myelin are altered, and myelin production ceases. This disruption to normal neurological functioning eventually reaches an extent to which vital functions of the body can no longer be carried out. The condition is fatal.[24]

Multiple sclerosis is a disease that most often appears for the first time during the young adult years—the traditional college years. After its onset, the disease progresses off and on over the next 20 to 25 years. The initial symptoms of the condition are often visual impairment, prickling and burning in the extremities, or an altered **gait.** Deterioration of nervous system function occurs in various forms during the course of MS. In the disease's most advanced stages, movement is

greatly impaired, and mental deterioration may be present.

Treatment for MS involves attempts to reduce the severity of the symptoms and extend the periods of remission. Today a variety of therapies are used, including steroid drugs, drugs to relieve muscle spasms, injections of **nerve blockers,** and physical therapy.

Most recently, the development of a new drug, Betaseron, represents the most promising treatment for MS. A genetically engineered form of interferon, it is not a cure for MS but is the first drug in decades to effectively treat the disease itself and not just the symptoms. Psychotherapy is also an important addition to the treatment of MS. Profound periods of depression often accompany the initial diagnosis of this condition. Emotional support is helpful in dealing with the progressive impairment associated with the condition.

The cause of MS is not fully understood. Research continues to focus on virus-induced **autoimmune** mechanisms in which T-cells attack viral-infected myelin-producing cells and on the role of genetic alterations in myelin production.

Asthma

Bronchial asthma is a chronic respiratory disease characterized by acute attacks of breathlessness and wheezing caused by narrowing of the bronchioles.

Two main types of asthma have been identified: *extrinsic* and *intrinsic.* In extrinsic asthma, allergens such as pollen, house dust, house-dust mites, animal fur, and feathers produce sudden and extensive bronchoconstriction that narrows the airways. Increased sputum production further narrows the bronchioles and restricts the passage of air. This narrowing fosters the development of chronic inflammation of the airways, which is the most damaging aspect of asthma. Wheezing is most pronounced when the victim attempts to exhale air through the narrowed air passages. For many asthmatics, exercise, cigarette smoke, and particular foods or drugs can cause an asthma attack.

Intrinsic asthma, the least common form, displays similar symptoms but is caused by stress or is a consequence of frequent respiratory tract infections. Allergens as such are not involved in this form of asthma.

Prevention of extrinsic asthma is sometimes possible through the use of immunotherapy, in which the victim is desensitized through injections of weakened allergens. Perhaps more successful in preventing attacks is the careful use of corticosteroid drugs several times per day to reduce inflammation.

Once an attack has started, asthmatics now routinely use bronchodilator drugs delivered through an inhaler. After inhalation, normal breathing is restored within several minutes. Each year in this country, however, several thousand persons die as the result of asthma attacks. Some experts believe that this number could be reduced if physicians were more aggressive in their treatment of the bronchial inflammation component of the condition.

Regardless of the potential seriousness, most children with asthma can be managed with the proper use of medication and may experience less asthma, or none at all, as they reach adulthood.

> **gait (gate)** pattern of walking.
>
> **nerve blockers** drugs that can stop the flow of electrical impulses through the nerves into which they have been injected.
>
> **autoimmune (awe** toe im **yoon)** immune response against the cells of a person's own body.

Summary

✔ Regulatory genes, tumor suppressor genes, protooncogenes, and oncogenes play an important role in the development of cancer.

✔ Carcinogens may stimulate the formation of oncogenes.

✔ Cigarette smoking and perhaps having a genetic predisposition are both related to the development of lung cancer.

✔ Breast cancer demonstrates clear familial patterns that suggest a genetic predisposition.

✔ Mammograms are recommended as an important component of breast cancer identification.

✔ The PSA test improves the ability to diagnose prostate cancer.

✔ Skin cancer prevention requires protection from excessive sun exposure.

✔ Regular use of Pap tests is related to the early detection of uterine (cervical) cancer.

✔ Regular self-examination of the testicles leads to early detection of testicular cancer.

✔ Ovarian cancer is often "silent" in its presentation of symptoms.

✔ Conventional and alternative treatment methods can be used to treat cancer.

✔ Cancer risk reduction techniques should be practiced on a regular basis.

✔ Diabetes mellitus, in both noninsulin-dependent and insulin-dependent forms, is a chronic condition reflecting the body's inability to use blood glucose in a normal manner.

✔ Multiple sclerosis involves the autoimmune destruction of the insulating cover of neurons.

✔ Asthma may be a response to extrinsic factors such as pollen and dust or intrinsic factors such as stress and chronic respiratory system infections.

Review Questions

1. What is the relationship between regulatory genes and tumor suppressor genes in the development of cancer? Why are regulatory genes called both protooncogenes and oncogenes?

2. What are some of the major types of cancer, based on the tissues in which they originate?

3. What are the principal factors that contribute to the development of lung cancer? Or breast cancer?

4. When should regular use of mammography begin, and which women should begin using it earliest?

5. How does the PSA test contribute to the early detection of prostate cancer?

6. What signs indicate the possibility that a skin lesion has become cancerous?

7. What important information can be obtained with the use of Pap tests?

8. What are the steps for effective self-examination of the breasts and testicles?

9. Why is ovarian cancer described as a "silent" cancer?

10. What are the conventional and alternative cancer treatments most often used in the treatment of cancer?

11. What are the risk reduction activities identified in this chapter?

12. How do noninsulin-dependent and insulin-dependent diabetes mellitus differ? How are they the same?

13. What is the role of the immune system in multiple sclerosis?

14. How do extrinsic and intrinsic asthma differ?

Think about This . . .

✔ Do you believe you could cope with a significant health problem at this time in your life?

✔ Do you know anyone who has or has had cancer? How did cancer affect that person's life?

✔ How regularly do you perform either breast or testicular self-examination?

✔ If you were diagnosed as having a terminal illness, how willing would you be to serve as a subject in a research project that tested a potentially toxic experimental drug?

✔ Which conditions in this chapter are you likely to develop, and which are you not likely to develop?

REAL LIFE REAL CHOICES

YOUR TURN

▼ What health risks does Tina Mavrakos face as a consequence of her prolonged exposure to the sun?

▼ Is it safe for darker-skinned people like Tina to swim and sunbathe without using a sunscreen? Why or why not?

▼ What are the ABCD guidelines for detecting melanomas?

AND NOW, YOUR CHOICES . . .

▼ Have you ever gotten a severe sunburn? If so, did you change your attitude and behavior related to sunbathing?

▼ If you were a friend of Tina's, what do you think would be the most helpful advice you could give her? ▼

References

1. US Bureau of the Census: *Statistical abstract of the United States, 1993,* annual ed 113, Washington, DC, 1993, US Department of Commerce.

2. Fisher W: Oncologist, personal interview, Oct 1992.

3. Fisher R, Lescoe M, Rao M, et al: The human mutator gene homolog MSH2 and its association with hereditary nonpolyposis colon cancer, *Cell* 75:1027-1038, Dec 3, 1993.

4. Leach F, Nicholas N, Papadopouloa N, et al: Mutations of a mutS homolog in hereditary nonpolyposis colorectal cancer, *Cell* 75:1215-1225, Dec 17, 1993.

5. Bronner C, Baker S, Morrison P, et al: Mutation in the DNA mismatch repair gene homologue hMLH1 is associated with hereditary nonpolyposis colon cancer, *Nature* 368:258-261, March 17, 1994.

6. American Cancer Society: *Cancer facts and figures: 1993,* Atlanta, 1993, The Society.

7. Sellers TA, et al: Evidence of Mendelian inheritance in the pathogenesis of lung cancer, *J Natl Cancer Inst* 82(15):1272-1279, 1990.

8. Seller TA, et al: Effect of family history, body fat distribution, and reproductive factors on the risk of postmenopausal breast cancer, *N Engl J Med* 326(20):1323-1329, 1992.

9. Ballard-Barbash R, et al: Body fat distribution and breast cancer in the Framingham study, *J Natl Cancer Inst* 82(24):1943-1944, 1990.

10. Willett W, Hunter D, Stampfer M, et al: Dietary fat and fiber in relation to risk of breast cancer: an 8-year follow-up, *JAMA* 268(15):2037-2044, 1992.

11. Eddy D: Screening for cervical cancer, *Ann Intern Med* 113(7):560-561, 1990.

12. Eads MD: *If it runs in your family: breast cancer: reducing your risk,* New York, 1991, Bantam Books.

13. Richardson G: Ovarian cancer (editoral), *JAMA* 269(9):1163, 1993.

14. Carter BS, Beaty TH, Steinberg GD, et al: Mendelian inheritance of familial prostate cancer, *Proc Natl Acad Sci USA* 89:3367-3371, 1992.

15. Giovannucci E, Rimm E, Colditz G, et al: A prospective study of dietary fat and risk of prostate cancer, *J Natl Cancer Inst* 85(19):1571-1579, 1993.

16. Johansson JE, et al: High 10-year survival rate in patients with early, untreated prostatic cancer, *JAMA* 267(16):2191-2196, 1992.

17. Giovannucci E, Rimm E, Stampfer M, et al: A prospective study of cigarette smoking and risk of colorectal adenoma and colorectal cancer is US men, *J Nat Cancer Inst* 86(3)183-191, 1994.

18. Winawer S, Zauber A, May N, et al: Prevention of colorectal cancer by colonoscopic polypectomy, *N Engl J Med* 329(27):1977-1981, 1993.

19. Thun M, Namboodiri M, Calle E, et al: Aspirin use and risk of fatal cancer, *J Cancer Res* 53:1322-1327, March 15, 1993.

20. Friend T: Vaccine battles melanoma, *USA Today,* March 29, 1993, 1A.
21. Koh H, Lew R: Sunscreens and melanoma: implications for prevention (editoral), *J Natl Cancer Inst* 86(2):78, 1994.
22. Friend T: Fear of cancer deters detection, *USA Today,* March 31, 1993, 1D.

23. Bryant J: NIH panel reviews "unconventional" medical practices, *The NIH Record* 44(14):1, 1992.
24. Crowley LV: *Introduction to human disease,* Boston, 1992, Jones and Bartlett Publishers.

Suggested Readings

Dravecky D: *Comeback,* San Francisco, 1990, Zondervan Books/Harper & Row.

The heroic chronicles of a major league baseball pitcher who developed bone cancer in his pitching arm. Dravecky shows that with faith and determination, the fear of cancer can be overcome.

Schapiro R: *Multiple sclerosis: a rehabilitation approach to management,* New York, 1991, Demos Publications.

A highly authoritative book dealing with all aspects of rehabilitation for people with MS. Written with 12 other contributors who are experienced in this field, the author describes not only rehabilitation strategies but *also the underlying neurological basis of each.*

Siegel BS: *Peace, love, and healing,* New York, 1990, Perennial Library/Harper & Row.

Bestselling author (Love, Medicine and Miracles) and surgeon, Siegel explores the concepts of self-healing by explaining the body-mind interaction capabilities. Siegel believes that diseases can cause people to love themselves and others and to live life to the fullest. Siegel is convinced that "wonder drugs" reside with each person. This book provides a positive, optimistic look at illness.

12

Infectious Diseases

A Shared Concern

The information sticker we sometimes see attached to the door of restroom stalls succeeds in identifying the important concept underlying the study of infectious diseases:

GONORRHEA: THE GIFT THAT KEEPS ON GIVING

We can see how this message can extend to other infectious diseases. Infectious diseases are, in a sense, "gifts" from people that we may pass on to other people. In this chapter we explore the basic processes underlying the causes and management of several of today's important infectious diseases.

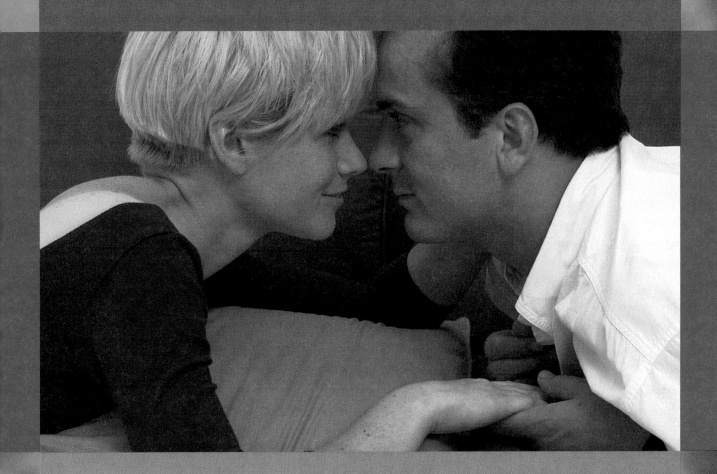

INFECTIOUS DISEASES

The following objectives are covered in this chapter:

▼ Reduce to zero the indigenous cases of the following vaccine-preventable diseases: diphtheria and tetanus (among people aged 25 and under), polio, measles, rubella, and congenital rubella syndrome. (Baseline 1988: diphtheria [1 case], tetanus [3 cases], polio [0 cases], measles [3058 cases], rubella [225 cases], congenital rubella syndrome [6 cases]; p. 513.)

▼ Reduce cases of mumps to 500 and cases of pertussis to 1000. (Baseline 1988: mumps cases [4866] and pertussis cases [3450]; p. 513.)

▼ Confine the prevalence of HIV infection to no more than 800 per 100,000 people. (Baseline: an estimated 400 per 100,000 in 1989; p. 483.)

▼ Increase to at least 50% the proportion of sexually active, unmarried people who used a condom at last sexual intercourse. (Baseline: 19% of sexually active, unmarried women aged 15 through 44 reported that their partners used a condom at last sexual intercourse in 1988; p. 485.)

▼ Reduce Chlamydia trachomatis infections, as measured by a decrease in the incidence of nongonococcal urethritis to no more than 170 cases per 100,000 people. (Baseline: 215 per 100,000 in 1988; p. 498.)

REAL LIFE
REAL CHOICES

AIDS in the Workplace: Fact versus Fear

▼ Name: Chris Karasawa
▼ Age: 53
▼ Occupation: Electrical engineer

"What if he uses my coffee mug?" "He shouldn't be allowed in our restroom." "I don't want him working anywhere near me."

Those are just a few of the comments Chris Karasawa has heard from some of his employees since the beginning of this week when he interviewed a young engineer for a newly created position in his department. Of all the candidates Chris has met with, John Travers is by far the best qualified for the position Chris has been seeking to fill for the past 2 months. He graduated summa cum laude from one of the top engineering programs in the country, has impeccable references, is enthusiastic, energetic—and openly gay. His partner recently died of AIDS, and John (who has consistently tested negative for the HIV virus) wants to relocate from the West Coast to this New England city.

Those of Chris's employees who object to his hiring John know intellectually that he won't inevitably contract AIDS. They also know that HIV isn't spread by casual contact, so even if a co-worker did have AIDS, the risk to fellow employees is extremely low.

Overall, the people on Chris's staff are a diverse and tolerant group who attach little importance to differences in race, sex, religion, and lifestyle. Chris knows, however, that when it comes to AIDS, reasonable and accepting people with otherwise open minds often slam the door shut. AIDS thus far is a fatal disease, and it's most prevalent among gay men. John Travers is gay, his partner died of AIDS, and therefore some of Chris's staffers perceive his presence as a threat to their physical and their emotional well-being.

As you study this chapter, think about Chris Karasawa's challenges and choices in hiring John Travers, and prepare yourself to answer the questions in **Your Turn** at the end of the chapter. ▼

INFECTIOUS DISEASES IN THE 1990s

Before the turn of the twentieth century infectious diseases were the leading cause of death. These deaths came after exposure to the organisms that produced such diseases as smallpox, tuberculosis, influenza, whooping cough, typhoid, diphtheria, and tetanus. However, since the early 1990s improvements in public sanitation, the widespread use of antibiotic drugs as a treatment method, and vaccinations as preventive therapy considerably reduced the numbers of persons dying from infectious diseases. People now die from chronic, long-term disease processes. We die from complications of cardiovascular disease, cancer, diabetes, liver damage, kidney disease, or other conditions.

Perhaps because of this shift in the causes of death, we recently went through a period in which we did not think much about infectious diseases. Many people could not imagine that an infectious disease might ever really jeopardize their health or threaten their lives. Who had ever heard of someone dying from whooping cough? Few people could say they knew someone who was debilitated after having had measles, mumps, or even a sexually transmitted disease. We just did not believe that these could affect us in the high-tech world we live in.

Today, however, we have a new respect for infec-

tious diseases. We have learned that AIDS threatens millions of people in many areas of the world. We are witnessing the resurgence of tuberculosis (TB). We recognize the role of pelvic infections in infertility. We also know that people vaccinated for measles between 1963 and 1967 may need a second immunization to be fully protected.[1] Finally, we know that failure to fully immunize children has laid the groundwork for a return of whooping cough (pertussis), a serious childhood bacterial infection. This chapter will make you more aware of some of the potentially serious infectious diseases, their causes, treatments, and methods of prevention. You can use this information to keep yourself healthier and more productive throughout the rest of your life.

INFECTIOUS DISEASE TRANSMISSION

Infectious diseases can generally be transferred from person to person, although there is not always a direct transfer from one person to another. Infectious diseases can be especially dangerous because of their ability to spread to large numbers of people, producing **epidemics** or **pandemics.**

Pathogens

For a disease to be transferred, a person must come into contact with the disease-producing agent, or

TABLE 12-1 Pathogens and Common Infectious Diseases

Pathogen	Description	Representative disease processes
Viruses	Smallest common pathogens; nonliving particles of genetic material (DNA) surrounded by a protein coat	Rubeola, mumps, chickenpox, rubella, influenza, warts, colds, oral and genital herpes, shingles, AIDS, genital warts
Bacteria	One-celled microorganisms with sturdy, well-defined cell walls; three distinctive forms: spherical (cocci), rod shaped (bacilli), and spiral shaped (spirilla)	Tetanus, strep throat, scarlet fever, gonorrhea, syphilis, chlamydia, toxic shock syndrome, Legionnaires' disease, bacterial pneumonia, meningitis, diphtheria, food poisoning, Lyme disease
Fungi	Plantlike microorganisms; molds and yeasts	Athlete's foot, ringworm, histoplasmosis, San Joaquin Valley fever, candidiasis
Protozoa	Simplest animal form, generally one-celled organisms	Malaria, amebic dysentery, trichomoniasis, vaginitis
Rickettsia	Viruslike organisms that require a host's living cells for growth and replication	Typhus, Rocky Mountain spotted fever, rickettsialpox
Parasitic worms	Many-celled organisms; represented by tapeworms, leeches, and roundworms	Dirofilariasis (dog heartworm), elephantiasis, onchocerciasis

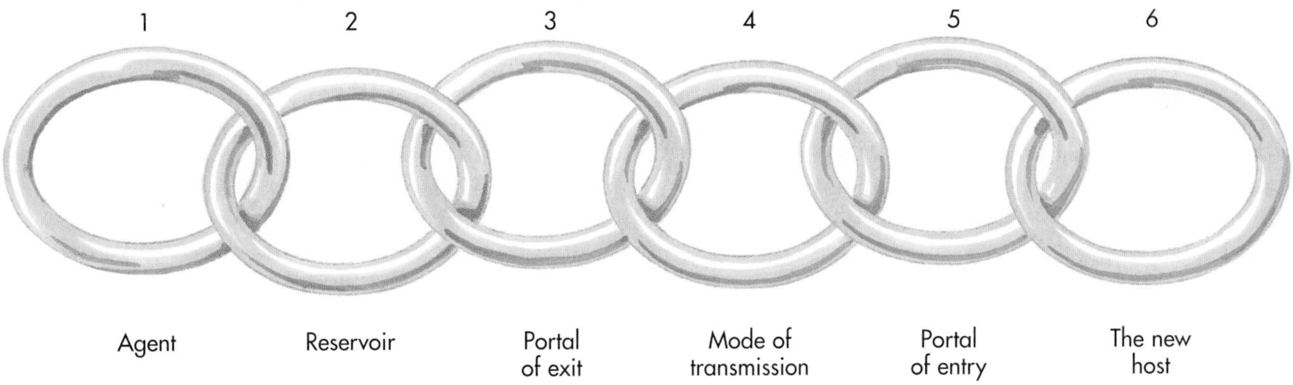

1	2	3	4	5	6
Agent	Reservoir	Portal of exit	Mode of transmission	Portal of entry	The new host

Figure 12-1 The chain of infection.

pathogen, such as viruses, bacteria, or fungi. When pathogens enter our bodies, they are sometimes able to resist our body defense systems, flourish, and produce an illness. We commonly call this an *infection*. Because of their small size, pathogens are sometimes referred to as microorganisms, microbes, or germs. Table 12-1 describes the more familiar infectious disease agents and some of the illnesses they produce.

Chain of Infection

The transmission of a pathogenic agent through the various links in the chain of infection (Figure 12-1) forms the basis for an understanding of how diseases spread.[2] Not every pathogenic agent will move all of the way through the chain of infection, because various links in the chain can be broken. Therefore the presence of a pathogen creates only the potential for a disease.

AGENT

The first link in the chain of infection is the disease-causing **agent**. Whereas some agents are very **virulent** and cause serious infectious illnesses such as HIV,

epidemic (ep a **dem** mick) rapid spread of a disease among individuals within a given area or within a given population.

pandemic (pan **dem** mick) spread of a disease process over a wide geographical area.

pathogen (**path** oh jen) disease causing agent.

agent causal pathogen of a particular disease.

virulent (**veer** yuh lent) capable of causing disease.

which causes AIDS, others produce far less serious infections, as in the common cold. Through mutation, some pathogenic agents, particularly viruses, become more virulent than they once were.

RESERVOIR

For infectious agents to survive they must have the support and protection of a favorable environment. This environment forms the second link in the chain of infection and is referred to as the *reservoir* where the agent resides. In many of the most common infectious diseases the reservoirs in which the pathogenic organisms live are the bodies of already infected persons. Here the agents thrive before being spread to others. These infected persons are, accordingly, the hosts for particular disease agents.

For other infectious diseases, however, the reservoirs in which the agents are maintained are the bodies of animals. Rabies is among the most familiar of the animal-reservoir diseases. Not in all cases will the animals be sick or show symptoms similar to those seen in infected persons.

The third type of reservoir in which disease-causing agents can reside is on or in nonliving environments such as the soil. (The spores of the tetanus bacterium can survive in soil for up to 50 years, entering the human body in a puncture wound.) Warm and moist locker room floors are another example of this environment because the fungi that cause ringworm and jock itch can survive here.

PORTAL OF EXIT

For pathogenic agents to cause diseases and illnesses in others, it is necessary that they leave the security of their reservoirs. The third link in the chain of infection is the *portal of exit*, or the point at which agents leave their reservoirs.

Particularly in terms of infectious diseases that involve human reservoirs, the principal portals of exit are familiar—the digestive system, urinary system, respiratory system, reproductive system, and the blood.

Infected body wastes, including urine and feces, leave the bodies of infected people and eventually may have contact with healthy people through contaminated water and food. Respiratory infections are spread when contaminated materials are discharged with coughing, forceful speaking, or hand contact with mucuslike discharges from the nose or mouth. Pathogenic agents that reside in the reproductive system exit through the openings of the penis and vagina (condoms collect infected ejaculate from the penis), and infected blood exits the body through the use of needles or with injuries that require care.

MODE OF TRANSMISSION

The fourth link in the chain of infection is the *mode of transmission*, or the way that pathogens are passed from reservoirs to susceptible hosts. Two principal methods seen are *direct transmission* and *indirect transmission*.

Three types of direct transmission are observed in human-to-human transmission. These include contact between body surfaces (such as kissing, touching, and sexual intercourse), droplet spread (inhalation of contaminated air droplets), and fecal-oral spread (feces on the hands are brought into contact with the mouth).

Indirect transmission occurs between infected and uninfected persons when infectious agents travel by means of nonhuman materials. Vehicles of transmission include inanimate objects such as water, food items, soil, towels, items of clothing, and eating utensils. Today, great effort is made to minimize the spread of infectious agents through indirect transmission. Food and milk processing, waste disposal, and general environmental hygiene are employed to minimize the role of nonliving objects in the indirect transmission of pathogenic agents.

A second method of indirect transmission of infectious agents occurs in conjunction with vectors. The term *vector* is related to living things, such as insects, birds, and other animals that carry diseases from human to human. Perhaps no vector is in the news more at this time than the deer tick that transmits Lyme disease.

Airborne indirect transmission involves the inhalation of infected particles that have been suspended in an air source for an extended period. Unlike droplet transmission, in which both infected and uninfected persons must be in close physical proximity, noninfected persons can become infected through airborne transmission by sharing air with infected persons who were in the same room hours earlier. Viral infections such as German measles may be spread in this manner.

PORTAL OF ENTRY

The fifth link in the chain of infectious disease is the *portal of entry*. As with the portals of exit, there are three primary portals of entry for pathogenic agents to enter the bodies of uninfected persons. These are through the digestive system, respiratory system, and reproductive system. In addition, the broken skin resulting from an injection into the circulatory system provides another portal of entry. In the majority of infectious conditions, the portals of entry prove to be within the same systems as the portals of exit were for the infected persons: digestive to digestive, respiratory to respiratory, and reproductive to reproductive. In the case of HIV, however, cross-system transmission is observed. Oral and anal sex allow for infectious agents to pass between warm, moist tissues of the reproductive and digestive systems.

THE NEW HOST

All persons are, in theory, at risk for contracting infectious diseases and thus could be identified as *suscepti-*

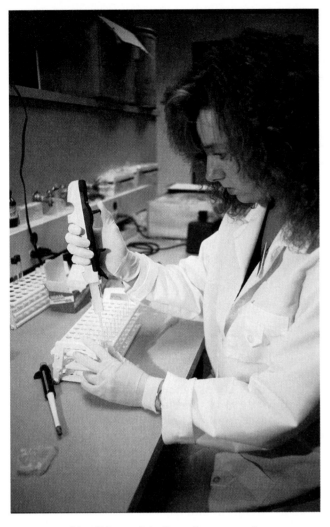

Identifying an infectious disease agent.

ble hosts. In practice, however, factors such as overall health, acquired immunity, health care services, and health-related behaviors can influence susceptibility to infectious diseases. In the remainder of this chapter, we examine some of these factors to reduce the likelihood that you will have contact with infectious agents and the diseases they produce.

Stages of Infection

When a new host is assaulted by a pathogenic agent, a reasonably predictable sequence of events takes place. That is, the disease moves through four rather distinctive stages.[2] You may be able to recognize these five stages of infection each time you catch a cold.

1. *The incubation stage.* This stage lasts from the time a pathogen enters the body until it multiplies enough to produce signs and symptoms of the disease. The length of this stage can vary from a few hours to many months, depending on the virulence of the organisms, the concentration of organisms, the host's level of immune responsiveness, and other health problems. This stage has been called a silent stage. Transmission of the pathogen to a new host is possible but not probable during this stage. Thus a host may be infected during this stage, but not infectious. HIV infection is an exception to this rule.

2. *The prodromal stage.* The stage of incubation is followed by a short period during which the host may experience a variety of general signs and symptoms. Watery eyes, runny nose, slight fever, and overall tiredness (malaise, apathy) are signs of this stage. These symptoms are nonspecific in nature and may not be so overwhelming that the host is forced to rest. During this stage, the pathogenic agent continues to multiply. Now the host is capable of transferring this pathogen to a new host. Self-imposed isolation should be practiced during this stage to protect others.

3. *The clinical stage.* This stage, also called the *acme* or *acute stage,* is often the most unpleasant stage for the host. At this time, the disease reaches its highest point of development. All of the clinical signs and symptoms for the particular disease can be seen or analyzed by appropriate laboratory tests. The likelihood of transmitting the disease to others is highest during the peak stage. During this peak stage, all of our available defense mechanisms are in the process of resisting further damage from the pathogen. For most of us, our body defense systems are sufficient to provide over 70 years of protection over invading microorganisms. We may harbor some infections throughout our lives, but never totally lose a battle.

4. *The decline stage.* During this stage the first signs of recovery occur. The infection is ending or, in some cases, being reduced to a subclinical level. Relapse may occur if people overextend themselves.

5. *The recovery stage.* Also called the *convalescence stage,* this stage is characterized by apparent recovery from the invading agent. Disease transmission during this stage is possible but not probable. Until the host's overall health has been strengthened, he or she may be especially susceptible to another (perhaps different) disease pathogen. Fortunately, after the recovery stage, further susceptibility to the pathogenic agent should be reduced because of the body's buildup of immunity. This buildup of immunity is not always permanent. For example, many sexually transmitted diseases can be contracted repeatedly.

BODY DEFENSES: MECHANICAL AND CELLULAR IMMUNE SYSTEMS

Much as a military installation is protected by a series of defensive alignments, so too is the body. These defenses can be classified as being either mechanical or

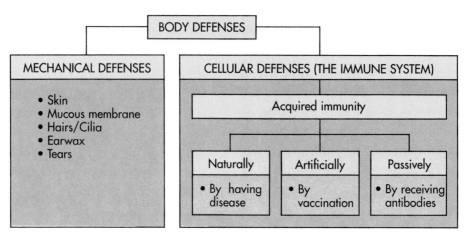

Figure 12-2 The body has a variety of defenses against invading organisms. Mechanical defenses are the body's first line of defense. Cellular defenses include chemicals and specialized cells that provide immunity against subsequent infections.

cellular (Figure 12-2). *Mechanical* defenses are first line defenses, since they physically separate the internal body from the external environment. Included among these are the skin, the mucous membranes that line the respiratory and gastrointestinal tracts, ear wax, the tiny hairs and cilia that filter incoming air, and even tears. These defenses serve primarily as a shield against foreign materials that may contain pathogenic agents.

The second component of the body's protective defenses is the *cellular* system or, more commonly, the **immune system.** The immune system is, in comparison to the mechanical system, far more specific, with the elimination of microorganisms, foreign proteins, and cells foreign to the body as its primary mission. Collectively, the triggers that activate the cells of the immune system are identified as *antigens.*[3]

Divisions of the Immune System

Closer examination of the immune system reveals two separate but highly cooperative groups of cells. One group of cells has its origins in the fetal thymus gland and thus has become known as *T-cell–mediated immunity,* or simply *cell-mediated immunity.* The second group of cells that make up cellular immunity are the B-cells that are the working units of *humoral immunity.*[3] Cellular elements of both cell-mediated and humoral immunity can be found within the bloodstream, the lymphatic tissues of the body, and the fluid that surrounds body cells.

Although we are born with the structural elements of both cell-mediated and humoral immunity, the development of an immune response requires that components of these cellular systems encounter and successfully defend against specific antigens. Once this has occurred, the immune system is primed to respond quickly and effectively should the same antigens be encountered again. This confrontation results in the development of a state of **acquired immunity**

(AI). As seen in Figure 12-2, the development of AI can occur in different ways.

▼ **Naturally acquired immunity (NAI)** occurs when the body is exposed to infectious agents. Thus when we catch an infectious disease, we fight the infection and in the process become immune (protected) from developing illness again should reinfection occur.

▼ **Artificially acquired immunity (AAI)** occurs when the body is exposed to infectious agents introduced through vaccination or immunization. As in NAI, the body engages the infectious agents, as well as produces a record of how to fight the same battle again. Young children, older adults, and adults in higher risk occupations should consult their physicians about immunizations for flu, hepatitis B, pneumonia, and other infectious diseases. Table 12-2 shows a schedule for immunization.

▼ **Passively acquired immunity (PAI),** a third form of immunity, results when **antibodies** are introduced into the body. These antibodies are for a variety of specific infections and are produced outside the body (either in animals or by the genetic manipulation of microorganisms). When introduced into the human body, they provide immediate protection until a more natural form of immunity can be developed.

Collectively, these forms of immunity can provide important protection against infectious disease.

Immunizations

Although the incidence of several childhood communicable diseases is at or near the lowest level ever, the risk of a resurgence of diseases such as measles, polio, diphtheria, and rubella could occur in the not too distant future. This possible upturn in childhood infectious illnesses is based on the disturbing finding that fewer than half of American preschoolers are adequately immunized.

★ Rheumatoid Arthritis

A commonly recognized form of arthritis is rheumatoid arthritis. Unlike osteoarthritis (see Chapter 20), rheumatoid arthritis is not the result of wear and tear but rather is caused by an autoimmune response. For unknown reasons the body's immune system attacks perfectly good cells in virtually all of the joints in the body. Approximately 2% of the population above the age of 15 has some degree of rheumatoid arthritis. Early in the condition, stiffness and joint pain are relatively common characteristics. When the condition is more advanced, swelling, redness, throbbing pain, muscle atrophy, joint deformity, and limited mobility are often reported. Significantly greater numbers of women than men develop this form of arthritis.

Interestingly, a traumatic or stressful event often triggers the onset of rheumatoid arthritis. In many cases the first symptoms are noticed in the days after a fall or a car accident. The possibility of a genetic predisposition for developing this form of arthritis is being explored. ★

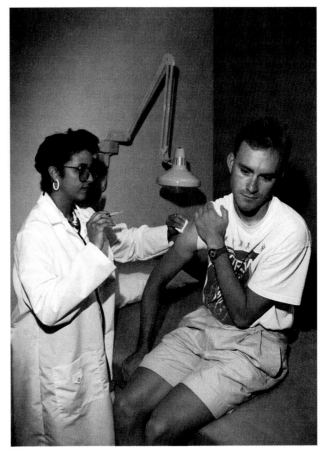

Vaccination provides artificially acquired immunity.

Today a concerted effort is underway to raise the level of immunization to 90% of all children under the age of 2 years. Congress has recently authorized over $800 million to provide immunizations to children on Medicaid and to Native American children, improve immunization clinic availability, inform physicians of the opportune time to vaccinate, and help states purchase vaccines at lower prices.[4,5] Currently the full-fee cost for all recommended immunizations averages $280 per child. Availability and cost aside, however, the principal reason for the lower level of immunization seen today is a failure on the part of many parents to complete their children's immunization programs.

On the basis of current technology, vaccinations against several potentially serious infectious conditions are available. These include the following:

▼ *Diphtheria:* a potentially fatal illness that leads to inflammation of the membranes that line the throat, and to swollen lymph nodes, and heart and kidney failure
▼ *Whooping cough (pertussis):* a bacterial infection of the airways and lungs that results in deep, noisy breathing and coughing
▼ *Hepatitis B:* a viral infection that can be transmitted sexually or through the exchange of blood or body fluids and causes serious liver damage
▼ *Haemophilus influenzae type B:* a bacterial infection that can damage the heart and brain, resulting in meningitis, and can produce profound hearing loss

immune system (im **yoon**) system of cellular elements that protect the body from invading pathogens and foreign materials.

acquired immunity (AI) major component of the immune system associated with the formation of antibodies and specialized blood cells that are capable of destroying pathogens.

naturally acquired immunity (NAI) type of acquired immunity resulting from the body's response to naturally occurring pathogens.

artificially acquired immunity (AAI) type of acquired immunity resulting from the body's response to pathogens introduced into the body through immunizations.

passively acquired immunity (PAI) temporary immunity achieved by providing antibodies to a person exposed to a particular pathogen.

antibodies (**an** ti bodies) chemical compounds produced by the body's immune system to destroy antigens and their toxins.

TABLE 12-2 Recommended Immunization Schedule*,†

	Months							Years
	Birth	1-2	2	4	6	6-18	12-15	6
Diphtheria/pertussis/ tetanus (DPT)			X	X	X		X‡	X
Polio (OPV)			X	X	X			X
Measles/mumps/ rubella (MMR)						X		X
Haemophilus influenzae (Hib)			X	X	X§		X	
Hepatitis B¶ (Hep B)	X	X				X		
or:		X		X		X		

*Foreign travelers: renew immunizations for diseases prevalent in the countries of travel.

†Influenza: yearly for elderly adults, in occupations (such as health care workers and teachers) exposed to infected persons, and for all adults with chronic respiratory and heart disease.

‡As early as 12 months, as long as at least 6 months since last DTP dose.

§May not be required, depending on which Hib vaccine is used.

¶Anyone exposed to infected individuals or contaminated food and water, and foreign travelers and health care workers.

For referral to an immunization clinic or for other information, contact the Centers for Disease Control and Prevention National Immunization Program: (800) 232-2522 in English or TDD; (800) 232-0233 in Spanish.

▼ *Tetanus:* a fatal infection caused by bacteria found in the soil that damage the central nervous system

▼ *Rubella (German measles):* a viral infection of the upper respiratory tract that can cause damage to a developing fetus when the mother contracts the infection during the first trimester of pregnancy

▼ *Measles (red measles):* a highly contagious viral infection leading to a rash, high fever, and other upper respiratory tract symptoms

▼ *Polio:* a viral infection capable of causing paralysis of the large muscles of the extremities

▼ *Mumps:* a viral infection of the salivary glands

Parents of newborns should take their infants to their family care physicians, pediatricians, or well-baby clinics operated by county health departments to begin the immunization schedule. The schedule shown in Table 12-2 is followed by most physicians. It is hoped that a single immunization to protect children against all of the infectious childhood illnesses will soon be available. Such a vaccine is perhaps only 10 years away. However, until then, VariVax, a vaccine against chickenpox, may be the next vaccine ready for wide-scale use. If it is approved, another childhood infectious illness could vanish from the scene.

THE IMMUNE RESPONSE

To fully understand the function of the immune system requires a substantial understanding of human biology and is beyond the scope of this text. Figure 12-3 provides an easily understood view of the immune response.

When antigens (whether microorganisms, foreign substances, or abnormal cells) are discovered within the body, they are confronted by macrophages (large white blood cells), and their number is initially reduced by the destructive action of the macrophages. At the same time macrophages call in *helper T-cells* (components of cell-mediated immunity) to assist in marshalling yet other components of the immune system.

Once activated by the presence of the antigens, helper T-cells notify a second component of cellular immunity, the *killer T-cells,* and a component of humoral immunity, *B-cells.* Killer T-cells produce powerful chemical messengers that activate specific white blood cells that are capable of destroying antigens. At the same time, B-cells are transformed into specialized cells capable of producing *antibodies,* the highly specific molecules that are capable of inactivating antigens by clumping them into groups and attacking them with chemical agents.

At the same time that helper T-cells and killer T-cells are engaged in destroying invading antigens, two additional components of cellular immunity are formed: *memory T-cells* and *suppressor T-cells.* As the name suggests, the memory T-cells remember the immune system's responses so that reinfections can be encountered even more quickly and decisively. Suppressor T-cells are specialized T-cells that moderate B-cell activity by offsetting the action of helper T-cells. Their action allows the production of antibodies to be reduced once it is apparent that the immune system has won its battle.

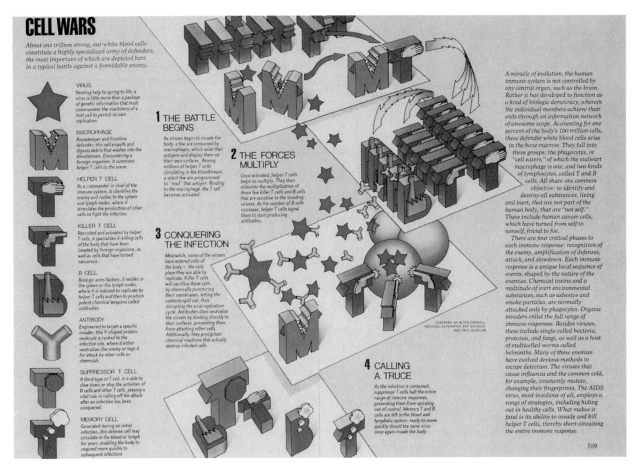

Figure 12-3 The four phases of the immune system and how they function.

People who have allergies have abnormal body reactions to certain substances called *antigens* or *allergens*. These might include certain molds, foods, plant pollens, drugs, animal hair, and insect stings. When exposed to antigens, people display allergic reactions including nasal congestion; red, swollen, watery eyes; and sneezing. Itching of the ears, nose, throat, and mouth is often reported.

The cause of allergies lies in a disturbance in the immune system. For unknown reasons, after initial exposure to a particular antigen, some individuals' bodies prepare an overly elaborate defense system to counter later exposures to that antigen. These people have developed a hypersensitivity to the antigen. In certain extreme cases a person's body may react overwhelmingly to an antigen and produce such congestion that anaphylactic shock, asphyxiation, and death may result.

Once the antigens are identified, people can attempt to avoid exposure to them, control the symptoms if an allergic response occurs, and undergo preventive treatment called *desensitization* or *immunotherapy.* ★

On this basis, the complex and highly integrated interplay of cell-mediated immunity and humoral immunity can be seen. Clearly, without a normal immune system, we would quickly become the victims of serious and life-shortening infections and malignancies.

CAUSES AND MANAGEMENT OF SELECTED INFECTIOUS DISEASES

This section focuses on some of the common infectious diseases as well as some that, although less common, are serious when contracted. We hope this information provides some reference points you can use to judge your own disease susceptibility.

The Common Cold

The common cold, an acute, upper respiratory tract infection, must reign as humankind's supreme infectious disease. Also known as **acute rhinitis,** this highly contagious viral infection is caused by one of the nearly 200 known rhinoviruses.[6] College students are easily at risk because they expose themselves to large numbers of people in crowded classrooms.

Health ACTION Guide

Tips for Self Care When You Have a Cold

When you have a cold, follow these guidelines:

▼ Stay away from others
▼ Rest
▼ Drink fluids
▼ Eat moderately
▼ Wash hands frequently
▼ Use disposable tissues
▼ Do not use over-the-counter remedies for more than a few days
▼ Contact your physician if symptoms persist

The signs and symptoms of a cold are fairly predictable. Runny nose, watery eyes, general aches and pains, a listless feeling, and a slight fever may all accompany your cold in its early stages. Eventually your nasal passages swell and the inflammation may spread to the throat. Stuffy nose, sore throat, and coughing may follow. Since your senses of taste and smell are blocked, you probably will not feel like eating very much.

With the onset of symptoms, management of a cold should begin promptly. After a few days, most of the cold's symptoms subside. In the meantime, isolate yourself from others, drink plenty of fluids, eat moderately, and rest. Keep in mind that antibiotics are effective only against bacterial infections—not viral infections.

Your management of a cold can be aided by using some of the many over-the-counter cold remedies. These remedies will not cure your cold but may lessen the discomfort associated with it. Nasal decongestants, **expectorants,** cough syrups, and aspirin (or acetaminophen) can all provide some temporary relief. Use of some of these products for more than a few days is not recommended, however, since a **rebound effect** may occur.

If your cold appears to become more persistent, as evidenced by prolonged chills, noticeable fever above 103° F, chest heaviness or aches, shortness of breath, coughing up rust-colored mucus, or persistent sore throat or hoarseness, you should contact a physician.

Unfortunately, it appears to be nearly impossible to prevent colds. Since colds are now thought to be transmitted most readily by hand contact, frequent handwashing and the use of tissues are recommended.

Influenza

Influenza is also an acute, contagious disease caused by viruses. Some influenza outbreaks have produced widespread death, as seen in the influenza pandemics of 1889-1890, 1918-1919, and 1957. The viral strains

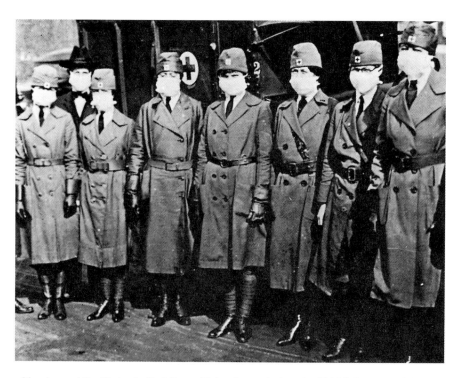

Members of the St. Louis Red Cross Motor Corps during the 1918 influenza epidemic.

What's the Difference?

DIFFERENCE	COLD	FLU
Cause	200+ viruses	Three influenza viruses
Transmission	Contact with contagious people, hand and air-borne	Airborne
Onset	Several days	A few hours
Duration	1 to 2 weeks	3 to 5 days
Symptoms	Throat soreness and irritation, sneezing, runny nose	Temperature elevation, headache, congestion, coughing, fatigue
Treatment	Symptoms relieved with over-the-counter medications	If symptoms are immediately recognized, amantadine (a prescription drug) can be taken for type-A flu
Prevention	Avoid contagious people, wash hands frequently	Flu vaccinations are 60% to 70% effective for one flu season only

that produce this infectious disease (for example, Hong Kong, Asian, Victorian, swine, and influenza A, B, and C strains) have the potential for more severe complications than the viral strains that produce the common cold. The viral strain for a particular form of influenza enters the body through the respiratory tract. After brief incubation and prodromal stages, the host develops signs and symptoms not just in the upper respiratory tract but throughout the entire body. These symptoms include fever, chills, cough, sore throat, headache, gastrointestinal disturbances, and muscular pain.

Except for possible *secondary bacterial infections,* antibiotics are not generally prescribed for people with influenza. Your physician may recommend only aspirin, fluids, and rest. Of course, parents are reminded not to give aspirin to children. Some antiviral drugs, such as amantadine, have been developed but their use is limited. (See the box above for a comparison of influenza with the common cold.)

Most young adults can cope with the milder strains of influenza that are prevalent each winter or spring season. Although we may be very uncomfortable for a while, most of us can return to our normal activities in about a week. However, pregnant women and older people—especially older people with additional health complications (heart disease, kidney disease, emphysema, chronic bronchitis)—are not so capable of handling this viral attack. They may quickly develop secondary bacterial complications (especially pneumonia), which can prove fatal. Each year in the United States, about 10,000 people die of flu and its resultant complications. In severe seasons the death toll has reached 40,000.[7] Susceptible people must attempt to prevent an influenza infection from ever reaching them in the first place. Therefore flu vaccinations are routinely recommended for older people.

For strains that appear to be especially dangerous, most health authorities recommend that all of us re-

ceive a flu vaccination. This preventive approach attempts to confer artificially acquired immunity by inoculating us with the specific (though noninfectious) viral antigen. Some inoculations may include antigens for more than one strain of virus. These are the *polyvalent vaccines.*

Tuberculosis (TB)

Until recently tuberculosis, a bacterial infection of the lungs resulting in chronic coughing, weight loss, and even death, was considered to be under control in this country. Today, however, there is renewed concern that major outbreaks (26,283 cases in 1992) of TB are underway,[8] many of which are drug resistant.

Because tuberculosis is spread through coughing, the disease thrives in crowded places where infected people are in constant contact with others. Prisons, hospitals, public housing units, and even college residence halls are places where close day-to-day contact occurs. In such settings a single infected person can spread the TB agents to many others.

When healthy people are exposed to TB agents, their immune systems generally are able to contain the bacteria in a way that both prevents the development of symptoms and reduces the likelihood of infecting others. However, when the immune system may be damaged, such as in the elderly, the malnourished,

acute rhinitis (uh **cute** rye **nye** tis) the common cold; the sudden onset of nasal inflammation.

expectorants (x **peck** tor ants) drugs that help bring mucus and phlegm up from the respiratory system.

rebound effect excessive congestion that results from the overuse of nosedrops and sprays.

and those who are HIV infected, the disease can become established and eventually be transmitted to other persons at risk.

A new form of TB is also evident—*multiple drug-resistant (MDR) TB.* Increasingly prevalent in this country, MDR is the result of patient inability to follow physician instructions when initially treated (for whatever reason), inadequate treatment by physicians, and increased exposure of HIV-infected persons to TB. Only 50% of people with this form of TB can be cured. Some believe that MDR is the next epidemic to be expected in this country.

Health officials are again requesting that TB testing programs be implemented and that those infected, once found, be isolated and brought into treatment. Every dollar spent on prevention will save $5 to $10 on treatment. Unfortunately, even as TB rates rise, major cities are cutting back on prevention and treatment programs.[9]

Pneumonia

Pneumonia is a general term under which a variety of infectious respiratory conditions can be placed. Bacterial, viral, fungal, rickettsial, mycoplasmal, and parasitic forms of pneumonia exist.[10] However, bacterial pneumonia is the most common form and is often seen in conjunction with other illnesses that weaken the body's immune system. This is why even healthy young people should consider colds and flu as potentially serious and treat them properly. In fact, pneumonia is so common in the frail elderly that it is often the specific condition causing death. *Pneumocystis carinii* pneumonia, a parasitic form, is of great importance today since it is a condition associated with the diagnosis of AIDS in HIV-infected persons.

Among older adults with a history of chronic obstructive lung disease, cardiovascular disease, diabetes, or alcoholism, a midwinter form of pneumonia known as *acute community-acquired pneumonia* is often a serious health problem.[10] The sudden onset of chills, chest pain, and a cough producing sputum are characteristics of this condition. Additionally, a symptom-free form of pneumonia known as *walking pneumonia* is also commonly seen in adults and can become serious without warning. Individuals with the illnesses listed above should be watched carefully during the high-risk season of the year and provided with effective treatment should symptoms develop.

Mononucleosis

Of all the common infectious diseases that a college student can contract, **mononucleosis (mono)** can force a lengthy period of bed rest during a semester or quarter when you can least afford it. Other common diseases that can attack you can be managed with minimal amounts of disruption. However, the overall weakness and fatigue seen in many people with mono

Health ACTION Guide

Tips for Avoiding Mononucleosis

Although no vaccine is currently available to avoid contracting mononucleosis, following these preventive measures will help you avoid this disease:

▼ Eat a well-balanced diet
▼ Exercise regularly
▼ Obtain adequate amounts of sleep
▼ Have regular health care checkups
▼ Avoid direct contact with infected individuals

sometimes require a month or two of rest and recuperation.

Mono is a viral infection in which the body produces an excess number of *mononuclear leukocytes.* After uncertain, perhaps lengthy, incubation and prodromal stages, the acute symptoms of mono can appear, including weakness, headache, low-grade fever, swollen lymph glands (especially in the neck), and sore throat. Mental fatigue and depression are sometimes reported as side effects of mononucleosis. Usually after the acute symptoms disappear, the weakness and fatigue remain—perhaps for a few months. Mono is diagnosed on the basis of characteristic symptoms. Also, the Monospot blood smear can be used to determine the prevalence of abnormal white blood cells. In addition, an antibody test can detect activity of the immune system that is characteristic of the illness.

Since this disease is caused by a virus (Epstein-Barr virus), antibiotic therapy is not recommended. Treatment most often includes bed rest and the use of over-the-counter remedies for fever (aspirin or acetaminophen) and sore throat (lozenges). In extreme cases corticosteroid drugs can be used. Appropriate fluid intake and a well-balanced diet are also important in the recovery stages of mono. Fortunately, the body tends to develop naturally acquired immunity (NAI) to the mono virus, so subsequent infections of mono are unusual.

For years mono has been labeled the "kissing disease"; however, mono is not highly contagious and is known to be spread by direct transmission in ways other than kissing. At this time no vaccine has been developed to confer artificially acquired immunity (AAI) for mononucleosis. The best preventive measures include the steps that you can take to increase your resistance to most infectious diseases: (1) eat a well-balanced diet, (2) exercise regularly, (3) sleep sufficiently, (4) use health care services appropriately, and (5) live in a reasonably healthful environment.

Chronic Fatigue Syndrome (CFS)

Perhaps the most perplexing "infectious" condition seen by physicians is **chronic fatigue syndrome.** First identified in 1985, this mononucleosis-like condition was most commonly seen in women in their thirties and forties. Its victims, many of whom were busy professional people, reported flulike symptoms, including severe exhaustion, fatigue, headaches, muscle aches, fever, inability to concentrate, allergies, intolerance to exercise, and depression. Examinations done on its first victims revealed antibodies to the Epstein-Barr virus. Thus it was assumed to be an infectious viral disease (and initially called chronic Epstein-Barr syndrome).

In the near decade since its first appearance, the condition has received a great deal of attention that has resulted in considerable confusion over its exact nature. Today, opinions vary widely as to whether the condition is (1) an Epstein-Barr viral infection, (2) a herpes virus type-6 infection, (3) an HTLV-II virus infection, or (4) a complex condition that involves both viral infections and nonviral components.[11] Some physicians may even view CFS as a psychological disorder.

Regardless of its cause(s), CFS is extremely unpleasant for its victims. Certainly, those experiencing the symtoms over an extended time need to be seen by a physician experienced in dealing with CFS.

Measles

Thought to be only a childhood disease, red measles (also called **rubeola** or common measles) has recently been seen in large numbers on some American college campuses. Red measles is the highly contagious type of measles characterized by a short-lived, relatively high fever (103° to 104° F) and a whole-body red spotty rash that lasts about a week. The other type of measles, *German measles* (**rubella,** or 3-day measles), is a much milder form of measles that has serious implications for newborn babies of mothers who contracted this disease during pregnancy.[12] Highly successful vaccines are now available for both varieties of measles and are usually given in the same injection. Women should receive these vaccinations *before* they become pregnant.

The outbreak of red measles among college students during each of the last several school years points to the fact that our society mistakenly believes that most infectious diseases have now been eliminated. Public health experts now realize that those who contracted the disease either had never been vaccinated or had been vaccinated with a killed variety vaccine used before 1969. Only students who had al-

ready had red measles as children or who had been vaccinated with a live virus were guaranteed full immunity against the red measles virus. Nontraditional college students in particular should attempt to determine whether their immunization status is based on use of the older, less effective, vaccine.

In addition to the college students who lack protection from measles, a second segment of the population is of great concern to health personnel. As mentioned earlier in the chapter, today a large percentage of preschoolers are unvaccinated and therefore unprotected. Of the more than 25,000 cases of measles in 1990, over half were among preschool children.

Today, most public school systems are requiring documented proof of immunization from a physician or clinic before children can attend classes. As educated parents, you should be conscientious about adhering to immunization schedules for your children. In fact, measles immunization efforts have increased so effectively because of school and public health department involvement that measles is now virtually on the edge of extinction.[13]

Mumps

Mumps is one of the more familiar childhood infectious diseases. A viral illness, mumps is characterized by inflammation and swelling in one or both salivary glands at the angle of the jaw. Fever, pain, and difficulty swallowing are common symptoms associated with mumps. Treatment involves fluids, bed rest, painkillers, and, in children, a few day's absence from school.[6]

When mumps occurs in older male children, adolescents, and adults, the likelihood of infection to the testicles increases. A less common condition is inflammation of the pancreas, with abdominal pain and vomiting.

Today, protection against mumps is available with the standard childhood immunization series, MMR. Those who contract mumps will develop a naturally acquired immunity to the disease.

---

mononucleosis ("mono") (mon oh nook lee **oh** sis) viral infection characterized by weakness, fatigue, swollen glands, and low-grade fever.

chronic fatigue syndrome (kron ick) illness that causes severe exhaustion, fatigue, aches, and depression; mostly affects women in their thirties and forties.

rubeola (roo be **oh** luh) red or common measles.

rubella (roo **bell** uh) German or 3-day measles.

Lyme Disease

An infectious disease that is becoming increasingly common in eastern, southeastern, upper midwestern, and west coast states is **Lyme disease.** This bacterial disease results when infected deer ticks, usually in the nymph state (Figure 12-4), attach to the skin and inject the infectious agent as they feed on a host's blood. Deer ticks become infected by feeding on infected white-tailed deer or white-footed mice.[14]

The symptoms of Lyme disease are variable but generally first appear within 30 days as small red bumps surrounded by a circular red rash at the site of bites. In conjunction with this phase I stage, flulike symptoms may appear, including chills, headaches, muscle and joint aches, and low-grade fever. For approximately 20% of infected persons, a phase II stage develops in which nervous system or heart disorders may occur. For those who remain untreated even to this stage, a phase III stage can develop in which chronic arthritis, lasting up to 2 years, can occur. Fortunately, Lyme disease can be treated with antibiotics. Unfortunately, however, no immunity develops, so subsequent infections can occur.[14] Although not yet available, a Lyme disease vaccine has been successfully tested on animals. Experts project its availability for human use by the mid-1990s.[15]

For persons living in susceptible areas, outdoor activities can expose them to the nearly invisible tick nymphs that have fallen from deer into the grass. Thus persons who are active outdoors should check themselves frequently to be sure that they are tick free.

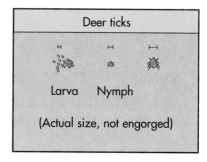

Figure 12-4 Developmental stages of deer ticks.

Shirts should be tucked into pants, pants tucked into socks, and gloves and hats worn when possible. It is also helpful to shower after coming in from outdoors and to check clothing for evidence of ticks. Pets can carry infected ticks into the house. If ticks are found, they should be carefully removed from the skin with tweezers and the affected area washed. A physician should be consulted if symptoms appear or you are concerned that you might have been exposed.

Hantavirus Pulmonary Syndrome

Since 1993 a small but rapidly expanding number of people have died of extreme pulmonary distress caused by the leakage of plasma into the lungs. In all of the initial cases the people lived in the Southwest, had been well up until they began developing flulike symptoms over 1 or 2 days, then quickly experienced difficulty breathing, and died only hours later. Epidemiologists quickly suspected a viral agent such as the hantavirus known to exist in Asia and, to a lesser degree, in Europe. Exhaustive laboratory work led to the culturing of the virus and confirmed that all of the victims had been infected with an American version of the hantavirus. The latest infectious condition, *hantavirus pulmonary syndrome*, was identified.

Today the hantavirus disease described above has been reported in areas beyond the Southwest, including most of the western states and in some of the eastern United States. The common denominator in all areas in which the hantavirus infection has occurred is the presence of deer mice. It is now known that this common rodent serves as the reservoir for the virus.

The mode of transmission of the virus from deer mice to humans involves the inhalation of dust contaminated with dried virus-rich rodent urine or saliva-contaminated materials, such as nests. In areas with deer mice populations (most of the United States), health experts are now warning people to be extremely careful when cleaning houses and barns in which deer mice droppings are likely to be found. Should it be necessary to remove rodent nests, wear rubber gloves, pour Lysol or bleach on the nests and soak them thoroughly, and finally, pick up nests with

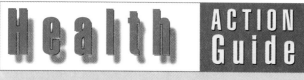

Tips for Avoiding Lyme Disease

Since Lyme disease is transmitted by the deer tick, check yourself for ticks when you have been outdoors, especially if you live in or near areas where Lyme disease has occurred. Also, follow these simple steps:

▼ Check yourself and your clothing frequently to be sure you are tick free
▼ Keep shirts tucked in, and tuck pants into socks
▼ Wear gloves and hats
▼ Shower when you come inside
▼ Check your pets for ticks, and immediately remove any that are found
▼ Consult your physician if you have any symptoms or think you may have been exposed to Lyme disease

shovels and burn or bury them in holes that are several feet deep. If done properly, these procedures should greatly minimize the airborne spread of the viral particles.[16]

To date there is no vaccine for hantavirus pulmonary syndrome, although the illness is now more quickly recognized. As a result of awareness of the importance of early evaluation of flulike symptoms, the death rate has begun to fall.

Toxic Shock Syndrome

Toxic shock syndrome (TSS), first reported in 1978, made front-page headlines in 1980, when it was reported by the Centers for Disease Control and Prevention (CDCP) that there was a connection between TSS and the presence of a specific bacterial agent *(Staphylococcus aureus)* in the vagina associated with the use of tampons. A 1980 CDCP epidemiological study indicated that 98% of 928 women who developed TSS did so during a menstrual period. The highest incidence of TSS was in females in the 15 to 19 age group.

TSS presents the signs and symptoms listed in the box on the right. Superabsorbent varieties of tampons apparently can irritate the vaginal lining three times more quickly than regular tampons. This vaginal irritation is enhanced when the tampons remain in the vagina for a long time (over 5 hours). Once this irritation has begun, the staphylococcal bacteria (which are commonly present in the vagina) have relatively easy access to the victim's bloodstream. Proliferation of these bacteria in the circulatory system and their resultant toxins produce the toxic shock syndrome. Left untreated, the victim can die—usually as a result of cardiovascular failure. Fortunately, less than 10% of women diagnosed as having TSS actually die.

Although the extent of this disease is still quite limited (only about 3 to 6 cases per 100,000 women per year) and the mortality figures are low (comparable to

---

★ **Could You Have Toxic Shock Syndrome? Recognize Its Symptoms**

★ **Fever (102° or above)**

★ **Headache**

★ **Vomiting**

★ **Sore throat**

★ **Diarrhea**

★ **Muscle aches**

★ **Sunburnlike rash**

★ **Low blood pressure**

★ **Bloodshot eyes**

★ **Disorientation**

★ **Reduced urination**

★ **Peeling of skin on the palms and soles of the feet**

---

those in women who use oral contraceptives), each woman should still exercise reasonable caution in the use of tampons during her period. Recommendations are that (1) women should not use only tampons during their menstrual periods, and (2) women should not leave tampons in place for too long a time. Women should change tampons every few hours and intermittently use sanitary napkins. Tampons should not be used during sleep. Because the use of highly absorbent tampons increases the risk of TSS by 10 times over the use of regular tampons, medical experts now recommend that women use the least absorbent tampon that fits their needs.[17] Some physicians recommend that all tampon use be curtailed if a woman wants to be extraordinarily safe from TSS.

The incidence of TSS has dropped significantly since the early 1980s. Possible reasons for this decrease are the removal of some superabsorbent tampons from the market and the standardization of the labels for junior, super, and super-plus tampons that began in 1990.[18]

Health ACTION Guide

Tips for Avoiding Toxic Shock Syndrome

Although toxic shock syndrome occurs infrequently, these steps should be followed when using tampons:

▼ Change tampons every few hours.
▼ Intermittently substitute sanitary napkins.
▼ Use sanitary napkins at night.
▼ Use the least absorbent tampon that fits your needs.

Lyme disease bacterial infection transmitted by deer ticks.

toxic shock syndrome (TSS) potentially fatal condition resulting from the proliferation of certain bacteria in the vagina that enter the general blood circulation.

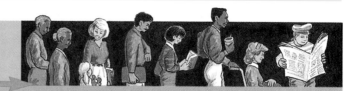

Learning FROM ALL Cultures

Hepatitis B

Because of the AIDS epidemic, some serious diseases get little attention from the media. Hepatitis B is one of these potentially dangerous diseases. It is estimated that 200 million people in the world are chronic carriers and can therefore infect others. The virus is transmitted through blood, sexual contact, and from mother to infant.

Some people who contract hepatitis B develop chronic health problems, such as cirrhosis of the liver or liver cancer. In Asia and Africa the hepatitis B virus is believed to be a major cause of liver cancer. The chronic effects of this virus are considered a major world health problem. A vaccine to prevent the virus is available, but for people in developing countries it is not widely administered.

Treatment for limiting liver damage caused by hepatitis B is currently being researched. Some folk medicines, such as the extracts of tropical weeds, are being tested. In some parts of the world these extracts are used to treat jaundice caused by some type of illness involving the liver. At the present time treatments like this are being used on patients in India.

Considering that hepatitis B is potentially preventable, why does it remain such a worldwide health concern? What do you think the focus of research should be on hepatitis B: prevention, treatment, or cure? ●

Hepatitis

Hepatitis is an inflammatory process in the liver and can be caused by several viruses. Types A, B, C (once called non-A and non-B), and D have been recognized. Additionally, hepatitis can result from abuse of alcohol and other drugs. General symptoms of hepatitis include fever, nausea, loss of appetite, abdominal pain, and jaundice (yellowing of the skin and eyes).[14]

Type A hepatitis is often associated with eating of fecally contaminated food, such as raw shellfish, or water. Poor sanitation, particularly with the handling of food, has led to outbreaks associated with restaurants, while diaper-changing activities have resulted in outbreaks in child-care centers.

Type B (HBV) hepatitis is spread in various ways including sexual contact, intravenous drug use, tattooing, and through medical and dental practice. Once spread principally through blood transfusions, this route no longer exists because of the use of effective screening tests. Chronic HBV infection has been associated with liver cirrhosis and liver cancer. Type C hepatitis is contracted in similar ways as HBV (sexual contact, tainted blood, and shared needles).

The newly identified type D (delta) hepatitis has proven very difficult to treat but is almost only found in persons already suffering from type B hepatitis. Transmission of this virus, along with type B hepatitis and HIV, makes unprotected sexual contact very risky in today's world.[14]

Acquired Immune Deficiency Syndrome (AIDS)

Acquired immune deficiency syndrome (AIDS) is rapidly becoming the most devastating infectious disease to have occurred in modern times (Table 12-3). On the basis of current data, since the initial reporting of the disease in 1981, through June 1994, 401,749 Americans have been diagnosed with AIDS and 243,423 have died from the disease.[19] Furthermore, it is estimated that by the year 2000, $13.1 billion in health insurance claims will be paid for AIDS-related illnesses.[20] Today the cost of treating one AIDS patient is $119,000: $50,000 before the onset of AIDS and $69,000 thereafter.[21] The toll in human lives and the financial burden AIDS will place on our health care system make AIDS a frightening disease.

Health ACTION Guide

Tips for Avoiding Hepatitis

▼ Use good personal hygiene habits, including careful washing of your hands.

▼ Do not use illegal drugs.

▼ Should you need to inject drugs for medical reasons, do not share needles.

▼ Avoid sexual behaviors that may put you at risk. Follow safer sex practices.

▼ If you think you may have been exposed to hepatitis, contact your physician immediately.

TABLE 12-3 The Scope of the Problem	
According to the Centers for Disease Control and Prevention, the persons most likely to develop AIDS are homosexual or bisexual males and intravenous drug users. As of June 1994, the breakdown of AIDS cases was as follows:	
Men who have sex with men	47%
Injection drug use	28%
Heterosexual contact	9%
Risk not identified	9%
Men who have sex with men and inject drugs	5%
Recipients of blood products or tissue	1%
Hemophilia or other coagulation disorders	1%
TOTAL	100%

CAUSE OF AIDS

AIDS is caused by a virus (human immunodeficiency virus, or HIV) that attacks the helper T-cells of the immune system (see p. 302). This virus has been called HTLV-III (human T-lymphotropic virus, type III), but HIV (human immunodeficiency virus) is now the more commonly recognized name.

When HIV attacks helper T-cells, the individual loses the ability to fight off a variety of infections that a person with a normal immune system could destroy. HIV-infected patients become vulnerable to infection by bacteria, protozoa, fungi, and a number of viruses and malignancies. Such infections are called *opportunistic infections,* since they develop when the immune system is weakened.

During the initial years of the AIDS epidemic the presence of specific diagnosable conditions formed the basis of receiving the clinical label of HIV + w/AIDS. Among these were *Pneumocystis carinii* pneumonia, and *Kaposi's sarcoma,* a rare but deadly form of skin cancer. Gradually additional conditions were recognized as being associated with advancing deterioration of the immune system and thus were added to the list of AIDS conditions. Eventually this list contained over 25 definitive conditions with more conditions being added as they became apparent. Among the conditions found on the current version of the list are *toxoplasmosis* within the brain, *cytomegalovirus retinitis* with loss of vision, *lymphoma* involving the brain, recurrent *salmonella septicemia,* and a *wasting syndrome* including invasive cervical cancer, recurrent pneumonia, and recurrent tuberculosis. Today, however, there is a growing tendency to assign the label of HIV + w/AIDS to HIV-infected persons when their level of T-helper cells drops below 200 cells per cubic millimeter, regardless of whether specific conditions are present.

HOW IS HIV SPREAD?

HIV cannot be contracted easily. The chances of contracting HIV through casual contact with HIV-infected patients at work, school, or at home are extremely rare or nonexistent. HIV is known to be spread only by direct sexual contact involving the exchange of body fluids (including blood, semen, and vaginal secretions),

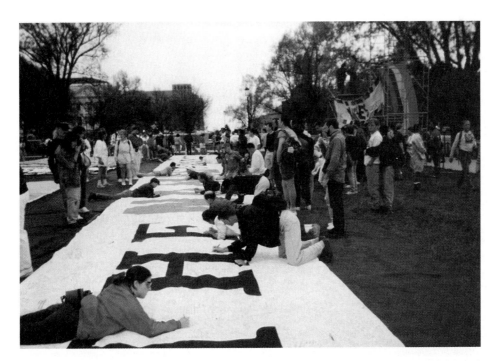

Signing of the AIDS quilt in Washington, D.C., demonstrates community support for AIDS education.

the sharing of hypodermic needles, transfusion of infected blood or blood products, and perinatal transmission (from an infected mother to a fetus or newborn baby). For HIV to be transmitted, it must enter the bloodstream of the noninfected person. HIV enters the bloodstream of noninfected persons through contaminated blood or needles and tears in body tissues lining the rectum, mouth, and reproductive system. Current research also indicates that HIV is not transmitted by sweat, saliva, or tears.

Women are at much greater risk (12 times the risk) than men for the heterosexual transmission of HIV because of the higher concentration of HIV in semen than in vaginal secretions.[22]

WHAT ARE THE SIGNS AND SYMPTOMS OF HIV INFECTION?

Most persons infected with HIV initially feel well and have no symptoms (are asymptomatic). The incubation period for HIV infection is generally considered to be from 6 months to 10 or more years, with the average being approximately 6 years. Despite the lengthy period between infection and the first clinical observation of damage to the immune system, antibodies to HIV may appear within several weeks to 3 months of contracting the virus. Of course, relatively few persons are tested for HIV infection during the incubation period. Thus infected persons could remain in the asymptomatic state (more currently referred to as HIV+ without symptoms) and be carriers of HIV for years before they would experience signs of illness sufficient enough to warrant a physical examination.

In the absence of symptoms for immune system deterioration and for AIDS testing results, sexually active people need to redefine the meaning of monogamous. Today it is very possible that two people need to account for the sexual partners that they both have had over a 10-year period before it is completely safe to assume that there have been no other partners involved in their special relationship.

Virtually all persons infected with HIV eventually develop signs and symptoms of a more advanced stage of the disease. These signs and symptoms include tiredness, fever, loss of appetite and weight, diarrhea, night sweats, and swollen glands (usually in the neck, armpits, and groin). At this point they are said to have HIV+ with symptoms. (Previously this was called ARC, for AIDS-related complex.)

Table 12-4 indicates that these persons are infectious and have damage to the immune system.

It is estimated that given sufficient time, perhaps even as long as twenty years, the vast majority (90% to 95%) of infected persons will move beyond HIV+ with symptoms to develop one or more of the over 25 conditions whose presence leads to the label HIV w/AIDS or *AIDS* being applied.

As mentioned earlier, in addition to being labeled *AIDS* on the basis of being HIV+ and having one or more of the conditions, the label is also applied to those persons whose helper T-cell count falls below 200 per cubic millimeter. A normal helper T-cell range is 800 to 1000. Therefore, even in the absence of specific conditions, some people will qualify for the label AIDS because of the degree of damage already done to their immune systems.

TABLE 12-4   Spectrum of HIV Infection

	HIV+ without symptoms (asymptomatic)	HIV+ with symptoms	HIV+ with AIDS
External signs	No symptoms Looks well	Fever Night sweats Swollen lymph glands Weight loss Diarrhea Minor infections Fatigue	Kaposi's sarcoma *Pneumocystis carinii* pneumonia and/or other predetermined illnesses Neurological disorders One or more of an additional 25 + diagnosable conditions or a T4 helper cell count falls below 200 per cubic milliliter
Incubation	Invasion of virus to 10 years	Several months to 10 or more years	Several months to 10-12 or more years
Internal level of infection	Antibodies are produced Immune system remains intact Positive antibody test	Antibodies are produced Immune system weakened Positive antibody test	Immune system deficient Positive antibody test
Infectious?	Yes	Yes	Yes

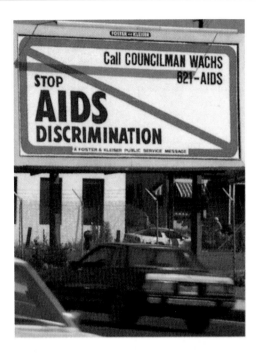

HOW IS HIV INFECTION DIAGNOSED?

The Centers for Disease Control and Prevention have established specific criteria that physicians and researchers use to define HIV infection. In addition to a clinical examination and laboratory tests for accompanying infections, HIV infection is diagnosed by the use of an initial screening test, the *enzyme-linked immunosorbent assay (ELISA)*. If antibodies to HIV are identified, a confirming test, the *western blot,* can be performed. It is estimated that 1.5 to 3 million people in this country have been infected with HIV.

TREATMENT FOR AIDS

There is no cure for HIV infection and AIDS. However, several drugs may be effective in reducing the rate at which helper T-cells are destroyed by HIV. Among these immune system–supporting medications are AZT (azidothymidine), DDI (didanosine) and ddC (didoxycytidine). Unfortunately, in comparison to other prescription medications, the cost of these new experimental AIDS drugs is very high.

Most recently the effectiveness of AZT has come under closer scrutiny. Several studies have concluded that, although AZT delays the onset of diagnosable diseases associated with AIDS (see p. 311), the harshness of the drug's side effects may so weaken its users that their real gain in life expectancy is much less than was once anticipated.[23] Regardless, AZT in combination with the other drugs mentioned above remains in the forefront of AIDS treatment. Also, a new class of HIV-influencing drugs, the proteinase inhibitors, is in

the earliest stages of development. There drugs are intended to alter the virus's ability to introduce its genetic material into the DNA of the host helper T-cell.

In addition to these drugs, physicians have a variety of medications that can be used in treating the symptoms associated with various infections and malignancies that comprise AIDS. As with AZT, DDI, and ddC, these drugs cannot reverse the victims' HIV+ status or cure AIDS.

In addition to the development of drugs to treat HIV and AIDS, research continues into the development of vaccines to prevent HIV infection. To date, no effective vaccine has been developed for humans. This inability to develop a safe, effective, and affordable vaccine (such as those that have been developed for other infectious diseases) is the result of the unique ability of HIV to alter its outer coat, quickly incorporate its genetic material into the host's T-helper cell's genetic material, and thus deprive the immune system of the ability to develop immune recognition.[24] This ability of the virus to change its appearance is so prolific that dozens of strains of HIV exist at all times in the United States. There may even be more than one version of HIV within a single individual. In ongoing trials, some volunteers who received the vaccine are now HIV+. However, why these individuals are now HIV+ cannot be conclusively determined since some of them could nave been infected shortly before being innoculated. To date over 20 killed-virus vaccines have been developed, but none has proven effective against this rapidly changing virus. A live-virus vaccine, although effective in animal studies, is still considered too dangerous for trials involving uninfected humans.

AIDS IN THE HEALTH-CARE SETTING

For students pursuing careers in health-care fields, the risk of HIV transmission is no doubt of interest. To date the news is good—with precautions the risk of infection is relatively low.

Through July 1993, health-care workers have documented occupational transmission of HIV: 8 have developed AIDS, and 78 have possibly been infected with HIV in conjunction with their work. Nurses and clinical laboratory technologists appear to be at the highest risk.[25]

Because HIV exposure is of some risk to health-care workers, universal precautions for invasive procedures and for the handling of spilled blood and body fluids have been formulated. In addition, a wide array of protective clothing to be worn during patient contact has also been developed. Policies regarding mandatory testing of all hospital patients remain under consideration.

Conversely, only five persons are known to have contracted HIV from an infected health-care worker (all were patients of the same dentist in Florida).[26] In

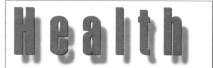

Reduce Your Risk

It is important to keep in mind that sexual partners may not reveal their true sexual history or drug habits. If you are sexually active, you can lower your risk of infection with HIV, as well as other STDs, by adopting the following safer sex practices.

▼ Learn the sexual history and HIV status of your sex partner.
▼ Limit your sex partners.

▼ Always use condoms correctly and consistently.
▼ Avoid contact with body fluids, feces, and semen.
▼ Curtail use of drugs that impair good judgment.
▼ Never share hypodermic needles.
▼ Refrain from sex with known injectable drug abusers.*
▼ Avoid sex with HIV-infected patients, those with signs and symptoms of AIDS, and the partners of high-risk individuals.*
▼ Get regular tests for STD infections.
▼ Do not insert any foreign objects into the rectum.
▼ Practice proper hygiene (shower before and after sex).

How easy will it be to adopt these behaviors? How real is your risk of becoming HIV positive? ▼

*Recent studies indicate that the elimination of high-risk persons as sexual partners is the single most effective safer sex practice that can be implemented.

an ongoing study of 15,795 persons known to have been treated by HIV+ health-care workers, no cases of HIV transmission have yet been substantiated.

PREVENTION OF HIV INFECTION

Can HIV infection be prevented? The answer is a definite "yes." There are a number of steps an individual can take to reduce the risk of contracting and transmitting HIV. All of these steps involve understanding one's behavior and the methods by which HIV can be transmitted. The U.S. Public Health Service has provided recommendations (1) for the general public, (2) for persons at increased risk of infection (including health-care workers), and (3) for persons with a positive HIV antibody test. The Public Health Service has a toll-free AIDS telephone hotline (1-800-342-AIDS), and local or state hotlines may exist. Keep informed about HIV infection and AIDS!

Although HIV infection rates on college campuses are thought to be low (approximately 0.2%), students can be at risk. The Health Action Guide above details several behaviors that, if implemented, will significantly reduce even this relatively low level of risk. If high-risk behavior has already occurred, then modifying your behavior and eventual testing are of extreme importance, not only for yourself but for others as well.

SEXUALLY TRANSMITTED DISEASES

Sexually transmitted diseases (STDs) were once referred to as venereal diseases (for Venus, the Roman goddess of love). Today the term *venereal disease* has been superseded by the broader term sexually transmitted disease. The current emphasis is on the successful prevention and treatment of STDs rather than on the ethics of sexuality. These diseases are, first and foremost, medical problems—problems that have the potential for causing infertility, birth defects, and long-term disability.

This section focuses on the STDs most frequently diagnosed among college students (chlamydia, gonorrhea, human papillomavirus infection, herpes simplex, syphilis, and pubic lice). A short section follows covering common vaginal infections, some of which may occur without sexual contact. Also, refer to the Health Action Guide above for safer sex practices.

Chlamydia (Nonspecific Urethritis)

Chlamydia is considered the most prevalent STD in the United States today. Chlamydial infections occur an estimated 5 times more frequently than gonorrhea and up to 10 times more frequently than syphilis. However, since physicians are not required to report cases of chlamydia to the Centers for Disease Control and Prevention, the true extent of the disease is not known.

Chlamydia trachomatis is the bacterial agent that causes the chlamydial infection. Chlamydia is the most common cause of nonspecific urethritis (NSU).[27] NSU refers to infections of the **urethra** and surrounding tissues that are not caused by the bacterium responsible for gonorrhea. Only when a culture smear test for suspected gonorrhea proves negative do clinicians diagnose NSU, usually by calling it chlamydia. Although not as accurate, new diagnostic tests, such as Test Pack, should allow a diagnosis to be made more quickly. About 80% of men with chlamydia indicate gonorrhea-like signs and symptoms, including painful urination and a whitish pus discharge from the penis. As in gonorrheal infections and many other STDs, most women report no overt signs or symptoms. A few women might exhibit a mild urethral discharge, painful urination, and swelling of *vulval* tissues.

Whereas oral forms of penicillin are used in the treatment of gonococcal infections, oral tetracycline or doxycycline is prescribed for chlamydia and other NSUs.

As with all STDs, both sexual partners should receive treatment to avoid the Ping-Pong effect. This effect refers to the back-and-forth reinfection that occurs among couples when only one partner receives treatment. Furthermore, as with other STDs, having chlamydia does not effectively confer immunity.

Unresolved chlamydia can lead to the same negative health consequences that result from untreated gonorrheal infections. Initially your body's immune system might contain the infection to a subclinical level, where you temporarily exhibit no ill effects. However, in men the pathogens can invade and damage the deeper reproductive structures (the prostate gland, the seminal vesicles, and Cowper's glands). Sterility can result. The pathogens can spread further and produce joint problems (arthritis) and heart complications (damaged heart valves, blood vessels, and heart muscle tissue).

In women the pathogens enter the body through the urethra or the cervical area. If not properly treated, the invasion can reach the deeper pelvic structures, producing a syndrome called **pelvic inflammatory disease (PID).** The inner uterine wall (endometrium), the fallopian tubes, and any surrounding structures may be attacked to produce this painful syndrome. A variety of further complications can result, including sterility and **peritonitis.** Infected women can transmit a chlamydial infection to the eyes and lungs of newborns during a vaginal birth. For both men and women the early detection of chlamydia and other NSUs is of paramount concern.

Human Papillomavirus (HPV)

With all of the concern about HIV and other STDs, the presence of an additional STD is unwanted news. Nevertheless, such is the case with **human papillomavirus (HPV).** Because HPV infections are generally asymptomatic, the exact extent of the disease is unknown. In a study with a group of sexually active college women, HPV infection was found in approximately 20% of the women. In 1988, nearly 500,000 office visits for STD diagnosis and treatment were related to HPV infection. HPV-related changes to the cells of the cervix have been found in nearly 5% of the Pap smears taken from women under the age of 30. It is currently believed that for women, risk factors for HPV infection include (1) sexual activity before age 20, (2) intercourse with three or more partners before age 35, and (3) intercourse with a partner that has three or more partners.[28] The extent of HPV infection in males is even less clearly known, but it is likely widespread.

The concern about HPV infections is centered around the ability of some forms of the virus to foster precancerous changes in the cervix. (There are more than 50 forms of HPV.) In addition, HPV is associated with the development of genital warts (*Condyloma acuminata*). These pinkish white lesions may be found in raised clusters that resemble tiny heads of cauliflower. Found most commonly on the penis, scrotum, labia, cervix, and around the anus, genital warts are the most common symptomatic viral STD in this country. Although most genital wart colonies are small, they may become very large and block the anus or birth canal during pregnancy.

Treatment for HPV, including genital warts, may include burning, freezing, removal with the CO_2 laser, or the use of various medications. Regardless of treatment, however, return of the viral colonies will most likely occur. Condom use should be encouraged in an attempt to slow transmission of HPV.

Gonorrhea

Another extremely common STD, gonorrhea is caused by a bacterium (*Neisseria gonorrhoae*). In men this bacterial agent can produce a milky-white discharge from the penis accompanied by painful urination. About 80% of men who contract gonorrhea report varying degrees of these symptoms. This figure is approximately reversed for women: only about 20% of women are *symptomatic* and thus report varying degrees of frequent, painful urination, with a slimy yellow-green discharge from the vagina or urethra. Oral sex with an infected partner can produce a gonorrheal infection of

---

sexually transmitted diseases (STDs) infectious diseases that are spread primarily through intimate sexual contact.

chlamydia (kla **mid** e uh) the most prevalent sexually transmitted disease. Caused by a nongonococcal bacterium.

urethra (yoo **ree** thra) passageway through which urine leaves the urinary bladder.

pelvic inflammatory disease (PID) acute or chronic infection of the peritoneum or lining of the abdominopelvic cavity; associated with a variety of symptoms and a potential cause of sterility.

peritonitis (pare it ton **eye** tis) inflammation of the peritoneum or lining of the abdominopelvic cavity.

human papillomavirus (HPV) (pap ill **oh** ma) sexually transmitted virus capable of causing precancerous changes in the cervix; causative agent for genital warts.

shingles viral infection affecting the nerve endings of the skin.

What Is Your Risk of Contracting a Sexually Transmitted Disease?

PERSONAL ASSESSMENT

A variety of factors interact to determine your risk of contracting a sexually transmitted disease (STD). This inventory is intended to provide you with an estimate of your level of risk.

Circle the number of each row that best characterizes you. Enter that number on the line at the end of the row (points). After assigning yourself a number in each row, total the number appearing in the points column. Your total points will allow you to interpret your risk for contracting an STD.

Age   **Points**

1	3	4	5	3	2	
0-9	10-14	15-19	20-29	30-34	35 +	_____

Sexual Practices

0	1	2	4	6	8	
Never engage in sex	One sex partner	More than one sex partner but never more than one at a time	Two to five sex partners	Five to ten sex partners	Ten plus sex partners	_____

Sexual Attitudes

0	1	8	1	7	8	
Will not engage in nonmarital sex	Premarital sex is okay if it is with future spouse	Any kind of premarital sex is okay	Extramarital sex is not for me	Extramarital sex is okay	Believe in complete sexual freedom	_____

Attitudes Toward Contraception

1	1	6	5	4	8	
Would use condom to prevent pregnancy	Would use condom to prevent STDs	Would never use a condom	Would use the birth control pill	Would use other contraceptive measure	Would not use any-thing	_____

Attitudes Toward STD

3	3	4	6	6	6	
Am not sexually active so I do not worry	Would be able to talk about STD with my partner	Would check an infection to be sure	Would be afraid to check out an infection	Can't even talk about an infection	STDs are no problem—easily cured	_____

YOUR TOTAL POINTS _____

INTERPRETATION

5-8   Your risk well below average
9-13   Your risk is below average
14-17 Your risk is at or near average
18-21 Your risk is moderately high
22+   Your risk is high

TO CARRY THIS FURTHER . . .

Having taken this Personal Assessment, were you surprised at your level of risk? What is the primary reason for this level? How concerned are you and your classmates and friends about contracting an STD?

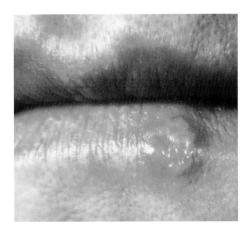

Oral herpes.

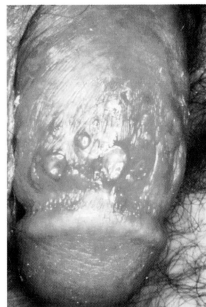
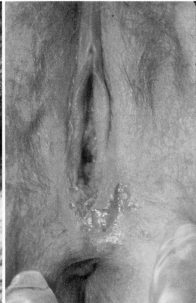

Genital herpes.

the throat (pharyngeal gonorrhea). Gonorrhea can also be transmitted to the rectal areas of both men and women.

Diagnosis of gonorrhea is made by culturing the bacteria. Antibiotic treatment regimens included use of penicillin, tetracycline, ampicillin, or other drugs. Some strains of gonorrhea (penicillin-resistant strains) are much more difficult to treat than others.

Transmission of gonorrhea is included as a part of prenatal care so that infections in mothers can be treated before birth. Should the birth canal be infected, newborns could easily contract the infection in the

mucous membrane of the eye. Most states still require that drops be placed in the eyes of all newborns to prevent this infection.

Herpes Simplex Infections

Public health officials think that the sexually transmitted genital herpes virus infection rivals chlamydia as the most prevalent STD. Recent studies show that about 16% of the adult population is infected with genital herpes virus, although most people are asymptomatic for genital herpes. Herpes is really a family of over 50 viruses, some of which produce recognized

---

Health ACTION Guide

Tips About Herpes

Although herpes rarely has serious consequences, the lesions are infectious and tend to reappear. It is important to talk openly with your partner about this sexually transmitted disease. Here are some tips to make things easier:

▼ *Educate yourself.*
   Be aware that herpes is rarely dangerous.
   Learn when the disease is most contagious (during the eruption and blister stage) and when sex is safest.

▼ *Choose the right time to talk.*
   Discuss herpes with your partner only after you have gotten to know each other.
▼ *Listen to your partners.*
   Be prepared to answer any questions that he or she may have.
▼ *Together, put things in perspective.*
   Keep a positive outlook
   Remember that you are not alone.
   Be aware that using a condom and abstaining from coitus during the most infectious period can prevent transmission of the disease.
   Although there is no known cure, research continues on an antiviral drug.
   Join a local support group together.

diseases in humans (chickenpox, **shingles,** mononucleosis, and others). One subgroup called *herpes simplex 1 virus* (HSV-1) produces an infection called *labial herpes* (oral or lip herpes). Labial herpes produces common fever blisters or cold sores seen around the lips and oral cavity. Herpes simplex 2 virus (HSV-2) is a different strain that produces similar clumps of blisterlike lesions in the genital region. Lay persons have referred to this second type of herpes as the STD type, although both types produce identical clinical pictures. Both forms can exist at either site. Oral-genital sexual practices have resulted in genital herpes cases now being caused by HSV-1.

Herpes appears as a single sore or as a small cluster of blisterlike sores. These sores burn, itch, and (for some) become quite painful. The infected person might also report swollen lymph glands, muscular aches and pains, and fever. Some patients feel weak and sleepy when blisters are present. The lesions may last from a few days to a few weeks. A week is the average time for active viral shedding. Then the blisters begin scabbing, and new skin is formed.

Herpes is an interesting virus for several reasons. It can lie dormant for extended periods. However, for reasons not well understood but perhaps related to stress, diet, or overall health, the viral particles can be stimulated to travel along the nerve pathways to the skin and then create an active infection. Thus herpes can be considered a recurrent infection. Fortunately for most people, recurrent infections are less severe than the initial episode and do not last as long. Herpes is also interesting because, unlike most STDs, no treatment method has been successful at killing the virus. Acyclovir (Zovirax), in oral, ointment, and intravenous forms, has been used successfully in reducing the number and length of genital herpes infections in certain groups of patients.[29] There are also some medications that may provide symptomatic relief. Diagnosis of genital herpes is almost always made by a clinical examination.

The best prevention against ever getting a herpes infection is to avoid all direct contact with a person who has an active infection. Do not kiss someone with a fever blister—or let them kiss you (or your children) if they have an active lesion. Do not share drinking glasses or eating utensils. Check your partner's genitals. Do not have intimate sexual contact with someone who displays the blisterlike clusters or rash. (Condoms are only marginally helpful and cannot protect against lesions on the female vulva or the lower abdominal area of the male.) Be careful not to inoculate yourself by touching a blister and then touching any other part of your body.

Newborn babies are especially susceptible to the virus should they come into contact with an active lesion during the birth process. Newborns have not developed the defense capabilities to resist the invasion.

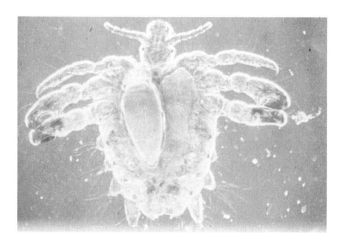

Pubic louse.

They can quickly develop a systemic, general infection (neonatal herpes) that is often fatal, or local infections that produce permanent brain damage or blindness. Fortunately, most of these possible problems can be prevented through proper prenatal care. If there is any chance that the viral particles may be present at birth, a *cesarean delivery* will be performed. This may reduce the likelihood of herpes transmission.

Syphilis

Like gonorrhea, syphilis is caused by a bacterium (*Treponema pallidum*) and is transmitted almost exclusively by sexual intercourse. The incidence of syphilis, a CDCP-reportable disease, is far lower than that of gonorrhea. However, the incidence of syphilis has risen steadily over the last several years and is now at a 40-year high. Estimated cases for 1989 were 44,000. An alarming number of these cases were also HIV+. More information of this once nearly defeated disease is presented in the box on p. 319. An alarming increase in infant syphilis has been noted in children born to mothers who use drugs and support their habit through sexual activity.

Pubic Lice

Three types of lice infect humans: the head louse, the body louse, and the pubic louse all feed on the blood of the host. Except for the relatively uncommon body louse, these tiny insects do not carry diseases. They are, however, quite annoying.

Pubic lice, also called *crabs,* attach themselves to the base of the pubic hairs, where they live and attach their eggs (nits). These eggs move into a larval stage after 1 week, and after 2 more weeks develop into mature adult crab lice.

People usually notice they have a pubic lice infestation when they are confronted with intense itching in the genital region. Fortunately, both prescription and over-the-counter creams, lotions, and shampoos are

Syphilis: The On-Again, Off-Again STD

Although we may think less often of syphilis than other sexually transmitted diseases, it remains a serious disease that if left untreated is capable of causing death. The chance of contracting syphilis during a single sexual encounter with an infected partner is now about 30%. The course taken by syphilis is well established once it is contracted.

INFECTION

The bacterium of syphilis, *Treponema pallidum,* a spirochete, is transmitted from infected person to new host through intimate contact. Moist, warm tissue, such as that lining the reproductive, urinary, and digestive systems, offers an ideal environment for the agent.

INCUBATION

After infection, an asymptomatic incubation period of from 10 to 90 days gives way to the characteristic first stage of the disease.

PRIMARY STAGE

Lasting 1 to 5 weeks, the first stage of syphilis is associated with the formation of a small, raised, painless sore called a *chancre.* In 90% of women and 50% of men this highly infectious lesion is not easily identified, thus treatment is generally not sought. The chancre heals in 4 to 8 weeks.

SECONDARY STAGE

The extremely contagious second stage of the disease is seen 6 to 12 weeks after initial infection. Because the infectious agents are now systemic, symptoms may include a generalized body rash, a sore throat, or a patchy loss of hair. A blood test (VDRL) will be positive, and treatment can be effectively administered. If untreated, the second stage will subside within 2 to 6 weeks. This is a stage during which syphilis can easily be transmitted by a pregnant woman to her fetus. Congenital syphilis often results in stillbirth or an infant born with a variety of life-threatening complications. Early treatment of infected pregnant women can prevent congenital syphilis.

LATENT STAGE

After the secondary stage subsides, an extended period of noninfectiousness is seen. The infectious agents remain dormant within the body cells, and few clinical signs exist during this stage.

LATE STAGE

Syphilis can recur for a third time 15 to 25 years after initial contact. In late stage syphilis, tissue damage will be profound and irreversible. Damage to the cardiovascular system, central nervous system, eyes, and skin occurs, and death from the effects of the disease is likely.

TREATMENT

Syphilis is treated with penicillin, tetracycline, or erythromycin. Such treatment can kill the pathogen at any stage of the infection, but it cannot reverse the physical damage caused during the late stage of syphilis. ★

---

extremely effective in killing both the lice and their eggs.

Lice are not transmitted exclusively through sexual contact, but also by contact with bedsheets and clothes that may be contaminated. Should you inadvertently develop a pubic lice infestation, you will have to treat yourself, your clothes, your sheets, and your furniture.

Vaginal Infections

Two common pathogens produce uncomfortable vaginal infections in women. The first is the yeast or fungus pathogen *Candida (Monilia) albicans,* which produces the yeast infection often called *thrush.* These organisms, commonly found in the vagina, seem to multiply rapidly when some unusual stressor (pregnancy, use of birth control pills, diabetes, use of antibiotics) affects a woman's body. This infection, called *candidiasis,* is easily noticed by a white or cream-colored vaginal discharge that resembles cottage cheese. Vaginal itching and swelling are also commonly reported. Treatment often consists of an oral antibiotic or antibiotic douche to reduce the organisms to a normal level. Recently introduced OTC drugs for vaginal yeast infections allow for effective home treatment. Initial consultation with a physician is recommended before using these new products for the first time. (Men rarely report this monilial infection, although some may report mildly painful urination or a mild discharge at the urethral opening or beneath the foreskin of the penis.)

A second common agent that produces a vaginal infection is the protozoan *Trichomonas vaginalis.* This parasite can be transmitted through sexual intercourse or by contact with contaminated (often damp) objects, such as towels, clothing, or toilet seats that may contain some vaginal discharge. In women, this "trich" infection produces a foamy, yellow-green, foul-smelling discharge that may be accompanied by itching, swelling, and painful urination. Treatment consists of a 2-week course of oral medication that helps to kill the parasite. Men infrequently contract this infection (trichomoniasis) but may harbor the organisms without realizing it.

Since the vagina is warm, dark, and moist, it is an ideal breeding environment for a variety of organisms. Normal hygienic measures seem to help keep vaginal infections at a minimum. Unfortunately, use of some highly promoted commercial products seem to lead to increased incidences of vaginal infections. Among these are tight pantyhose (without cotton panels), which tend to increase the vaginal temperature, and commercial vaginal douches, which can alter the acidic level of the vagina. Use of both of these products might promote infections. Women are advised to wipe from front to back after every bowel movement to reduce the opportunity for direct transmission of pathogenic agents from the rectum to the vagina. The avoidance of public bath facilities is also a good suggestion. Of course, if you notice any atypical discharge from the vagina, you should report this to your physician.

Cystitis and Urethritis

Cystitis, an infection of the urinary bladder, and *urethritis,* an infection of the urethra, are conditions that can be caused by a sexually transmitted organism. Other modes of transmission are also associated with cystitis and urethritis, including infection with the organisms that cause vaginitis and organisms found in the intestinal tract. A culture is required to determine the specific pathogen associated with a particular case of cystitis or urethritis. The symptoms include pain when urinating, the need to urinate frequently, a dull aching pain above the pubic bone, and the passing of blood-streaked urine.

Cystitis and urethritis can be easily treated with antibiotics when the specific organism has been identified. Few complications result from infections that are treated promptly. If cystitis and urethritis are left untreated, the possibility exists for the infectious agents to move upward in the urinary system and produce an infection of the ureters and kidneys. These upper urinary tract infections are more serious and require more extensive evaluation and aggressive treatment. It is therefore very important to obtain medical care upon noticing symptoms.

Prevention of cystitis and urethritis depends on some degree on the source of the infectious agent. In a general sense, however, the incidence of infection can be lowered by urinating completely (to fully empty the urinary bladder) and by drinking ample quantities of fluids to flush the urinary tract. Whether the drinking of cranberry juice helps reduce urinary tract infections is a debatable issue.

Summary

✔ A variety of agents are responsible for infectious conditions.

✔ A chain of infection with six links characterizes every infectious condition.

✔ Infectious conditions progress through four distinct stages.

✔ The body possesses mechanical defenses designed to prevent infectious agents from gaining entry.

✔ The immune response to infection relies on cellular and humoral elements.

✔ The common cold and influenza display many similar symptoms but differ in terms of infectious agents, incubation period, prevention, and treatment.

✔ Tuberculosis and pneumonia are potentially fatal infections of the respiratory system.

✔ Mononucleosis and chronic fatigue syndrome are viral infections that both result in chronic tiredness.

✔ Measles and mumps are childhood infections that can be potentially harmful when contracted during adulthood.

✔ Lyme disease is a bacterial infection contracted in conjunction with outdoor activities.

✔ Hantavirus pulmonary syndrome is caused by a virus carried by deer mice.

✔ Hepatitis B (serum hepatitis) is a bloodborne infectious condition that can lead to serious liver damage. Hepatitis A, C, and D also exist.

✔ HIV/AIDS is a widespread, incurable viral disease transmitted through sexual activity, intravenous drug use, the use of infected blood products, or across the placenta during pregnancy.

✔ The definitive definition of AIDS can be based on the presence of specific conditions or the diminished number of helper T-cells.

✔ Effective treatment of AIDS is limited, and prevention through the use of an effective vaccine is nonexistent.

✔ A variety of sexually transmitted conditions exists, many of which are asymptomatic in most infected females and many infected males.

✔ Safer sex practices can reduce the risk of contracting STDs.

Review Questions

1. What are the agents responsible for the most familiar infectious conditions?
2. What are the six links that form the chain of infection?
3. What are the four stages that characterize the progression of infectious conditions?
4. What are the two principal components of the immune system, and how do they cooperate to protect the body from infectious agents and abnormal cells?
5. How are the common cold and influenza similar, yet how do they differ in terms of causative agents, incubation period, prevention, and treatment?
6. What symptoms make mononucleosis and chronic fatigue syndrome similar? What aspects of each are different?
7. Why are mumps and measles more serious conditions when they develop in adults?
8. Why is outdoor activity a risk factor in contracting Lyme disease?
9. How is hepatitis B transmitted, and which occupational group is at greatest risk of contracting this infection? How do forms A, C, and D compare to hepatitis B?
10. How is HIV transmitted? To what extent is the treatment of AIDS effective? What is meant by the term *safer sex*?
11. What specific infectious diseases could be classified as being STDs?
12. Why are females more often asymptomatic for STDs than males?
13. To what extent and in what manner can STD transmission be prevented?

Think about This . . .

✔ How do you feel when a classmate or co-worker comes to class or work ill? Is it fair to expose you to his or her illness?
✔ Which infectious disease have you had in the recent past? What impact did this infection have on your day-to-day activities?
✔ What diseases have you been immunized against?
✔ How do you feel about parents who do not have their children immunized?
✔ What would your initial reaction be if you found out that someone close to you had a sexually transmitted disease?

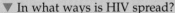

REAL LIFE REAL CHOICES

YOUR TURN

▼ In what ways is HIV spread?
▼ What are some ways in which Chris Karasawa can deal with his employees' fear of working with John Travers?
▼ To what degree do you think hospital patients and health care providers should be required to undergo HIV testing?

AND NOW, YOUR CHOICES . . .

▼ If John Travers were your classmate or co-worker, how would you feel about him and behave toward him?
▼ If you were in John Travers' situation, how would you respond to the concerns of prospective co-workers? ▼

References

1. Creager J, Black J, Davinson V: *Microbiology—principles and applications,* Englewood Cliffs, NJ, 1990, Prentice Hall.
2. Hamann B: *Disease—identification, prevention, and control,* St Louis, 1994, Mosby.
3. Moffett D, Moffett S, Schauf C: *Human physiology: foundations and frontiers,* St Louis, 1993, Mosby.
4. Salsberry PJ, Nickel JT, Mitch R: Immunization status of 2-year-olds in middle/upper—and lower-income populations: a community survey, 11(1):17-23, 1994
5. Zell ER, Vance D, Stevenson J, et al: Low vaccination levels of US preschool and school-age children, *JAMA* 271(11):833-839, 1994
6. Clayman C, editor: *The American Medical Association home medical encyclopedia,* New York, 1989, Random House.
7. Advisory Committee on Immunization Practices: Prevention and control of influenza, *MMWR* 36:373, 1987.
8. Manning A: Speeding up diagnosis of drug-resistant TB, *USA Today,* May 11, 1993.
9. Leff DR, Leff AR: Part I. Tuberculosis control policies in major metropolitan health departments in the United States, *Am Rev Respir Dis* 148(6):1530-1536, 1993.
10. Mandell G, Douglas GR, Bennett J: *Principles and practice of infectious diseases,* ed 3, New York, 1990, Churchill Livingstone.
11. Gold D et al: Chronic fatigue: a prospective clinical and virologic study, *JAMA* 264(1):48, 1990.
12. Lee S, Ewert D, Frederick P et al: Resurgence of congenital rubella syndrome in the 1990s: report on missing opportunities and failed prevention policies among women of childbearing age, *JAMA* 267(19):2616, 1992.
13. Manning A: Vaccinations whip measles epidemic, *USA Today,* May 5, 1993.
14. Crowly L: *Introduction to human disease,* ed 3, Boston, 1992, Jones & Bartlett.
15. Fikrig S et al: Protection of mice against the Lyme disease agent by immunizing with recombinant OspA, *Science* 250(4980):553, 1990.
16. Update: Hantavirus infection—United States, 1993, *MMWR* 42:517-519, 1993, as reported in *JAMA* 270(4):429-432, 1993.
17. U.S. Department of Health and Human Services, Public Health Service: Toxic shock syndrome is so rare you might forget it can happen, *DHHS Publication No. (FDA) 90-4192,* Rockville, MD, 1990.
18. Nightingala S: New requirement for tampon labeling, *Am Fam Physician* 41(3):990, 1990.
19. HOLDING FOR THE NEWEST HIV/AIDS SURVEILLANCE REPORT
20. Baumann M: AIDS cost to insurers (as reported by American Counsel of Life Insurers/Health Insurance Association of America), *USA Today,* April 15, 1991.
21. Hellinger FJ: The Lifetime cost of treating a person with HIV, *JAMA* 270(4):474-478,, 1993.
22. U.S. Department of Health and Human Services, Public Health Service, National Center for Infectious Diseases, Division of HIV/AIDS: *HIV/AIDS surveillance* (third quarter edition), Atlanta, 1993.
23. Cooper DA, Gatell JM, Kroon S, et al: Zidovudine in persons with asymptomatic HIV infection and CD4+ cell counts greater than 400 per cubic millimeter, *N Engl J Med* 329(5):297-303, 1993.
24. Bolognesi DP: A live-virus AIDS vaccine? Not yet, it is too early to consider use of a live-attenuated virus vaccine against HIV-1, *J NIH Res* 6:55-62, 1994.
25. U.S. Department of Health and Human Services, Public Health Service, National Center for Infectious Diseases, Division of HIV/AIDS: *HIV/AIDS surveillance* (second quarter edition), Atlanta, 1993.
26. Ciesielski C et al: Transmission of human immunodeficiency virus in a dental practice, *Ann Intern Med* 116(10):798, 1992.
27. Atlas RM: *Principles of microbiology,* St Louis, 1995, Mosby.
28. Ratcher R et al: *Contraceptive technology: 1990 to 1992,* ed 15, New York, 1990, Irvington Publishing.
29. Jackson J: *Wellness: AIDS, STD, and other communicable diseases,* Guilford, CT, 1992, Duskin Publishing.

Suggested Readings

Brandt A: *No magic bullet: a social history of venereal disease in the United States since 1880,* New York, 1987, Oxford University Press.
   A detailed history of the social and political factors related to sexually transmitted diseases with a chapter specifically on AIDS.
Nussbaum B: *Good intentions: how big business and the medical establishment are corrupting the fight against AIDS,* New York, 1990, Atlantic Monthly Press.
   Describes the difficulty of developing and introducing potentially beneficial drugs due to the lack of a unified effort against AIDS between the FDA and the pharmaceutical industry.
Stine GJ: *Acquired immune deficiency syndrome: biological, medical, social, and legal issues,* Englewood Cliffs, NJ, 1992, Prentice Hall.
   Written for the serious student of the AIDS epidemic. Content focuses on the entire AIDS picture, including immunology, treatment, prevention, social and legal aspects, and the pandemic scope of the disease.

Illness and major health problems influence the progress we make with respect to the five developmental tasks: identity, independence, responsibility, social skills, and intimacy. The reverse is also true. The progress we make regarding these developmental tasks has some bearing on our susceptibility to illness and our ability to recover from illness. Let us look more closely at each task.

Forming an Initial Adult Identity

Most of us probably go through life without really believing that we might one day become seriously ill. We prefer to imagine ourselves as always being free from major health problems. Our identity is based on a view of ourselves as being healthy. However, we encourage you to think occasionally about how your identity might be changed if you were to contract or develop a serious illness. What would the impact be on your view of yourself, your interactions with others, and your dreams for the future? We believe that such introspection is healthful, because it serves two purposes: it prepares us for the future and it allows us to appreciate the good health we have today.

Establishing Independence

As you move into and through adulthood, you will probably find yourself increasingly seeking ways of expressing individualism, freedom, your independence. In turn, the collective society expects you to balance this independence with some realism. You will be expected to manage finances, make academic and career decisions, and select friends according to your own criteria. Most college students relish these new opportunities.

Developing an independent lifestyle also means that you will be gradually moving away from those people you have regularly turned to for advice and support. With respect to the content in this unit, this emerging independence means that you may be forced to start experiencing illnesses all by yourself. The years of having others care for all of your health needs may nearly be over. Thus as an emerging independent adult you must become familiar with many techniques regarding self-care, prevention, and access to the health care system. Fortunately, you are the beneficiary of this growth process.

Assuming Responsibility

Nearly every day, we are being encouraged by health professionals to be active participants in the promotion of our health. We are asked to become more responsible for aspects of our health that we can control, such as our weight, alcohol and other drug use, fitness level, and dietary practices. Indeed, the collective society is losing patience with people who completely ignore the importance of living a healthful life.

Not only do irresponsible persons hurt themselves, but they also have a significant impact on the lives of others. Those who, by their own actions, are frequently ill and absent from work, overuse group health insurance protection, and place great burdens on family and friends can reduce the quality of life for everyone. Practicing preventive health measures enables you to be responsible to the collective society.

Developing Social Skills

The content in Chapters 10, 11, and 12 provides a large stage for the practice and rehearsal of social skills. From the social involvement with friends who have a chronic health condition to the intimate discussions couples have concerning possible STD transmission, it is important to feel comfortable while communicating with others. Interacting with sick people, their families, and members of the health care delivery system sometimes take persistence and a good deal of tact. For most persons, these social skills tend to develop with practice.

Developing Intimacy

Too frequently, chronic illness such as heart disease, cancer, degenerative conditions, and infections make intimacy difficult because of frequent hospitalizations, reduced energy, and the effects of medications and treatment.

In contrast though, a chronic illness can actually build a new dimension into an intimate relationship as it forces everyone to reassess their interactions with each other. For the ill person, there is greater reliance on the well partner. For the partner who is well, there is a greater than normal opportunity to express concern and give care. Although an illness can ultimately end a relationship, it can, for a while, enhance the quality of that very same relationship.

UNIT FIVE

Sexuality is an important part of our being. It colors the way in which we interact with the world around us and affects how we plan for our lives in terms of goals, relationships, reproductivity, and our role in society.

● Physical Dimension of Health

Sexuality is closely related to the physical dimension of health. Common physical changes related to sexuality include maturation at puberty, responses to sexual arousal, changes associated with contraception or pregnancy, and adjustments to increased age. How well we respond to these varied developmental processes may reflect our ability to feel comfortable about sexuality. Another point that connects sexuality and the physical dimension of health is that sexual experiences and relationships can be very demanding. Intense, pleasurable sexual experiences are fueled by energy and time. These experiences, and the relationships that accompany them, are enhanced when the body is well maintained, energized, and relatively free from illness and pain.

◆ Emotional Dimension of Health

As emerging adults, the gender images you are forming are, out of necessity, changing as your perceptions of being a woman or a man change. For example, few of you hold the same picture of femininity or masculinity today that you held when you were 14 years old. Your changing perceptions and priorities about being a man or a woman can be emotional stressors.

One of the most stressful aspects of living for many young adults concerns sexual intimacy. Feelings about your own sexually intimate behavior can range from exhilaration to ambivalence to depression. Being comfortable with your sexuality comes from acting on the basis of core values, recognizing when you are using someone or are being used by another, and being able to recover from disappointment.

■ Social Dimension of Health

As your adult sexuality emerges, interest in other people develops rapidly. Because sexuality often involves interactions with other persons, the development of social skills is imperative. For many, dating provides an excellent arena in which to establish a base of social skills. As dating relationships become more serious, skills in communication can grow significantly. These skills are, of course, important factors in the process of mate selection and marriage.

▲ Intellectual Dimension of Health

Within the context of a growing relationship, opportunities abound for individuals to contemplate, analyze, and interpret currently available information. Intellectual resources may be challenged when you examine information concerning reproductive anatomy, fertility, sexual response, contraception, and the birth process.

Sexual relationships are also valuable in providing the opportunity for the growth of the intellect through the process of introspection. Sexual relationships quickly force individuals to sort through their feelings, values, and past experiences to find guidance in pursuing a relationship.

● Spiritual Dimension of Health

Paired sexual experiences can provide you with an arena in which to serve others. In dating, courtship, and particularly in marriage, you are provided the opportunity to extend empathy, support, and love to another person. These responses reflect the highest spiritual values to which most aspire. The growth of a paired sexual relationship also presents an excellent opportunity for an individual to explore behavior and beliefs that relate to the spiritual dimension of health. Your sense of morality, the appropriateness of premarital sexual intimacy, and the value of fidelity within a marital relationship are specific touch points that you may wish to examine.

Sexuality

The Person, the Partner, the Parent

13

Sexuality

Biological and Psychosocial Origins

In the 1990s it seems that we have achieved balance in our ability to realize that both biological and psychosocial factors contribute to the complex expression of our *sexuality*. As a society we are now inclined to view human behavior in terms of a complex script written on the basis of both biology and conditioning. Reflecting this understanding is the way in which we use the words *male* and *female* to refer to the biological roots of our sexuality and the words man and woman to refer to the psychosocial roots of our sexuality. In this chapter we will explore human sexuality as it relates to the dynamic interplay of the biological base and the psychosocial base that form your *masculinity* or *femininity*.

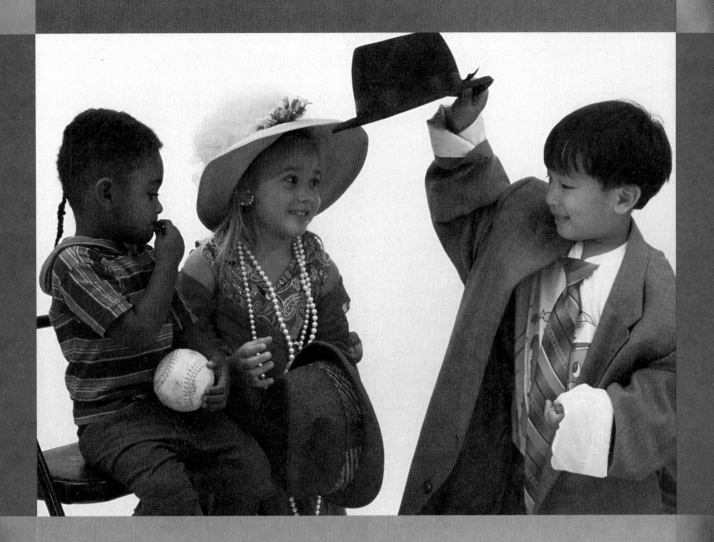

S E X U A L I T Y

The following objectives are covered in this chapter.

▼ Increase to at least 85% the proportion of people aged 10 through 18 who have discussed human sexuality, including values surrounding sexuality, with their parents or have received information through another parentally endorsed source, such as youth, school, or religious programs. (Baseline: 66% of people in 1986 aged 13 through 18 have discussed sexuality with their parents; p. 198.)

▼ Increase to at least 50% the proportion of post-secondary institutions with institution-wide health promotion programs for students, faculty, and staff. (Baseline: At least 20% of higher education institutions had offered health promotion activities for students in 1989-90; p. 256.)

▼ Increase to at least 50% the proportion of primary care providers who routinely review with patients cognitive, emotional, and behavioral functioning and the resources available to deal with problems that are identified. (Baseline data unavailable; p. 219.)

HEALTHY PEOPLE 2000 OBJECTIVES

REAL LIFE
REAL CHOICES
Sex Roles: Conflict and Change

▼ Name: Diana Schumacher Lutz and Jerry Lutz
▼ Age: 34 and 32
▼ Occupations: Diana, high school principal
  Jerry, insurance broker

"Sugar and spice and everything nice…" "Snips and snails and puppy dog tails…." In these words from an old nursery rhyme, it isn't hard to figure out which phrase applies to girls and which to boys. Girls are supposed to be sweet, quiet, and nice; boys are expected to be frisky, adventurous, and scruffy.

That's exactly how things were in both Diana and Jerry Lutz's families when they were growing up in a small, conservative farm town in western Kansas. The girls wore dresses, did housework, and tended the garden while the boys cared for livestock, fished and hunted, and tinkered with old cars.

When Diana won a full scholarship to a prestigious out-of-state university, she entered a radically different world where many women wore jeans, majored in engineering, and left dishes in the sink, while men often baked bread, raised herbs, and cleaned house—and where everyone felt free to do some, all, or none of

these activities without regard to their traditional sex-based roles.

That's the way Diana wants to bring up her and Jerry's children: Jenny, 9 and Richard, 6. But Jerry is adamantly opposed to the idea of his son baking cakes and his daughter playing rugby. He's far less stern than his parents, but he still believes in the traditional sex roles with which both he and Diana grew up. He's proud of Jenny's school record but is uncomfortable with her enthusiastic talk of being an astronaut or an architect. First-grader Richard can already name more than 20 flowering plants and loves to help his mother in the garden, but Jerry tries to distract him by suggesting they practice batting or toss the football.

Diana and Jerry don't argue or contradict each other in front of the kids, but everyone's aware of the tension caused by their conflict over appropriate sex roles.

As you study this chapter, think about the issues that confront the Lutzes, and prepare yourself to answer the questions in **Your Turn** at the end of the chapter. ▼

THE BIOLOGICAL BASES OF HUMAN SEXUALITY

Within a few seconds after the birth of a baby, someone (a doctor, nurse, or parent) emphatically labels the child:

"It's a boy," or "It's a girl." For the parents, and the society as a whole, the child's **biological sexuality** is being displayed and identified. Another male or female enters the world.

Genetic Basis

At the moment of conception a Y-bearing or an X-bearing sperm cell joins with the X-bearing ovum to establish the true basis of biological sexuality.[1] A fertilized ovum with sex chromosomes XX is a biological female, and the fertilized ovum bearing the XY sex chromosomes is a biological male. Genetics forms the most basic level of an individual's biological sexuality.

Gonadal Basis

The gonadal basis for biological sexuality refers to the growing embryo's development of **gonads.** Male embryos develop testes about the seventh week after con-

ception, and female embryos develop ovaries about the twelfth week after conception.[2]

Structural Development

The development of male or female reproductive structures is initially determined by the presence or absence of hormones produced by the developing testes—androgens and müllerian-inhibiting substance (MIS).[2] With these hormones present, the male embryo starts to develop male reproductive structures (penis, scrotum, vas deferens, seminal vesicles, prostate gland, and Cowper's glands).

Since the female embryo is not exposed to these male hormones, it develops the characteristic female reproductive structures. These structures include the uterus, fallopian tubes, vagina, labia, and clitoris.

Biological Sexuality and the Childhood Years

The growth and development of the child in terms of reproductive organs and physiological processes have traditionally been thought to be latent during the childhood years. However, a gradual degree of growth occurs in both the female and male child. The reproductive organs, however, undergo more greatly accel-

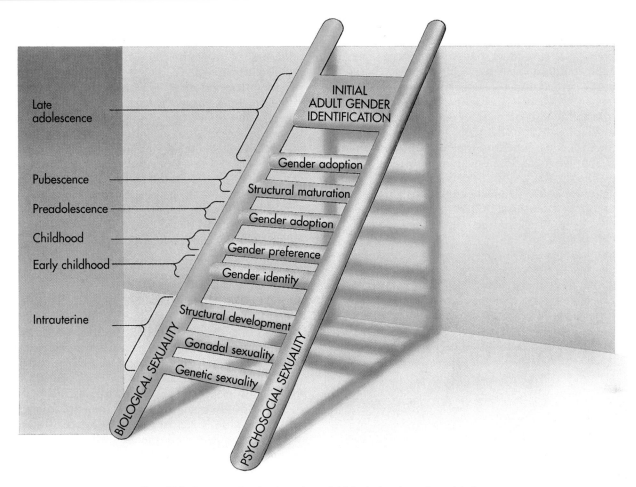

Figure 13-1 Our sexuality develops through biological and psychosocial stages.

erated growth at the onset of **puberty** and achieve their adult size and capabilities shortly thereafter.

Puberty

The entry into puberty is a gradual maturing process for young females and males. For young girls, the onset of menstruation, **menarche,** occurs around age 13, but may come somewhat earlier or later.[2] Early menstrual cycles tend to be **anovulatory.** Menarche is usually preceded by a growth spurt that includes the budding of breasts and the growth of pubic and underarm hair.[3]

Young males follow a similar pattern of maturation, including a growth spurt followed by gradual sexual maturity. However, this process takes place about 2 years later than in young females. Genital enlargement, underarm and pubic hair growth, and a lowering of the voice commonly occur. The male's first ejaculation is generally experienced by the age of 14, most commonly through **nocturnal emission** or masturbation. For many young boys, fully mature sperm do not develop until about age 15.

Reproductive capability only gradually declines over the course of the adult years. In the female, however, the onset of **menopause** signals a more direct turning off of the reproductive system than is the case for the adult male. By the early to mid 50s, virtually all women have entered a postmenopausal period,[4] but for males, relatively high-level **spermatogenesis** may continue for a decade or two.

The story of sexual maturation and reproductive maturity cannot, however, be soley focused on the changes that take place in the body. Now we will discuss the psychosocial processes that accompany the biological changes.

THE PSYCHOSOCIAL BASES OF HUMAN SEXUALITY

If growth and development of our sexuality were to be visualized as a step ladder (Figure 13-1), then one vertical rail of the ladder would represent our biological sexuality. Arising at various points along this rail would be rungs representing the sequential unfolding of the genetic, gonadal, and structural components.

Because humans, more so than any other life forms, have the ability to rise above a life centered on reproduction, a second dimension or rail to our sexuality exists—our **psychosocial sexuality.** As to why we possess the ability to be more than reproductive beings is a question to direct to the theologian or philosopher. The fact remains, however, that we are considerably more complex than those functions determined by biology. The process that transforms a male into a man and a female into a woman begins at birth and continues to influence us through the course of our lives.

Gender Identity

Although parents awaiting the birth of a baby may hold a preference for a baby of one **gender** over the other, they frequently must wait until the birth of the baby to have their question answered. The answer, in the form of an emotionally charged statement, "It's a girl!" or "It's a boy!" occurs within seconds of the delivery. At that moment expectations and aspirations

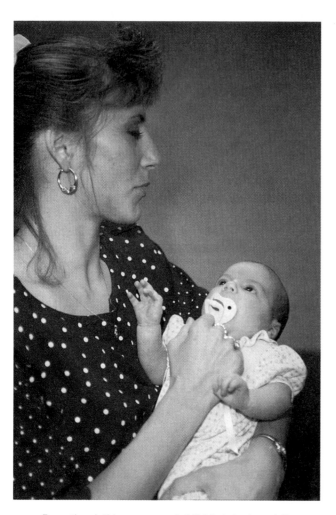

From the clothing, can you tell if this baby is a girl?

for the baby close or remain open on the basis of the child's gender. External genitals "cast the die," and femininity or masculinity begins to receive its traditional reinforcement.

During the first year and a half, the effects of parenting practices begin to inform children of the gender to which they have been assigned. Toy selection, room decorations, clothing selection, language use, and the type of physical contact employed by the parents effectively educate a child's subconscious as to what gender he or she is. By the eighteenth month, typical children have both the language and the insight to correctly identify their gender. They have established a **gender identity.**[5] The first rung rising from the psychosocial rail of the ladder (see Figure 13-1) has been climbed.

Gender Preference

During the preschool years children receive the second component of the *scripting* required for the full development of psychosocial sexuality—the desire to prefer the gender to which they have been assigned. The process whereby **gender preference** is transmitted to the child is more than likely a less subtle form of the practices observed during the gender identity period (the first 18 months). Many parents begin to actively control the child's exposure to experiences traditionally reserved for children of the opposite sex. Particularly for boys, parents will stop play activities they perceive as being too feminine.

With the recent acceleration in the importance of competitive sports for women, many of the skills and experiences once reserved for boys are now being fostered in young girls. What effect, if any, this movement will have on the speed at which gender preference is reached will be a topic of further research.*

Gender Adoption

The process of reaching an initial adult gender identification requires a considerable period of time. The specific knowledge, attitudes, and behaviors characteristic of adults must be observed, analyzed, and practiced. The process of acquiring and personalizing these insights about how men and women think, feel, and act is reflected by the term **gender adoption,** the first and third rungs below the initial adult gender identification rail of the ladder in Figure 13-1.

In addition to the construction of a personalized version of an adult sexual identity, it is important that the child and particularly the adolescent construct a *gender schema* for a member of the *opposite sex*. Clearly, the world of adulthood, with its involvement with intimacy, parenting, and employment requires that men know women and women know men. Gender adop-

*If you want to test the existence of gender preference, ask a group of first or second grade boys or girls if they would be happier being a member of the opposite sex. Be prepared for some frank replies.

tion provides an opportunity for young persons to begin to assemble this equally valuable picture of what the other sex is like.

Comprehensive sexuality programs delivered through school, youth, or religious programs can contribute greatly to a young person's efforts at gender adoption. An increase in sexuality education programs will help the U.S. reach its Healthy People 2000 objectives.

Initial Adult Gender Identification

By the time young adults have climbed all of the rungs of the sexuality ladder, they have arrived at the chronological point in the life cycle when they are charged to construct an initial adult **gender identification.** If this label seems remarkably similar to the terminology used in identifying one of the developmental tasks being used in this textbook, your observation is accurate. In fact, the task of forming an initial adult identity is closely related to developing an initial adult self-image of oneself as a man or a woman. Although most of us currently support the concept of "person" in many gender-neutral contexts (for some very valid reasons), we still must identify ourselves as either a man or a woman.

ANDROGYNY: SHARING THE PLUSES

Over the last 15 years our society has increasingly accepted an image of a person who possesses both masculine and feminine qualities. This accepted image has taken years to develop, because our society traditionally has reinforced rigid masculine roles for males and rigid feminine roles for females.

In the past, from the time a child was born, we assigned and reinforced only those roles and traits that were thought to be directly related to his or her biological sex. Boys were not allowed to cry, play with dolls, or help in the kitchen. Girls were not encouraged to become involved in sports; they were told to learn to sew, cook, and babysit. Males were encouraged to be strong, expressive, dominant, aggressive, and career oriented, while females were encouraged to be weak, shy, submissive, passive, and home oriented.

These traditional biases have resulted in some interesting phenomena related to career opportunities. Women were denied jobs requiring above-average physical strength, admittance into professional schools (law, medicine, and business) requiring high intellectual capacities, and entry into most levels of military participation. Likewise, men were not encouraged to enter traditionally feminine careers such as nursing, clerical work, and elementary school teaching.

For a variety of reasons, the traditional picture has changed. **Androgyny,** or the blending of both feminine and masculine qualities, is more clearly evident in our society now than ever before. Today it is perfectly acceptable to see men involved in raising children (in-

cluding changing diapers) and doing routine housework. On the other hand, it is also acceptable to see women entering the workplace in jobs traditionally managed by men and participating in sports traditionally played by men. Men are not scoffed at when they are seen crying after a touching movie. Women are not

---

sexuality (sex you **al** ih tee) the quality of being sexual; can be viewed from many biological and psychosocial perspectives.

masculinity (mas kyou **lin** ih tee) behavioral expressions traditionally observed in males.

femininity (fem in **nin** ih tee) behavioral expressions traditionally observed in females.

biological sexuality male and female aspects of sexuality.

gonads (**go** nads) male or female sex glands; testes produce sperm and ovaries produce ova (eggs).

puberty (**pyoo** ber tee) achievement of reproductive ability.

menarche (muh **nar** key) time of a female's first menstrual cycle.

anovulatory (an **oh** vyu luh tory) not ovulating; refers to a time period when the ovaries repeatedly fail to release an ovum.

nocturnal emission (nock **turn** al ee mish un) ejaculation that occurs during sleep; wet dream.

menopause (**men** oh pause) decline and eventual cessation of hormone production by the reproductive system.

spermatogenesis (sper mat oh **jen** uh sis) process of sperm production.

psychosocial sexuality (psy cho **so** shul) masculine and feminine aspects of sexuality.

gender (**jen** der) general term reflecting a biological basis of sexuality; the male gender or the female gender.

gender identity recognition of one's gender.

gender preference emotional and intellectual acceptance for the gender that one is.

gender adoption lengthy process of learning the behaviors that are traditional for one's gender.

gender identification achievement of a personally satisfying interpretation of one's masculinity or femininity.

androgny (an **droj** en ee) the blending of both masculine and feminine qualities.

Learning FROM ALL Cultures

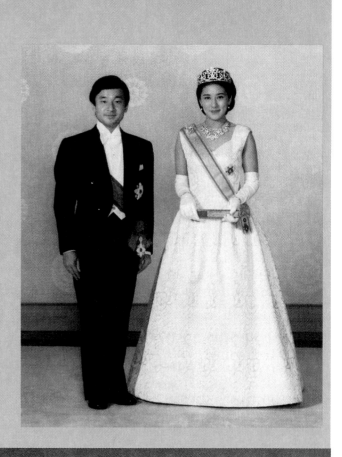

Japan's New Princess

There was a time when many little girls grew up dreaming about marrying a prince and living happily ever after. A few little girls do grow up to become princesses, but because of today's changing attitudes about the roles of men and women, being a princess may not be as desirable as it once may have been.

Japan has a new princess. Masako Owada, who became the wife of Crown Prince Naruhito. Masako Owada could be described as a modern woman; she attended Harvard and Oxford universities, speaks five languages, and until recently worked in trade relations for her government. As the new princess, life will be very different. Owada will have to live according to the traditions of Japanese royalty; ladies-in-waiting will take care of her needs, and others will manage her schedule. She will have to abide by rules and limitations. For example, if she wants to invite her friends to her home, she must attain approval from a special agency.[6]

Some would say she is taking a trip back through time. Others suggest that she will have more freedom than other Japanese princesses or empresses have ever had and that she will accomplish many things with that freedom. Has the princess given up her identity by taking on this new role, or is she embarking on a new and exciting challenge? How would you feel if you found yourself confronting a similar challenge? ●

laughed at when they choose to assert themselves. The disposal of numerous sexual stereotypes has probably benefitted our society immensely by relieving persons of the pressure to be 100% "womanly" or 100% "macho."

Research data suggest that androgynous people are more flexible, have greater self-esteem, and show more social skills and motivation to achieve.[4] This should encourage you to be unafraid to break the sex role stereotype occasionally.

THE REPRODUCTIVE SYSTEMS

The most familiar aspects of biological sexuality are the structures that compose the reproductive systems. Each structure contributes in unique ways to the reproductive process. Thus with these structures males have the ability to impregnate. Females have the ability to become pregnant, give birth, and nourish infants through breast-feeding. In addition, many of these structures are associated with nonreproductive sexual behaviors (see Chapter 14).

The Male Reproductive System

The male reproductive system consists of external structures or genitals (the penis and scrotum), and internal structures (the testes, various passageways or ducts, seminal vesicles, the prostate gland, and Cowper's glands) (Figure 13-2, *A*). The *testes* (also called *gonads* or *testicles*) are two egg-shaped bodies that lie within a saclike structure called the *scrotum*. During most of fetal development the testes lie within the abdominal cavity. They descend into the scrotum during the last 2 months of fetal life. The testes are housed in the scrotum because a temperature lower than the body core temperature is required for adequate sperm development. The walls of the scrotum are composed of contractile tissue and have the ability to draw the testes closer to the body during cold temperatures (and sexual arousal) and to relax during

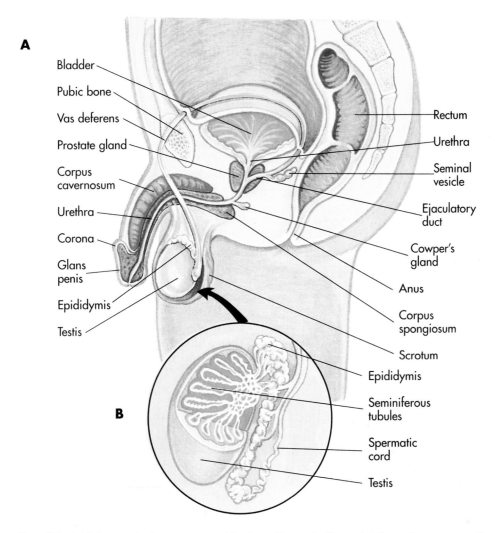

Figure 13-2 **A,** Male reproductive structures, side views. The production and delivery of sperm, as well as the production of the sex hormone testosterone, are accomplished by the male reproductive structures. **B,** Cross section of the testis.

warm temperatures. Scrotal contraction and relaxation allow a constant, productive temperature to be maintained in the testes.

A cross-sectional view of a single testis reveals an intricate network of structures called *seminiferous tubules* (Figure 13-2, *B*). It is within these 300 or so seminiferous tubules that the process of sperm production (*spermatogenesis*) takes place. Sperm cell development starts at about age 11 in boys and is influenced by the release of the hormone **ICSH (interstitial cell stimulating hormone)** from the pituitary gland. ICSH does primarily what its name suggests: it stimulates specific cells (called *interstitial cells*) within the testes to begin producing the male sex hormone *testosterone*. Testosterone in turn is primarily responsible for the gradual development of the male secondary sex characteristics at the onset of puberty. By the time a boy is approximately 15 years old, sufficient levels of testosterone exist so that the testes become capable of full spermatogenesis.

Before the age of about 15, most of the sperm cells produced in the testes are incapable of fertilization. The production of fully mature sperm (*spermatozoa*) is triggered by another hormone secreted by the brain's pituitary gland—**FSH (follicle stimulating hormone).** FSH influences the seminiferous tubules to begin to produce spermatozoa that are capable of fertilization.

ICSH (interstitial cell stimulating hormone) (in ter **stish** ul) a gonadotropic hormone of the male required for the production of testosterone.

FSH (follicle stimulating hormone) (**fol** ick uhl) a gonadotropic hormone required for initial development of ova (in the female) and sperm (in the male).

Spermatogenesis takes place around the clock, with hundreds of millions of sperm cells produced daily. The sperm cells do not stay in the seminiferous tubules, but rather are transferred through a system of ducts that lead into the *epididymis,* a tubular coil that attaches to the back side of each testicle. These collecting structures house the maturing sperm cells for 2 to 3 weeks. During this period the sperm finally become capable of motion, but they remain inactive until they mix with the secretions from the accessory glands (the seminal vesicles, prostate gland, and Cowper's glands).

Each epididymis leads into an 18-inch passageway known as the *vas deferens.* Sperm, moved along by the action of hairlike projections called *cilia,* can also remain in the vas deferens for an extended time without losing their viability.

The two vas deferens extend into the abdominal cavity, where each meets with a *seminal vesicle*—the first of the three accessory structures or glands. Each seminal vesicle contributes a clear, alkaline fluid that nourishes the sperm cells with fructose and permits the sperm cells to be suspended in a movable medium. The fusion of a vas deferens with the seminal vesicle results in the formation of a passageway called the *ejaculatory duct.* Each ejaculatory duct is only about 1 inch long and empties into the final passageway for the sperm—the urethra.

This juncture takes place in an area surrounded by the second accessory gland—the *prostate gland.* The prostate gland secretes a milky fluid containing a variety of substances, including proteins, cholesterol, citric acid, calcium, buffering salts, and various enzymes. The prostate secretions further nourish the sperm cells and also raise the pH level, making the mixture quite alkaline. This alkalinity permits the sperm greater longevity as they are transported during ejaculation through the urethra, out of the penis, and into the highly acidic vagina.

The third accessory glands, *Cowper's glands* (also called bulbourethral glands), serve primarily to lubricate the urethra with a clear, viscous mucus. These paired glands empty their small amounts of preejaculatory fluid during the arousal stage of the sexual response cycle. Alkaline in nature, this fluid also neutralizes the acidic level of the urethra. It is hypothesized that viable sperm cells can be suspended in this fluid and can enter the female reproductive tract before full ejaculation by the male.[3] This may account for many of the failures that accrue to users of the withdrawal method of contraception.

The sperm cells, when combined with secretions from the seminal vesicles and the prostate gland, form a sticky substance called **semen.** Interestingly, the microscopic sperm actually make up less than 5% of the seminal fluid discharged at ejaculation. Contrary to popular belief, the paired seminal vesicles contribute about 60% of the semen volume, whereas the prostate gland adds about 30%.[7] Thus the fear of some men that a **vasectomy** will destroy their ability to ejaculate is completely unfounded (see Chapter 15).

During *emission* (the gathering of semen in the upper part of the urethra) a sphincter muscle at the base of the bladder contracts and inhibits semen from being pushed into the bladder and urine from being deposited into the urethra.[3] Thus semen and urine rarely intermingle, even though they leave the body through the same passageway.

Ejaculation takes place when the semen is forced out of the penis through the urethral opening. The involuntary, rhythmic muscle contractions that control ejaculation result in a series of pleasurable sensations known as *orgasm.*

The urethra lies on the underside of the *penis* and extends through one of three cylindrical chambers of erectile tissue (two cavernous bodies and one spongy body). Each of these three chambers provides the vascular space required for sufficient erection of the penis. When a male becomes sexually excited, these areas become congested with blood *(vasocongestion).* After ejaculation or when a male is no longer sexually stimulated, these chambers release the blood into the general circulation and the penis returns to a **flaccid** state.

The *shaft* of the penis is covered by a thin layer of skin that is an extension of the skin that covers the scrotum. This loose layer of skin is sensitive to sexual stimulation and extends over the head of the penis, except in males who have been circumcised. The *glans* (or head) of the penis is the most sexually sensitive (to tactile stimulation) part of the male body. Nerve receptor sites are especially prominent along the *corona* (the ridge of the glans) and the *frenulum* (the thin tissue at the base of the glans).

The Female Reproductive System

The external structures (genitals) of the female reproductive system consist of the mons pubis, labia majora, labia minora, clitoris, and vestibule (Figure 13-3). Collectively these structures form the *vulva* or vulval area. The *mons pubis* is the fatty covering over the pubic bone. The mons pubis (or mons veneris or mound of Venus) is covered by pubic hair and is quite sensitive to sexual stimulation. The *labia majora* are large longitudinal folds of skin that cover the entrance to the vagina, the *labia minora* are the smaller longitudinal skin folds that lie within the labia majora. These hairless skin folds of the labia minora join at the top to form the *prepuce.* The prepuce covers the glans of the *clitoris,* which is the most sexually sensitive part of the female body.

A rather direct analogy can be made between the clitoris and the penis. In terms of tactile sensitivity, both structures are the most sensitive parts of the male and female genitals. Both contain a glans and a shaft

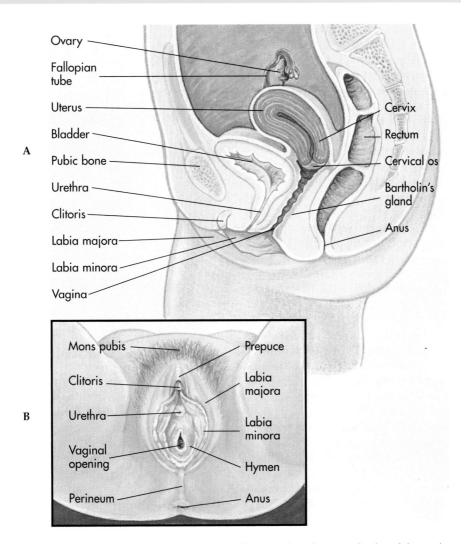

Figure 13-3 A, Female reproductive structures, side view. The formation of ova, production of the sex hormones estrogen and progesterone, and support for the developing fetus are functions of the structures of the female reproductive system. **B,** External view of female genitals.

(although the clitoral shaft is beneath the skin surface). Both organs are composed of erectile tissue that is capable of becoming engorged with blood. Both are covered by skin folds (the clitoral hood of the female and the foreskin of the male), and both can collect **smegma** beneath these tissue folds.[4]

The *vestibule* is the region enclosed by the labia minora. Evident here are the urethral opening and the entrance to the vagina (or vaginal orifice). Also located at the vaginal opening are *Bartholin's glands,* which secrete a minute amount of lubricating fluid during sexual excitement.

The *hymen* is a thin layer of tissue that stretches across the opening of the vagina. Once thought to be the only indication of virginity, the intact hymen rarely covers the vaginal opening entirely. Openings in the hymen are necessary for the discharge of menstrual fluid and vaginal secretions. Many hymens are stretched or torn to full opening by adolescent physi-

semen (see men) secretion containing sperm and other nutrients discharged from the urethra at ejaculation.

vasectomy (va sek ta me) surgical procedure in which the vas deferens are cut to prevent the passage of sperm from the testicles; the most common form of male sterilization.

flaccid (flak sid) nonerect; the state of erectile tissue when vasocongestion is not occurring.

smegma (smeg ma) cellular discharge that can accumulate beneath the clitoral hood and the foreskin of an uncircumcised penis.

cal activity or by the insertion of tampons. In women whose hymens are not fully ruptured, the first act of sexual intercourse will generally accomplish this purpose. Pain may accompany first intercourse in females with relatively intact hymens.

The internal reproductive structures of the female include the vagina, uterus, fallopian tubes, and ovaries. The *vagina* is the structure that accepts the penis during sexual intercourse. Normally the walls of the vagina are collapsed, except during sexual stimulation, when the vaginal walls widen and elongate to accommodate the erect penis. Only the outer third of the vagina is especially sensitive to sexual stimulation. In this location, vaginal tissues swell considerably to form the **orgasmic platform.** This platform constricts the vaginal opening and, in effect, grips the penis—regardless of its size.[4] Thus the belief that a woman receives considerably more sexual pleasure from men with large penises is not supported from an anatomical standpoint.

The *uterus* (or *womb*) is approximately the size and shape of a small pear. This organ is a highly muscular organ capable of undergoing a wide range of physical changes, as evidenced by its enlargement during pregnancy, its contractions during menstruation and labor, and its movement during the orgasmic phase of the female sexual response cycle. The primary function of the uterus is to provide a suitable environment for the possible implantation of a fertilized ovum, or egg. This implantation, should it occur, will take place in the innermost lining of the uterus—the *endometrium.* In the mature female the endometrium undergoes cyclic changes as it prepares a new lining on a near-monthly basis.

The lower third of the uterus is called the *cervix.* The cervix extends slightly into the vagina. Sperm can enter the uterus through the cervical opening, or *cervical os.* Mucous glands in the cervix secrete a fluid that is thin and watery near the time of ovulation. Mucus of this consistency apparently facilitates sperm passage into the uterus and deeper structures. However, cervical mucus is much thicker during portions of the menstrual cycle when pregnancy is improbable and during pregnancy, when bacterial agents and other substances are especially dangerous to the developing fetus.

The upper two thirds of the uterus constitute the *corpus* or *body.* This is where implantation of the fertilized ovum generally takes place. The upper portion of the uterus opens into two *fallopian tubes* (or *oviducts*)— each about 4 inches long. Each fallopian tube is directed toward an *ovary.* They serve as a passageway for the ovum in its week-long voyage toward the uterus. In most cases conception takes place in the upper third of the fallopian tubes.

The ovaries are analogous to the testes in the male. Their function is to produce the *ova,* or eggs. Usually one ovary produces and releases just one egg each month. Approximately the size and shape of an un-

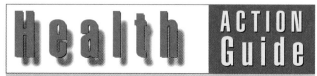

Self-Examinations

Having read about your reproductive structures, you should have a reasonable grasp of the names and locations of your genital structures. As part of a preventive health plan, most human sexuality books recommend that you routinely conduct a self-examination of your genitals. To do this:

▼ Carefully examine your genitals. Use a mirror to see structures that are difficult to see.
▼ Become familiar with your body. Learn the names of the various structures and note their typical appearance.
▼ Use your sense of touch to explore. Discover the locations that are especially sensitive.

shelled almond, an ovary produces viable ova in the process known as *oogenesis.* The ovaries also produce the female sex hormones through the efforts of specific structures within the ovaries. These hormones play multiple roles in the development of female secondary sex characteristics, but their primary function is to prepare the endometrium of the uterus for possible implantation of a fertilized ovum. In the average healthy female, this preparation takes place about 13 times a year for about 35 years. At menopause, the ovaries shrink considerably and stop nearly all hormone production.

The Menstrual Cycle

Each month or so, the inner wall of the uterus prepares for a possible pregnancy. When a pregnancy does not occur (as is the case throughout most months of a woman's fertile years), this lining must be released and a new one prepared. The breakdown of this endometrial wall and the resultant discharge of blood and endometrial tissue is known as *menstruation* (or *menses*) (Figure 13-4). The cyclic timing of menstruation is governed by hormones released from two sources: the pituitary gland and the ovaries.

Girls generally have their first menstrual cycle *(menarche)* sometime between 12 and 14 years of age. Body weight, nutrition, heredity, and overall health are factors that are related to menarche. Interestingly, after a girl first menstruates, she may be anovulatory for a year or longer before she releases a viable ovum during her cycle. She will then continue this cyclic activity until about age 45 to 55.

For purposes of explanation, this text refers to a menstrual cycle that lasts 28 days. Be assured that few

Menstrual cycle

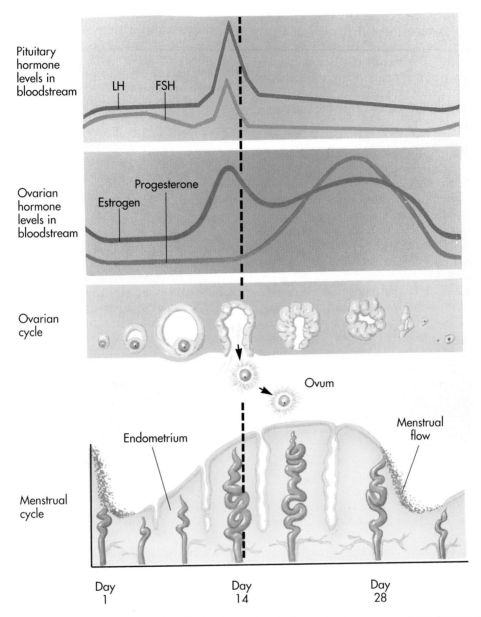

Pituitary hormone levels in bloodstream

LH   FSH

Ovarian hormone levels in bloodstream

Progesterone

Estrogen

Ovarian cycle

Ovum

Menstrual flow

Endometrium

Menstrual cycle

Day 1

Day 14

Day 28

Figure 13-4 The menstrual cycle involves the development and release of an ovum, supported by hormones from the pituitary, and the buildup of the endometrium, supported by hormones from the ovaries, for the purpose of establishing a pregnancy.

women display absolutely perfect 28-day cycles. Most women fluctuate by a few days to a week around this 28-day pattern. Some women vary extremely from this average cycle.

Your knowledge about the menstrual cycle is critical for your understanding of pregnancy, contraception, menopause, and issues related to the overall health and comfort of women. Although at first it may sound like a complicated process, each segment of the cycle can be studied separately for better understanding.

The menstrual cycle can be thought of as occurring in three segments or phases. The first is the menstrual phase (lasting about 1 week); the second is the proliferative phase (also lasting about 1 week); and the third is the secretory phase (lasting about 2 weeks). Day 1 of this cycle starts with the first day of bleeding, or menstrual flow.

orgasmic platform (or **gaz** mick) expanded outer third of the vagina that during the plateau phase of the sexual response pattern grips the penis.

The *menstrual phase* signals the woman that a pregnancy has not taken place and that her uterine lining is being sloughed off. During a 5- to 7-day period, a woman discharges about one-fourth to one-half cup of blood and tissue. (Only about 1 ounce of the menstrual flow is actual blood.) The menstrual flow is heaviest during the first days of this phase. Since the muscular uterus must contract to accomplish this tissue removal, some women experience uncomfortable cramping during menstruation. Most women, however, report more pain and discomfort during the few days before the first day of bleeding. (See the discussion of premenstrual syndrome [PMS] below.)

Modern methods of absorbing menstrual flow include the use of internal tampons and external pads. Caution must be exercised by the users of tampons to prevent the possibility of toxic shock syndrome (TSS) (see Chapter 12). Since menstrual flow is a positive sign of good health, women are encouraged to be normally active during menstruation.

The *proliferative phase* of the menstrual cycle starts about the time menstruation stops. Lasting about 1 week, this phase is first influenced by the release of follicle stimulating hormone (FSH) from the pituitary gland. FSH circulates in the bloodstream and directs the ovaries to start the process of maturing approximately 20 primary ovarian *follicles.* Thousands of primary egg follicles are present in each ovary at birth. These follicles resemble shells that house immature ova. As these follicles ripen under FSH influence, they release the hormone *estrogen.* Estrogen's primary function is to direct the endometrium to start the development of a thick, highly vascular wall. As the estrogen levels increase, the pituitary gland's secretion of FSH is reduced. Now the pituitary gland prepares for the surge of the **luteinizing hormone (LH)** required to accomplish ovulation.[8]

In the days immediately preceding ovulation, one of the primary follicles (called the *graafian follicle*) matures fully. The other primary follicles degenerate and are absorbed by the body. The graafian follicle moves toward the surface of the ovary. When LH is released in massive quantities about day 14, the graafian follicle bursts to release the fully mature ovum. The release of the ovum is called **ovulation.**

The ovum is quickly captured by the fingerlike projections (*fimbriae*) of the fallopian tubes. In the upper third of the fallopian tubes, this ovum is capable of being fertilized for a period of 24 to 36 hours. If the ovum is not fertilized by a sperm cell, it will begin to degenerate and eventually be absorbed by the body.

After ovulation, the *secretory phase* of the menstrual cycle starts when the remnants of the graafian follicle restructure themselves into a **corpus luteum.** The corpus luteum remains inside the ovary secreting estrogen as well as a fourth hormone—*progesterone.* Progesterone (literally meaning "for pregnancy") continues

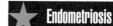

★ Endometriosis

Endometriosis is a condition in which endometrial tissue that normally lines the uterus is found growing within the pelvic cavity. Because the tissue remains sensitive to circulating hormones, it is the source of pain and discomfort during the latter half of the menstrual cycle. Endometriosis is most commonly found in younger women and is frequently related to infertility.

In addition to discomfort before menstruation, the symptoms of endometriosis include low back pain, pain during intercourse, and a variety of lower digestive tract symptoms such as diarrhea and constipation. As with the general pain and discomfort of endometriosis, these symptoms are also more noticeable during the latter weeks of the cycle.

Treatment of endometriosis depends to a large degree on its extent. Drugs to suppress menstruation, including birth control pills, may be helpful in mild cases. For more severe cases, surgical removal of the tissue or a hysterectomy may be necessary. For some women, endometriosis is suppressed during pregnancy and does not return after pregnancy. ★

to direct the endometrial buildup. If pregnancy occurs, the corpus luteum monitors progesterone and estrogen levels throughout the pregnancy. If pregnancy does not occur, high levels of progesterone signal the pituitary to stop the release of LH and the corpus luteum starts to degenerate on about day 24. When estrogen and progesterone levels diminish significantly by day 28, the endometrium is discharged from the uterus and out the vagina. The secretory phase ends and the menstrual phase begins. The cycle is complete.

PREMENSTRUAL SYNDROME (PMS)

Premenstrual syndrome (PMS) is characterized by psychological (depression, lethargy, irritability, aggressiveness) and somatic (headache, backache, asthma, acne, epilepsy) symptoms that recur in the same phase of each menstrual cycle, followed by a symptom-free phase in each cycle. Some of the more frequently reported symptoms of PMS include tension, tender breasts, fainting, fatigue, abdominal cramps, and weight gain.

The cause of PMS appears, most likely, to be hormonal. Perhaps a woman's body is insensitive to a normal level of progesterone, or her ovaries fail to produce a normal amount of progesterone. These reasons seem plausible because PMS-type symptoms do not occur during pregnancy, a time during which natural progesterone levels are very high, and because women with PMS seem to feel much better after receiving high doses of natural progesterone in suppository form. When using oral contraceptives that supply synthetic progesterone at normal levels, many women report relief from some symptoms of PMS. At the time of this writing however, the effectiveness of the most frequently used form of treatment, progesterone suppositories, is being questioned.

Until the effectiveness of progesterone has been fully researched, it is unlikely that the medical community will deal with PMS through any approach other than a relatively conservative treatment of symptoms through the use of *analgesic drugs* (including *prostaglandin inhibitors*), diuretic drugs, dietary modifications (including restriction of caffeine and salt), vitamin B$_6$ therapy, exercise, and stress-reduction exercises. The exact nature of PMS has been further complicated by the classification of severe PMS as a mental disturbance by some segments of the American Psychiatric Association.

FIBROCYSTIC BREAST CONDITION

In some women, particularly those who have yet to experience pregnancy, stimulation of the breast tissues by estrogen and progesterone during the menstrual cycle results in an unusually high degree of secretory activity by the cells lining the ducts. The fluid released by the secretory lining finds its way into the fibrous connective tissue areas in the lower half of the breast, where in pocketlike cysts the fluid presses against neighboring tissue. Excessive secretory activity produces in many women, a fibrocystic breast condition characterized by swollen, firm or hardened, tender breast tissue before menstruation.

Women who experience a more extensive fibrocystic condition can be treated with drugs that have a calming effect on progesterone production. In addition, occasional draining of the fluid-filled cysts can bring relief.

ADDITIONAL ASPECTS OF HUMAN SEXUALITY

Earlier in this chapter, we identified the biological and psychosocial bases of our sexuality. In this section we explore three additional aspects of our sexuality—reproductive, genital, and expressionistic—around which many of our important decisions in life are made.* With these new perspectives in mind, you will be better able to see the complexity associated with our development as productive and satisfied beings.

Reproductive Sexuality

Of these three aspects of sexuality, *reproductive sexuality* reflects the most basic level of sexuality over which

*We cite no specific source for the terms *reproductive sexuality, genital sexuality,* and *expressionistic sexuality.* They are labels we and our colleagues use in instructional units associated with human sexuality.

the adult must exercise direction and display insight. Simply stated, reproductive sexuality is related to your knowledge of, desire for, and ability to participate in the act of *procreation.* Pregnancy, delivery, natural childbirth, breast-feeding, fertility control, and pregnancy termination are terms related to this dimension of sexuality. Demographic data indicate that most (but not all) of you will choose to be active in this dimension of your sexuality by becoming parents.

Genital Sexuality

Genital sexuality refers to the nonreproductive use of the reproductive organs. In comparison with the concept of reproductive sexuality, genital sexuality implies *recreation* and *communication* rather than procreation. The behaviors and meanings associated with the terms orgasm, having sex, making love, oral-genital sex, prostitution, and sexual responsiveness are genital in their orientation.

In the most positive sense, sexual experiences that are genitally oriented should be sensual, erotic, and stimulating, and should give the individual a sense of release. Genital sexuality reflects our gift to ourselves and to our partners as well. However, many forms of genital sexuality may not be condoned by certain groups of people or religions.

For some genital sexuality can be a volatile experience. Far too frequently a genitally centered sexual experience results in an unanticipated and unwanted pregnancy. In such circumstances the couple, or more often the female acting alone, is forced to make decisions that could significantly influence the future. An unexpected pregnancy, even for the relatively mature college person, may result in a series of necessary compromises. Also, the close association between genital sexuality and sexually transmitted diseases (including HIV infection) makes some sexual activities potentially dangerous.

For some people genital sexuality becomes the mode of communication with which they feel most comfortable. In such cases, partners may be known only in a very limited way. Growth in sexual technique may readily occur within the context of a genitally cen-

luteinizing hormone (LH) (loo tee en eye zing) a gonadotropic hormone of the female required for fullest development and release of ova; ovulating hormone.

ovulation (ov you **lay** shun) the release of a mature egg from the ovary.

corpus luteum (kore pus loo **tee** um) cellular remnant of the graafian follicle after the release of an ovum.

PERSONAL ASSESSMENT

Respond to each of the following statements by selecting a numbered response (1-5) that most accurately reflects you feelings. Circle the number of your selection. At the end of the questionnaire, total these numbers for use in interpreting your responses.

1. Agree strongly
2. Agree moderately
3. Uncertain
4. Disagree moderately
5. Disagree strongly

Men and women have greater differences than they have similarities.	①	2	3	4	5
Homosexuality and bisexuality are immoral and unnatural.	1	2	3	4	⑤
Our society is too sexually oriented.	①	2	3	4	5
Pornography encourages sexual promiscuity.	1	②	3	4	5
Children know far too much about sex.	1	②	3	4	5
Education about sexuality is solely the responsibility of the family.	①	2	3	4	5
Dating begins far too early in our society.	①	2	3	4	5
Sexual intimacy before marriage leads to emotional stress and damage to one's reputation.	1	2	③	4	5
Sexual availability is far too frequently the reason that people marry.	1	2	③	4	5
Reproduction is the most important reason for sexual intimacy during marriage.	1	2	3	④	5
Modern families are too small.	1	2	③	4	5
Family planning clinics should not receive public funds.	1	2	3	4	⑤
Contraception is the woman's responsibility.	1	2	3	4	⑤
Abortion is the murder of an innocent child.	1	2	3	4	⑤
Marriage has been weakened by the changing role of women in society.	1	2	③	4	5
Divorce is an unacceptable means of resolving marital difficulties.	1	②	3	4	5
Extramarital sexual intimacy will destroy a marriage.	①	2	3	4	5
Sexual abuse of a child does not generally occur unless the child encourages the adult.	1	2	3	4	⑤
Provocative behavior by the woman is a factor in almost every case of rape.	1	2	3	4	⑤
Reproduction is not a right but a privilege.	①	2	3	4	5

Your Total Points _____

INTERPRETATION

20-34 points   A very traditional attitude toward sexuality

35-54 points   A moderately traditional attitude toward sexuality

55-65 points   A rather ambivalent attitude toward sexuality

66-85 points   A moderately open attitude toward sexuality

86-100 points   A very open attitude toward sexuality

TO CARRY THIS FURTHER...

Were you surprised at your results? Compare your results with those of a roommate or close friend. How do you think your parents would score on this assessment?

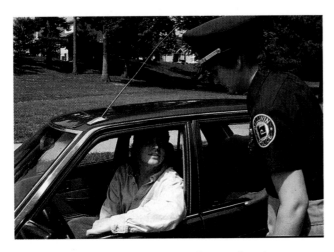

Ideas about traditional sex roles are changing.

tered relationship, but little in the way of a fully developed relationship will occur. Genitally based relationships are rarely elevated to a much higher level.

Expressionistic Sexuality

Expressionistic sexuality represents the most broadly based dimension of yourself as a man or woman. As its name implies, this is your expression of your current gender schema. Cognitively, **affectively,** and behaviorally, you are playing out your initial adult gender identification. The way you dress, the occupation you pursue, and the leisure activities you develop are all aspects of this dimension of your sexuality.

Expressionistic sexuality encompasses the reproductive and genital dimensions of your sexuality, but it is more. It is the sexuality that will serve you most fully for the rest of your life. Most adults probably are conventional in their patterns of expressionistic sexuality, yet a variety of additional patterns also exists (see Chapter 14).

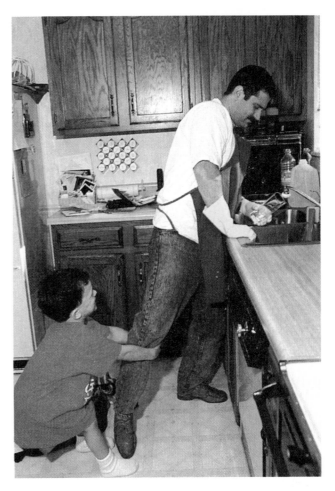

affective (af **feck** tive) pertaining to beliefs, values, and predispositions.

Summary

✔ Biological and psychosocial factors contribute to the complex expression of our sexuality.

✔ The genetic basis of biological sexuality begins at conception.

✔ The gonadal basis of biological sexuality begins with development of testes or ovaries.

✔ The structural basis of sexuality begins as the male or female reproductive structures develop in the growing embryo and fetus. Structural sexuality changes as one moves through adolescence and later life.

✔ The psychosocial processes of gender identity, gender preference, and gender adoption form the basis for an initial adult gender identification.

✔ Androgynous people seem better able to cope with life's stressors.

✔ The male and female reproductive structures are external and internal. The complex functioning of these structures is controlled by hormones.

✔ The menstrual cycle's primary functions are to produce ova and to develop a supportive environment in the uterus.

✔ FSH and LH are hormones from the pituitary gland that influence the menstrual cycle. Estrogen and progesterone influence the menstrual cycle but come from the ovaries.

✔ Premenstrual syndrome and fibrocystic breast condition are health concerns that are related to hormonal changes during the menstrual cycle.

Review Questions

1. Explain the following bases of our biological sexuality: genetic, gonadal, and structural development.

2. Explain the role of the male hormones in the structural development in female and male embryos.

3. Describe the physical changes that take place in both males and females during puberty.

4. Define and explain the following terms: gender identity, gender preference, gender adoption, gender schema, and initial adult gender identification.

5. Define androgyny. What are the advantages of an androgynous lifestyle? What are the disadvantages?

6. Identify the major components of the male and female reproductive systems. Explain the structure of each component and its function in the reproductive process.

7. Trace the passageways for sperm and ova.

8. Explain the menstrual cycle. Identify and describe the three stages of the menstrual cycle.

9. Differentiate between reproductive, genital, and expressionistic aspects of sexuality.

10. Which hormones are thought to be responsible for the development of PMS and fibrocystic breast condition?

Think about This . . .

✔ How would you summarize your feelings about the changes in your body that took place during puberty?

✔ What kinds of activities were you encouraged to participate in during your early years?

✔ Do you feel your character is mostly masculine, mostly feminine, or androgynous?

✔ To what extent do you believe that PMS is primarily a physical problem?

REAL LIFE, REAL CHOICES

YOUR TURN

▼ What is the term used to describe the blending of male and female qualities?

▼ Do you identify more strongly with Jerry or with Diana? Why?

▼ How do you think Diana and Jerry can resolve their conflict over appropriate sex roles for their children?

AND NOW, YOUR CHOICES...

▼ What were your parents' attitudes about sex roles when you were growing up? Were you comfortable with their treatment of you and your siblings in this respect?

▼ If you are now a parent or plan to have children, do you or will you use your parents' approach to sex roles, or something different? In each case, give reasons for your answer. ▼

References

1. Moffett D, Moffett S, Schauf C: *Human physiology,* ed 2, St Louis, 1993, Mosby.
2. Hyde JS: *Understanding human sexuality,* ed 5, New York, 1994, McGraw-Hill.
3. Haas K, Haas A: *Understanding sexuality,* ed 3, St Louis, 1993, Mosby.
4. Crooks R, Baur K: *Our sexuality,* ed 5, Menlo Park, CA, 1993, Benjamin-Cummings.
5. Strong B, DeVault C: *Human sexuality,* Mountain View, CA, 1994, Mayfield.
6. Powell B: The reluctant princess, *Newsweek,* pp. 28-39, May 24, 1993.
7. Thibodeau GA: *Structure and function of the body,* ed 10, St Louis, 1993, Mosby.
8. Hatcher RA et al: *Contraceptive technology 1994-1996,* ed 16, New York, 1994, Irvington Publishers.

Suggested Readings

Belliotti RA: *Good sex: perspectives on sexual ethics,* Lawrence, KS, 1993, University Press of Kansas.
An in-depth exploration of the ethical dimensions of human sexuality. A professor of philosophy, Belliotti draws upon history, philosophy, and current social criticism to explore social, moral, and political perspectives of sexuality.

Haas A, Haas K: *Understanding sexuality,* ed 3, St Louis, 1993, Mosby.
A college-level textbook suitable for an introductory human sexuality course, this book presents a comprehensive overview of issues and scientific topics related to sexuality.

Salcedo H: *The prostate: facts and misconceptions,* New York, 1993, Birch Lane Press.
This physician writes about common diseases that affect the prostate gland, including benign hypertrophy and prostatitis. Designed to ease men's fears and encourage prostate awareness. Includes many diagrams, charts, and drawings.

14

Sexuality

A Variety of Behaviors and Relationships

The focus of Chapter 14 is on sexuality as it relates to your experiences in paired relationships. In light of the American College Health Association's listing of sexual issues as the most critical health area for college students in the 1990s,[1] the topics of sexual responsiveness, patterns of sexual behavior, dating, mate selection, marriage, alternatives to marriage, and sexual orientations and variations are explored.

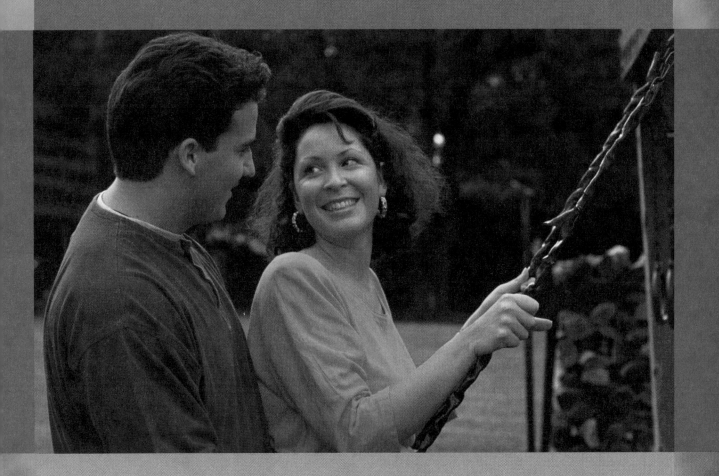

BEHAVIORS AND RELATIONSHIPS

The following objectives are covered in this chapter:

▼ Reduce the proportion of adolescents who have engaged in sexual intercourse to no more than 15% by age 15 and no more than 40% by age 17. (Baseline: 27% of girls and 33% of boys by age 15; 50% of girls and 66% of boys by age 17; reported in 1988; p. 484.)

▼ Increase to at least 40% the proportion of ever sexually active adolescents age 17 and younger who have abstained from sexual activity for the previous 3 months. (Baseline: 26% of sexually active girls ages 15 through 17 in 1988; p. 195.)

▼ Increase to at least 75% the proportion of people age 10 and older who have discussed issues related to nutrition, physical activity, sexual behavior, tobacco, alcohol, other drugs, or safety with family members on at least one occasion during the preceding month. (Baseline data available in 1991; p. 260.)

▼ Reduce to no more than 30% the proportion of all pregnancies that are unintended. (Baseline: 56% of pregnancies in the previous 5 years were unintended, either unwanted or earlier than desired, in 1988; p. 191.)

REAL LIFE
REAL CHOICES

I Love You, But... Running from the "M" Word

▼ Name: Kim Hendricks
▼ Age: 22
▼ Occupation: Law Student

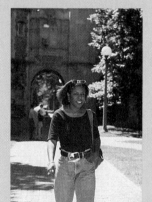

"Love and marriage, love and marriage/Go together like a horse and carriage..." So went the lyrics to a popular song of the early 1950s, when most Americans still believed that true love always led to the exchange of vows to love, honor, and cherish till death do us part.

But although lifelong commitments offer comfort and security to many people, there are those, like Kim Hendricks, to whom weddings, rings, and promises are a cruel hoax. Her parents were divorced when she was in the first grade, and she and her older brothers not only had to deal with shuttling between two households but also had to adjust to a bewildering succession of new stepparents and siblings as their parents continued their pattern of marrying, divorcing, and remarrying. Every time, Kim recalls, she and her brothers heard the same refrain from a parent: "This is really the one, kids. This won't be like it was with Bob (or Irene). We're finally going to be a real family."

Despite these promises and each parent's good intentions, however, somehow the happy, stable, "forever" family scene never made it to real life. Kim's parents weren't promiscuous or abusive—they just kept repeating their old mistakes and dragging their children into each new "dream" marriage.

As a teenager, Kim enjoyed dating and the usual round of high school social activities; but no matter how much she liked and was attracted to a boy, she never wanted to get serious or talk about the future. When she was applying to colleges, she chose schools that were far from her home town, which not only enabled her to get away from her parents' tangled lives but also made it easier to break up with her high school boyfriend.

Kim worked hard to obtain a scholarship during her undergraduate years. Now busy with her studies, Kim is very involved with the pressures and demands of law school, as well as occasionally tutoring students for extra income. She talks with her parents and brothers on the phone but rarely visits, always claiming to be too swamped at school. She's comfortable with her sexuality and twice has been in love, but at the first mention of a long-term commitment, she runs fast the other way rather than get tangled up in the sad chaos typical of her parents' marriage-go-round.

As you study this chapter, think about Kim's childhood experiences and resulting feelings, and prepare yourself to answer the questions in **Your Turn** at the end of the chapter. ▼

THE HUMAN SEXUAL RESPONSE PATTERN

Genital sexuality—the sexuality of recreation, communication, and performance—exists because of the ability of the human body to respond to erotic stimuli. Rooted in biological function, sexual responsiveness links the biologically based reproductive sexuality with the psychosocially conditioned expressionistic sexuality. Genital sexuality can be an important component in human relationships. The healthy adult can take pleasure in the fact that there is an easily accessible pathway whereby arousal, release, and intense satisfaction can come from structures whose primary purpose is reproduction.

Although history has many written and visual accounts of the human's ability to be sexually aroused, it was not until the pioneering work of Masters and Johnson[2] that the events associated with arousal were clinically documented. Five questions posed by these researchers gave direction to a series of studies involving the scientific evaluation of human sexual response.

1. Is there a predictable pattern associated with the sexual response of males and females?
2. Is the sexual response pattern stimulus specific?
3. What differences occur in the sexual response patterns of males and females? What differences might be found among members of the same sex? Within a given individual?
4. What are the basic physiological mechanisms underlying a sexual response pattern?
5. What role is played by specific organs and organ systems within the sexual response pattern?

Question 1—a Predictable Response Pattern

The answer to the first question posed by the researchers was an emphatic "yes." A predictable sexual response pattern was identified.[2] The sexual response pattern consists of an initial **excitement stage,** a **plateau stage,** the **orgasmic stage,** and a **resolution stage.** Each stage involves predictable changes in the structural characteristics and physiological function of reproductive and nonreproductive organs in both the male and female. These changes are shown in the box on pp. 348-349.

Question 2—Stimulus Specificity

The research of Masters and Johnson[2] clearly established a "no" answer to the second question concerning stimulus specificity. Their findings demonstrated that numerous sensory modalities can supply the stimuli necessary for initiating the sexual response pattern. Although tactile stimuli might initiate arousal in most people and maximize it for the vast majority, in both males and females visual, olfactory, auditory, and *vicariously formed stimuli* can accomplish the same sexual arousal patterns.

Question 3A—Male versus Female Response Pattern

In response to the third question, several differences are observable when comparing the sexual response patterns of males and females:

▼ With the exception of some late adolescent males, the vast majority of males are not multiorgasmic. The **refractory phase** of the resolution stage prevents most males from experiencing more than one orgasm in a short period, even though sufficient stimulation is available.

▼ Females possess a **multiorgasmic capacity.** As many as 10% to 30% of all adult females routinely experience multiple orgasms.[2]

▼ Although they possess multiorgasmic potential, Masters and Johnson found that about 10% of all adult females are *anorgasmic*—that is, they never experience an orgasm.[2] For many anorgasmic females orgasms can be experienced when masturbation, rather than **coitus,** provides the stimulation.

▼ When measured during coitus, males generally reach orgasm more quickly than do females. However, when masturbation is the source of stimulation, females reach orgasm as quickly as do males.[2]

More important than any of the differences pointed out is the finding that the sexual response patterns of males and females are far more alike than they are different. Not only do males and females experience the four basic stages of the response pattern, but they also have similar responses in specific areas, including the **erection** and *tumescence* of sexual structures; the ap-

pearance of a **sex flush;** the increase in cardiac output, blood pressure, and respiratory rate; and the occurrence of *rhythmic pelvic thrusting.*

Question 3B—Variation: Within a Same-Sex Group

When a group of subjects of the same sex was studied in an attempt to answer questions about similarities and differences in the sexual response pattern, Masters and Johnson noted considerable variation. Even when variables such as age, race, education, and general health were held constant, the extent and duration of virtually every stage of the response pattern varied.

Question 3C—Variation: Within the Same Individual

For a given person, the nature of the sexual response pattern does not remain constant, even when observed over a relatively short period. A variety of internal and external factors can alter this pattern. The aging process, changes in general health status, levels of stress, altered environmental settings, use of alcohol and other drugs, and behavioral changes in a sexual partner or a relationship can cause one's own sexual response pattern to change from one sexual experience to another.[3]

---

excitement stage initial arousal stage of the sexual response pattern.

plateau stage (plah **toe**) second stage of the sexual response pattern; a leveling off of arousal immediately before orgasm.

orgasmic stage (or **gaz** mick) third stage of the sexual response pattern; the stage during which neuromuscular tension is released.

resolution stage fourth stage of the sexual response pattern; the return of the body to a pre-excitement state.

refractory phase (re **frac** tor ee) that portion of the male's resolution stage during which sexual arousal cannot occur.

multiorgasmic capacity potential to have several orgasms within a single period of sexual arousal.

coitus (**co** ih tus) penile-vaginal intercourse.

erection (e **rek** shun) the engorgement of erectile tissue with blood; characteristic of the penis, clitoris, nipples, labia minora, and scrotum.

sex flush the reddish skin response that results from increasing sexual arousal.

Sexual Response Pattern

UNAROUSED STAGE

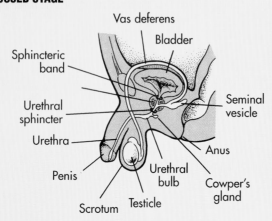

Vas deferens
Bladder
Sphincteric band
Urethral sphincter
Urethra
Penis
Scrotum
Testicle
Urethral bulb
Cowper's gland
Anus
Seminal vesicle

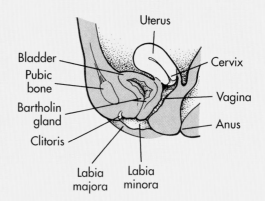

Uterus
Bladder
Pubic bone
Bartholin gland
Clitoris
Labia majora
Labia minora
Cervix
Vagina
Anus

EXCITEMENT STAGE

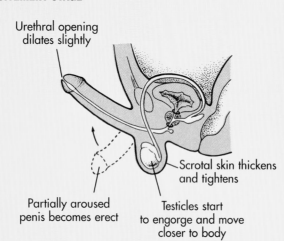

Urethral opening dilates slightly
Partially aroused penis becomes erect
Scrotal skin thickens and tightens
Testicles start to engorge and move closer to body

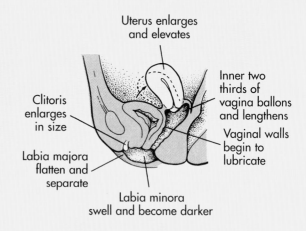

Uterus enlarges and elevates
Clitoris enlarges in size
Labia majora flatten and separate
Inner two thirds of vagina ballons and lengthens
Vaginal walls begin to lubricate
Labia minora swell and become darker

PLATEAU STAGE

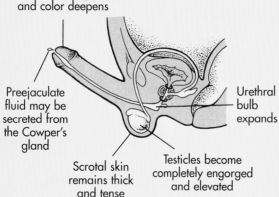

Glans enlarges and color deepens
Preejaculate fluid may be secreted from the Cowper's gland
Scrotal skin remains thick and tense
Testicles become completely engorged and elevated
Urethral bulb expands

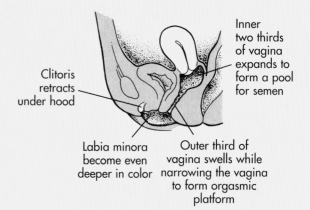

Clitoris retracts under hood
Labia minora become even deeper in color
Outer third of vagina swells while narrowing the vagina to form orgasmic platform
Inner two thirds of vagina expands to form a pool for semen

ORGASMIC STAGE

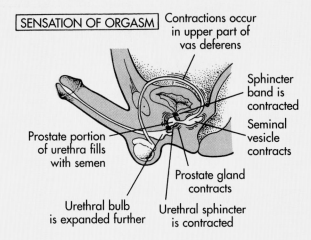

SENSATION OF ORGASM
Contractions occur in upper part of vas deferens

Sphincter band is contracted

Seminal vesicle contracts

Prostate portion of urethra fills with semen

Prostate gland contracts

Urethral bulb is expanded further

Urethral sphincter is contracted

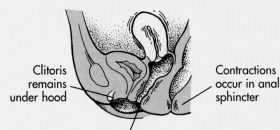

Uterine contractions occur

Clitoris remains under hood

Contractions occur in anal sphincter

Contractions in outer third of the vagina occur rhythmically 3 to 15 times; the first of these contractions are spread at 0.8-second intervals; latter contractions are weaker and occur more slowly

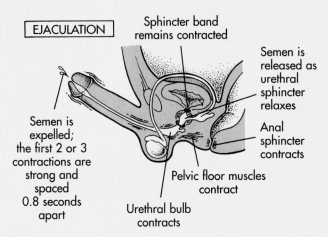

EJACULATION

Sphincter band remains contracted

Semen is released as urethral sphincter relaxes

Anal sphincter contracts

Semen is expelled; the first 2 or 3 contractions are strong and spaced 0.8 seconds apart

Pelvic floor muscles contract

Urethral bulb contracts

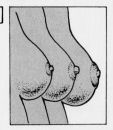

BREAST CHANGES

1. *Unaroused stage*

2. *Excitement stage*
   Breast size increases; nipples become erect; veins become more visible

3. *Plateau and orgasmic stages*
   Breast size increases more; areola increases in size (making nipples appear less erect); skin color may become flushed from vasocongestion

RESOLUTION STAGE

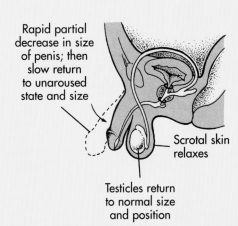

Rapid partial decrease in size of penis; then slow return to unaroused state and size

Scrotal skin relaxes

Testicles return to normal size and position

Uterus returns to normal position

Cervical canal enlarges

Clitoris quickly returns to normal position and slowly returns to unaroused state

Inner two thirds of vagina returns to normal in 5 to 8 minutes

Vaginal lips slowly return to unaroused position and color

Outer third of vagina quickly returns to normal

Question 4—Physiological Mechanisms Underlying the Sexual Response Pattern

The basic mechanisms in the fourth question posed by Masters and Johnson are now well recognized. One factor, *vasocongestion,* or the retention of blood or fluid within a particular tissue, is of major importance in the development of physiological changes that promote the sexual response pattern. The presence of erectile tissue underlies the changes that can be noted in the penis, breast, and scrotum of the male, and the clitoris, breast, and labia minora of the female.

A second mechanism now recognized as necessary for the development of the sexual response pattern is that of *myotonia,* or the buildup of *neuromuscular tonus* within a variety of body structures. At the end of the plateau stage of the response pattern a sudden release of the accumulated neuromuscular tension gives rise to the rhythmic muscular contractions and muscular spasms that constitute orgasm as well as ejaculation in the male.

Question 5—Role of Specific Organs in the Sexual Response Pattern

The fifth question posed by Masters and Johnson concerning the role played by specific organs and organ systems during each stage of the response pattern can be readily answered by referring to the material presented in the preceding box. As you study this box, remember that direct stimulation of the penis and either direct or indirect stimulation of the clitoris are the principal avenues toward orgasm. Also, intercourse represents only one activity that can lead to orgasmic pleasure.[4]

PATTERNS OF SEXUAL BEHAVIOR

Whereas sex researchers may see sexual behavior in terms of the human sexual response pattern just described, most people are more interested in the observable dimensions of sexual behavior. We begin by discussing celibacy and end with heterosexual coital behavior.

Celibacy

Celibacy can be defined as the self-imposed avoidance of sexual intimacy. Celibacy is synonymous with sexual abstinence. There are many reasons why people could choose not to have a sexually intimate relationship. For some, celibacy is part of a religious doctrine. Others might be afraid of sexually transmitted diseases. For the majority, however, celibacy is preferred simply because it seems appropriate for them. Celibate persons certainly have deep, intimate relationships with other people—just not sexual relationships. Celibacy may be short term or last a lifetime, and no identified physical or psychological complications appear to result from a celibate lifestyle.

Masturbation

Throughout recorded history, **masturbation** has been a primary method of achieving sexual pleasure. Through masturbation, people can explore their sexual response patterns. Traditionally, some societies and religious groups have condemned this behavior based on the belief that intercourse is the only acceptable sexual behavior. With sufficient lubrication, masturbation cannot do physical harm. Today masturbation is considered by most sex therapists and researchers to be a normal source of self-pleasure.[5]

Fantasy and Erotic Dreams

The brain is the most sensual organ in the body. In fact, many sexuality experts classify **sexual fantasies** and **erotic dreams** as forms of sexual behavior. Particularly for people whose verbal ability is highly developed, the ability to create rich vicarious scenes enriches other forms of sexual behavior.

Sexual fantasies are generally found in association with some second type of sexual behavior. When occurring before coitus or masturbation, fantasies prepare a person for the behavior that will follow. As an example, fantasies experienced while reading a book may focus your attention on sexual activity that will occur later in the day.

When fantasies occur in conjunction with another form of sexual behavior, the second behavior may be greatly enhanced by the supportive fantasy. Both females and males fantasize during foreplay and coitus.[6] Masturbation and fantasizing are inseparable activities.

Erotic dreams occur during sleep in both men and women. The association between these dreams and ejaculation resulting in a nocturnal emission (wet dream) is readily recognized in males. In females, erotic dreams can lead not only to vaginal lubrication, but to orgasm as well.

Shared Touching

Virtually the entire body can be an erogenous zone when sensual contact between partners is involved. A soft light touch, a slight application of pressure, the brushing back of a partner's hair, and gentle massage are all forms of communication that heighten sexual arousal.

Genital Contact

Two important uses can be identified for the practice of stimulating a partner's genitals. The first is that of being the tactile component of **foreplay.** Genital contact, in the form of holding, rubbing, stroking, or caressing, heightens arousal to a level that allows for progression into intercourse.

The second role of genital contact is that of *mutual masturbation* to *orgasm.*[6] Stimulation of the genitals so that both partners experience orgasm is a form of sex-

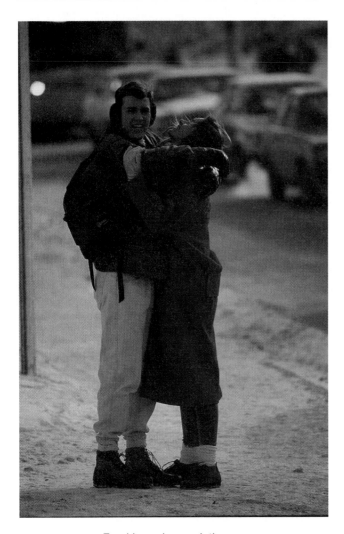
Touching enhances intimacy.

ual behavior practiced by many persons as well as couples during the late stage of a pregnancy. For couples not wishing a pregnancy, the risk of pregnancy is virtually eliminated when this becomes the form of sexual intimacy practiced.

As is the case of other aspects of intimacy, genital stimulation is best enhanced when partners can talk about their needs, expectations, and reservations. Practice and communication can shape this form of contact into a pleasure-giving approach to sexual intimacy.

Oral-Genital Stimulation

Oral-genital stimulation brings together two of the body's most erogenous areas: the genitalia and the mouth. Couples who engage in oral sex consistently report that this form of intimacy is highly satisfactory. Some persons have experimented with oral sex and found it unacceptable, and some have never experienced this form of sexual intimacy. Some couples pre-

fer not to participate in oral sex because they consider it immoral (according to religious doctrine), illegal (which it is in some states), or unhygienic (because of a partner's unclean genitals). Some couples may refrain because of the mistaken belief that oral sex is a homosexual practice. Regardless of the reason, a person who does not consider oral sex to be pleasurable should not be coerced into this behavior.

Because oral-genital stimulation can involve an exchange of body fluids, the risk of disease transmission is real. Small tears of mouth or genital tissue may allow transmission of disease-causing pathogens. Only couples who are absolutely certain that they are free from all sexually transmitted diseases (including HIV infection) can practice unprotected oral sex. Couples in doubt should refrain from oral-genital sex or carefully use a condom (on the male) or a latex square to cover the female's vulval area. Increasingly, latex squares (dental dams) can be obtained from drugstores or pharmacies. (Dentists may also provide you with dental dams, or you can make your own latex square by cutting a condom into an appropriate shape.)

Three basic forms of oral-genital stimulation are practiced by both heterosexual and homosexual couples.[7] **Fellatio,** in which the penis is sucked, licked, or kissed by the partner, is the most common of the three. **Cunnilingus,** in which the vulva of the female is kissed, licked, or penetrated by the partner's tongue, is only slightly less frequently practiced.

Mutual oral-genital stimulation, the third form of oral-genital stimulation, combines both fellatio and cunnilingus. When practiced by a heterosexual couple, the female partner performs fellatio on her partner, while her male partner performs cunnilingus on her. Homosexual couples can practice mutual fellatio or cunniligus.

masturbation (mas ter **bay** shun) self-stimulation of the genitals.

sexual fantasies fantasies with sexual themes; sexual daydreams or imaginary events.

erotic dreams (er **ot** ick) dreams whose content elicits a sexual response.

foreplay (**four** play) activities, often involving touching and caressing, that prepare individuals for sexual intercourse.

fellatio (fuh **lay** she oh) oral stimulation of the penis.

cunnilingus (kun uh **ling** gus) oral stimulation of the vulva or clitoris.

Sexual Performance Difficulties and Therapies

For all of the predictability of the human sexual response pattern, many people find that at some point in their lives they are no longer capable of responding sexually. The inability of a person to perform adequately is identified as a sexual difficulty or dysfunction. Sexual difficulties can have a corrosive influence on a person's sense of sexual satisfaction and on a partner's satisfaction. Fortunately, most sexual difficulties can be resolved through strategies that use individual, couple, or group counseling. Most sexual performance difficulties stem from psychogenic factors.

Difficulty	Possible causes	Therapeutic approaches
WOMEN		
Orgasmic difficulties		
Inability to experience orgasm	Anxiety, fear, guilt, anger, poor self-concept; lack of knowledge about female responsiveness; inadequate sexual arousal; interpersonal problems with partner	Counseling to improve a couple's communication; educating a woman and her partner about female responsiveness; teaching a woman how to experience orgasm through masturbation
Vaginismus		
Painful, involuntary contractions of the vaginal muscles	Previous traumatic experiences with intercourse (rape, incest, uncaring partners); fear of pregnancy; religious prohibitions; anxiety about vaginal penetration of any kind (including tampons)	Counseling to alleviate psychogenic causes; gradual dilation of the vagina with woman's fingers or dilators; systematic desensitization exercises; relaxation training
Dyspareunia		
Painful intercourse	Insufficient sexual arousal; communication problems with partner, infections, inflammations; structural abnormalities; insufficient lubrication	Individual and couple counseling with a focus on relaxation and communication; medical strategies to reduce infections and structural abnormalities
MEN		
Erectile Dysfunction		
Inability to achieve an erection (impotence)	Chronic diseases (including diabetes, vascular problems, and chemical dependencies); trauma; numerous psychogenic factors (including anxiety, guilt, fear, poor self-concept)	Medical intervention (including possible vascular surgery or the use of penile implants); couple counseling using sensate focusing, pleasuring, and relaxation strategies
Rapid Ejaculation		
Ejaculating too quickly after penile penetration; premature ejaculation	Predominantly psychogenic; a male's need to prove his sexual prowess; anxiety associated with previous sexual experiences	Counseling to free the man from the anxiety associated with rapid ejaculation; altering coital position; masturbation prior to intimacy; use of the squeeze technique as orgasm approaches
Dyspareunia		
Painful intercourse	Primarily physical in origin; inability of the penile foreskin to retract fully; urogenital tract infections; scar tissue in seminal passageways; insufficient lubrication	Medical care to reduce infection or repair damaged or abnormal tissue; additional lubrication

Intercourse

Sexual intercourse (coitus) refers to the act of inserting the penis into the vagina. Intercourse is the sexual behavior that is most directly associated with **procreation.** For some, intercourse is the only natural and appropriate form of sexual intimacy.

The incidence of sexual intercourse is a much-studied topic. Information concerning the percentages of persons who have engaged in intercourse is readily available in textbooks used in sexuality courses. Data concerning sexual intercourse among college students may be changing somewhat because of concerns about HIV infection and other STDs, but a reasonable estimate of the percentage of college students reporting sexual intercourse is between 65% and 80%.

These percentages reflect two major concepts about the sexual activity of college students. The first is that a large majority of college students are having intercourse. The second major concept is that a sizable percentage (20% to 35%) of students are choosing to refrain from intercourse. Indeed, the belief that "everyone is doing it" may be a bit shortsighted. From a public health standpoint, we believe it is important to provide accurate health information to protect those who choose to have intercourse and to actively support a person's right to choose not to have intercourse. (This position is supportive of the Healthy People 2000 objectives.)

Couples need to share their expectations concerning techniques and the desired frequency of intercourse. Even the "performance" factors, such as depth of penetration, nature of body movements, tempo of activity, and timing of orgasm are of increasing importance to many couples. Issues concerning sexually transmitted diseases (including HIV infection) are also critical for couples who are contemplating intercourse. These factors also need to be explored through open communication.

A variety of books (including textbooks) provide written, as well as visually explicit, information on intercourse positions. The four basic positions for intercourse—*male above, female above, side by side,* and *rear entry*—offer relative advantages and disadvantages.

THREE-STAGE DATING—MATE SELECTION MODEL

Although a dating–mate selection sequence involving casual dating, steady dating, and engagement is very familiar to you, the process that propels two persons along this continuum may be unfamiliar. Therefore we present a three-stage model to account for this movement. We recognize, of course, that a model can be nothing more than a word picture to describe how a process might occur. Your experiences are the criteria on which you can judge your relationships. Also, it is

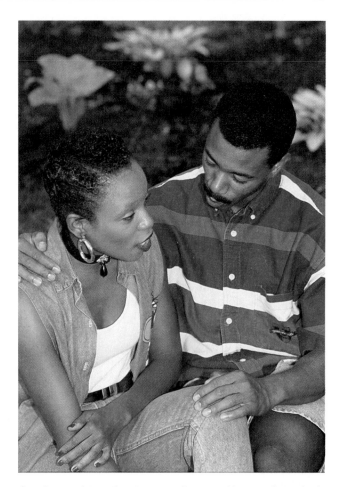

Couples need to arrive at a mutually agreeable sexual standard.

important to remember that many couples might be dating just for companionship, not as part of a mate selection process.

Stage 1—the Marketing Stage

The earliest stage of dating begins when, after meeting a new person, you construct an ideal image of yourself that you want to transmit to this person. The very same process is, of course, being undertaken by the new partner. You become the recipient of a carefully constructed facade. You both are "putting your best foot forward." **Infatuation** with your partner may be strong during this stage.

In this initial stage of dating, and at each of two remaining stages, both you and your partner are operating on the basis of personal gains and losses. Relationships continue at one level so long as gains at that level

---

procreation (pro kree **a** shun) reproduction.

infatuation (in fat you **a** shun) an often shallow, intense attraction to another person.

are deemed sufficient. Relationships progress when both partners wish to experience new and more highly valued gains and are willing to risk greater losses. Difficulties begin when partners progress at different rates in their desire for greater gains.

For most young adults, dating at this marketing stage may last only a relatively short time as both partners quickly tire of dealing with shallow "perfection" and begin to want to know what exists beyond the partner's titles, memberships, clothes, or physical appearance. For these individuals, dating will progress to the second level of our dating–mate selection model.

Stage 2—the Sharing Stage

The second stage in the progression from casual dating to marriage is made possible by a desire of the partners to explore the underlying belief systems that account for the compatibility found during the latter portion of the marketing stage. The fact that two persons appear to have things in common and appear to enjoy each other is no longer a good enough reason for continuing a relationship. Maturity and self-awareness urge couples to discover why the relationship seems to be headed in the direction of increased commitment and permanence. Infatuation declines as the relationship deepens.

The sharing stage of the dating–mate selection model can occur only when the two partners are willing to act on their interest in knowing more about each other. A commitment to engaging in the verbal exchange of ideas and information is critical. Open and honest discussions about future hopes, priorities, beliefs, and concerns must occur regularly.

Health ACTION Guide

"Dos and Don'ts" About Dating

▼ Do convey your honest feelings.
▼ Do discuss contraception and STDs before having any sexual contact.
▼ Do offer to pay for some expenses.
▼ Do be courteous and try to have a good time.
▼ Do respect the feelings and wishes of your date.
▼ Don't break a date unless absolutely necessary.
▼ Don't gossip about your date.
▼ Don't use your date to hurt other people.
▼ Don't allow yourself to be pressured into sex.
▼ Don't lie to your date.

Can you add anything else to this list? ▼

This stage of the dating–mate selection process will more than likely be labeled by the observer as steady dating. As the relationship grows in its depth of understanding, the movement toward permanence becomes more evident. Time alone cannot, however, sustain the growth of a relationship if the exchange of value-centered information by both partners does not take place. And certainly an enjoyable sexual relationship cannot alone substitute for meaningful communication.

As was the case in the cautious stage of the dating–mate selection process, both partners must feel they are making sufficient gains to justify their continued participation. Particularly because of the need to be increasingly open and honest with yourself and your partner, feelings of vulnerability are common during this stage.

Indeed, the sharing stage of the dating–mate selection process is critical. If you marry after moving through only the marketing stage of the process, the marriage's stability will be extremely questionable. A marriage after you move through the second stage of the process should be much better equipped to handle the demands of marriage.

Stage 3—the Behavior Stage

As you might well have determined by now, the third stage of the dating–mate selection process centers around the ability of you and your partner to transfer values into consistently observable behaviors. For you or your partner to have discussed these values during the sharing stage is, of course, important to the maturing of your relationship. In the third stage, however, you must now determine whether your behaviors are consistent with the values you shared in the second stage. The mate selection process will not be fully completed until this stage has been undertaken.

LOVE

Love may be one of the most elusive, yet widely recognized, concepts that describe some level of emotional attachment to another. Haas and Haas[3] describe five forms of love, including erotic, friendship, devotional, parenteral, and altruistic love. Other behavioral scientists have focused primarily on two types of love most closely associated with dating and mate selection: *passionate love* and *companionate love*.[4]

Passionate love, also described as romantic love or infatuation, is a "state of extreme absorption in another. It is characterized by intense feelings of tenderness, elation, anxiety, sexual desire, and ecstasy."[4] Often appearing early in a relationship, passionate love typically does not last very long. Passionate love is driven by the excitement of being closely involved in a relationship with a person whose character is not fully known.

How Compatible Are You?

This quiz will help test how compatible you and your partner's personalities are. You should each rate the truth of these 20 statements based on the following scale. Circle the number that reflects your feelings. Total your scores and check the interpretation following the quiz.

1 Never true
2 Sometimes true
3 Frequently true
4 Always true

We can communicate our innermost thoughts effectively.	1	2	3	4
We trust each other.	1	2	3	4
We agree on whose needs come first.	1	2	3	4
We have realistic expectations of each other and of ourselves.	1	2	3	4
Individual growth is important within our relationship.	1	2	3	4
We will go on as a couple even if our partner doesn't change.	1	2	3	4
Our personal problems are discussed with each other first.	1	2	3	4
We both do our best to compromise.	1	2	3	4
We usually fight fairly.	1	2	3	4
We try not to be rigid or unyielding.	1	2	3	4
We keep any needs to be "perfect" in proper perspective.	1	2	3	4
We can balance desires to be sociable and the need to be alone.	1	2	3	4
We both make friends and keep them.	1	2	3	4
Neither of us stays down or up for long periods.	1	2	3	4
We can tolerate the other's mood without being affected by it.	1	2	3	4
We can deal with disappointment and disillusionment.	1	2	3	4
Both of us can tolerate failure.	1	2	3	4
We can both express anger appropriately.	1	2	3	4
We are both assertive when necessary.	1	2	3	4
We agree on how our personal surroundings are kept.	1	2	3	4

YOUR TOTAL POINTS _____

INTERPRETATION

20-35 points You and your partner seem quite incompatible. Professional help may open your lines of communication.

36-55 points You probably need more awareness and compromise.

56-70 points You are highly compatible. But be aware of the areas where you can still improve.

71-80 points Your relationship is very fulfilling.

TO CARRY THIS FURTHER...

Ask your partner to take this test too. You may have a one-sided view of a "perfect" relationship. Even if you scored high on this assessment, be aware of areas where you can still improve.

Health ACTION Guide

Some Tips for Partners

▼ Take the time and make the effort to show you care for your partner.
▼ Share plans, activities, and friendships.
▼ Listen to your partner; find out what is important to him or her.
▼ Tell your partner what is important to you.
▼ Don't expect your partner to fulfill all your needs.
▼ Try to accept your partner's shortcomings.
▼ Don't blame your partner for all your problems; learn to see when you are at fault.
▼ Learn to compromise.
▼ Handle conflicts at the earliest opportunity; find a solution that benefits both of you.
▼ Keep a sense of humor; have fun together. ▼

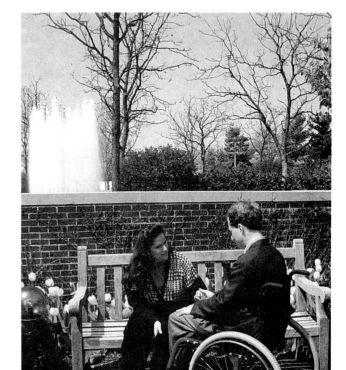

People develop attachments through familiarity and understanding.

If a relationship progresses into the sharing stage of the dating and mate selection model, passionate love is gradually replaced by companionate love. This type of love is "a less intense emotion than passionate love. It is characterized by friendly affection and a deep attachment that is based on extensive familiarity with the loved one."[4] This is a love that is enduring and capable of sustaining long-term, mutual growth. Central to companionate love are feelings of empathy, support, and tolerance of the partner.

FRIENDSHIP

One of the exciting aspects of college life is that you will probably meet many new people. Some of these people will become your best friends. Because of your common experiences, it is likely that you will keep in contact with a few of these friends for a lifetime. Close attachments to other people can have a major influence on all of the dimensions of your health.

What is it that draws people together in a relationship characterized by friendship? With the exception of physical intimacy, many of the same growth experiences seen in the dating and mate selection model are also seen in the development of friendships. Think about how you and your best friend developed the relationship you now have. You probably became friends when you shared similar interests and experiences. Your friendship progressed (and even faltered at times) through personal gains or losses. In all likelihood, you cared about each other and learned to share your deepest beliefs and feelings. Last, you cemented your friendship by transferring your beliefs into behaviors.

Throughout development of a deep friendship, the qualities of trust, tolerance, empathy, and support must be demonstrated. Otherwise the friendship can fall apart. You may have noticed that the qualities seen in a friendship are very similar to the qualities noted in the description of companionate love. In both cases, people develop deep attachments through extensive familiarity and understanding.

INTIMACY

When they hear the word **intimacy** most people immediately think about physical intimacy. They think

> **intimacy** (**in** tim uh see) any close, mutual verbal or nonverbal behavior within a relationship.

about shared touching, kissing, and even intercourse. However, sexuality experts and family therapists prefer to view intimacy more broadly. They see intimacy as any close, mutual verbal or nonverbal behavior within a relationship. In this sense, intimate behaviors can range from sharing deep feelings and experiences with a partner to sharing profound physical pleasures with a partner.

Intimacy is present in both love and friendship relationships. You have likely shared intimate feelings with your closest friends, as well as with those you love. Intimacy helps us feel connected to others and allows us to feel the full measure of our own self-worth.

MARRIAGE

Just as there is no single way for two persons to move through dating and mate selection, marriage is an equally variable undertaking. In marriage, two persons join their lives in a way that affirms each as an individual and both as a legally constituted pair. However, for a large percentage of couples, the demands of marriage are too rigorous, confining, and demanding. They will find resolution for their dissatisfaction through divorce or extramarital affairs. However, for the majority, marriage will be an experience that alternates periods of happiness, productivity, and admiration with periods of frustration, unhappiness, and disillusionment with the partner. Each of you who marries will find the experience unique in every regard.

As we move through the mid-1990s, certain trends regarding marriage are evident. The most obvious of these is the age at first marriage. Today men are waiting longer than ever to marry. Now the average age at first marriage for men is 26 years.[8] In addition, these new husbands are better educated than in the past and are more likely to be established in their careers.

Women are also waiting longer to get married and tend to be more educated and career oriented. Recent statistics indicate that the average age at first marriage is 24 years.[8]

Marriage still appeals to the majority of adults. Currently, 77% of adults age 18 and older are either married, widowed, or divorced. Thus only about one fifth of today's adults have not married. Singlehood and other alternatives to marriage are discussed later in this chapter.

FORMS OF MARRIAGE

To describe the nature of marital relationships, we use the classic categories of marital relationships advanced by Cuber and Harroff.[9] The marriage types described should not be viewed as being either good or bad. Rather, you should recognize one simple reality: these marriages are routinely found and apparently meet the needs of the individuals involved. Some of the types of marriages we present began in the form in which they are being described. Others, however, evolved into their present form, having once been a very different type of marital relationship.

Conflict-Habituated Marriage

"We fought on our first date, our honeymoon was a disaster, and we've disagreed on everything of importance ever since." This frank description of a marital relationship characterized by confrontation, disagreement, and perhaps physical abuse reflects a *conflict-habituated marriage*. The central theme of this type of marital relationship is conflict, and its continous presence suggests that no attempt at resolution is actively sought. Couples in conflict-habituated marriages agree to disagree and, on this basis, the relationship takes its form.

Devitalized Marriage

In the same way a dying person is said to possess failing signs, a *devitalized marriage* has lost its signs of life. Unlike the conflict-habituated marriage, which since its beginning was chronically impaired, the devitalized marriage was once a more active and satisfying marital relationship. For some reason, however, one or both partners have lost their desire to maintain the marriage in its original, dynamic state.

The future of a devitalized marriage is difficult to predict. Some marriages of this type can be revitalized. Effective marriage counseling, a new job, or moving to a new community can rekindle a relationship. Other

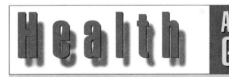

Ending Conflict

Here are some successful ways to resolve conflicts:

▼ Show mutual respect.
▼ Identify and resolve the real issue.
▼ Seek areas of agreement.
▼ Mutually participate in decision-making.
▼ Be cooperative and specific.
▼ Focus on the present and future—not the past.
▼ Don't try to assign blame.
▼ Say what you are thinking and feeling.
▼ When talking, use sentences that begin with "I."
▼ Avoid using sentences that start with "You" or "Why."
▼ Set a time limit for discussing problems.
▼ Accept responsibility.
▼ Schedule time together. ▼

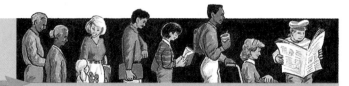

Learning FROM ALL Cultures

Marriage Customs

The institution of marriage is found in many societies, although the rules, practices, and laws can be very different. In the United States and other Western nations, marriage is a reflection of the Judeo-Christian heritage. Monogamy is practiced, fidelity is emphasized, and the permanency of marriage is stressed.[14]

In primitive societies, marriage practices greatly vary. Some accepted forms are arranged marriages, bride abductions, and bride payments. Polygyny (having two or more wives) is common, although monogamy is also practiced, especially when eco-

nomic conditions make it difficult for a man to have more than one wife.[14]

In nations in which the Islamic faith is practiced, polygyny is accepted. In countries such as India and China, parents choose marriage partners for their children or the unions are arranged. The practice of choosing one's own mate, however, is becoming more acceptable in those countries.[14]

In view of the high divorce rate in the United States, are arranged marriages any less successful than our own practices? How can men and women make wise choices in deciding upon a marriage partner? ●

---

devitalized marriages are able to remain intact because one or both partners find vitality through an extramarital relationship. Some devitalized marriages persist at low levels of involvement and commitment with little hope for improvement. We would not be surprised that, for those of you who have witnessed the dissolution of your parents' marriage, devitalization was an important factor in its ending.

Passive-Congenial Marriage

Passive refers to a low level of commitment or involvement, and the word *congenial* suggests warmth and friendliness. When these two familiar words are combined as they are in *passive-congenial marriage,* they describe perfectly the type of marital relationship sought by some couples.

For some of today's young professionals, the passive-congenial marriage offers a safe harbor from the rigors encountered in the world of corporate positions and professional practices. Children may not be valued "commodities" in the passive-congenial marriage. The added financial and personal stressors that are related to child rearing could compromise an already established lifestyle. You may be able to construct an image of a passive-congenial couple if you can picture two people meeting after work for a quiet dinner at a small restaurant, talking in muffled tones about their corporate battles, and planning their winter cruise.

Maintaining a passive-congenial marriage requires less time and energy than other forms of marriage. For two persons who feel certain that their major contributions to society will be made principally through their efforts in the workplace, this marraige may be ideal. Certainly you may know many couples who are choosing this increasingly popular form of marriage.

 Improving Marriage

Few marital relationships are "perfect." All marriages are faced with occasional periods of strain or turmoil. Even marriages that do not exhibit major signs of distress can be improved, mostly through better communication. Marriage experts suggest that implementing some of these patterns can strengthen marriages:

★ Problems that exist within the marriage should be brought into the open so that both partners are aware of the difficulties.

★ Balance should exist between the needs and expectations of each partner. Decisions should be made jointly. Partners should support each other as best they can. When a partner's goals cannot be actively supported, he or she should at least receive moral support and encouragement.

★ Realistic expectations should be estimated. Partners should negotiate areas in which disagreement exists. They should work together to determine the manner in which resources should be shared.

★ Participating in marriage counseling and marriage encounter groups can be helpful.

Beyond the patterns listed above, a sense of permanence helps sustain a marriage over the course of time. If the partners are convinced that their relationship can withstand difficult times, then they are more likely to take the time to make needed changes. Couples can develop a sense of permanence by implementing some of the patterns described above. ★

Total Marriage

In the *total marriage* little remains of the unique identities that existed between two people before their marriage took place. For reasons that are probably lost to the subconscious mind, two persons possessing individual personalities use marriage to fuse their identities into one identity—the total pair.

The total marriage requires that the individual partners set aside all aspirations for individual growth and development. Decisions are not made with "me" or even "you" as the focus of attention. Rather, energies are directed to what is best for "us." Life outside of the marital relationship and partner's presence does not exist, at least figuratively speaking. Eventually outsiders, when talking about these individuals, can no longer truly speak about the man or the woman, but are limited to speaking about the couple.

Vital Marriage

The *vital marriage* is undertaken with the intent that it will serve as an arena for the growth of both the individuals and of the pair. The concepts of "my growth," "your growth," and "our growth" prevail. In a vital marriage, personal goals may at times be subordinated for the good of the partner or the paired relationship.

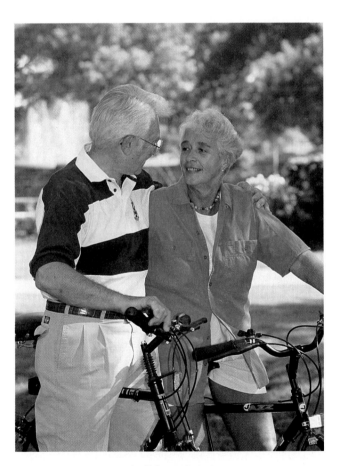

A vital marriage.

Yet both the man and woman (and the children) know that when it is possible and desirable, those once-subordinated goals will assume top priority. Equality of opportunity exists.

In describing the vital marriage, we must point out that this type of marital relationship is not perfect, nor is it appropriate for all couples. In today's complex society, the vital marriage may be especially difficult to maintain.

ALTERNATIVES TO MARRIAGE

Although the great majority of you have experienced or will experience marriage, alternatives to marriage certainly exist. This section briefly explores divorce, singlehood, cohabitation, and single parenthood.

Divorce

Marriage relationships, like many other kinds of interpersonal relationships, can end. Today, marriages—relationships begun with the intent of permanence "until death do us part"—end nearly as frequently as not.

Why should approximately half of marital relationships end in divorce? Unfortunately, marriage experts cannot provide one clear answer to this question. Rather, they suggest that divorce is a reflection of unfulfilled expectations for marriage on the part of one or both partners, including:

▼ The belief that marriage will ease your need to deal with your own faults and that your failures can be transferred to the shoulders of your partner
▼ The belief that marriage will change faults that you know exist in your partner
▼ The belief that the high level of romance of your dating and courtship period will be continued through marriage
▼ The belief that marriage can provide you with an arena for the development of your personal power, and that once married you will not need to compromise with your partner
▼ The belief that your marital partner will be successful in meeting all of your needs

If these expectations seem to be ones you anticipate through marriage, then you may find that disappointments will abound. To varying degrees, marriage is a partnership that requires much compromise and cooperation. Marriage can be a complicated proposition. Because of the high expectations that many people hold for marriage, the termination of marriage can be an emotionally difficult process to undertake.

When divorce occurs among people with children, concern is frequently voiced over the well-being of the children. Included among these factors are the sex of the children, the age of the children, custodial arrangements, financial support, and the remarriage of one or both partners. For many children, adjustments must

Health ACTION Guide

Coping with Breakup

The end of a relationship is always a wrenching and painful experience. The following tips suggest both alternatives to breakup and ways to cope with it.

▼ *Talk first.* Try to deal effectively and directly with the conflicts. The old theory said that it was good for a couple to fight. But anger can cause anger and even lead to violence. Freely venting anger is as likely to damage a relationship as to improve it. Therefore, cool off first, then discuss issues fully and freely.

▼ *Trial separation.* Sometimes only a few weeks apart can convince a couple that it is far better to work together than to go it totally alone. It is generally better to establish the rules of such a trial quite firmly. Will the individuals see others? What are the responsibilities if children are involved? There should also be a time limit, perhaps a month or two, after which the partners reunite and discuss their situation again.

▼ *Obtain help.* The services of a *qualified* counselor, psychologist, or psychiatrist may help a couple resolve their problems. Notice the emphasis on the word *qualified*. Some people who have little training or competence represent themselves as counselors. For this reason a couple should insist on verifying the counselor's training and licensing.

▼ *Allow time for grief and healing.* When a relationship ends, people are often tempted to immediately become as socially and sexually active as possible. This can be a way to express anger and relieve pain. But it can also cause frustration and despair. A better solution for many is to acknowledge the grief the breakup has caused and allow time for healing. Up to a year of continuing one's life and solidifying friendships typically helps the rejected partner establish a new equilibrium. ▼

be made to accept their new status as a member of a blended family.

Singlehood

An alternative to marriage for adults is *singlehood*. For many people, being single is a lifestyle that affords the potential for pursuing intimacy, if desired, and provides an uncluttered path for independence and self-directedness. Other persons, however, are single because of divorce, separation, death, or the absence of an opportunity to establish a partnership. The U.S. Bureau of the Census indicates that 41% of women and 37% of men over the age of 18 are currently single.[8]

Many different living arrangements are seen among singles. Some single persons maintain separate residences and choose not to share a household. Other arrangements for singles include cohabitation, periodic cohabitations, singlehood during the week and cohabitation on the weekends or during vacations, or the **platonic** sharing of a household with others. Among young adults, large percentages of single males and females live with their parents (Table 14-1).

Like habitation arrangements, the sexual intimacy patterns of singles are individually tailored. Some singles practice celibacy, others pursue heterosexual or homosexual intimate relationships in a **monogamous** pattern, and others may have multiple partners. As in all interpersonal relationships, including marriage, the levels of commitment are as variable as the persons involved.

TABLE 14-1   Percent of Young Adults Living with Their Parents: 1970 and 1992[8]*

	Age 18-24		Age 25-34	
	1970	1992	1970	1992
Male	54%	60%	10%	15%
Female	41%	48%	7%	9%
Total	47%	54%	8%	12%

*Includes unmarried college students living in dormitories.

platonic (pluh **ton** ick) describing a close association between two people that does not include a sexual relationship.

monogamous (ma **nog** ah mus) describing a paired relationship with one partner.

If You Are Single

Is your life on hold just because you are single? Are you living in limbo instead of making a real home for yourself?

To see if you're taking good care of yourself as a single "nester," try this quiz from Janice Harayda, adapted from her book, *The Joy of Being Single*. Total your yes responses, and check the interpretation after the quiz.

	Yes	No
Do you sleep on a real bed rather than a convertible sofa or a mattress on the floor?	_____	_____
Would you feel comfortable buying such items as monogrammed towels or antiques if you liked them and could afford them?	_____	_____
Do you have at least one specialty that you can cook with pride for friends?	_____	_____
Do you already own a condo, co-op, or house? If not, are you saving up for one?	_____	_____
Do you have family pictures displayed in your home?	_____	_____
Do you participate in at least one community or neighborhood group, such as a block association, a tennis committee, or the Jaycees?	_____	_____
Could you invite your boss to your home without feeling embarrassed?	_____	_____
Do you put up decorations on important holidays?	_____	_____
Do you occasionally give sit-down dinner parties instead of having the gang over for pizza and beer?	_____	_____
Do you look forward to coming home from work each night?	_____	_____
YOUR TOTAL POINTS	_____	_____

INTERPRETATION

1-2 Your place probably feels more like a sensory deprivation chamber than a real home.

3-7 You are well on the way to creating a real home and a real life for yourself.

7+ Congratulations. You have a strong sense of who you are and aren't afraid to let your place show it.

TO CARRY THIS FURTHER...

How does your residence compare with those of your other single friends? Can you learn anything from their arrangements?

PERSONAL ASSESSMENT

Cohabitation

Cohabitation, or the sharing of living quarters by unmarried persons, represents yet another alternative to marriage. According to the U.S. Bureau of the Census, the number of unmarried, heterosexual couples living together has doubled between 1980 and 1992, from 1.5 million to over 3 million couples.[8]

Although cohabitation may seem to imply a vision of sexual intimacy between male and female roommates, several forms of shared living arrangements can also be viewed as cohabitation. For some couples cohabitation is only a part-time arrangement for weekends, during summer vacation, or on a variable schedule. In addition, platonic cohabitation can exist when a couple shares living quarters but does so without establishing a sexual relationship. Close friends, persons of retirement age, and homosexuals might all be included in a group called "cohabitants."

A typical cohabitation arrangement is the couple who has drifted into cohabitation as the result of a dating relationship in which sexual intimacy and occasional "overnighting" have already occurred. In the living arrangement that follows, both material possessions and emotional support are generally shared. Only occasionally is a contractual relationship established. Monogamy usually exists. About half of cohabitation relationships disband, and the persons involved depart with the feeling that they would cohabit again if it appears desirable. Finally, cohabitation is neither more nor less likely to lead to marriage than is a more traditional dating relationship. It is, in fact, only an alternative to marriage.

Single Parenthood

The situation in which an unmarried young woman becomes pregnant and becomes a single parent is a continuing reality in this country. A new and significantly different form of single parenthood is, however, also a reality in this country. It is the planned entry into a single parenthood by older, better educated people, the vast majority of whom are women.

In contrast to the teenage girl who becomes a single parent through an unplanned pregnancy, the more mature woman who desires single parenting has usually planned carefully for the experience. She has explored several important concerns, including questions regarding how she will become pregnant (with or without the knowledge of a male partner or through artificial insemination), the need for a father figure for the child, the effect of single parenting on her social life, and, of course, its effect on her career development. Once these questions have been resolved, no legal barriers stand in the way of her becoming a single parent.

A very large number of women, and a growing number of men, are also actively participating in single parenthood in conjunction with a divorce settlement involving sole or joint custody of children. All told, over 7 million single women manage households with children under age 18. The number of single male parents, however, is on the rise.

In fact, between 1980 and 1992 the greatest change in the type of family in the U.S. was the 108% increase in households with children under age 18 headed by single men.[8] In 1992, 1,283,000 males were single and heading up households. Studies are ongoing concerning the effect that being reared by a single parent has on the school performance and social adjustment of these children.

A few single parents have been awarded children through adoption. Given the limited pool of adoptable children, the likelihood of a single person's receiving a child is small, but more persons have been successful recently in single-parent adoptions.

SEXUAL ORIENTATION AND VARIANT SEXUAL BEHAVIORS

People express their sexuality in many ways. Sexual orientation and variant sexual behaviors are described in this section.

Homosexuality

Sexual orientation refers to the sex to which one is attracted.[4] Homosexual orientation (or homosexuality) refers to an attraction toward same-sex partners. Heterosexual orientation (or heterosexuality) refers to an attraction to opposite-sex partners. *Bisexual* orientation (or bisexuality) refers to an attraction to both same-sex and opposite-sex partners.

The term *homosexuality* comes from the Greek word *homos,* meaning same. The word homosexuality may be used with regard to males or females. Thus we use the terms homosexual males and homosexual females. Frequently the word *gay* is used to refer to homosexual orientation in both males and females. *Lesbianism* is also commonly used to refer to the sexual attraction between females. This word stems from the Island of Lesbos, which the Greek poet Sappho described as an island for women in love.

The distinctions among the categories of sexual object preference are much less clear than their definitions might suggest. Most people probably fall somewhere along a continuum between exclusive heterosexuality and exclusive homosexuality. Kinsey in 1948 presented just such a continuum.[10] Any distinctions become further clouded when one considers that the definitions refer to sex object preference, not just to sexual behavior. Thus males who are sexually attracted to other males but never pursue a relationship with a male might be considered homosexual.

Why does a given individual have a homosexual orientation? Theories regarding the cause of homosex-

Gays in the Military

In February 1994, under pressure from President Clinton, the U.S. Congress implemented a new policy concerning homosexuals in the military services. The new guidelines (nicknamed "Don't ask, don't tell, don't pursue") permit gays to serve in the military as long as they keep their sexual orientation private, do not engage in homosexual conduct, and do not act in a manner that calls attention to their sexual orientation.[15]

Before the new policy, homosexuals were not permitted to serve in the military. In fact, military recruiters were required to ask recruits about sexual orientation during the enlistment process. Admitted homosexuals could not enter the military. Servicemen and women who were later discovered to be homosexual were discharged from the armed forces.

At the time of this writing, it is too early to tell how the new guidelines are working in actual practice. Some believe that the policy has encouraged a more tolerant atmosphere in the military. However, there is some preliminary speculation that the new policy may have inadvertently polarized attitudes about gays and made it easier for antigay personnel to enforce the policy in an overly aggressive fashion.[15] It could take years to determine the actual effects of this new policy. ★

uality have focused on psychoanalytical factors, family environment factors, genetic factors, hormonal factors, and behavioral (social learning) factors. In the 1960s and 1970s, the behavioral theory (positive homosexual experiences reinforce continued homosexual behavior) and the family environment theory (dominant mother and detached father) received much support. In the late 1980s, a biological theory based on a genetic/hormonal predisposition gained some acceptance for exclusive homosexuality.[4]

In the mid-1990s, some studies are pointing to differences in the sizes of certain brain structures (especially the hypothalamus, an area concerned with sexual function, and the anterior commissure bands of nerve fibers that connect the hemispheres of the brain) as a possible biological basis for homosexuality.[11,12] However, for sexual orientation in general, no one theory has emerged that fully explains this developmental process. Regardless of cause, however, reversal to heterosexuality generally does not occur.

The extent of homosexuality in our society is a debatable issue. Undoubtedly, gathering valid information of this kind is difficult. The extent of homosexual orientation is probably much greater than many het-

erosexuals realize. Furthermore, many persons refuse to reveal their homosexuality and thus prefer to remain "in the closet."

Although operational definitions of homosexuality may vary from researcher to researcher, Kinsey estimated that about 2% of American females and 4% of American males were exclusively homosexual.[10,13] More recent estimates place the overall combined figure of predominantly homosexual people at about 10% of the population.[4] Clearly the expression of same-sex attraction is not uncommon in our society.

Bisexuality

People whose attraction for sexual partners includes both sexes are referred to as bisexuals. Bisexuals may fall into one of three groups: those who are (1) genuinely attracted to both sexes, (2) homosexual but also feel the need to behave heterosexually, (3) aroused physically by the same sex but attracted emotionally to the opposite sex. Some persons participate in a bisexual lifestyle for extended periods, whereas others move quickly to a more exclusive orientation. Little research has been conducted on bisexuality, and thus the size of the bisexual population is not accurately known.

A particularly pressing reason for learning more about the bisexual lifestyle is its relationship to the transmission of HIV infection. Next to intravenous drug users and their partners, bisexuals hold the greatest potential for extending HIV infection into the heterosexual population. Since the prevalence of bisexuality is unknown, the consistent use of safer sex practices becomes more important than ever.

Transsexualism

Transsexualism refers not to a type of sexual orientation but rather a sexual identity difficulty. Transsexualism represents a complete rejection by an individual of his or her biological sex. The transsexual male believes that he is a female and desires to be the woman that he knows he is. The female transsexual believes that she is a male and thus desires to become the man that she knows she should be.

For transsexuals, the period of gender adoption is perplexing as they attempt, with limited success, to resolve the contrast between what their mind tells them is true and what their body displays. Adolescent and young adult transsexuals often cross-dress, undertake homosexual relationships (which they view as being heterosexual relationships), experiment with hormone

cohabitation (koe hab ih **tay** shun) sharing of a residence by two unrelated, unmarried people; living together.

replacement therapy, and in some cases actively pursue a **sex reassignment operation.** Several thousand of these operations have been performed at some of the leading medical centers in the United States.

An interesting point that emerges from the study of transsexualism is that concerning the most basic indicator of gender. Does a deeply held belief of being a male or female constitute the basis of gender? Does removal of external genitalia and the construction of new genitals change a person from one gender to another? Can a court of law accomplish this conversion?

Biologically the answers to these questions must be "no." Regardless of what can be accomplished through surgical, psychiatric, or legal intervention, the fact remains that the transsexual still possesses the XY or XX chromosomal benchmarks of his or her original gender.

Variant Sexual Behaviors

It seems fairly simple to suggest that any sexual behavior not engaged in by a majority of people could be labeled a **variant** behavior. However, since the culture we live in is dynamic and thus changes constantly, getting a handle on what is normal and what is variant is difficult at best. For example, such behaviors as *masturbation* and *oral-genital stimulation,* which were considered variant a few decades ago, are now practiced by a majority of sexually active people.

As we move closer to the twenty-first century, some behaviors that today appear to be variant may be considered socially or culturally acceptable behaviors in the future. Other variant behaviors, such as incest and pedophilia, are not likely to ever be considered culturally or socially acceptable.

The following is a list of variant sexual behaviors.

▼ Fetishism: an obsession with a body part or inanimate object as the primary focus of sexual excitement
▼ Transvestism: sexual excitement gained from cross-dressing, or wearing the clothes of another gender
▼ Exhibitionism: the display of one's genitals to an involuntary observer
▼ Voyeurism: observing unsuspecting persons removing their clothes or engaging in sexual activity

▼ Masochism: obtaining sexual excitement from receiving pain
▼ Sadism: obtaining sexual excitement from causing pain to another person
▼ Sadomasochism: obtaining sexual excitement by both causing and receiving pain
▼ Zoophilia: sexual excitement through contact with animals; also called *bestiality*
▼ Pedophilia: sexual contact with children
▼ Incest: marriage or sexual contact with a close relative

COMMERCIALIZATION OF SEX

We live in a society that places a great deal of importance on sexuality. We are expected to be interesting, alluring, and provocative, particularly with regard to interpersonal relationships. It is not surprising, therefore, that a commercial side to sexuality has emerged over the course of time. To some extent, this commercialization of sex affects everyone.

As a direct consequence of certain forms of sexual commercialization, many people have become victimized, such as the prostitute and his or her client, the runaway teenager, the aspiring actress or actor, and the victim of child pornography. In a less detrimental way, few of us can make a consumer decision that is not in some way influenced by a sexual message. The car, the alcoholic beverage, the perfume, and the clothes we purchase are sold to us through sexually alluring commercials. Do you envision any change in our collective consciousness that will diminish the emphasis on the commercialization of sex?

---

sex reassignment operation surgical procedures designed to remove the external genitalia and replace them with genitalia appropriate to the opposite sex.

variant (**var** ee ant) different from the statistical average.

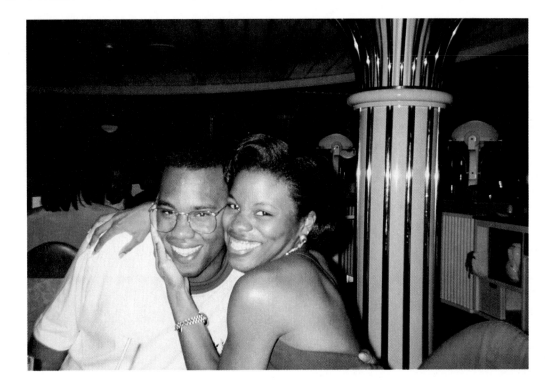

Summary

✔ The sexual response pattern consists of four stages: excitement, plateau, orgasmic, and resolution stages.

✔ Males and females show similarities and differences in sexual response.

✔ There is a wide variety of human sexual behaviors, including celibacy, masturbation, sexual fantasy, erotic dreams, shared touching, genital contact, oral-genital sexual stimulation, and intercourse.

✔ A dating–mate selection model was presented that consisted of three stages: marketing, sharing, and behavior stages.

✔ Passionate and companionate love are described.

✔ The age of first marriage continues to rise,.

✔ Alternatives to marriage include divorce, singlehood, cohabitation, and single parenthood.

✔ No single theory fully explains the development of a person's sexual orientation.

✔ Variant sexual behaviors are those not engaged in by a majority of people.

Review Questions

1. Identify the four stages of the human sexual response pattern. Describe the changes that occur during each stage.
2. What differences exist between the sexual response patterns of males and females?
3. Define celibacy, masturbation, sexual fantasies, erotic dreams, shared touching, genital contact, oral-genital stimulation, and sexual intercourse.
4. Approximately what percentage of today's college students report having experienced sexual intercourse?
5. What are the three stages that couples generally move through from dating to marriage? Describe what takes place during each stage.
6. Identify and describe the five forms of marriage presented in this chapter.
7. Approximately what percentage of marriages are likely to end in divorce?
8. Discuss some of the trends in the areas of singlehood, cohabitation, and single parenthood.
9. Explain the differences between homosexuality and bisexuality. How common are these orientations in the United States?
10. Identify the term "variant sexual behavior." What are some of the variant sexual behaviors listed in this chapter?

Think about This . . .

✔ What are your perceptions of the percentages of males and females at your college or university who have had sexual intercourse?

✔ Do you think a celibate lifestyle is possible or practical in the late 1990s? Why or why not?

✔ If you are currently dating someone, which of the three stages presented in this chapter are you currently in?

✔ If you are married, which of the five types of marriage (listed in this chapter) best reflects your marriage? Your parents' marriage?

✔ In comparison to a decade ago, are heterosexuals generally more comfortable with homosexuals in our society? Support your answer with specific examples.

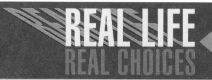

YOUR TURN

▼ Do you identify in any way with Kim Hendricks's feelings about commitment and marriage? Why or why not?

▼ How do you feel about the conviction expressed in the lyric "Love and marriage go together like a horse and carriage"?

▼ In what ways are your attitudes about commitment and marriage (1) similar to and (2) different from those of your parents?

AND NOW, YOUR CHOICES...

▼ Have you ever been in a relationship where one of you wanted to make a serious commitment and the other one didn't? If so, what was your position, why, and how did you handle the conflict?

▼ If you were in Kim's situation, would you try to change your attitude toward commitment and marriage, or would you deal with your feelings as she does, or in another way? Give reasons for your answer. ▼

References

1. Guyton R et al: College students and the national health objectives for the year 2000: a summary report, *J Am College Health Assoc* 38:9, 1989.
2. Masters W, Johnson V: *Human sexual response,* Boston, 1966, Little, Brown.
3. Haas K, Haas A: *Understanding sexuality,* ed 3, St Louis, 1993, Mosby.
4. Crooks R, Baur K: *Our sexuality,* ed 5, Menlo Park, Calif, 1993, Benjamin-Cummings.
5. Strong B, DeVault C: *Human sexuality,* Mountain View, Calif, 1994, Mayfield.
6. Hyde JS: *Understanding human sexuality,* ed 5, New York, 1994, McGraw-Hill.
7. Rathus SA, Nevid JS, Fichner-Rathus L: *Human sexuality in a world of discovery,* Needham Heights, Mass, 1993, Allyn & Bacon.
8. U.S. Bureau of the Census: *Statistical abstract of the United States: 1993,* ed 113, Washington, DC, 1993, US Government Printing Office.
9. Cuber J, Harroff P: *Sex and the significant Americans,* Baltimore, 1965, Penguin Books.
10. Kinsey A, Pomeroy W, Martin C: *Sexual behavior in the human male,* Philadelphia, 1948, WB Saunders.
11. Allen LS, Gorski RA: Sexual orientation and the size of the anterior commissure in the human brain, vol 89, no 15, *Proceedings of the National Academy of Sciences of the United States of America* (August 1, 1992), 7199-7202.
12. LeVoy S: A difference in hypothalamic structure between heterosexual and homosexual men, *Science* 253:1034, 1991.
13. Kinsey A et al: *Sexual behavior in the human female,* Philadelphia, 1953, WB Saunders.
14. Fletcher R: Mating, the family, and marriage: a sociological view. In Reynolds V, Kellet J, editors: *Mating and marriage,* Oxford, 1991, Oxford University Press.
15. Schmitt E: Military gays say new policy often misused, (New York Times News Service), Lexington Herald-Leader, May 9, 1994, p. A-1.

Suggested Readings

1. Marcus E: *Is it choice?* San Francisco, 1993, Harper Collins.
   Provides answers to 300 wide-ranging questions about homosexuality. Questions about relationships, spiritual contexts, sexual behaviors, discrimination, and coming out are covered. "Dear Abby" recommends this book as an excellent resource.
2. Nolan M, Sarrett E: *I'm so tired of other people, I'm dating myself: an insider's guide to being single,* Nashville, Tenn, 1993, Janet Thoma Books.
   A humorous look at life in the world of the single person.
3. Page S: *Now that I'm married, why isn't everything perfect? The eight essential traits of couples who thrive,* Boston, 1994, Little, Brown.
   Written by a well-known author and former campus minister, this book contains exercises, examples, and stories about how to have a successful, long-term partnership. The author believes that marital problems have more to do with unrealistic expectations than with irreconcilable differences.
4. Rhodes R: *Making love: an erotic odyssey,* New York, 1992, Simon & Schuster.
   Discusses the author's growth as a sexual being, from his early sexual experiences to his current love relationship. Describes activities that have led him to develop sexual intensity.

15

Fertility Control

Responsible Choices for Your Future

How you decide to control your *fertility* will have a major impact on your future. Your understanding of information and issues related to fertility control should help you make responsible decisions in this complex area. Now more than ever before, couples must remember that sexual activity can be closely related to risks of sexually transmitted diseases, as well as possible pregnancy.

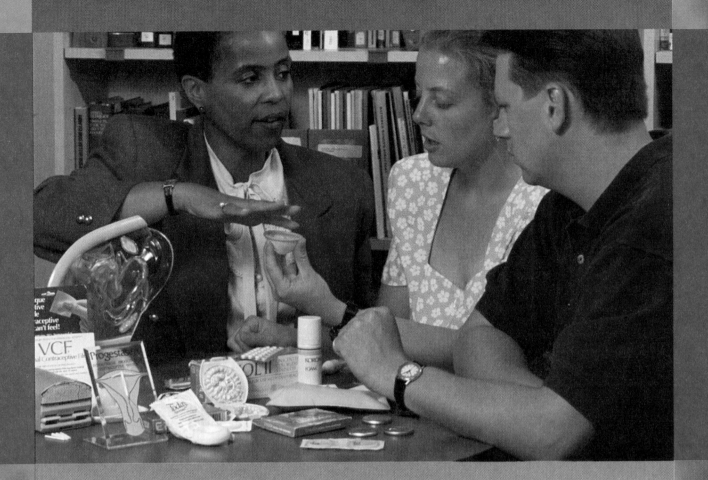

FERTILITY MANAGEMENT

The following objectives are covered in this chapter.

▽ Increase to at least 90% the proportion of sexually active, unmarried people aged 19 and younger who use contraception, especially combined method contraception that both effectively prevents pregnancy and provides barrier protection against disease. (Baseline: 78% at most recent intercourse and 63% at first intercourse; 2% used oral contraceptives and a condom at most recent intercourse among young women aged 15 through 19 reporting in 1988; p. 196.)

▽ Reduce to no more than 30% the proportion of all pregnancies that are unintended. (Baseline: 56% of pregnancies in the previous 5 years were unintended, either unwanted or earlier than desired, in 1988; p. 191.)

▽ Increase the effectiveness with which family planning methods are used, as measured by a decrease to no more than 5% in the proportion of couples experiencing pregnancy despite use of a contraceptive method. (Baseline: Approximately 10% of women using reversible contraceptive methods experienced an unintended pregnancy in 1982; p. 197.)

▽ Increase to at least 50% the proportion of sexually active, unmarried people who used a condom at last sexual intercourse. (Baseline: 19% of sexually active, unmarried women aged 15 through 44 reported that their partners used a condom at last sexual intercourse in 1988; p. 503.)

REAL LIFE
REAL CHOICES
The Morning After: Choice and Conflict

▼ **Names:** Laurie and Todd Lindemark
▼ **Ages:** 28 and 33
▼ **Occupations:** Laurie, symphony cellist
Todd, architect

"Everything was so perfect—why couldn't it stay that way?"

To everyone who knows them, Laurie and Todd Lindemark seem to have a life that's about as close to perfect as it could be. That's what Laurie and Todd thought, too, until a call from Laurie's gynecologist last week confirmed that, as she'd suspected, she's almost 4 weeks pregnant.

I can't be, she'd thought, as the phone slid from her nerveless fingers. Not now, not when I've just been asked to go on the symphony's European tour, not when Todd has just quit his job to start his own firm, not when we've just bought this condo . . . later, when we're settled, when we have more money saved, when we're ready to move to the suburbs . . . but not now.

It's been just 3 days since Laurie and Todd got the news, and it's been 72 hours of almost round-the-clock agonizing, debating, agreeing, we'll have the baby, we won't, we have to, we can't, until they're both wrung out, exhausted, incapable of making the hardest decision they may ever confront: whether to terminate their first pregnancy.

Like many couples, Laurie and Todd didn't plan to start a family until they'd become established in their professions and begun to build a stable financial base for their life together. Their long years of study, work,

and practice are finally beginning to produce results, and they'd just worked out a plan for accelerating the repayment of their student loans.

They've always been scrupulous about using birth control, and if their situation weren't so serious, it would almost be funny, because there was just that one night after Don's party, that one extra glass of wine, that one time they left the package of condoms in the bedside table drawer.

Both Laurie and Todd are pro choice and believe in a woman's right to reproductive freedom. Now that a formerly abstract issue has become reality, however, Todd tends to favor having the baby. He remembers the anguish of his sister and her husband when they decided to terminate their first pregnancy so they could both finish law school. Not only do they still mourn the loss of their unborn child, but they've spent the last 4 years unsuccessfully trying to have another.

Laurie leans more toward ending the pregnancy, partly because she really feels unprepared to deal with the major changes to her body and her life. And also because she has a former college roommate who, in the same situation, chose to have the baby and is now the frazzled mother of a rambunctious 2-year-old. Her former roommate is light years away from the career she'd planned in cancer research.

As you study this chapter, think about the choice that confronts Laurie and Todd, and prepare yourself to answer the questions in **Your Turn** at the end of the chapter. ▼

BIRTH CONTROL VERSUS CONTRACEPTION

Any discussion about the control of your fertility should start with an explanation of the subtle differences between the terms **birth control** and **contraception**.[1] Although many persons use the words interchangeably, they reflect different perspectives about fertility control. "Birth control" is an umbrella term that refers to all of the procedures you might use to prevent the birth of a child. Birth control includes all available contraceptive measures, as well as sterilization, use of the intrauterine device (IUD), and abortion procedures.

"Contraception" is a much more specific term for any procedure you or your partner might use to pre-

vent the fertilization of an ovum. Contraceptive measures vary widely in the mechanisms they use to accomplish this task. They also vary considerably in their method of use and their rate of success in preventing conception. A few examples of contraceptive methods are condoms, oral contraceptives, spermicides, and diaphragms.

Beyond the numerous methods mentioned above, could it also be possible that certain forms of sexual behavior not involving intercourse be considered forms of contraception? For example, mutual masturbation by couples substantially reduces the likelihood of pregnancy. This practice, as well as additional forms of sexual expression other than intercourse (such as kissing, touching, and massage), have been given the generic term **outercourse**.[2] Not only does outercourse

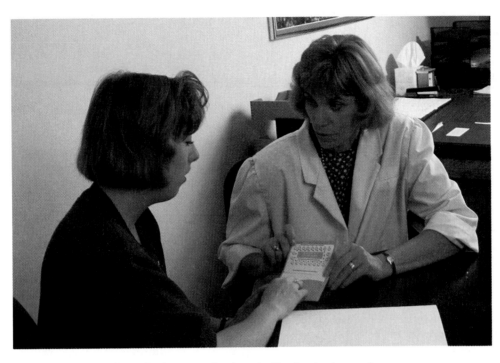

Reproductive counseling is part of family planning services.

protect against unplanned pregnancy, but it also may significantly reduce the transmission of sexually transmitted diseases, including HIV infection.

REASONS FOR CHOOSING TO USE BIRTH CONTROL

People choose to use birth control for a variety of reasons. Many career-minded individuals carefully plan the time and spacing of children so that they can best provide for the children's financial support without sacrificing their own job status. Others choose methods of birth control to ensure that they will never have children. Some use birth control methods to permit safe participation in a wide variety of sexual behaviors. Fear of contracting a sexually transmitted disease prompts some people to use specific forms of birth control.

Financial and legal considerations can be significant factors in the use of certain birth control methods. Many people must, by necessity, take the cost of a method into account when selecting an appropriate birth control. The cost of sterilization and abortion can prohibit some low-income persons from choosing these alternatives, especially since federal funds do not support such procedures. A number of states have established statutes and policies that make contraceptive information and medical services relatively difficult to obtain.

Another important consideration in the use of birth control methods is the availability of professional services. An example of the impact of this factor may be the selection of birth control methods by college students. Some colleges and universities provide contraceptive services through their student health centers. Students enrolled in these schools have easy access to low-cost, comprehensive contraceptive services. Students enrolled in colleges that do not provide such complete services may find that access to accurate information and clinical services is difficult and that private professional services are expensive.

For many persons religious doctrine will be a factor in the selection of a birth control method. This influence can be seen in the Roman Catholic Church's ban on the use of all forms of contraception other than periodic abstinence and in the condemnation of abortion by certain religious groups.

fertility (fur **til** ih tee) ability to reproduce.

birth control all of the procedures that can prevent the birth of a child.

contraception (con tra **sep** shun) any procedure that prevents fertilization.

outercourse (**ow** ter korse) sexual behaviors that do not involve intercourse.

PERSONAL ASSESSMENT

Developing Your Personal Life Plan

Your decisions concerning children and birth control must be made within the broad context of your reproductive life plan. To help you develop this plan, ask yourself each of the following questions.

1 Do I wish to marry?
2 At what age would I like to marry?
3 How many years of formal education would I like to complete?
4 When, during or after my education, would I like to marry?
5 Would I like to wait until I'm married to start having intercourse?
6 Would I like to have children one day?
7 How old would I like to be when I have my first child?
8 How concerned would I be if I (or my partner) were to become pregnant before we were married?
9 If I (or my partner) were to become pregnant when we did not want to be pregnant, what would I do? Raise the child? Adoption? Abortion?
10 How many children would I like to have?
11 Will I be able to support this family emotionally and financially?
12 How would I feel if I were not able to have *any* children?
13 Would I consider adoption if I were unable to become pregnant?
14 What kind of obligation, if any, do I feel toward limiting the size of my family to help reduce the pressure of overpopulation?
15 Would I like to work when my children are toddlers? When my children are in their childhood years? When my children are no longer in the home?
16 How do I expect my partner to participate in child rearing?
17 Of all the things I could do in my life, probably the most important thing would be . . .
18 This life goal would be affected by marriage in the following ways: . . . By child rearing in the following ways: . . .
19 What would it mean to me if my marriage were to end in divorce?
20 Would I like to have sexual intercourse with the person I marry before that marriage occurs?
21 How would I feel if my spouse were to have an intimate sexual relationship outside of our marriage?
22 How would my spouse feel if I were to have an intimate sexual relationship outside of our marriage?
23 How would I feel if I were to have an intimate sexual relationship outside my marriage?
24 How does my life plan thus far fit in with my spiritual beliefs, with the beliefs of the family and society in which I live, and with my personal code of ethics? How does it fit in with what I feel is spiritually or ethically right or wrong *for me*? If my actions are in conflict with what I feel is right for me to be doing, how can I eliminate this potential conflict that may lead to loss of self-respect?

TO CARRY THIS FURTHER...

To more fully develop your reproductive life plan, discuss these questions with your partner or trusted friend.

THEORETICAL EFFECTIVENESS VERSUS USE EFFECTIVENESS

Persons considering the use of a contraceptive method need to understand the difference between the two effectiveness rates given for each form of contraception. *Theoretical effectiveness* is a measure of a contraceptive method's ability to prevent a pregnancy when the method is used precisely as directed during every act of intercourse. *Use effectiveness,* however, refers to the effectiveness of a method in preventing conception when used in the way it is used by the general public. Use effectiveness rates take into account factors that lower effectiveness below that based on "perfect" use. Failure to follow proper instructions, illness of the user, physician or pharmacist error, forgetfulness, and a subconscious desire to experience risk or even pregnancy are but a few of the factors that can lower the effectiveness of even the most theoretically effective contraceptive technique.

Effectiveness rates are often expressed in terms of the percentage of women users of childbearing age who do not become pregnant while using the method for 1 year. For some methods the theoretical and use effectiveness rates are vastly different; the theoretical rate is always higher than the use rate. Table 15-1 presents data concerning estimated effectiveness rates, advantages, and disadvantages of many birth control methods.

SELECTING YOUR CONTRACEPTIVE METHOD

In this section we discuss some of the many factors that should be important to you as you consider selecting a contraceptive method. Remember that no method possesses equally high marks in all of the following areas. It is important that you and your partner select a contraceptive method that is both acceptable and effective, as determined by your unique needs and expectations.

For a contraceptive method to be acceptable to those who wish to exercise a large measure of control over their fertility, the following should be given careful consideration.

▼ *It should be safe.* The contraceptive approach you select should not pose a significant health risk for you or your partner.
▼ *It should be effective.* Your approach must have a high success rate in preventing pregnancy.
▼ *It should be reliable.* The form you select must be able to be used over and over again with consistent success.

▼ *It should be reversible.* Couples who eventually want to have a family should select a method that can be reversed.
▼ *It should be affordable.* The cost of a particular method must fit comfortably into a couple's budget.
▼ *It should be easy to use.* Complicated instructions or procedures can make a method difficult to use effectively.
▼ *It should not interfere with sexual expression.* An ideal contraceptive fits in comfortably with a couple's intimate sexual behaviors.

CURRENT BIRTH CONTROL METHODS

Withdrawal

Withdrawal or **coitus interruptus,** is the contraceptive practice in which the erect penis is removed from the vagina just before ejaculation of semen. Theoretically this procedure prevents sperm from entering the deeper structures of the female reproductive system. The use effectiveness of this method, however, reflects how unsuccessful this method is in actual practice (see Table 15-1).

To be more effective, this method requires a considerable amount of discipline on the part of the users. Withdrawing the penis before ejaculation is a physical maneuver quite contrary to most couples' intercourse behavior. Men generally prefer deep penetration at the moment of ejaculation. Women generally prefer consistent thrusting movements, which tend to trigger their orgasms. Withdrawal tends to inhibit complete sexual enjoyment—especially for the woman.[3]

There is strong evidence to suggest that clear, preejaculate fluid that helps to neutralize and lubricate the male urethra can contain *viable* (capable of fertilizing) sperm.[2] This sperm can be deposited near the cervical opening before withdrawal of the penis. This phenomenon may in part explain the relatively low use effectiveness of this method. Furthermore, withdrawal does not protect users from the transmission of STDs.

Periodic Abstinence

There are four approaches included in the birth control strategy called **periodic abstinence:** (1) the calendar method, (2) the basal body temperature (BBT) method, (3) the Billings cervical mucus method, and (4) the symptothermal method.[3] All four methods attempt to

---

coitus interruptus (withdrawal) (**co** ih tus in ter **rup** tus) a contraceptive practice in which the erect penis is removed from the vagina before ejaculation.

TABLE 15-1   Effectiveness Rates of Birth Control for 100 Women During 1 Year of Use

| Method | Estimated Effectiveness | | Advantages | Disadvantages |
	Theoretical	Use		
No method (chance)	15%	15%	Inexpensive	Totally ineffective
Withdrawal	85%	75%-80%	No supplies or advance preparation needed; no side effects; men share responsibility for family planning	Interferes with coitus; may be difficult to use effectively; women must trust men to withdraw as orgasm approaches
Contraceptive sponge	90%	75%-85%	Continuous protection for 24 hours; effective immediately after insertion; may help protect against some STDs	Must be moistened before insertion; some women may find it awkward or embarrassing to use; may cause vaginal irritation in some users; sometimes difficult to insert and remove; relatively expensive
Periodic abstinence Calendar Basal body temperature Cervical mucus method Symptothermal	90%-98%	75%-85%	No supplies needed; no side effects; men share responsibility for family planning; women learn about their bodies	Difficult to use, especially if menstrual cycles are irregular, as is common in young women; abstinence may be necessary for long periods; lengthy instruction and ongoing counseling may be needed
Cervical cap	94%	82%	No health risks; helps protect against some STDs and cervical cancer	Limited availability
Spermicide	97%-98%	75%-85%	No health risks; helps protect against some STDs; can be used with condoms to increase effectiveness considerably	Must be inserted 5 to 30 minutes before coitus; effective for only 30 to 60 minutes; some women may find them awkward or embarrassing to use
Diaphragm with spermicide	97%-98%	80%-90%	No health risks; helps protect against some STDs and cervical cancer	Must be inserted with jelly or foam before every act of coitus and left in place for at least 6 hours after coitus; must be fitted by health care personnel; some women may find it awkward or embarrassing to use; may be inconvenient to clean, store, and carry
Male condom and male condom with spermicide	98% 99%	80%-90% 95%	Easy to use; inexpensive and easy to obtain; no health risks; very effective protection against some STDs; men share responsibility for family planning	Must be put on just before coitus; some men and women complain of decreased sensation
Female condom	90%+	74%-79%	Relatively easy to use; no prescription required; polyurethane is stronger than latex; provides some STD protection; silicone-based lubrication provided; useful when male will not use a condom	Contraceptive effectiveness and STD protection not as high as with male condom; couples may be unfamiliar with a device that extends outside the vagina; more expensive than male condoms

TABLE 15-1 **Effectiveness Rates of Birth Control for 100 Women During 1 Year of Use—cont'd**

Method	Estimated Effectiveness		Advantages	Disadvantages
	Theoretical	Use		
IUD	99%	95%-98%	Easy to use; highly effective in preventing pregnancy; does not interfere with coitus; repeated action not needed	May increase risk of pelvic inflammatory disease (PID) and infertility in women with more than one sexual partner; not usually recommended for women who have never had a child; must be inserted by health care personnel; may cause heavy bleeding and pain in some women
Combined pill (Estrogen-progestin) Triphasic pill	99%	97%-98%	Easy to use; highly effective in preventing pregnancy; does not interfere with coitus; regulates menstrual cycle; reduces heavy bleeding and menstrual pain; helps protect against ovarian and endometrial cancer	Must be taken every day; requires medical examination and prescription; minor side effects such as nausea or menstrual spotting; possibility of circulatory problems, such as blood clotting, strokes, and hypertension, in a small percentage of users
Minipill (progestin only)	99%	96%-97%		
Depo-Provera	99%+	99%+	Easy to use; highly effective for 3-month period; continued use prevents menstruation	Requires supervision by a physician; administered by injection; some women experience irregular menstrual spotting in early months of use
Subdermal implants (progestin only)	99%+	99%+	Highly effective for 5-year period; helps prevent anemia, and regulates menstrual cycle	Requires minor surgery; some women experience irregular menstrual spotting
Tubal ligation	99%+	99%+	Permanent; removes fear of pregnancy	Surgery-related risks; generally considered irreversible
Vasectomy	99%+	99%+	Permanent; removes fear of pregnancy	Generally considered irreversible

determine the time a woman ovulates. Figure 15-1 shows a day-to-day fertility calendar used to calculate fertile periods. Most research indicates that an ovum is viable for only about 24 to 36 hours after its release from the ovary. (Once inside the female reproductive tract, some sperm can survive up to a week.) When a woman can accurately determine when she ovulates, she must refrain from intercourse long enough for the ovum to begin to disintegrate. Fertility awareness, rhythm, natural birth control, and natural family planning are terms interchangeable with periodic abstinence. Remember that periodic abstinence methods *do not* provide protection against the spread of STDs, including HIV infection.

Periodic abstinence is the only acceptable method edorsed by the Roman Catholic Church. For some persons who have deep concerns for the spiritual dimensions of their health, the selection of a contraceptive method other than periodic abstinence may indicate a major compromise on their part.

The **calendar method** requires close examination of a woman's menstrual cycle for at least eight cycles.

periodic abstinence (peer ee **od** ick **ab** stih nence) birth control methods that rely on a couple's avoidance of intercourse during the ovulatory phase of a woman's menstrual cycle; also called fertility awareness or natural family planning.

calendar method form of periodic abstinence in which the variable lengths of a woman's menstrual cycle are used to calculate her fertile period.

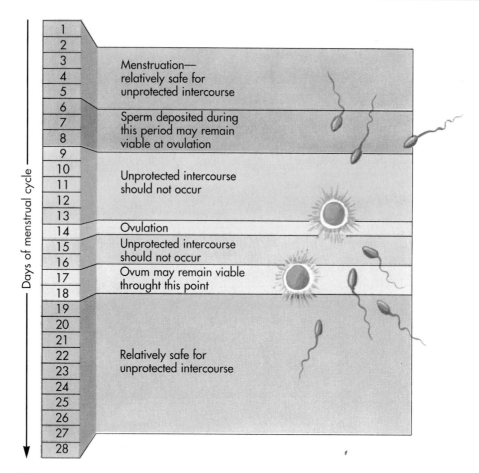

Days of menstrual cycle

Day	
1	
2	
3	Menstruation— relatively safe for unprotected intercourse
4	
5	
6	
7	Sperm deposited during this period may remain viable at ovulation
8	
9	
10	Unprotected intercourse should not occur
11	
12	
13	
14	Ovulation
15	Unprotected intercourse should not occur
16	
17	Ovum may remain viable throught this point
18	
19	
20	
21	
22	Relatively safe for unprotected intercourse
23	
24	
25	
26	
27	
28	

Figure 15-1 Periodic abstinence (fertility awareness or natural family planning) can combine use of the calendar, basal temperature, and Billings mucus techniques to identify the fertile period. Remember that most women's cycles are not consistently perfect 28-day cycles as shown in most illustrations.

Records are kept of the length (in days) of each cycle. A *cycle* is defined as the number of days from the first day of bleeding of one cycle to the first day of bleeding of the next cycle.

To determine the days she should abstain from intercourse, a woman should subtract 18 from her shortest cycle. This is the first day she should abstain from intercourse. Now she should subtract 11 from her longest cycle: this is the last day she must abstain from intercourse.[3]

The *basal body temperature method* requires a woman (for about 3 or 4 successive months) to take her body temperature every morning before she rises from bed. A finely calibrated thermometer, available in many drugstores, is used for this purpose. The theory behind this method is that a distinct correlation exists between body temperature and the process of ovulation. Just before ovulation, the body temperature supposedly dips and then rises about 0.5° to 1.0° F for the rest of the cycle. The woman is instructed to refrain from intercourse during the interval when the temperature change takes place.

Drawbacks of this procedure include the need for consistent, accurate readings and the realization that all women's bodies are different. Some women may not fit the temperature pattern projection because of biochemical differences. Also, body temperatures can fluctuate because of a wide variety of illnesses and physical stressors.

The *Billings cervical mucus method* is another periodic abstinence technique. Generally used with other periodic abstinence techniques, this method requires a woman to evaluate the daily mucous discharge from her cervix. Users of this method become familiar with the changes in both appearance (from clear to cloudy) and consistency (from watery to thick) of their cervical mucus throughout their cycles. Women are taught that the unsafe days are when the mucus becomes clear and is the consistency of raw egg whites. Such a technique of ovulation determination must be learned from a physician or family planning professional.

The *symptothermal method* of periodic abstinence combines the use of the basal body temperature method and the cervical mucus method.[3] Of course,

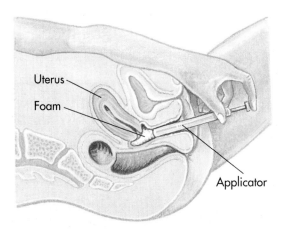

Health ACTION Guide

Determining Your Cycle

Even if you are not sexually active or are not planning to use periodic abstinence, you will find it helpful to use the calendar method of calculations to find the days in your cycle on which you are most fertile. (Hopefully, you are already keeping a record of your cycles on a calendar. This is a good addition to your health history.)

Subtract 18 from your shortest cycle. Subtract 11 from your longest cycle. The days in between are your unsafe days. Record your results.

What is your first unsafe day? What is your last unsafe day?

Can you identify the approximate time during your unsafe days that ovulation actually takes place?

Figure 15-2 Spermicidal foams and suppositories are placed deep into the vagina in the region of the cervix no longer than 30 minutes before intercourse.

couples using the symptothermal method are already using a calendar to chart the woman's body changes. Thus, some family planning professionals consider the symptothermal method a combination of all of the periodic abstinence approaches.

Vaginal Spermicides

Although they are not recommended as your primary form of fertility control, spermicidal agents are often recommended to be used with other forms of birth control. Alone, **spermicides** offer a reasonable amount of contraceptive protection for the woman who is sexually active on an *infrequent* basis. Spermicides containing nonoxynol-9 provide some protection (but *not full* protection) against STDs and HIV infection.

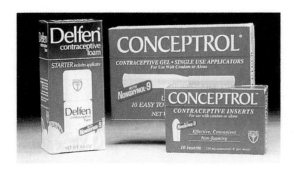

Vaginal spermicide.

Modern spermicides are safe, reasonably effective, reversible forms of contraception that can be obtained without a physician's prescription; they can be purchased in most drugstores and in many supermarkets. Like condoms, spermicides are relatively inexpensive. When used together, spermicides and condoms provide a high degree of contraceptive protection and disease prevention.

Spermicides, which are available in foam, cream, paste, or film form, are made of water-soluble bases with a spermicidal chemical incorporated in the base. The base material is designed to liquefy at body temperature and distribute the spermicidal component in an even layer over the tissues of the upper vagina (Figure 15-2). The star box on p. 378 describes a newly developed film-type spermicide.

Spermicides are not specific to sperm cells; they also attack other cells and thus may provide the woman with some additional protection against many sexually transmitted diseases and **pelvic inflammatory disease (PID)**. However, when used alone, spermicides do not provide sufficient protection against most pathogens, including the virus that causes AIDS.

---

spermicides (**sper** mih sides) chemicals capable of killing sperm.

pelvic inflammatory disease (PID) (in **flam** ah tory) generalized infection of the pelvic cavity that results from the spread of an infection through a woman's reproductive structures.

★ Vaginal Contraceptive Film (VCF)

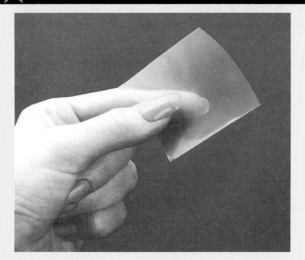

A unique spermicide delivery system developed in England is vaginal contraceptive film (VCF). Vaginal contraceptive film is a nonoxynol-9 impregnated sheet that is inserted over the cervical opening. Shortly after insertion of the VCF, it dissolves into a gel-like material that clings to the cervical opening. The VCF can be inserted up to an hour before intercourse. Over the course of several hours, the material will be washed from the vagina in the normal vaginal secretions.

This spermicide is a nonprescription form of contraception that is as effective as other spermicidal foams and jellies. A box of 12 sheets costs about $7. Like other spermicidal agents, VCF may also help in minimizing the risk of STDs and PID. ★

★ Reality—The Female Condom

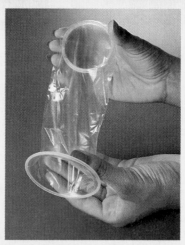

In April 1993, the Wisconsin Pharmacal Company finally gained approval to market a female condom called RE-ALITY. This device consists of a soft, loose-fitting polyurethane sheath and two flexible rings (see photo). REALITY is inserted like a tampon and lines the inner contours of the vagina. The device extends outside the vagina and covers the labia.

REALITY does not require a physician's prescription. This device is prelubricated and is intended for one-time use. Manufacturer's studies have shown that female condoms have fewer leaks and less slippage and dislodgement, and they provide less risk of exposure to semen than do male condoms. The polyurethane used is stronger and more resistant to oils than is the latex membrane used for condoms.

Despite these claims, the FDA contends that male latex condoms provide greater contraceptive protection and protection from STDs than female condoms.[5] Each REALITY sells for about $2.50 and will be available to the public in August, 1994. ★

Condom

Colored or natural, smooth or textured, straight or shaped, plain or reservoir-tipped, dry or lubricated—the condom is approaching an art form. Exaggerated? Perhaps. Nevertheless, the familiar **condom** remains a safe, effective, reversible contraceptive device. All condoms manufactured in the United States must be approved by the Food and Drug Administration.[4]

For couples who are highly motivated in their desire to prevent a pregnancy, the effectiveness of a condom can approach that of the oral contraceptive—especially if condom use is combined with a spermicide. (Some lubricated condoms now also contain a spermicide.) For couples who are less motivated or who use condoms on an irregular basis, the condom can be considerably less effective. This readily available and inexpensive method of contraception requires responsible use if it is to achieve a high level of effectiveness.

The condom offers a measure of protection against sexually transmitted diseases. For both the man and the woman, chlamydial infections, gonorrhea, HIV infection, and other sexually transmitted diseases are less likely to be acquired when the condom is used. When combined with a spermicide containing nonoxynol-9, condoms may become even more effective against the spread of sexually transmitted diseases. Although advertisements suggest that condoms provide protection against the transmission of genital herpes, users of condoms must remember that this protection is limited to the penis and vagina—not to the surrounding genital region, where significant numbers of lesions are found. Like other barrier methods of contraception, the condom is a reasonable choice for couples who are motivated in their desire to prevent a pregnancy and who are willing to assume the level of responsibility required.

Health ACTION Guide

How Can the Condom Be Used to Maximize Its Effectiveness?

These simple directions, in combination with your motivation and commitment to regular use, should provide you with reasonable protection:

▼ Keep a supply of condoms at hand. Condoms should be stored in a cool, dry place so that they are readily available at the time of intercourse. Condoms that are stored in wallets or automobile glove compartments may not be in satisfactory condition when they are used. Temperature extremes are to be avoided. Check the condom package for the expiration date.

▼ Do not test a condom by inflating or stretching it. Handle it gently, and keep it away from sharp fingernails.

▼ For maximum effectiveness, put the condom on before genital contact. Either the man or the woman can put the condom in place. Early application is particularly important in the prevention of sexually transmitted diseases. Early application also lessens the possibility of the release of preejaculate fluid.

▼ Unroll the condom on the erect penis. For those using a condom without a reservoir tip, a ½-inch space should be left to catch the ejaculate. To leave this space, pinch the tip of the condom as you roll it on the erect penis. Do not leave any air in the tip of the condom (Figure 15-3).

▼ Lubricate the condom if this has not already been done by the manufacturer. When doing this, be certain to use a water-soluble lubricant and not a petroleum-based product, such as petroleum jelly. Petroleum can deteriorate the latex material. Other oil-based lubricants, such as mineral oil, baby oil, vegetable oil, shortening, and certain hand lotions, can quickly damage a condom. Use water-based lubricants only!

▼ After ejaculation, be certain that the condom does not become dislodged from the penis. Hold the rim of the condom firmly against the base of the penis during withdrawal. Do not allow the penis to become flaccid (soft) while still in the vagina.

▼ Inspect the condom for tears before throwing it away. If the condom is damaged in some way, immediately insert a spermicidal agent into the vagina. ▼

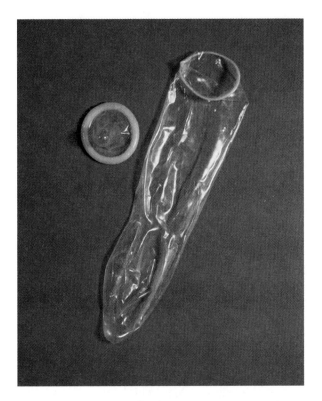

Condoms.

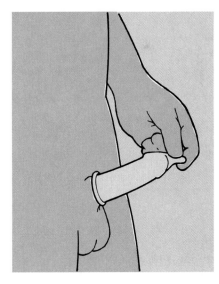

Figure 15-3 Pinch the tip of the condom and leave one-half inch of empty space at the tip.

---

condom (**con** dum) latex shield designed to cover the erect penis and retain semen upon ejaculation; "rubber."

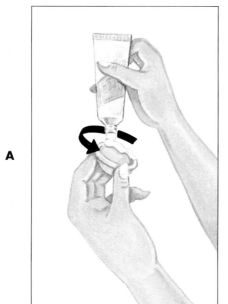

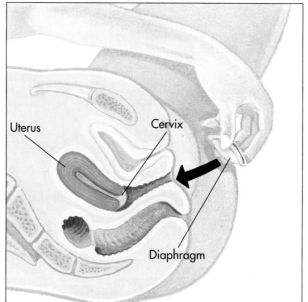

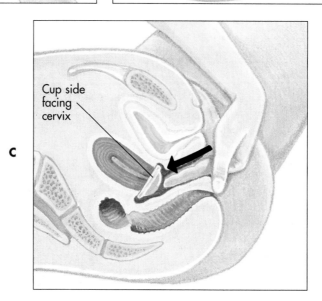

Figure 15-4 **A,** Spermicidal cream or jelly is placed into the diaphragm. **B,** The diaphragm is folded lengthwise, inserted into the vagina. **C,** The diaphragm is then placed against the cervix so that the cup portion with the spermicide is facing the cervix. The outline of the cervix should be felt through the central part of the diaphragm.

Diaphragm

The **diaphragm** is a soft rubber cup with a springlike metal rim that, when properly fitted and properly inserted by the user, rests in the top of the vagina. In its proper position the diaphragm covers the cervical opening (Figure 15-4). During intercourse the diaphragm stays in place quite well and cannot usually be felt by either the man or the woman.

The diaphragm is always used in conjunction with a spermicidal cream or jelly. The diaphragm should be covered with an adequate amount of spermicide inside the cup and around the rim. When used properly with a spermicide, the diaphragm is a relatively effective contraceptive, and when combined with the man's use of a condom, its effectiveness is even greater.

Diaphragms must always be fitted and prescribed by a physician. The cost of obtaining a diaphragm and keeping a supply of spermicide may be higher than that of other methods. Also, a high level of motivation to follow the instructions *exactly* is important.

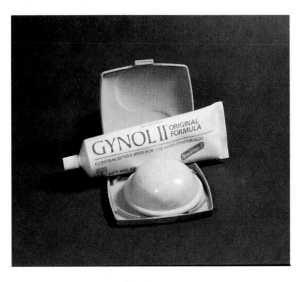

Diaphragm.

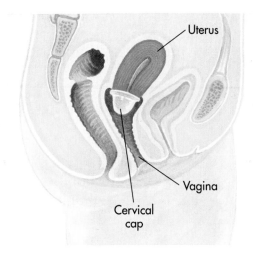

Figure 15-5 After the spermicidal cream or jelly is placed in the cervical cap, the cap is inserted into the vagina and placed against the cervix.

Diaphragms and other vaginal barrier methods (the cervical cap or the contraceptive sponge) provide some protection against STDs, including gonorrhea and chlamydia, PID, and cervical cancer. However, the ability of diaphragms and other vaginal barrier methods to provide protection against HIV infection, for either partner, is not known. If you are concerned about possible HIV infection, either avoid sexual activity or use a latex condom and spermicide in combination.[3]

Cervical Cap

The **cervical cap** is a small thimble-shaped device that fits over the entire cervix. Resembling a small diaphragm, the cervical cap is placed deeper than the diaphragm. The cap is held in place by suction rather than by pushing against anatomical structures (Figure 15-5). As with the diaphragm, a spermicide is used with the cervical cap. Thus it requires many of the same skills for insertion and care as does the di-

aphragm. The use effectiveness of the cervical cap appears to be approximately equal to that of the diaphragm. These devices are distributed in the United States through prescription by a physician.

Contraceptive Sponge

The **contraceptive sponge** is an over-the-counter product that consists of a soft, spongy, disklike object that is moistened and inserted over the cervical area. The contraceptive sponge contains 1 g of the spermicide nonoxynol-9. Thus this device both blocks sperm from entering the uterus and kills sperm. Each sponge is effective for about 14 hours and is not reusable. The safety and use effectiveness of this product are approximately equal to that of the diaphragm but only among users who have not had children. Among women who have had children, the use effectiveness drops considerably.[3] There is some indication that use of the sponge decreases the risk of contracting chlamydia and gonorrhea infections.

A small percentage of women experience unpleasant side effects and complications from the use of the sponge. Among these are vaginal irritation or allergic reactions, difficulty in sponge removal, tearing of the sponge into fragments, and increased vaginal dryness.[3]

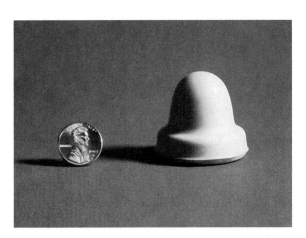

Cervical cap.

---

diaphragm (**dye** a fram) soft rubber cup designed to cover the cervix.

cervical cap (**sir** vick al) small thimble-shaped device designed to fit over the cervix.

contraceptive sponge soft, spongy disk that is moistened and inserted over the cervical area.

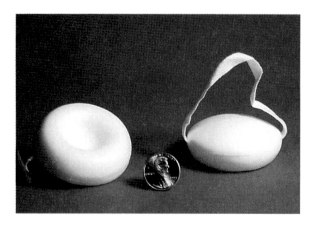

Contraceptive sponge.

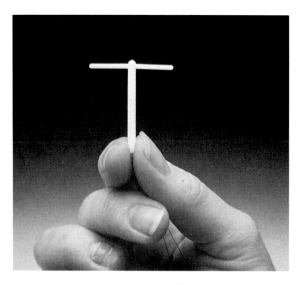

Progestasert IUD.

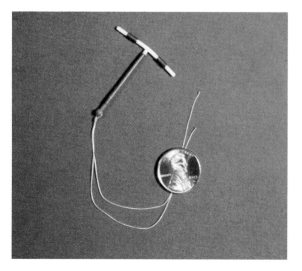

Copper T 380A (ParaGard) IUD.

Intrauterine Device

The **intrauterine device (IUD)** is a method of birth control that works by reducing the chances that a fertilized ovum will be able to implant itself into the uterus. Most health professionals believe that the IUD does not prevent conception; thus in a technical sense the IUD is not a contraceptive device but rather a birth control device.

Two types of IUDs are available in the United States: the Progestasert (A T-shaped IUD containing progestin) and the Copper T 380-A (Para Gard), a T-shaped IUD wrapped with copper wire. Photographs of these IUDs are on the left. The Progestasert must be replaced every year, but the Copper T 380-A can remain in place for up to 4 years. Only a physician can prescribe and insert an IUD. As with many other forms of contraception, IUDs do not offer protection against STDs, including the AIDS virus.

As Table 15-1 indicates, IUDs are very effective birth control devices, surpassed in effectiveness only by abstinence, sterilization, and oral (or implanted) contraceptives. Some women using IUDs experience increased menstrual bleeding and cramping. Two uncommon but potentially serious side effects of IUD use are uterine perforation (in which the IUD embeds itself into the uterine wall) and PID. PID is a life-threatening infection of the abdominal cavity. However, one recent study by the World Health Organization indicates that today's IUDs do not increase the risk of pelvic infection, except in the early weeks after the insertion.[6]

A woman deciding whether to use an IUD must discuss any concerns openly with her physician. One expert panel of physicians has suggested that the IUD is an acceptable form of contraception, especially for women who are in their middle to late reproductive years, unable to take birth control pills, in a stable monogamous relationship, and not at risk for STDs.[7]

Oral Contraceptives

Developed in the 1950s, the **oral contraceptive pill** provides the highest effectiveness rate of any single reversible contraceptive method commonly used today. The pill is the method of choice for nearly 14 million users in the United States.[3]

Use of the pill requires a physician's examination and prescription. Since oral contraceptives are available in a wide range of formulas, follow-up examinations are important to ensure that a woman is receiving an effective dosage with as few side effects as possible. Matching the right prescription with the woman may require a few consultations.

All oral contraceptives contain synthetic (laboratory-made) hormones. The *combined pill* uses both synthetic estrogen and synthetic progesterone in each of 21 pills. In 1984 *triphasic pills* were introduced in the United States. In these pills the level of synthetic pro-

Morning-After Pill

A "morning-after pill" is an oral contraceptive a woman can take to reduce the possibility of pregnancy after unprotected intercourse. The FDA has not officially approved any oral contraceptive that could be used in this fashion. Formerly, the drug DES (diethylstilbestrol) was used as a type of morning-after pill, although it was primarily for women who were victims of rape. Because of its potentially dangerous side effects, DES was removed from the market. A relatively high-dose combined oral contraceptive (Ovral) is now "unofficially" the drug of choice as a morning-after pill.

Physicians, who have the right to prescribe drugs for purposes other than those specifically indicated by the FDA, are now prescribing Ovral for patients who have unprotected mid-cycle intercourse. Some physicians prefer not to use Ovral in this fashion. In taking this drug, a woman must take two Ovral pills within 3 days of unprotected intercourse (preferably within 12 to 24 hours). Then she must take two more Ovral pills 12 hours after her first dose of pills. The use of Ovral will start menstrual flow within a few weeks.[3]

The use of a morning-after pill in cases of rape or contraceptive failure is understandable. However, frequent use in cases of unprotected intercourse seems to many people to be a reflection of irresponsibility. What do you think? ★

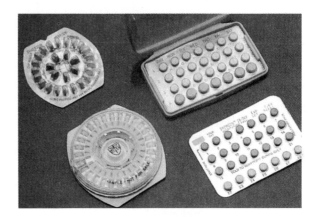

Oral contraceptives.

menstrual cramping is reduced, and the resultant menstrual flow is diminished. Research indicates that oral contraceptive use may provide protection against anemia, PID, noncancerous breast tumors, recurrent ovarian cysts, ectopic pregnancy, endometrial cancer, and cancer of the ovaries.[3] No conclusive evidence has been found that links oral contraceptive use to breast cancer, despite a well-publicized 1989 British study.

The negative side effects of the oral contraceptive pill can be divided into two general categories: (1) unpleasant and (2) potentially dangerous. The unpleasant side effects generally subside within 2 or 3 months for most women. A number of women report some or many of the following symptoms:

▼ Tenderness in breast tissue
▼ Nausea
▼ Mild headaches
▼ Slight, irregular spotting
▼ Weight gain
▼ Fluctuations in sex drive
▼ Mild depression
▼ More frequent vaginal infections

The potentially dangerous side effects of the oral contraceptive pill are most often seen in the cardiovas-

gesterone varies every 7 days during the cycle.[3] Estrogen levels remain constant during the cycle. As with many forms of contraception, it must be emphatically stated that *oral contraceptives do not provide protection from the transmission of STDs, including HIV infection.* Furthermore, the use of antibiotics lowers the pill's contraceptive effectiveness.

Oral contraceptives function in several ways. The estrogen in the pill tends to reduce ova development and ovulation. The progesterone in the pill helps reduce ovulation (by lowering the release of luteinizing hormone). The progesterone in the pill also causes the uterine wall to develop inadequately and helps to thicken cervical mucus, thus making it difficult for sperm to enter the uterus.

The physical changes produced by the oral contraceptive provide some beneficial side effects in women. Since the synthetic hormones are taken for 21 days and then are followed by **placebo pills** or no pills for 7 days, the menstrual cycle becomes regulated. Even women who have irregular cycles quickly become regular. Since the uterine lining is not developed to the extent seen in a non-pill taking woman, the uterus is not forced to contract with the same amount of vigor. Thus

intrauterine device (IUD) (in tra **yoo** ter in) small, plastic, medicated or unmedicated device that, when inserted in the uterus, prevents continued pregnancy.

oral contraceptive pill pill taken orally, composed of synthetic female hormones that prevent ovulation or implantation; "the pill."

placebo pills (pla **see** bo) pills that contain no active ingredients.

cular system. Blood clotting, strokes, hypertension, and heart attack all seem to be associated with the estrogen component of the combined pill. When compared to nonusers, the risk of dying from cardiovascular complications is only slightly increased among healthy, young oral contraceptive users. Nevertheless, the risks that are associated with pregnancy and childbirth are still much greater than those associated with oal contraceptive use.

There are some **contraindications** for the use of oral contraceptives. If you have a history of blood clotting, migraine headaches, liver disease, a heart condition, high blood pressure, obesity, diabetes, epilepsy, anemia, or if you have not established regular menstrual cycles, the pill probably should not be your contraceptive choice. A thorough health history is important before a woman starts to take the pill.

Two additional contraindications are receiving considerable attention by the medical community. Cigarette smoking and advancing age are highly associated with an increased risk of potentially serious side effects. Increasing numbers of physicians are not prescribing oral contraceptives for their patients who smoke. The risk of cardiovascular-related deaths is greatly enhanced in women over age 35. The risk is even higher in female smokers over 35. The data are quite convincing.[3]

For the vast majority of women, however, the pill, when properly prescribed, is safe and effective. Careful scrutiny of one's health history and careful follow-up examinations when a problem is suspected are essential elements that can provide a margin of safety. The ease of administration, the relatively low cost, and the effectiveness of the pill make it a sound choice for many women.

MINIPILLS

Some women prefer not to use the combined oral contraceptive pill. Thus to avoid some of the potentially serious side effects of the combined pill, some physicians are prescribing **minipills.** These oral contraceptives contain no estrogen—only low-dose progesterone. The minipill is taken daily, with no pill-free intervals.[3] The minipill seems to work by making an unsuitable environment for the transportation and implantation of the fertilized ovum. The effectiveness of the minipill is slightly lower than that of the combined pill. *Breakthrough bleeding* and **ectopic pregnancy** are more common in minipill users than in combined-pill users.

DEPO-PROVERA

In late 1992 the FDA approved a form of synthetic progesterone called *Depo-Provera.* This contraceptive is injectable and provides an extremely high degree of effectiveness for a 3-month period. The success rate for

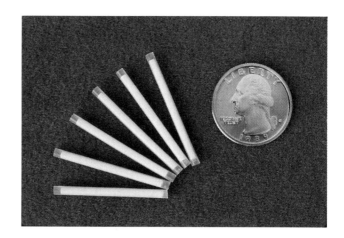

The Norplant subdermal implant.

Depo-Provera is higher than 99%. For women who prefer not to take daily birth control pills or use the Norplant implants described below, Depo-Provera may provide a good alternative.

Although this drug has been used in over 80 countries worldwide, the FDA took 25 years to finally approve its use in the United States. Concerns over possible increased rates of a variety of cancers in users of Depo-Provera were ultimately not substantiated by research. New users of Depo-Provera report occasional breakthrough bleeding as the most common unpleasant side effect.[3] Once the woman's body becomes adjusted to the presence of this drug, breakthrough bleeding is reduced considerably. After this time, the most commonly reported side effect is amenorrhea (the absence of periods). This absence is understandable, since the drug inhibits ovulation. Many women consider amenorrhea to be a desirable effect of Depo-Provera use. Unlike users of oral contraceptives and subdermal implants who return to fertility a few months after stopping their use, women who stop using Depo-Provera may experience infertility for a period of up to 1 year.[3]

Subdermal Implants

In late 1990 subdermal implants (Norplant) were approved for use in the United States. This form of contraception uses six silicone rods filled with synthetic progesterone. Using a local anesthetic, the physician implants these rods just beneath the skin of the woman's upper or lower arm. They release low levels of hormone for 5 years. An extremely effective contraceptive, subdermal implants appear to produce minimal side effects. Irregular patterns of menstrual bleeding are the most common side effect. Norplant implants cost approximately $600 to $800 for a 5-year supply.[7]

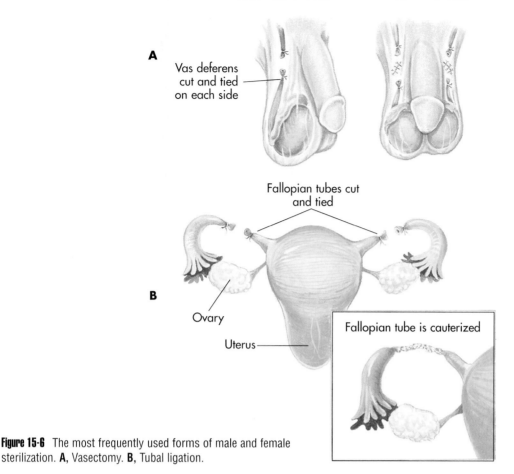

A

Vas deferens
cut and tied
on each side

Fallopian tubes cut
and tied

B

Ovary

Uterus

Fallopian tube is cauterized

Figure 15-6 The most frequently used forms of male and female sterilization. **A**, Vasectomy. **B**, Tubal ligation.

Sterilization

All of the contraceptive mechanisms or methods already discussed have one quality in common; they are reversible. Although microsurgical techniques are providing medical breakthroughs, **sterilization** should still be considered an irreversible procedure.[8] When you decide to use sterilization, you no longer control your own fertility because you no longer will be able to produce offspring.

For this reason, couples considering sterilization procedures usually must undergo extensive discussions with a physician or family planning counselor to identify their true feelings about this finality. People must be aware of the possible changes in self-concept they might have after sterilization. If you are a man who equates fertility with masculinity, you may have trouble accepting your new status as a sterile male. If you are a woman who equates motherhood with femininity, you might have adjustment problems after sterilization.

The male sterilization procedure is called a *vasectomy*. Accomplished with local anesthesia in a physician's office, this 20- to 30-minute procedure consists of the surgical removal of a section of each vas deferens. After a small incision is made through the scro-

tum, the vas deferens is located and a small section removed. The remaining ends are either tied or *cauterized* (Figure 15-6, *A*).

Immediately after a vasectomy, sperm may still be present in the vas deferens. A backup contraceptive is recommended until a physician microscopically examines a semen specimen. This examination usually occurs about 6 weeks after the surgery. After a vasec-

contraindications (**con** tra in di **cay** shuns) factors that make the use of a drug inappropriate or dangerous for a particular person.

minipills low-dose progesterone oral contraceptives.

ectopic pregnancy (ec **top** ick) a pregnancy wherein the fertilized ovum implants at a site other than the uterus, typically in the fallopian tubes.

sterilization (ster il iz **ay** shun) generally permanent birth control techniques that surgically disrupt the normal passage of ova or sperm.

tomy, men can still produce male sex hormones, get erections, have orgasms, and ejaculate. (Recall that sperm account for only a small portion of the semen.) Some men even report increased interest in sexual activity, since their chances of impregnating a woman are virtually nonexistent.

What happens to the process of spermatogenesis within each testicle? Sperm cells are still being produced, but they are destroyed by specialized white blood cells called *phagocytic leukocytes.*

The most common method of female sterilization is *tubal ligation.* During this procedure, the fallopian tubes are cut and the ends tied back. Some physicians cauterize the tube ends to ensure complete sealing (Figure 15-6, *B*).

The fallopian tubes are usually reached through the abdominal wall. In a *minilaparotomy,* a small incision is made through the abdominal wall just below the navel. The resultant scar is quite small and is the basis for the term *band-aid surgery.*

Female sterilization requires about 20 to 30 minutes, with the patient under a local or general anesthetic. The use of a *laparoscope* has made female sterilization much simpler than in the past. The laparoscope is a small tube equipped with mirrors and lights. Inserted through a single incision, the laparoscope locates the fallopian tubes before they are cut, tied, or cauterized. When a laparoscope is used through an abdominal incision, the procedure is called a *laparoscopy.*

Women who are sterilized still produce female hormones, ovulate, and menstruate. The ovum cannot move down the fallopian tube, however. Within a day of its release, the ovum will start to disintegrate and be absorbed by the body. Freed of the possibility of becoming pregnant, many sterilized women report an increase in sex drive and activity.

Two other procedures produce sterilization in women. *Ovariectomy* (the surgical removal of the ovaries) and *hysterectomy* (the surgical removal of the uterus) accomplish sterilization. However, these procedures are used to remove diseased (cancerous, cystic, or hemorrhaging) organs and are not primarily considered sterilization techniques.

Abortion

Regardless of the circumstance under which pregnancy occurs, women may now choose to terminate their pregnancies. No longer must women who do not want to be pregnant seek potentially dangerous, illegal abortions. This formerly weak link in the fertility control chain has now been strengthened. On the basis of current technology and legality, women need never experience childbirth. The decision will be theirs to make.

Abortion should never be considered a first-line, preferred form of fertility control. Rather, abortion is a final, last-chance undertaking. It should be used only when responsible control of one's fertility could not be

★ Unwanted Pregnancy

A woman who is pregnant with an unwanted child faces a difficult decision. Available options for the pregnant woman include keeping the child, placing the child in foster care until it can be cared for by the mother or placed for adoption, placing the child for immediate adoption, or terminating the pregnancy. The decision between immediate adoption and terminating the pregnancy is, perhaps, the most difficult.

The decision to carry an unwanted pregnancy to term and then place the child for immediate adoption is appealing to many for two reasons: (1) it protects the life of the developing fetus, and (2) it provides a child for people who wish to adopt. Advocates of this choice would attempt to convince the pregnant woman that the short length of pregnancy, the low risk of delivery, the freedom from the guilt that may be associated with abortion, and the happiness of the adopting family outweigh the convenience of terminating the pregnancy.

In contrast to placing the child for adoption, women have the legal right to end an unwanted pregnancy—regardless of the reason. Once the decision to have an abortion is reached, women need only act within the time frame established by the *Roe v. Wade* decision. Advocates of this freedom of choice position remind women that they need not function as "baby factories" purely to meet the demands of the adoption market. Further, women who do not want to spend time being pregnant and face the risks of labor and delivery have the right to terminate the pregnancy.

Which position do you support? What is the basis of your choice? ★

achieved. The decision to abort a fetus is a highly controversial, personal one—one that needs serious consideration by each woman.

On the basis of the landmark 1973 U.S. Supreme Court case *Roe v. Wade,* the United States joined many of the world's most populated countries in legalizing abortions within the following guidelines.

1. For the first 3 months of pregnancy (first trimester), the decision to abort lies with the woman and her doctor.
2. For the next 3 months of pregnancy (second trimester), state law may regulate the abortion procedure in ways that are reasonably related to maternal health.
3. For the last weeks of pregnancy (third trimester) when the fetus is judged capable of surviving if born, any state may regulate or even prohibit abortion except where abortion is necessary to preserve the life or health of the mother. If a pregnancy is terminated during the third trimester, a viable fetus would be considered a live birth and would not be allowed to die.

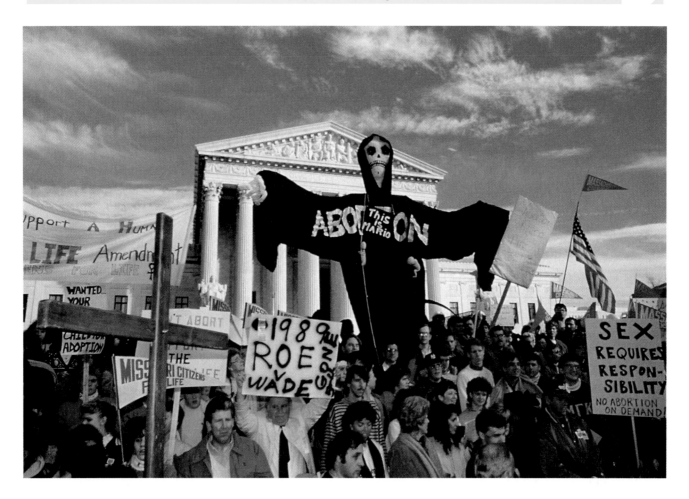

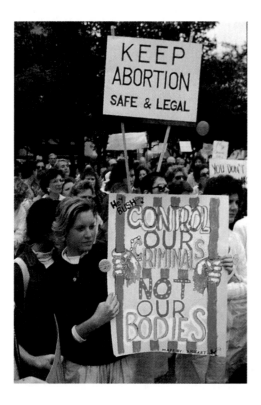

Each year approximately 1.5 million women make the decision to terminate a pregnancy in the United States. Thousands of additional women probably consider abortion but elect to continue their pregnancies.

Clearly, abortion is a political issue. During the 1980s and early 1990s, significant legislative efforts to restrict abortions were undertaken in numerous states. Questions over issues such as when life begins, the viability of the fetus, whether to inform parents about minors seeking abortions, using state employees to perform abortions, waiting periods, and abortion counseling in federally funded clinics were hot topics for the abortion debate. Those who were against abortion had support from both the Reagan and Bush administrations.

However, with the election of Bill Clinton to the United States Presidency in 1992, executive support to restrict abortion eased considerably. On January 22, 1993 (20 years to the day after the famous *Roe v. Wade*

abortion (a **bor** shun) induced premature termination of a pregnancy.

Which Birth Control Method Is Best for You?

PERSONAL ASSESSMENT

To assess which birth control method would be best for you, answer the following questions, and check the interpretation below.

	Do I:	*Yes*	*No*
1.	Need a contraceptive right away?	____	____
2.	Want a contraceptive that can be used completely independent of sexual relations?	____	____
3.	Need a contraceptive only once in a great while?	____	____
4.	Want something with no harmful side effects?	____	____
5.	Want to avoid going to the doctor?	____	____
6.	Want something that will help protect against sexually transmitted diseases?	____	____
7.	Have to be concerned about affordability?	____	____
8.	Need to be virtually certain that pregnancy will not result?	____	____
9.	Want to avoid pregnancy now but want to have a child sometime in the future?	____	____
10.	Have any medical condition or lifestyle that may rule out some form of contraception?	____	____

INTERPRETATION

If you checked *yes* to number:

1. Condoms, sponges, and spermicides may be easily purchased without prescription in any pharmacy.
2. Sterilization, oral contraceptives, hormone implants or injections, cervical caps, and periodic abstinence techniques do not require that anything be done just before sexual relations.
3. Diaphragms, condoms, sponges, and spermicides can be used by people who have coitus only once in a while. Periodic abstinence techniques may also be appropriate but require a high degree of skill and motivation.
4. IUDs should be carefully discussed with your physician. Sometimes the use of oral contraceptives or hormone products results in some minor discomfort and may have harmful side effects.
5. The sponge, condom, and spermicides do not require a prescription from a physician.
6. The condom and, to a lesser extent, spermicides and the other barrier methods may help protect against some sexually transmitted diseases. No method (except abstinence) can guarantee complete protection.
7. Be a wise consumer: check prices, ask pharmacists and physicians. The cost of sterilization is high, but there is no additional expense for a lifetime.
8. Sterilization provides near certainty. Oral contraceptives, hormone implants or injections, and a diaphragm-condom-spermicide combination also give a high measure of reliable protection. Periodic abstinence, withdrawal, and douche methods should be avoided. Outercourse may be a good alternative.
9. Although it is sometimes possible to reverse sterilization, it requires surgery and is more complex than simply stopping use of any of the other methods.
10. Smokers and people with a history of blood clots should probably not use oral contraceptives or other hormone approaches. Some people have an allergic reaction to a specific spermicide and should experiment with another brand. Some women cannot be fitted with a diaphragm or cervical cap because of the position of the uterus. The woman and her health care provider will then need to select another suitable means of contraception.

TO CARRY THIS FURTHER . . .

There may be more than one method of birth control suitable for you. Always consider how a method you select can also help you avoid an STD. Study the methods suggested above, and consult Table 15-1 to determine what techniques may be most appropriate.

Supreme Court decision legalizing abortion), President Clinton signed executive orders to do the following:

▼ Permit abortion counseling in federally funded clinics

▼ Permit research using fetal tissue from abortions

▼ Permit abortions at military hospitals

▼ Review the ban against the importation of RU-486, the French abortion pill

It will be interesting to see how future abortion-related decisions unfold. Special interest groups on both sides of the issues, the Supreme Court, state legislatures, federal agencies (such as the FDA and the Department of Health and Human Services), the Congress, and the President will all have a say in the abortion debate in this country. Regardless of the eventual outcomes of this debate, here are the present abortion procedures available in the United States.

FIRST TRIMESTER ABORTION PROCEDURES
Menstrual extraction

Also referred to as menstrual regulation, menstrual induction, and preemptive abortion, menstrual extraction is a process carried out between the fourth and sixth week after the last menstrual period (or in the days immediately after the first missed menstrual period). Generally performed in a physician's office under a local or *paracervical anesthetic*, a small plastic *cannula* is inserted through the undilated cervical canal into the cavity of the uterus. Once the cannula is in position, a small amount of suction is applied by a handheld syringe. By rotating and moving the cannula across the uterine wall, the physician can withdraw the endometrial tissue.

Vacuum aspiration

Induced abortions undertaken during the sixth through ninth week of pregnancy are generally done through a procedure of *vacuum aspiration* of the uterine contents. Vacuum aspiration is the most commonly performed abortion procedure. This procedure is similar in nature to menstrual extraction. Unlike menstrual extraction, however, vacuum aspiration may require **dilation** of the cervical canal and the use of a local anesthetic. In this more advanced stage of pregnancy, a larger cannula must be inserted into the uterine cavity. This process can be accomplished by using metal dilators of increasingly larger sizes to open the canal. After aspiration by an electric vacuum pump, the uterine wall may also be scraped to confirm complete removal of the uterine contents.

Dilation and curettage (D & C)

When a pregnancy is to be terminated during the ninth through fourteenth weeks, vacuum aspiration gives way to a somewhat similar procedure labeled **dilation and curettage,** or more familiarly, D & C. D & C

usually requires a general anesthetic, not a local anesthetic.[3]

Like vacuum aspiration, the D & C involves the gradual enlargement of the cervical canal through the insertion of increasingly larger metal dilators. When the cervix has been dilated to a size sufficient to allow for the passage of a *curette,* the removal of the endometrial tissue can begin. The curette is a metal instrument resembling a spoon, with a cup-shaped cutting surface on its end. As the curette is drawn across the uterine wall, the soft endometrial tissue and fetal parts are scraped from the wall of the uterus. (The D & C is also used in the medical management of certain health conditions of the uterine wall, such as irregular bleeding or the buildup of endometrial tissue.)

As in the case of menstrual extraction, both vacuum aspiration and D & C are very safe procedures for the woman. The need to dilate the cervix more fully in a D & C increases the risk of cervical trauma and the possibility of perforation, but these risks are reported to be low. Bleeding, cramping, spotting, and infections present minimal controllable risks when procedures are done by experienced clinicians under clinical conditions.

The abortion pill

The Roussel-UCLAF company in Paris, France, has produced a very controversial form of birth control, RU-486 (mifepristone). RU-486 is controversial because it is designed to produce an abortion. This drug is a pill that blocks the action of progesterone. When three 200-mg RU-486 pills are taken and followed 48 hours later by an injection (or vaginal suppository) of prostaglandin, menstruation begins, usually within 5 hours. According to a research report in the *New England Journal of Medicine,* RU-486 is effective in 96% of cases when taken within 49 days of a missed period. Few side effects were noticed.[9] In France, RU-486 is used in about 30% of abortion cases. RU-486 is also approved for use in China and West Germany.

In May 1994, Roussel-UCLAF, agreed to give its patent rights for RU-486 to the Population Council, a New York–based, international, nonprofit contraceptive research organization. This action paved the way for the Population Council to test this drug on U.S. women in the fall of 1994. If the testing indicates that RU-486 is as safe and effective as that found in the 150,000 women who have used the drug in Europe,

dilation (di **lay** shun) gradual expansion of an opening or passageway.

dilation and curettage (D & C) (kyoor i **tazh**) surgical procedure in which the cervical canal is dilated to allow the uterine wall to be scraped.

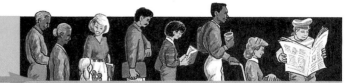

Learning FROM ALL Cultures

Controlling Birth Rates

Most Asian governments are trying to curb their population growth. China has been fairly successful in implementing its suggested policy of one child per couple. The government offers incentives for couples who have only one child and also imposes penalties, like taxation, on couples who produce more children.[10]

Malaysia, like other countries in the region, also promoted the small family policy until recently. The government is now encouraging Malaysian couples to have more children; as many as five. The aim is to increase the population, which will decrease to 70 million by the year 2100.[10]

The primary reason for this push for population growth is economic. Today in Malaysia there are labor shortages in certain areas in the economy. Also, the country is becoming more industrialized and will require a larger workforce, not to mention more people to whom products can be sold. The country's challenge and goal are to increase population while maintaining or improving the standard of living.[10]

Childbearing and raising a family today in some countries are not only personal choices. The decision to have children and how many to have is strongly influenced by some governments. Is government interference justified for this aspect of people's lives? How influenced would you be if your government strongly encouraged you to either limit or expand your family? ●

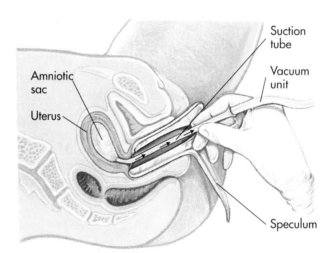

Figure 15-7 During dilation and evacuation, the cervix is dilated, and the contents of the uterus are aspirated. This procedure is used to perform abortions up to 16 weeks of gestation.

then the FDA is likely to approve RU-486 as a prescription drug, perhaps as early as 1996.

SECOND TRIMESTER ABORTION PROCEDURES

When a woman's pregnancy continues beyond the fourteenth week of gestation, termination becomes a more difficult matter. The procedures at this stage become more complicated and take longer to be completed, and complications become more common.

Dilation and evacuation

Vacuum aspiration and D & C can be combined in a procedure called *dilation and evacuation (D & E)* during the earliest weeks of the second trimester (Figure 15-7). The use of D & E increases the likelihood of trauma and postprocedural complications, since larger instruments and greater dilation are required. After about 16 weeks, more intensive procedures will be required to terminate the late second trimester pregnancy.

Hypertonic saline procedure

From the sixteenth week of gestation to the end of the second trimester, intrauterine injection of a strong salt solution into the amniotic sac is the procedure frequently used. The administration of intrauterine **hypertonic saline solution** requires a skilled operator so that the needle used to introduce the salt solution does enter the amniotic sac. Once the needle is in place, some amniotic fluid is withdrawn, allowing the saline solution to be injected.

Some physicians support the saline procedure by dilating the cervix with *laminaria* or another dilatory product and administering the hormone oxytocin to stimulate uterine contractions. The onset of uterine contractions will expel the dehydrated uterine contents within 24 to 36 hours.

Prostaglandin procedure

The use of prostaglandin is the third type of abortion procedure used during the second trimester. Prostaglandins are hormonelike chemicals that have a variety of useful effects on human tissue. Produced naturally within the body, these substances influence the contractions of smooth muscle. Since the uterine wall is composed entirely of smooth muscle, it is particularly sensitive to the presence of prostaglandins. When prostaglandin is administered in sufficient quantity (through either a uterine intramuscular injection or through a vaginal suppository), uterine contractions become strong enough to expel the fetal contents.

THIRD TRIMESTER ABORTION PROCEDURES

Should termination of a pregnancy be required in the latter weeks of the gestational period, a surgical procedure in which the fetus will be removed (*hysterotomy*) or a procedure in which the entire uterus is removed (*hysterectomy*) can be undertaken. As one can imagine, these procedures are more complicated and involve longer hospitalization, major abdominal surgery, and an extended period of recovery.

> **hypertonic saline solution** (hy per **ton** ick **say** leen) salt solution with a concentration higher than that found in human fluids.

As We Go to Press...

On May 26, 1994, President Bill Clinton signed into law the Freedom of Access to Clinic Entrances Act, or FACE. FACE authorizes serious federal criminal penalties and civil remedies for incidents of violence and obstructive behavior aimed at reproductive health clinics. This new federal law was expressly intended to stop clinic blockades, invasions, violence, and threats directed at patients and employees of reproductive health clinics.

FACE does not prohibit peaceful protests against clinics that provide reproductive services. Peaceful picketing, singing, demonstrations, and praying are free speech rights protected under the First Amendment to the U.S. Constitution. However, acts related to force, the threat of force, physical obstruction, intimidation, interference, and destruction of property are covered under FACE.

FACE appears to be a result of increased violence and threats of violence directed toward the physical facilities, patients, and employees of abortion clinics. For example, at the time this text went to press, Paul Hill, well known abortion protestor, was being charged with murder for the summer 1994 shotgun deaths of a Pensacola, Florida abortion clinic physician and his bodyguard. What impact do you think FACE will have in the near future?

Summary

✔ Birth control refers to all the procedures that can prevent the birth of a child.

✔ Contraception refers to any procedure that prevents fertilization.

✔ Each birth control method has both a theoretical and a use effectiveness rate. For some contraceptive approaches these rates are similar (such as hormonal methods), and for others the rates are very different (such as condoms, diaphragms, and periodic abstinence).

✔ Many factors should be considered when deciding which contraceptive is best for you.

✔ Contraceptive users must also protect themselves from STDs, including HIV infection.

✔ The contraceptive methods most recently approved by the FDA are the female condom, subdermal implants, and Depo-Provera.

✔ Sterilization (vasectomy and tubal ligation) is usually considered an irreversible procedure.

✔ Currently, abortion remains a woman's choice under the guidelines of the 1973 *Roe v. Wade* decision and various state restrictions.

✔ Abortion procedures vary according to the length of the pregnancy.

Review Questions

1. Explain the difference between the terms *birth control* and *contraception*. Give examples of each.

2. Explain the difference between theoretical and use effectiveness rates. Which one is always higher? Why is it important to know the difference between these two rates?

3. Identify some of the factors that should be given careful consideration when selecting a contraceptive method. Explain each factor.

4. For each of the methods of birth control, explain how it works and its advantages and disadvantages.

5. Identify each of the components in the periodic abstinence method of contraception. How does each component function?

6. How do minipills differ from the combined oral contraceptive? What is a morning-after pill? How do subdermal implants (Norplant) differ from Depo-Provera?

7. Identify and describe the different abortion procedures that are used during each trimester of pregnancy. When is the safest time for an abortion?

Think about This . . .

✔ What factors are most important to you when it comes to selecting an appropriate contraceptive method?

✔ How well do you think college students understand that oral contraceptives do not protect against STDs?

✔ Will you or your partner someday undergo sterilization? If so, which of you will have the surgery?

✔ Under what circumstances do you believe that abortion is acceptable? Unacceptable?

✔ Can you identify locations at or near your college where professional family planning services are available?

REAL LIFE
REAL CHOICES

YOUR TURN

▼ What do you think about Laurie and Todd Lindemark's reasons for (1) wanting and (2) not wanting to have an unplanned child?
▼ Can you think of any additional factors they might consider in trying to reach a decision?
▼ Have you been in a situation similar to the Lindemarks', or do you know anyone who has? If so, what was the decision, and what were the results?

AND NOW, YOUR CHOICES...

▼ If you are a man, try to decide how you would handle this situation in the best interests of you, your spouse, and your unborn child.
▼ If you are a woman, try to make the best decision for yourself, your spouse, and your unborn child. ▼

References

1. Strong B, DeVault C: *Human sexuality,* Mountain View, Calif, 1994, Mayfield.
2. Crooks R, Baur K: *Our sexuality,* ed 5, Menlo Park, Calif, 1993, Benjamin-Cummings.
3. Hatcher RA et al: *Contraceptive technology,* ed 16, New York, 1994, Irvington Publishers.
4. Hyde JS: *Understanding human sexuality,* ed 5, New York, 1994, McGraw-Hill.
5. Goldberg MS: Choosing a contraceptive, *FDA Consumer* 27(7):18, 1993.
6. Farley TMM et al: Intrauterine devices and pelvic inflammatory disease: an international study, *Lancet* 339(8796):785, 1992.
7. Painter K: The imperfect state of birth control in the USA, *USA Today,* March 16, 1992, p. 4D.
8. Haas K, Haas A: *Understanding sexuality,* ed 3, 1993, Mosby.
9. Silvestre L et al: Voluntary interruption of pregnancy with mifepristone (RU 486) and a prostaglandin analogue, *N Engl J Med* 322(10):645, 1990.
10. Tyler C: Baby power, *Geographical magazine,* January 1992, p. 16.

Suggested Readings

Abortion: opposing viewpoints, San Diego, 1991, Greenhaven Press.
 A collection of writings from both sides of the abortion debate. Laypersons, theologians, feminists, and prominent organizations contribute essays on a variety of abortion issues.
Hager D, Joy D: *Women at risk: the real truth about sexually transmitted disease,* Lexington, Ky, 1993, Bristol Books.
 STD transmission can occur despite successful contraceptive protection. Case studies are used to discuss the dangers and treatments of nine common STDs. This book is written with a Christian perspective by a na-tional medical expert on STDs and a well-known counselor, teacher, and author.
Hatcher RA et al: *Contraceptive technology,* ed 16, New York, 1994, Irvington Publishers.
 Perhaps the best primary reference concerning birth control for physicians, family planning centers, and educators. Contributors include national experts and staff members of the Centers for Disease Control and Prevention.

16

Sexuality
Pregnancy and Childbirth

You may be surprised at the many diverse topics you will find in this chapter. Information ranges from parenthood, pregnancy, childbirth, and birth technology to infertility. The common thread throughout this chapter involves the choices you will make in terms of your reproductive sexuality.

Our students find these topics especially interesting. Most likely this is because the topics involve decisions nearly everyone must face. Many of our nontraditional students have already made parenting decisions. These students' experiences add insights that help our traditional students better see what lies ahead.

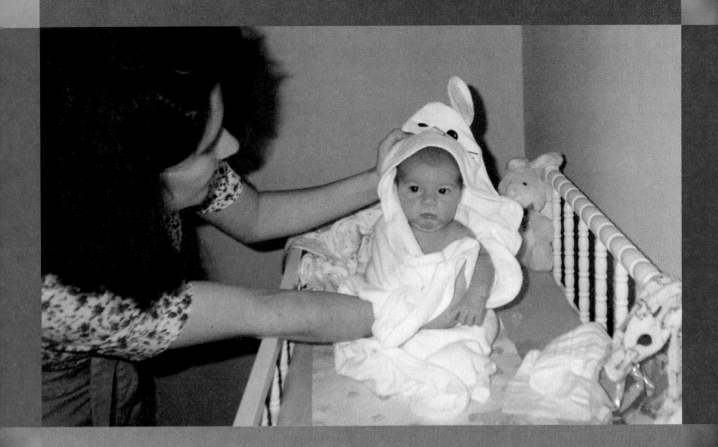

PREGNANCY AND CHILDBIRTH

The following objectives are covered in this chapter:

▽ Reduce the infant mortality rate to no more than 7 per 1000 live births. (Baseline: 10.1 per 1000 live births in 1987; p. 368.)

▽ Increase abstinence from tobacco use by pregnant women to at least 90% and increase abstinence from alcohol, cocaine, and marijuana by pregnant women by at least 20%. (Baseline: 75% of pregnant women abstained from tobacco use in 1985; p. 380.)

▽ Increase to at least 90% the proportion of all pregnant women who receive prenatal care in the first trimester of pregnancy. (Baseline: 76% of live births in 1987; p. 381.)

▽ Reduce the cesarean delivery rate to no more than 15 per 100 deliveries. (Baseline: 24.4 per 100 deliveries in 1987; p. 378.)

▽ Increase to at least 75% the proportion of mothers who breast-feed their babies in the early postpartum period and to at least 50% the proportion who continue breast-feeding until their babies are 5 to 6 months old. (Baseline: 54% at discharge from birth site and 21% at 5 to 6 months in 1988; p. 379.)

REAL LIFE
REAL CHOICES
Infertility: Ticking Clock, Tough Decisions

▼ **Names:** Susan Williams-Johnson and Gary Johnson
▼ **Ages:** 36 and 35
▼ **Occupations:** Susan, investment banker
Gary, plastic surgeon

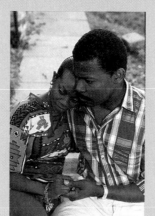

"Us? Infertile? But that's impossible!"

When Susan and Gary Johnson learned that it would be extremely difficult or even impossible for them to conceive a child, they were as stunned as if they'd been told that the Earth had fallen off its axis. Married for 12 years, much of it devoted to education and training, they'd faithfully used birth control and planned to have their first child a year after Gary completed his residency in plastic surgery. Susan had intended to resign her position at a major bank and, a year after having a baby, to become an independent investment consultant. Through some long lean years together, a major focus of this couple had been on *not* having a baby until they were sure they were ready emotionally and financially to be parents.

Now they're ready—but nature, apparently, is not.

After seemingly endless consultations and tests, a respected fertility specialist at Gary's hospital has told him and Susan that they belong to that small percentage of couples whose infertility has no detectable cause. She has explained to them the drug therapy, surgery, insemination, and fertilization procedures for which they may be candidates, but she has cautioned them that these procedures are likely to be time-consuming, expensive, and frustrating. And, there is no guarantee of success. In addition to these procedures, the specialist has suggested that Gary and Susan also may want to consider other options, such as adoption or surrogate parenting.

Still reeling from news they never expected to hear, feeling that their lives and plans have been turned upside down, Gary and Susan know they have some difficult and painful decisions to make.

As you study this chapter, think about Gary and Susan's situation and choices, and prepare yourself to answer the questions in **Your Turn** at the end of the chapter. ▼

BECOMING PARENTS

Although birth control is especially important for many young couples, most couples eventually want to have children and raise a family. Formerly, couples had their children very early after either high school or college. Now the trend seems to be to wait longer before having children. Most likely, educational, economic, contraceptive, and occupational factors have laid the groundwork for this trend. To the relief of many people, medical research indicates that women above the age of 30 or 35 are quite capable of having healthy babies.

Parenting Issues for Couples

Before deciding to have children, couples should have frank discussions about the impact that pregnancy and a newborn child will have on their lives. For those students contemplating single parenthood, we ask that you consider these issues as they relate to your particular situation and to excuse our consistent use of plural pronouns. In any event, some or all of the following basic considerations should be discussed:

▼ What impact will pregnancy have on us individually and jointly?
▼ Why do we want to have a child?
▼ What impact will a child have on the images we have constructed for ourselves as adults?
▼ Can we afford to have a child and provide for its needs?
▼ How will the responsibilities related to raising a child be divided?
▼ How will our professional careers be affected by the addition of a child?
▼ Are we ready now to accept the extended responsibilities that can come with a new child?
▼ How will we rear our child in terms of religious training, discipline, and participation in activities?
▼ Are we ready to part with much of the freedom associated with late adolescence and the early young adult years?
▼ How will we handle the possibility of being awakened by 6 AM each morning for the next couple of years?

▼ What plans have been made if we should discover that our baby (or fetus) is defective?

▼ Are we capable of handling the additional responsibilities associated with having a disabled child?

▼ Are we comfortable with the thought of bringing another child into an already overcrowded, violent, bigoted, and polluted world?

If these questions seem strikingly negative in tone, there is indeed a reason for this. We believe that all too frequently the "nuts and bolts" issues related to childbearing and parenting are ignored, or at least are placed on the back burner. Although it is important for future parents to consider how cute and cuddly a new baby will be, how enhanced holidays will be with a new child, and how pleased the grandparents will be, we would consider these issues secondary to the major realities of having a child enter your lives.

PREGNANCY: AN EXTENSION OF THE PARTNERSHIP

Pregnancy is a condition that requires a series of complex yet coordinated changes to occur in the female body. In this chapter pregnancy is followed from its beginning with fertilization to its conclusion with labor and childbirth.

Physiological Obstacles and Aids to Fertilization

Many sexually active young people believe that they will become pregnant (or impregnate someone) only when they want to, despite their haphazard contraceptive practices. Because of this mistaken belief, many young people are not sold on the use of contraceptives. It is important for young adults to remember that, from a species survival standpoint, our bodies were designed to promote pregnancy. It is estimated that about 85% of sexually active women of childbearing age will become pregnant within 1 year if they do not employ some form of contraception.[1]

With regard to pregnancy, each act of intercourse can be considered a game of physiological odds. There are obstacles that may reduce a couple's chance of pregnancy. The following is a list of some of these obstacles.

Obstacles to fertilization

1 *The acidic level of the vagina is destructive to sperm.* The low pH of the vagina will kill sperm that fail to enter the uterus quickly.

2 *The cervical mucus is thick during most of the menstrual cycle.* Sperm movement into the uterus is difficult except during the few days surrounding ovulation.

3 *The sperm must locate the cervical opening.* The cervical opening is small in comparison with the rest of the surface area where sperm are deposited.

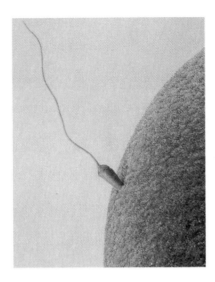

Fertilization of ovum by sperm.

4 *Half of the sperm travel through the wrong fallopian tube.* Most commonly, only one ovum is released at ovulation. The two ovaries generally take turns each month. The sperm have no way of knowing which tube they should enter. Thus it is probable that half will travel through the wrong tube.

5 *The distance sperm must travel is relatively long compared with the tiny size of the sperm cells.* Microscopic sperm must travel about 7 or 8 inches once they are inside the female.

6 *The sperm's travel is relatively upstream.* The anatomical positioning of the female reproductive structures necessitates an uphill movement by the sperm.

7 *The contoured folds of the tubal walls trap many sperm.* These folds make it difficult for sperm to locate the egg. Many sperm are trapped in this maze.

There are also a variety of aids that tend to help sperm and egg cells to join. Some of these are listed below.

Aids to fertilization

1 *An astounding number of sperm are deposited during ejaculation.* Each ejaculation contains about a teaspoon of semen.[2] Within this quantity are between 200 and 500 million sperm cells. Even with large numbers of sperm killed in the vagina, millions are able to move to the deeper structures.

2 *Sperm are deposited near the cervical opening.* Penetration into the vagina by the penis allows for the sperm to be placed near the cervical opening.

3 *The male accessory glands help make the semen nonacidic.* The seminal vesicles, prostate gland, and Cowper's glands secrete fluids that provide an alkaline environment for the sperm. This environment helps the sperm be better protected in the vagina until they can manage to move into the deeper, more alkaline uterus and fallopian tubes.

PERSONAL ASSESSMENT

Respond to each of the following items based on your own opinions about parenting. Circle the letters that best match your response (see explanation of these abbreviations below).

SA Strongly agree
A   Agree
U   Undecided
D   Disagree
SD Strongly disagree

1 One cannot parent successfully without, at the same time, being a generally successful adult member of the community.   SA   A   U   D   SD

2 It is inappropriate to view parenting as a method of achieving immortality.   SA   A   U   D   SD

3 Parenting requires that one be willing to make major personal sacrifices for the benefit of the child.   SA   A   U   D   SD

4 Parenting adds a large measure of vitality to an adult's life.   SA   A   U   D   SD

5 Parenting demands greater creativity than any other adult pursuit.   SA   A   U   D   SD

6 A person who cannot comfortably make decisions for others should not consider parenting.   SA   A   U   D   SD

7 A family cannot exist in the absence of children.   SA   A   U   D   SD

TO CARRY THIS FURTHER...

After completing this personal assessment, join three of your classmates in comparing and discussing your responses. What suggestions were made to help increase your awareness of all that parenting involves?

4 *Uterine contractions aid sperm movement.* The rhythmic muscular contractions of the uterus tend to cause the sperm to move in the direction of the fallopian tubes.[2]

5 *Sperm cells move rather quickly.* Despite their microscopic size, sperm cells can move relatively quickly—just about 1 inch per hour. Powered by sugar solutions from the male accessory glands and the whiplike movements of their tails, sperm can reach the distant third of the fallopian tubes in less than 8 hours as they swim in the direction of the descending ovum.

6 *Once inside the fallopian tubes, sperm can live for days.* Some sperm may be viable for up to a week after reaching the comfortable, nonacidic environment of the fallopian tubes. Most sperm, however, will survive an average of 48 to 72 hours in the fallopian tubes. Thus they can "wait in the wings" for the moment an ovum is released from the ovary.

7 *The cervical mucus is thin and watery at the time of ovulation.* This mucus allows for better passage of sperm through the cervical opening when the ovum is most capable of being fertilized.

Pregnancy Determination

For centuries the only way to find out that a woman had become pregnant was to see if she stopped menstruating (because continued progesterone secretion helps keep the endometrial wall from deteriorating) and her abdomen began to enlarge. Within a couple of months, pregnancy could be determined rather reliably. Although this method would still work in this era, most couples want to find out more quickly.

Earlier in this century a newer way of determining pregnancy was routinely used. In this pregnancy test, urine from the woman was injected into laboratory animals, most often rabbits, rats, or frogs. If the woman was pregnant, the hormone *human chorionic gonadotropin (HCG)* in her urine would stimulate ovulation in female animals and stimulate ejaculation in male animals. Of course, the female animals had to be sacrificed and analyzed for ovulation. (Thus the phrase "the rabbit died" was coined to indicate that this test determined that a woman was pregnant.) Positive readings were possible only if the woman had been pregnant for about 4 weeks and thereby had developed sufficiently high levels of HCG.

HCG is initially released in large quantities by embryonic cells that later form the fetal part of the placenta. For the first 6 weeks of pregnancy, HCG's primary function is to maintain the corpus luteum's continued release of estrogen and progesterone. By the beginning of the second trimester of pregnancy, estrogen and progesterone are produced mainly by the placenta.[3]

A wide array of pregnancy tests are now available for use by health care providers and as home preg-

★ Home Pregnancy Tests

Home pregnancy test kits have been available for many years. Using technology similar to that in the laboratory-based immune response tests, these pregnancy tests can be conducted in the privacy of one's home. Home pregnancy tests use a urine sample to identify the hormone HCG. The low cost and convenience make these tests attractive to many people.

Despite these advantages, home pregnancy tests are not nearly as accurate as laboratory-based ones. Manufacturers claim the tests to be 90% accurate, but research studies have found lower accuracy rates. Inaccuracies result not so much from the test itself, but from the difficulties some people have following directions and interpreting the results. The most common error stems from using the test kit too early in pregnancy, before the HCG can be detected.[1] Such an error (in this case, a false negative) could delay important prenatal care.

Most physicians will immediately order a more accurate test when a woman indicates she had a positive result on her home pregnancy test. This raises questions about duplication of health care costs. Nevertheless, the convenience and privacy provided by home tests continue to make them popular items for sexually active couples. ★

nancy tests. Although the specific technology varies from test to test, all pregnancy tests are based on the early and accurate identification of HCG through either urine or blood samples. Professional tests using urine samples are now as accurate as tests that use blood samples. Some tests available through professional clinics are highly accurate and can detect a pregnancy as early as 7 days after fertilization.[1]

With professionally administered pregnancy tests, the level of sensitivity is quite high. This sensitivity eliminates virtually all **false negatives** and nearly all **false positives.** If false negatives or false positives are suspected by the physician, a more highly sensitive test is recommended as a follow-up.

false negative in this case, a result that indicates "no pregnancy" when, in fact, there is a pregnancy.

false positive in this case, a result that indicates "pregnancy" when in fact, there is no pregnancy.

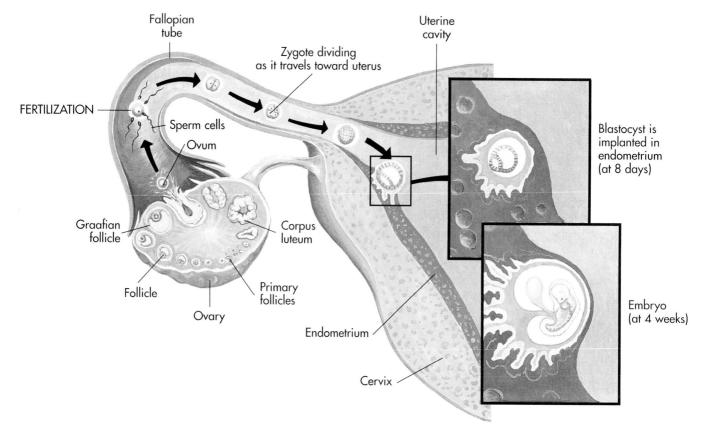

Figure 16-1   After its release from the follicle, the ovum begins its journey down the fallopian tube. Fertilization generally occurs in the outermost third of the tube. Now fertilized, the ovum progresses toward the uterus, where it imbeds itself in the endometrium. A pregnancy is established.

Signs of Pregnancy

Aside from pregnancy tests done in a laboratory, a woman can sometimes recognize early signs and symptoms. The signs of pregnancy have been divided into three categories.

Presumptive signs of pregnancy

Missed period after unprotected intercourse the previous month

Nausea upon awakening (morning sickness)

Increase in size and tenderness of breasts

Darkening of the areolar tissue surrounding the nipples

Probable signs of pregnancy

Increase in the frequency of urination (the growing uterus presses against the bladder)

Increase in the size of the abdomen

Cervix becomes softer by the sixth week (detected by a pelvic exam by clinician)

Positive pregnancy test

Positive signs of pregnancy

Determination of a fetal heartbeat

Feeling of the fetus moving (quickening)

Observation of fetus by ultrasound or optical viewers

Fetal Life

After fertilization occurs, the developing cell mass is called a *zygote*. Five to eight days will pass before the cell mass travels completely through the fallopian tube to the uterus (Figure 16-1). About a week after fertilization, the zygote will have undergone repeated cellular divisions and is now called a *blastocyst*. A day or two after entering the uterus, the blastocyst will implant itself into the endometrial wall. Once implanted, the cell mass is called an *embryo*. The **embryonic stage** of development lasts from the second through the eighth week of pregnancy. This stage is followed by the **fetal stage** (Figure 16-2).

Protected in its amniotic sac, the developing fetus is intimately connected to the mother by the *placenta*. The placenta is the organ of exchange between the mother and her fetus. Through the placenta, the fetus receives

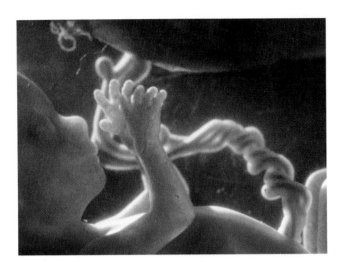

Figure 16-2 The fetus at 16 weeks gestation within the amniotic sac.

> ### ★ Warning: Acne, Accutane, and Birth Defects
>
> Accutane, manufactured by Roche Laboratories, may be the most effective prescription drug for severe cystic acne, a type of acne that often causes deep scarring. In 1988, the FDA reissued an earlier warning that pregnant women should not use this drug because it is capable of causing severe birth defects such as brain, skull, facial, and cardiac abnormalities. Women who use Accutane and are planning a pregnancy are encouraged to stop using the drug for two menstrual cycles before becoming pregnant. This gives the body time to clear Accutane from its system before conception. Some physicians recommend that women take a pregnancy test before beginning use of Accutane because of its severe effects on fetuses. ★

oxygen and nourishment from the mother's bloodstream and disposes of carbon dioxide and other waste products.[4] These exchanges take place through a *diffusion process* in the placenta, and the fetal and maternal blood never mix.

Multiple Births

The majority of pregnancies are single; however, some pregnancies lead to multiple births. The most common multiple birth is twins. On rare occasions, however, the birth of three, four, five, or more infants occurs (Table 16-1). The use of fertility drugs has increased the occurrence of multiple births.

In about one out of every 90 pregnancies, two babies will develop. These twin-multiple births are of two types, depending on the number of ova that have been fertilized.

Fraternal twins result when two separate ova are fertilized by different sperm (see Figure 16-3, *A*, p. 402). Fraternal twins can be of the same sex or opposite sex and are only slightly more similar in appearance than any two other siblings. Each fetus has its own placenta.

Identical twins result when only one ovum is fertilized but divides into two zygotes early in its development (Figure 16-3, *B*). Identical twins possess the same genetic background and share the same placenta.

These twins are always, of course, of the same sex.

In all multiple pregnancies, the developing infants must compete for space and, to some degree, must share nutrients. As a result, the incidence of prematurity is higher than in single pregnancies. Prematurity is higher for identical twins than for fraternal twins, perhaps because of the need to share a single placenta.

Agents That Can Damage a Fetus

A large number of agents that come into contact with a pregnant woman can affect fetal development.[5] Many of these (rubella and herpes viruses, tobacco smoke, alcohol, and virtually all other drugs) have been discussed in other chapters of this text. The best advice for a pregnant woman is to maintain close contact with her obstetrician during pregnancy and to consider carefully the ingestion of any over-the-counter drug (including aspirin, caffeine, and antacids) that could adversely harm the fetus. Abstinence from these products will help the nation achieve one of its important Healthy People 2000 objectives.

It is also important for any woman to avoid exposure to radiation during the pregnancy. Such exposure, most commonly through x-rays or radiation fallout from nuclear testing, can irreversibly damage fetal genetic structures. Epidemiological studies have shown

TABLE 16-1	Natural Occurrence of Multiple Births
Twins	1 in 90
Triplets	1 in 9,000
Quadruplets	1 in 900,000
Quintuplets	1 in 85,000,000

embryonic stage (em **bree on** ick) stage of human development from the second through the eighth week of pregnancy.

fetal stage (**fee** tul) stage of human development from the end of the eighth week of pregnancy until the time of birth.

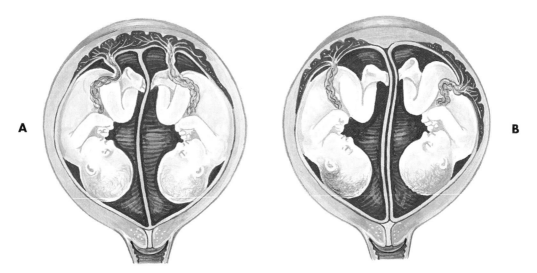

Figure 16-3 A, Identical twins. **B,** Fraternal twins. Note differences in construction of amniotic sacs.

that birth defects in the children of women exposed to radiation fallout are significantly higher than in the children of unexposed pregnant women. Pregnant women are advised to avoid unnecessary x-ray exposure during pregnancy.

CHILDBIRTH: THE LABOR OF DELIVERY

Determination of the Due Date

The day at which a pregnancy will come to term is called the *due date*. Nine months, 40 weeks, or 280 days is the average length of a human pregnancy. With this in mind, the due date can be calculated in a simple

Health ACTION Guide

The Well-Managed Pregnancy

▼ Determine the time of ovulation and the time of intercourse.
▼ Assume that conception has occurred.
▼ Avoid x-rays, unnecessary drugs, and exposure to infectious persons.
▼ Eat wholesome foods from the basic food groups.
▼ See your doctor as directed.
▼ Exercise as prescribed.
▼ Maintain appropriate weight. ▼

fashion by adding 7 days to the first day of the last menstrual period and then counting back 3 months. For example, let us say that you think you are pregnant and the first day of your last period was September 1. Adding 7 days to this will result in September 8. By counting back three months from September 8, you can determine a due date of June 8. There is about a 50/50 chance that the actual birth will occur within 1 week of this calculated date.

It is interesting to note that female babies tend to be born a few days earlier than male babies. Women who exercise regularly also tend to deliver earlier than women who do not exercise, and women who have relatively short menstrual cycles also tend to have shorter pregnancies.

Childbirth

Childbirth, or *parturition,* is one of the true peak experiences for both men and women. Most of the time childbirth is a wonderfully exciting venture into the unknown. For the parents, this intriguing experience can provide a stage for personal growth, maturity, and insight into a dynamic and complex world.

During the last few weeks of the third **trimester,** most fetuses will move deeper into the pelvic cavity in a process called *lightening*. During this movement, the fetus's body will rotate and the head will begin to engage more deeply into the mother's pelvic girdle. Many women will report that their babies have "dropped."

Another indication that parturition may be relatively near is the increased reporting of *Braxton Hicks contractions.* These uterine contractions, which are of mild intensity and often occur at irregular intervals, may be felt throughout a pregnancy. During the last few weeks of pregnancy *(gestation)*, these mild con-

Learning FROM ALL Cultures

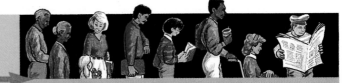

Maternal Deaths During Pregnancy and Childbirth

Throughout the world, one woman dies every minute due to pregnancy-related complications. Most of these deaths take place in developing countries among poor women who have little access to health care services. In developing countries pregnancy-related complications account for one fourth to one half of the deaths among women of reproductive age. Worldwide, approximately 500,000 women die each year because of pregnancy or childbirth complications.[11]

With the exception of women in China, a typical woman in the developing world has a one in 33 chance of dying from pregnancy or childbirth. In contrast, typical women in the developed world have only a one in 1500 chance of dying during pregnancy or childbirth.[11]

What makes pregnancy and childbirth so risky in developing countries? The major direct causes of

death are (1) hemorrhage (severe bleeding after childbirth, abortion, prolonged labor, or ectopic pregnancy), (2) infection (after childbirth or abortion, or related to STDs and resultant PID), and (3) eclampsia (high blood pressure during pregnancy).

What do you think are some of the obstacles that women face in developing countries that make them so vulnerable to this tragedy? Among these, consider issues such as the status of women, the health care delivery system, the age of marriage, prenatal care, and nutrition and health education efforts in developing countries. Do we face some of these same issues in North America? ●

---

tractions can occur more frequently and cause a woman to feel as if she were going into labor **(false labor)**.

Labor begins when uterine contractions become more intense and occur at regular intervals. The birth of a child can be divided into three stages: (1) *effacement* and dilation of the cervix, (2) delivery of the fetus, and (3) delivery of the placenta (see Figure 16-4, p. 404). For a woman having her first child, the birth process lasts an average of 12 to 16 hours. The average length of labor for subsequent children is much shorter—from 4 to 10 hours on the average. Labor is very unpredictable: labors that last between 1 and 24 hours occur daily at most hospitals.

STAGE ONE: EFFACEMENT AND DILATION OF THE CERVIX

In the first stage of labor the uterine contractions attempt to thin (*efface*) the normally thick cervical walls and to enlarge (*dilate*) the cervical opening. These contractions are directed by the release of *prostaglandins* and the hormone *oxytocin* into the circulating bloodstream. In women delivering first babies, effacement will occur before dilation. In subsequent deliveries, effacement and dilation usually occur at the same time.

The first stage of labor is often the longest of the three stages. The cervical opening must thin and dilate to a diameter of 10 centimeters before the first stage of labor is considered complete.[4] Often this stage begins

with the dislodging of the cervical mucous plug. The subsequent *bloody show* (mucous plug and a small amount of blood) at the vaginal opening may indicate that effacement and dilation have begun. Another indication of labor's onset may be the bursting or tearing of the fetal amniotic sac. "Breaking the bag of waters" is a reference to this phenomenon, which happens in various measures in expectant women. Some amniotic sacs burst with a large gush of clear amniotic fluid; some merely have a slight tear that trickles a small amount of fluid. Some women may even continue through the delivery of the baby before the sac is torn by the attending clinician or physician.

The pain of the uterine contractions becomes more intense as the woman moves through this first stage of labor. As the cervical opening effaces and dilates from 0 to 3 cm, many women report feeling happy, exhilarated, and confident. In the early phase of the first

---

trimester (try **mes** ter) three-month period of time; human pregnancies encompass three trimesters.

false labor conditions that tend to resemble the start of true labor; may include irregular uterine contractions, pressure, and discomfort in the lower abdomen.

A

FIRST STAGE

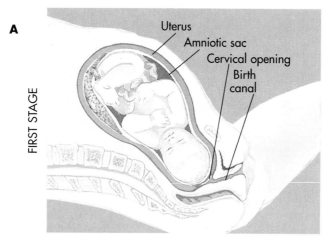

Uterus
Amniotic sac
Cervical opening
Birth canal

Uterine contractions thin the cervix and enlarge the cervical opening

B

SECOND STAGE

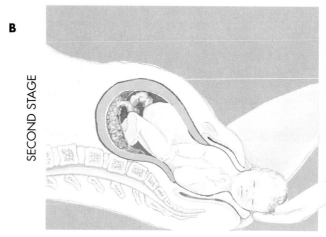

Uterine contractions are aided by mother's voluntary contractions of abdominal muscles

Fetus moves through dilated cervical opening and birth canal

C

THIRD STAGE

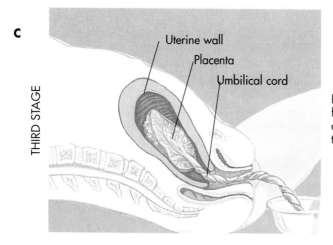

Uterine wall
Placenta
Umbilical cord

Placenta detaches from uterine wall and is delivered through the vagina

Figure 16-4 Labor, or childbirth, is a three-stage process. **A,** During effacement and dilation, the first stage, the cervical canal is gradually opened by contractions of the uterine wall. **B,** The second stage, birth of the baby, encompasses the actual delivery of the fetus from the uterus and through the birth canal. **C,** The delivery of the placenta, the third stage, empties the uterus, thus completing the process of childbirth.

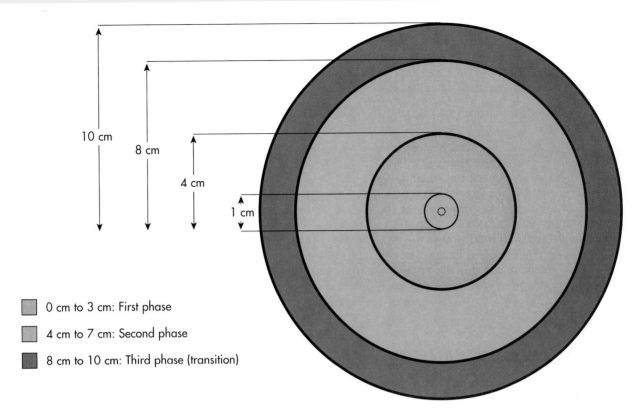

10 cm

8 cm

4 cm

1 cm

▢ 0 cm to 3 cm: First phase

▢ 4 cm to 7 cm: Second phase

▢ 8 cm to 10 cm: Third phase (transition)

Figure 16-5 Cervical dilation during the three phases of the first stage of labor.

stage of labor, the contractions are relatively short (lasting from 15 to 60 seconds) and the intervals between contractions range from 20 minutes to 5 minutes as labor progresses. However, these rest intervals will become shorter and the contractions more forceful when the woman's uterus contracts to dilate 4 to 7 cm.

In this second phase of the first stage of labor, the contractions usually last about 1 minute each, and the rest intervals drop from about 5 minutes to 1 minute over a period of 5 to 9 hours.

The third phase of the first stage of labor is called *transition*. During transition the uterus contracts to dilate the cervical opening to the full 10 cm required for safe passage of the fetus out of the uterus and into the birth canal (vagina). This period of labor is often the most painful part of the entire birth process. Fortunately, it is also the shortest phase of most labors. Lasting between 15 and 30 minutes, transition contractions often last 60 to 90 seconds each. The rest intervals between contractions are short and vary from 30 to 60 seconds.

An examination of the cervix by a nurse or physician will reveal whether full dilation of 10 cm has occurred. Until the full 10-cm dilation, women are cautioned not to push the fetus during the contractions (Figure 16-5). Special breathing and concentration techniques help many women cope with the first stage of labor.

STAGE TWO: DELIVERY OF THE FETUS

Once the mother's cervix is fully dilated, she enters the second stage of labor, the delivery of the fetus through the birth canal. Now the mother is encouraged to help push the baby out (with her abdominal muscles) during each contraction. In this second stage, the uterine contractions are less forceful than during the transition phase of the first stage of labor, and may last 60 seconds each with a 1- to 3-minute rest interval.

This second stage may last up to 2 hours in first births.[4] For subsequent babies this stage is usually much shorter. When the baby's head is first seen at the vaginal opening, *crowning* is said to have taken place. Generally the back of the baby's head appears first. (Infants whose feet or buttocks are presented first are said to be delivered in a *breech position*.) Once the head is delivered, the baby's body rotates upward to let the shoulders come through. The rest of the body follows quite quickly. The second stage of labor ends when the fetus is fully expelled from the vagina.

Newly delivered babies often look far different from the babies seen on television commercials. Their heads are often cone-shaped as a result of the compression of cranial bones that occurs during the delivery of the baby through the birth canal. Within a few days following birth, the newborn's head assumes a much more normal shape. Most babies (of all races) appear bluish at first, until they begin regular breathing. All babies are covered with a coating of *vernix,* a white, cheeselike substance that protects the skin.

STAGE THREE: DELIVERY OF THE PLACENTA

Usually within 30 minutes after the fetus is delivered, the uterus will again initiate a series of contractions to expel the placenta (or *afterbirth*). The placenta is examined by the attending physician to ensure that it was completely expelled. Torn remnants of the placenta could lead to dangerous *hemorrhaging* by the mother. Often the physician will perform a manual examination of the uterus after the placenta has been delivered.

Once the placenta has been expelled, the uterus will continue with mild contractions to help control bleeding and start the gradual reduction of the uterus to its normal, nonpregnant size. This final aspect of the birth process is called **post partum.** External abdominal massage of the lower abdomen seems to help the uterus contract, as does an infant's nursing at the mother's breast.

ADDITIONAL CONSIDERATIONS CONCERNING CHILDBIRTH

Medications

Despite the large movement toward prepared childbirth or natural childbirth methods of delivery, most women still receive some kind of medication during labor. The type of drug depends on the particular birth situation, physical preference, and pain tolerance of the mother. Since the use of any drug by the mother can potentially damage the fetus, the physician and mother need to discuss the use of any medications before the time of delivery.

Analgesics are drugs that are administered to reduce the mother's pain during labor. Analgesics are sometimes used with mild tranquilizers to reduce pain and encourage relaxation of the mother. *Anesthetics* are drugs that block off all sensations. *General anesthetics,* in the form of inhaled gases, were formerly used during the last 10 minutes or so of the second stage of labor. However, since it is now recognized that general anesthetics can damage a fetus and also do not allow the mother to participate actively in the final part of her delivery, general anesthetics are less commonly used, except in some cesarean deliveries.

Most anesthetics used today are regional or local anesthetics. *Regional anesthetics* are injected at specific points (near the spinal cord) and block off sensations in the body below the injection site. Some regional anesthetics can be injected that will allow a mother to use her muscles to assist in her delivery; other regional anesthetics prevent this. *Local anesthetics* are for smaller areas and help block sensations as the baby moves through the birth canal. Procaine (Novocain) is often injected near the vaginal opening if an *episiotomy*

has taken place. An episiotomy is an optional surgical procedure that enlarges the vaginal opening. Novocain permits the painless suturing of the episiotomy incision.

Cesarean Deliveries

A **cesarean delivery** (cesarean birth, cesarean section, C-section) is a procedure in which the fetus is surgically removed from the mother's uterus through the abdominal wall. Lasting up to an hour for the complete procedure, this type of delivery can be performed with the mother having a regional anesthetic or a general anesthetic.

In 1970, cesarean deliveries accounted for 6% of all deliveries. Currently, nearly 25% of all deliveries are by cesarean section.[6] The increase in the use of cesarean deliveries is questioned by some medical experts, although others point to the need for this kind of delivery when one or more of the following factors are present:

▼ The fetus is improperly aligned.
▼ The pelvis of the mother is too small.
▼ The fetus is especially large.
▼ The fetus shows signs of respiratory or cardiac distress.
▼ The umbilical cord is compressed.
▼ The placenta is being delivered before the fetus.
▼ The mother's health is at risk.

Although a cesarean delivery is considered major surgery, most mothers cope well with the delivery and postsurgical and postpartum discomfort. The hospital stay is usually a few days longer than for a vaginal delivery. The mother can still nurse her child and may still be able to have vaginal deliveries with later children. More and more hospitals are allowing the father to be in the operating room during cesarean deliveries. Fortunately, research indicates that early **bonding** between child, mother, and father can still occur with cesarean deliveries. Cesarean deliveries are much more expensive than vaginal deliveries.

Breast-feeding

For a variety of reasons, mothers of newborns are being encouraged to breast-feed (nurse) their babies.[1] The baby's nursing stimulates the release of the hormone oxytocin from the mother's pituitary gland. Oxytocin encourages the uterus to contract shortly after birth, but it also stimulates cells in the *mammary glands* of the breasts to release milk. This process is called *lactation*. Initially the child's sucking actions produce a watery clear fluid called *colostrum*, which is followed by milk in a couple of days.

Nursing has the advantage of providing a convenient, inexpensive, nutritionally complete diet for the infant. Furthermore, nursing provides the infant with an abundance of maternal antibodies that help fight infant infections and minimize allergic reactions—es-

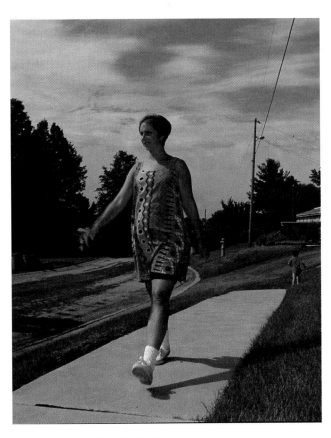

Keeping fit during pregnancy.

Health ACTION Guide

Physical Activity and Pregnancy

How much physical activity should a pregnant woman have? Follow these recommendations:

▼ Always check with your physician first to determine the right exercise program for your pregnancy status.

▼ Most pregnant women can participate in mild-to-moderate exercise. Strenuous exercise, contact sports, and highly competitive sports should be avoided.

▼ Recommended exercises are swimming, cycling (a stationary bike may be preferred to a standard one because of weight and balance shifts during pregnancy), walking, and low-impact aerobics.

▼ Running may be acceptable in the early months of pregnancy but is not generally recommended late in a pregnancy.

▼ The best rule of thumb is to get in shape before the pregnancy and continue your activities during pregnancy. ▼

pecially those of the digestive tract. Another advantage of breast-feeding is that it can provide a very close bonding experience between mother and child. Increasing breast-feeding is an important Healthy People 2000 Objective.

Possible disadvantages of breast-feeding include the passage of toxic substances to the infant (drugs, nicotine, alcohol) that are ingested by the mother, lack of freedom for the mother, discomfort caused by engorged breasts and sensitive nipples, and reduced time spent with the baby by the father. HIV-infected mothers should not breast-feed their infants, since HIV, the virus which causes AIDS, can be transmitted through breast milk.[1] Contrary to popular belief, breast-feeding is *not* an effective form of contraception. Backup methods of contraception should be used for couples having intercourse.

Clearly, whether to nurse or to bottle feed a baby depends on a host of factors that should be considered. Fortunately, most typical babies turn out to be healthy and happy regardless of how they were fed as infants. The choice is up to the parents.

Preparation for Birth

In the past, expectant mothers (and fathers) were somewhat restricted in their attempts to play a major role throughout the pregnancy and delivery of their child. As long as the physician's prenatal examinations

were normal, little information was given to the parents. Fathers were rarely seen in an obstetrician's office. Women were frequently told, "Everything is fine," and were instructed to come to the hospital as soon as they thought they were going into labor. At the hospital men sat anxiously in smoke-filled waiting rooms while their wives agonized through labor and then, often heavily sedated, delivered babies in sterile, impersonal surgical rooms. Indeed, the birthing process was perceived to be a painful, dreaded experience by many of its participants, except perhaps for the newborns, whose feelings could only be estimated.

Today expectant parents can elect to attend prepared childbirth classes during the last few months of their pregnancies. At these classes, parents can learn

post partum (post **par** tum) period of time after the birth of a baby during which the uterus returns to its prepregnancy size.

cesarean delivery (si **zare** ee an) surgical removal of a fetus through the abdominal wall.

bonding important, initial recognition established between the newborn and those adults on whom the newborn will be dependent.

not only about the biological events relating to childbirth, but also about appropriate techniques, exercises, and positions that will help to reduce the fear and therefore the pain surrounding childbirth. These classes often include lectures, discussions, films, demonstrations, and visits to hospital obstetrical units. Typically, a small fee is charged for prepared childbirth classes.

Most parents who deliver their children with this kind of training are overwhelmingly satisfied, even if their particular labor necessitated the use of medications or even an eventual cesarean delivery. The father's role appears to help establish an early bond between the *neonate* (newborn baby) and its father. Frequently the parents report their own relationship is stengthened as a result of a cooperative type of delivery.

Another trend with regard to childbirth is the use of **birthing rooms** in many hospitals. For many years, pregnant women progressed through the lengthy first stage of labor in *labor rooms* and were then transferred to surgically equipped *delivery rooms* for the second and third stages of labor. These transfers generally were seen as an uncomfortable break in the continuity of the birth experience. Birthing rooms allow women in labor to go through the entire labor and delivery in one room. Typically birthing rooms are decorated in a homelike way, with pictures, televisions, wall hangings, carpets, and lounge chairs present in the room. Depending on hospital policy, fathers, and sometimes entire families, can be present in birthing rooms.

Some hospitals permit mothers (and even families) to room in with newborn babies after they are delivered. Usually neonates are allowed to visit with their mothers and fathers only during limited hours. *Rooming in* allows unlimited (or near unlimited) visitation with newborns.

BIRTH TECHNOLOGY

Technological advances continue to occur in the field of *obstetrics*. Not only have new procedures been developed, but also some common procedures have been improved. Included among these are:

▼ *Sonography.* By using sound waves to produce images **(sonograms)** of fetuses, physicians can detect fetal abnormalities, determine fetal position, and monitor fetal growth. In the past, sonography was used mainly to determine the sex of a developing fetus or to take a first picture for the parents.

▼ *Amniocentesis.* The human fetus develops within a fluid-filled amniotic sac. Over the course of the pregnancy, cells and urine from the developing fetus accumulate within this fluid. Amniocentesis is a procedure in which a small quantity of amniotic fluid is drawn from the amniotic sac through a needle. The fluid is then analyzed for genetic abnor-

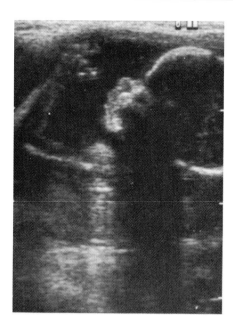

Sonogram.

malities. The procedure is generally done between the fourteenth and the sixteenth weeks of the pregnancy.[7] The results obtained by amniocentesis can help those involved make decisions about pregnancy termination or medical care of the fetus.

▼ *Chorionic villi sampling (CVS).* One of the most important technologies in the practice of obstetrics is chorionic villi sampling. CVS permits the microscopic examination of cells of the **chorionic villi** derived from the fetus. Chromosomes can be removed from these cells to be examined for genetic defects. Unlike amniocentesis, CVS can be performed during the first trimester, usually between 9 and 11 weeks after conception.[2] If serious defects are found, pregnancy termination becomes an option.

▼ *Amniotic fluid level assessment.* It is now known that many fetuses who are developing abnormally produce less amniotic fluid than do normally developing fetuses. Sonography assessment of amniotic fluid levels allows for earlier intervention by the physician.

Infertility

Most traditional-age college students are interested in pregnancy prevention. However, increasing numbers of other persons are trying to do just the opposite: they are trying to become pregnant. It is estimated that about one in six couples has a problem with *infertility.*[7] These couples wish to become pregnant but are unsuccessful.

Why are couples infertile? The reasons are about evenly balanced between males and females. About 10% of infertility cases have no detectable cause. The major male complication is insufficient sperm produc-

★ Sickle Cell Trait and Sickle Cell Disease

Of all the chemical compounds found within the body, few occur in as many forms as hemoglobin, which helps bind oxygen to the red blood cell. Two forms of hemoglobin are associated with sickle cell trait and sickle cell disease. African-Americans can be the recipients of either of these abnormal hemoglobin forms. Those who inherit the trait form do not develop the disease but are capable of transmitting the gene for abnormal hemoglobin to their offspring. Those persons who inherit the disease form face a shortened life characterized by periods of pain and impairment.

Approximately 8% of all African-Americans have the gene for sickle cell trait; they experience little impairment, and they can transmit the gene to their children.

For approximately 1.5% of African-Americans, sickle cell disease is a painful, incapacitating, and life-shortening disease. Red blood cells are elongated, crescent shaped (or sickled), and unable to pass through the body's minute capillaries. The body responds to the presence of these abnormal red blood cells by removing them very quickly. This sets the stage for anemia—thus the condition is often called *sickle cell anemia*. In addition to anemia, this form of the condition is associated with many serious medical problems including impaired lung function, congestive heart failure, gallbladder infections, bone changes, and possible abnormalities of the eye and skin. Living beyond early adulthood may not be possible.

If a key exists for preventing the occurrence of sickle cell trait and disease, it lies in the area of genetic counseling to help in making decisions regarding reproduction, including pregnancy termination. The decision to have children and perhaps risk passing on the gene for defective hemoglobin to the next generation is a decision that must be carefully made. ★

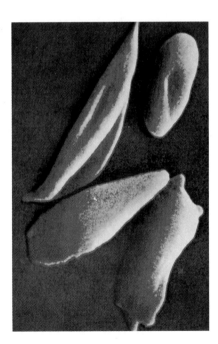

Sickled red blood cells.

Males can also collect (through masturbation) and save samples of their own sperm to use in a procedure called *artificial insemination by partner*. Near the time of ovulation, the collected samples of sperm are then deposited near the woman's cervical opening. In a related procedure called *artificial insemination by donor*, the sperm of a donor is used. Donor semen is screened for the presence of pathogens, including the AIDS virus.

Causes of infertility in females center mostly on obstructions in the female reproductive tract and the inability to ovulate. The obstructions frequently result from tissue damage (scarring) caused by infections. Unchecked chlamydial and gonorrheal infections often produce fertility problems. In certain women, the use of IUDs has produced infections and PID; both of these increase the chances of infertility. Other possible causes of structural abnormalities include scar tissue from previous surgery, fibroid tumors, polyps, and endometriosis. A variety of microsurgical techniques may correct some of these complications.

tion and delivery. A number of approaches can be used to increase sperm counts. Among the simple approaches are the application of periodic cold packs on the scrotum and the replacement of tight underwear with boxer shorts. When a structural problem reduces sperm production, surgery can be helpful. Opinion is divided concerning whether increased frequency of intercourse improves fertility. Most experts (fertility endocrinologists) do suggest that couples have intercourse at least a couple of times in the week preceding ovulation.

birthing rooms hospital facilities that serve as both a labor and a delivery room.

sonogram (**sahn** oh gram) images of internal structures produced by high-frequency sound waves; also called ultrasound and ultrasonography.

chorionic villi (core ee **on** ick **vill** eye) fingerlike extensions of the fetal portion of the placenta. These extensions carry fetal blood vessels close to the maternal blood vessels.

Where to Find Help

These agencies can provide you with information on fertility and give referrals to specialists in your area:

American Fertility Society
The Society for Reproductive Medicine
1209 Montgomery Highway
Birmingham, AL 35216-2809
(205) 978-5000

Planned Parenthood Federation of America
810 Seventh Avenue
New York, NY 10019
(212) 541-7800
(800) 829-7732

These agencies can provide help to prospective adoptive parents:

The National Adoption Center
1500 Walnut Street
Suite 701
Philadelphia, PA 19102
(215) 735-9988

The National Committee for Adoption
1930 17th Street, N.W.
Washington, DC 20009
(212) 328-8072

The North American Council on Adoptable Children
1821 University Avenue
Room N-498
St. Paul, MN 55104
(612) 644-3036

Adoptive Families of America, Inc.
3333 Highway 100 North
Minneapolis, MN 55422
(612) 535-4829
Publishes OURS Magazine (Organization for United Response)

One of the most recent innovative procedures involves the use of **transcervical balloon tuboplasty.**[8] In this procedure, a series of balloon-tipped catheters are inserted through the uterus into the blocked fallopian tubes. Once inflated, these balloon catheters help open the scarred passageways. A 1990 study in the *Journal of the American Medical Association* reported that one third of the infertile women who had their tubes opened by balloon tuboplasty were able to become pregnant within 1 year.[8]

When a woman has ovulation difficulties, pinpointing the specific cause can be very difficult. Increasing age produces hormone fluctuations associated with lack of ovulation. Being significantly overweight or underweight also has a major impact on fertility. However, in women of normal weight who are not approaching menopause, it appears that ovulation difficulties are caused by failure of syncronization between the hormones governing the menstrual cycle. Fertility drugs can help alter the menstrual cycle to produce ovulation. Clomiphene citrate (Clomid), in oral pill form, and injections of a mixture of LH and FSH taken from the urine of menopausal women (Pergonal) are the most common fertility drugs available. Both are capable of producing multiple ova at ovulation.

For couples who are unable to conceive following drug therapy, surgery, and artificial insemination, the use of *in vivo fertilization and embryo transfer (IVF-ET)* is another option. This method is sometimes referred to as the "test tube" procedure. Costing up to $10,000 per attempt, IVF-ET consists of surgically retrieving fertilizable ova from the woman and combining them in a glass dish with sperm. After several days, the fertilized ova are transferred into the uterus. The pregnancy success rate for a single treatment cycle is 19%.[9]

A newer test tube procedure is called *gamete intrafallopian transfer (GIFT)*. Similar to IVF-ET, this newer procedure deposits a mixture of retrieved eggs and sperm directly into the fallopian tubes. The pregnancy success rate for a single treatment cycle is 29%.[9]

Surrogate parenting is another option that has recently been explored, although the legal and ethical issues surrounding this method of conception are not fully resolved. Surrogate parenting exists in a number of forms. Typically, an infertile couple will make a contract with a woman (the surrogate parent) who will then be artificially inseminated with semen from the expectant father. In some instances the surrogate will receive an embryo from the donor parents. The surrogate will carry the fetus to term and return the newborn to the parents. Because of the concerns about true "ownership" of the baby, surrogate parenting may not be a particularly viable option for many couples. The box on p. 411 points out some serious questions raised by this issue.

The process of coping with infertility problems can be an emotionally stressful experience for a couple. Hours of waiting in physician's offices, having numerous examinations, scheduling intercourse, producing sperm samples, and undergoing surgical or drug treatments place multiple burdens on a couple. Knowing that other couples are able to conceive so effortlessly adds to the mental strain. Fortunately, support groups exist to assist couples with infertility problems. Some of these groups are listed in the box on the left.

What can one do to reduce the chances of developing infertility problems? Certainly the avoidance of infections in the reproductive organs is one crucial factor. Barrier methods of contraception (condom, diaphragm) with a spermicide reportedly cut the risk of developing infertility in half. The use of an IUD should

Surrogate Parenting: Unresolved Questions

Many important questions regarding surrogate parenting have been raised during the last decade. Among these are the following:

★ Does the surrogate mother sell a service or a product?

★ If a surrogate mother charges and is paid a fee, is this different from giving her service free of charge? Do her rights to the baby change?

★ Do the persons who receive the services of a surrogate mother have the right to reject the baby if it is disabled or otherwise unacceptable?

★ Does the surrogate mother have a right to keep the child?

★ Does the surrogate mother have visitation rights to the child?

★ Can the infertile couple require the surrogate mother not to consume alcohol, tobacco, or other dangerous products during the pregnancy?

★ How can the infertile couple monitor the pregnancy?

★ Who pays for long-term health care if the surrogate mother's health status is harmed by the pregnancy or delivery?

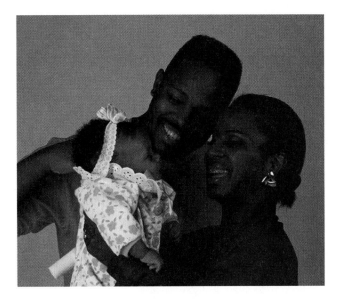

The new family.

be avoided, and the risk from multiple partners should be considered carefully. Men and women should be aware of the dangers of working around hazardous chemicals or consuming psychoactive drugs. Maintaining overall good health and having regular medical (and gynecological) checkups are also good ideas. Finally, since infertility is linked with advancing age, couples may not want to indefinitely delay having children.

A PARENTING PRESCRIPTION FOR THE EARLY YEARS

Dr. T. Berry Brazelton, internationally known pediatrician and child development specialist, realizes how difficult it is to raise children in the 1990s. Brazelton knows that trying to juggle employment, college work, and family life is especially difficult and can, at times, seem overwhelming. Firm in his belief that parents can be successful at coping with busy schedules and raising well-adjusted children, Brazelton has identified 14 key parenting points for families with young children.[10]

1. *Separate your home and work environments.* Try to keep the two separate as much as possible.
2. *Plan your daily separation from your children.* Don't just separate without a warm exchange.
3. *Realize that it is okay to feel sad about leaving your child.* This will encourage you to get the best child care available.
4. *Allow yourself to feel a measure of guilt.* In this case, guilt can be a powerful source for solving problems.
5. *Share your stress with friends or support groups.* Interacting with others can provide much needed support.
6. *Always include your spouse in family activities.* Let him or her have a major role in important decisions.
7. *Do not feel that you must be a "superparent" or that you must raise "superkids."* Don't hold yourself up to standards that are virtually impossible to reach. It's not fair to you or your kids.
8. *While at work, conserve some energy for your home life.* Plan your day so that you are ready to do more than collapse in front of the television when you get home.

transcervical balloon tuboplasty (trans **sir** vick al **tube** oh plas tee) the use of inflatable balloon catheters to open blocked fallopian tubes; a procedure used for some women with fertility problems.

9. *Be sure you understand all the parenting options available at your workplace.* Know the policies related to day care, flexible time schedules, shared-job possibilities, and sick leave if your child becomes ill.

10. *Prepare yourself for a bit of chaos when you return home after work.* Children often save some of their energy and feelings until they are back with their family.

11. *Hug or hold your young children for at least a few moments when you return from work.* Don't just come home and start your chores or housework without first making close contact with your children.

12. *Encourage your children to help you with your chores.* Most young children want to help. Be patient; encourage and praise their efforts.

13. *Make sure each child has some special time alone with each parent at least once every week.* This shows children that each child is important and deserves attention.

14. *Learn that stress is normal and that you can cope.* Solving problems together as a family can build warm and lasting relationships.

Summary

- ✔ Becoming pregnant and raising children will have a significant impact on the lives of parents.
- ✔ Without contraception, a high percentage of sexualy active women of childbearing age will become pregnant.
- ✔ A woman's natural defense system provides a number of obstacles to sperm cells. Among these are the acidic level of the vaginal secretions, the thickness of the cervical mucus, the relative distance to the fallopian tubes, and the anatomical positioning of the female reproductive structures.
- ✔ Numerous physiological mechanisms help sperm cells reach the ovum. Among these are the large number of sperm cells, the secretions of the male accessory structures, uterine contractions, changes in cervical mucus consistency, and the alkaline environment within the uterus and fallopian tubes.
- ✔ Professional pregnancy tests have high rates of accuracy. Home pregnancy tests are less accurate. Both kinds of tests search for the presence of the hormone HCG (human chorionic gonadotropin).
- ✔ Childbirth takes place in three distinct stages: effacement and dilation of the cervix, birth of the baby, and delivery of the placenta.
- ✔ Breast-feeding provides numerous health benefits for infants.
- ✔ Infertility is a major concern for some couples. Various technologies are improving infertile couples' chances of becoming pregnant.

Review Questions

1. Identify some basic concerns presented in the chapter that should be considered by an individual or couple planning parenthood.

2. What are some of the obstacles and aids to fertilization presented in the chapter? Can you think of others that were not presented?

3. What harmful agents can affect the fetus?

4. Identify and describe the events that occur during each of the three stages of labor. Approximately how long does each stage last?

5. What should a pregnant woman know about the following birth-related topics: anesthesia, medications, cesarean delivery, and breast-feeding?

6. Describe some of the recent advances in birth technology.

7. Distinguish between IVF-ET and GIFT procedures.

8. What can one do to reduce the chances of infertility?

Think about This . . .

✔ What effects do you think starting parenthood at a later age has? On the parent? On the child?

✔ Will you become a parent? If so, when?

✔ How do you feel about a couple's choice not to have children?

✔ If a woman should not smoke, drink, or use other drugs during pregnancy, should these limitations also be placed on the father? Why or why not?

✔ To what extent should fathers participate in the birth experience?

✔ Have you ever thought about how your current health behaviors could have an impact on your future fertility?

REAL LIFE REAL CHOICES

YOUR TURN

▼ What are the chief causes of (1) male and (2) female infertility?

▼ What procedures are used to correct causes of infertility and help women become pregnant?

▼ What is surrogate parenting, and what are the controversies that surround this issue?

AND NOW, YOUR CHOICES . . .

▼ If you plan to have children, how important is it to you that they be the biological offspring of you and your spouse? Give reasons for your answer.

▼ If you and your spouse, like Gary and Susan Johnson, very much wanted to have a child and found out in your later 30s that you had a serious fertility problem, what route would you choose: the available medical/surgical options, surrogate parenting, adoption, or another course of action (foster parenting, remaining childless)? Give reasons for your answer. ▼

References

1. Hatcher RA et al: *Contraceptive technology,* ed 16, New York, 1994, Irvington Publishers.
2. Hyde JS: *Understanding human sexuality,* ed 5, New York, 1994, McGraw-Hill.
3. Moffett DF, Moffett SB, Schauf CL: *Human physiology: foundations and frontiers,* ed 2, St Louis, 1993, Mosby.
4. Haas K, Haas A: *Understanding sexuality,* ed 3, St. Louis, 1993, Mosby.
5. Rayburn WF, Zuspan FP: *Drug therapy in obstetrics and gynecology,* ed 3, St Louis, 1992, Mosby.
6. U.S. Bureau of the Census: *Statistical abstract of the United States: 1993,* ed 113, Washington, DC, 1993, US Government Printing Office.
7. Crooks R, Baur K: *Our sexuality,* ed 5, Menlo Park, Calif, 1993, Benjamin-Cummings.
8. Confino E et al: Transcervical balloon tuboplasty: a multicenter study, *JAMA* 264(16):2079, 1990.
9. Medical Research International, Society for Assisted Reproductive Technology, The American Fertility Society: In-vitro fertilization-embryo transfer (IVF-ET) in the United States: 1990 results from the IVF-ET Registry. *Fertil Steril* 57(1):15, 1992.
10. Brazelton TB: Bringing up baby: a doctor's prescription for busy parents, *Newsweek,* February 13, 1989, p. 68.
11. Population Information Program: Mothers' lives matter: maternal health in the community, *Population Reports* 16:2, 1988; Series L: No 7, Center for Communications Programs; Johns Hopkins University.

Suggested Readings

Jones C: *Breastfeeding your baby: a guide for the contemporary family,* New York, 1993, Collins Books.

A certified childbirth educator covers practical advice on all aspects of breastfeeding. Topics include preventing and solving problems, how to combine breastfeeding and bottle-feeding, and how family and friends can help. Clear illustrations and straightforward advice.

Rosenberg HS, Epstein YM: *Getting pregnant when you thought you couldn't: the interactive guide that helps you up the odds,* New York, 1993, Warner Books.

A useful resource for infertile couples, and written by a nationally recognized married couple who have themselves struggled to conceive a child. Presents lots of information in a sensitive, thorough manner.

Sears W, Sears M: *The birth book: everything you need to know to have a safe and satisfying birth,* Boston, 1994, Little, Brown.

The authors are parents of eight children and are nationally renowned pediatric specialists. Gives expectant parents practical advice about every aspect of birthing, including preparing for birth, labor, and delivery. Issues of using technology, defining the father's role, and turning the surgical birth into a rewarding experience are discussed.

Walker M: *Sexual nutrition,* Garden City Park, NY, 1994, Avery Publishing Group.

An examination of factors related to fertility: nutrients and their relation to improved sex drive, stamina, and performance. A guide to enhance relationships through healthful changes in diet.

As you read through this unit, you probably saw connections between the nature of your own sexuality and the five developmental tasks: identity, independence, responsibility, social skills, and intimacy. If you are a traditional age student, these connections were probably based on personal experiences or those you expect in the future. Nontraditional students may have reflected on their past or current experiences, as well as those of their children.

Forming an Initial Adult Identity

In your search to accomplish this particular developmental task, the same question is repeated: "Who am I?" As a young adult, or as an older person looking back on this period, you see yourself engaged in writing a script about who you are and who you will become in the near future. Certainly, this script will include information about your sexuality. We would contend that to really know yourself, you must start to analyze the way you feel about aspects of your reproductive, genital, and expressionistic sexuality. Start asking yourself some important questions, such as: "What do I really want in a relationship?" "How much do I care about the feelings of my partner?" "Have I developed my personal code of ethics?" "Am I ready to become a parent?" "Am I happy with the way I express myself as a man or woman?" Answers to these kinds of questions will help you come to grips with your emerging adult identity.

Establishing Independence

For the majority of young adults, independence from the family encourages the freedom to live where you wish. This mobility provides the opportunity for experiences that allow you to achieve a fully developed adult gender identification. Living and working in new places and interacting with a variety of different individuals can help achieve this understanding of yourself. Being mobile allows you to see a wide range of masculine and feminine models. Some of these models you will appreciate more than others, yet we contend that you will learn something from them all. In much the same manner that college increases your pool of friends and presents alternative lifestyle experiences, your independence after college can further enhance this process.

Assuming Responsibility

Hand-in-hand with gaining independence goes the important task of increasing personal responsibility. In terms of a paired sexual relationship, how does one direct this responsibility? In our minds, the responsibility starts before the relationship begins. It is only beforehand that you have the opportunity to look carefully at intent regarding the sexual standards you will follow. You must ask yourself questions concerning personal standards and your ability to adhere to these standards. You must address questions concerning contraceptive effectiveness, the likelihood of STDs, and possible pregnancy. Ignoring these issues can lead to disappointment for yourself and frustration for others. Fortunately, many individuals want to share their responsibility with their partners.

Developing Social Skills

A discussion concerning paired sexual relationships and the development of social skills is very much like a description of the evolution of a friendship. In a growing friendship, new social skills are layered, level upon level. The evolving nature of the paired sexual relationship follows a similar pattern of growth and development in social skills.

A person engaged in dating relationships must develop insights, senstivities, and responses that will be of value not only through courtship but more important, in marriage. Social skills particularly relevant to mate selection include the ability to form and assess perceptions, to recognize the reward system around which you and your partner operate, to express your values, and to act on those values with honesty and consistency.

Developing Intimacy

To many, the word *intimacy* is inseparable from *sexual*, and only direct physical contact involving coital behavior or some from of erotic contact is considered intimate. They do not consider perceptions of femininity and masculinity, how people see themselves, and how they share with others. This narrow perspective diminishes the larger role that sexuality plays in structuring our intimate relationships. As the mate selection model presented in this section explains, for a lifelong relationship to prosper, the partners must feel comfortable with their own identities. Doing so provides greater opportunities for success in the relationships that you enjoy.

UNIT SIX

At first a unit that combines chapters on consumer health, the environment, and violence might seem unusual. Yet everything we do in life is in some way related to our environment. Each day we come into contact with our land, air, and water. Within our environment, we seek freedom from violence and make health-related consumer decisions. Unit VI focuses on these kinds of decisions because they affect the multiple dimensions of health.

● Physical Dimension of Health

In a variety of ways, the physical dimension of health can be immediately influenced by consumer decisions. Your choice of a particular physician, for example, is a good choice when you know that physician specializes in the services you require and is able to restore physical function within a few days. Similarly, the choices you make concerning where you live (perhaps in a location with clean air, clean water, and clean land) will have an impact on your physical health. And, of course, your ability to avoid violent persons reduces the chance of being harmed physically.

◆ Emotional Dimension of Health

The impact of an overcrowded, highly industrialized, and increasingly violent society on our emotional health is not as evident as the impact on our physical health. However, when we are able to spend a few days in a pristine environment, we begin to understand how our surroundings affect our mental health. We appreciate natural sounds and natural odors. We delight in the unspoiled beauty of an uncluttered forest or a sparkling clear stream. The psychological benefits are refreshing and may last months or years. On the other hand, emotional health can be damaged when we see an environment gradually overcome by society's greed and technological advancements. Even more powerful in influencing emotional health is the presence of violence in our day to day environment. Strong feelings can be harbored for years when you have been victimized by another person who intended to harm you. Further, the knowledge of your own violent behavior toward others may be the most corrosive force in your long-term emotional health.

■ Social Dimension of Health

Consumers are not born—they are made. They are shaped in part by their contact with others. The direction other people provide about the information, services, and products you use is a powerful factor in your development as a health-oriented consumer. Discussing health needs with parents, friends, or health care professionals can help you to quickly and efficiently meet those needs.

▲ Intellectual Dimension of Health

Understanding environmental concerns and consumer options is not a task for the unskilled mind. Trying to isolate causes of environmental pollution and preparing workable solutions are two extremely complicated tasks. Understanding the relationships among pollutants, humans, and our environment may require study in a variety of physical and biological sciences.

● Spiritual Dimension of Health

The study of consumer information and environmental issues that relate to our health can be viewed from a spiritual dimension. We frequently hold much faith in the health products and medical services that we select. When we are ill, we may hope that a higher power is capable of working through our physician to make a correct diagnosis. As our health improves, the beauty that we begin to notice in the world is a tribute to our unending search for a deeper meaning to life. As we search for solutions to complex environmental problems, we may be forced to make some difficult decisions. For example, will we someday force third world countries to use contraceptive measures or sterilization? Will we attempt to feed the world's hungry people? Will we continue to protect endangered species of plants and animals? Will we strive more forcefully for nuclear disarmament? To build a better world for future generations may be the biggest challenge in our spiritual commitment to serve others.

Consumerism and Environment

Outside Forces Shaping Your Health

Consumerism and Health Care

Making Sound Decisions

ealth care providers often evaluate you by criteria pertaining to their area of expertise. The nutritionist knows you by the food you eat. The physical fitness professional knows you by your body type and activity level. And in the eyes of the expert in health-related consumerism, you are the product of the health information you believe, the health-influencing services you use, and the products you consume. When your decisions about health information, services, and products are made after careful study and consideration, your health will probably be improved. However, when your decisions lack insight, your health, as well as your pocketbook, may suffer.

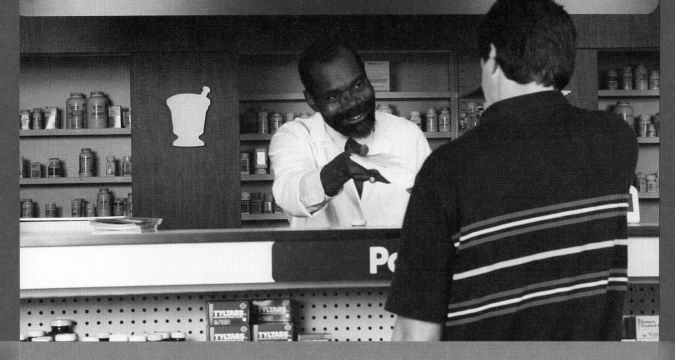

Medicine Shoppe® PRESCRIPTION CENTERS

C O N S U M E R I S M

The following objectives are covered in this chapter:

▽ Increase to at least 95% the proportion of people who have a specific source of ongoing primary care for coordination of their preventive and episodic health care. (Baseline: less than 82% in 1986, as 18% report having no physician, clinic, or hospital as a regular source of care; p. 535.)

▽ Improve financing and delivery of clinical preventive services so that virtually no American has a financial barrier to receiving, at a minimum, the screening, counseling, and immunization services recommended by the U.S. Preventive Services Task Force. (Baseline data unavailable; p. 536.)

▽ Increase to at least 75% the proportion of pharmacies and other dispensers of prescription medications that use linked systems to provide alerts to potential adverse drug reactions among medications dispensed by different sources to individual patients. (Baseline data unavailable; p. 344.)

▽ Increase the proportion of all degrees in the health professions and allied and associated health profession fields awarded to members of underrepresented racial and ethnic minority groups to these targets: degrees awarded to Blacks (8%), Hispanics (6.4%), and American Indians/Alaska Natives (0.6%). (Baseline percentages in 1985-86: Blacks (5%), Hispanics (3%), and American Indians/Alaska Natives (0.3%); p. 542.)

H E A L T H Y P E O P L E 2 0 0 0 O B J E C T I V E S

REAL LIFE
REAL CHOICES

Migraine Headache: Is the Consumer Right?

▼ **Name:** Ellen Gorman
▼ **Age:** 48
▼ **Occupation:** Graphic designer

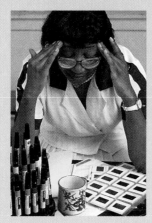

Flashing lights… pain like a steel vise tightening its grip on her skull…the agony of the slightest sound, the smallest movement.…Although she's experienced these symptoms for years, for Ellen Gorman there's no such thing as "just another migraine." Each episode is excruciating, usually involving 2 or 3 days of lying motionless in a darkened room with the phone turned off, unable to eat, snatching moments of sleep, and praying that no one comes to the door.

Ellen's had migraine headaches about once a month since she was in college, and she's pursued every mainstream medical option she could identify. She's had endless tests, including CAT scans, has consulted top neurologists, and has tried a pharmacy shelf full of prescription drugs. Sometimes she's achieved relief from a drug, but the temporary respite just isn't worth all the unpleasant side effects.

Ellen is an intelligent, talented, and highly successful graphic designer. She loves her work and is proud of her studio's excellent reputation among clients. Divorced and the mother of two grown children, Ellen enjoys a pleasant balance of work, friends, travel, and hobbies.

That is, she enjoys them when she's not totally incapacitated by a migraine headache. Tired of spending time and money in pursuit of traditional remedies that don't work, Ellen is now investigating a variety of alternative approaches to her problem. She's reading books about the Eastern-based philosophy of mind-body connection, about meditation, and about various botanical and herbal potions that have been used to treat migraine. Without telling her internist or neurologist, Ellen also has made appointments with an acupuncuturist and a naturopath. If a cure for migraine exists, she's determined to find it, even if it's not sanctioned by the practitioners of Western medicine.

As you study this chapter, think about Ellen's migraine condition and her methods of dealing with it, and prepare yourself to answer the questions in **Your Turn** at the end of the chapter. ▼

HEALTH-RELATED INFORMATION

The Informed Consumer

To be an informed consumer, you must learn about services and products that can influence health. Practitioners, manufactuers, advertisers, and sales personnel use a variety of approaches to transmit their messages regarding these products and services to you. Each approach is really an attempt to get you to buy a product or use a service. Because your health is potentially at stake when you "buy" into these messages, informed consumerism is important.

Sources of Information

The sources for information on a particular health topic are as diverse as the number of people you know, the number of publications you read, and the number of experts you see or hear. At present no single agency or profession regulates the quantity or quality of the health-related information you receive. Therefore you and the health community share the responsibility for using information in the most constructive way. If you fail to become a skilled and discriminating user of information, your health will always be at risk from those who purposefully or innocently disseminate information lacking accuracy. In contrast, once you are in a position as both an informed and critical consumer of information, you will quickly notice the various pitfalls that catch less prepared consumers which appear in advertisements and other sources of information.

Thirteen diverse sources of health-related information are presented in the following discussion. You should quickly recognize that all are familiar sources, that some provide more valid information than others, and that some require more effort to use effectively than others.

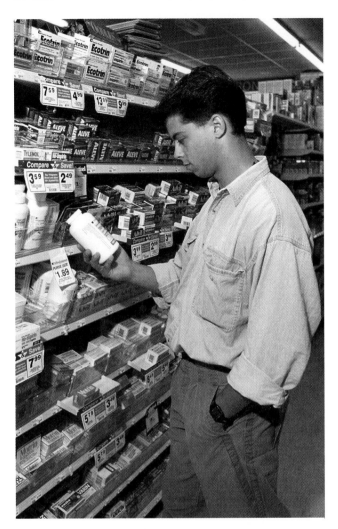

Reading the labels will keep you informed about the medications that you purchase.

Family and Friends

From a health consumerism point of view, the accuracy of information provided by a friend or family member may be questionable. Many persons are limited in their ability to understand or explain the application of technical information. Too often the information provided by family and friends is based on common knowledge that lacks technical accuracy. In addition, family members or friends may provide information they believe is in your best interests rather than providing factual information that may have a more negative impact on you.

Advertisements and Commercials

Many people spend a good portion of every day watching television, listening to the radio, and reading newspapers or magazines. Since many advertisements are health oriented, we should not be surprised to learn that these are major sources of information.

A Consumer Fraud

The story of Peroxy Gel and Peroxy Spray is an example of the potential fraud that can occur with health-related products, services, and sources of information.[1]

Vital Health Products in Minneapolis claimed that their hydrogen peroxide products, Peroxy Gel and Peroxy Spray (made with hydrogen peroxide and aloe vera), could do more than just lighten hair. According to the FDA, however, they cannot do what Vital Health Products claimed—treat AIDS, cancer, multiple sclerosis, emphysema, and heart disease. Neither could they detoxify the body, balance the body's pH, nor prevent the formation of free radicals thought to contribute to physical aging.

In response to these claims, the FDA sent the manufacturer a letter warning that these products made therapeutic claims "for which there was no scientific or medical evidence." Failure on the part of the manufacturer to discontinue sales of Peroxy Gel and Peroxy Spray resulted in an FDA request that the U.S. District Court for the Eastern District of Wisconsin issue an order to seize all products. On February 3, 1989, U.S. Marshalls seized all Peroxy Gel and Peroxy Spray from the manufacturer's home and subsequently destroyed it.

As recently as 1991 Vital Health Products, Ltd, attempted to market a line of newly developed drugs for the treatment and cure of all of the conditions just mentioned. Promotional literature in the form of a booklet titled "Hydrogen Peroxide Therapy" and a newsletter titled "Vital Health News" was also distributed by the company. The FDA initiated legal action and, despite challenges from the manufacturer, that action was upheld through various levels of the court system.[2]

As a consumer, you should be aware of the vulnerability that exists in health-related consumer markets. Individual awareness and collective action can make these markets more healthful for all consumers. ★

Although as consumers we may benefit from commercial messages, we should remember that the primary purpose of advertising is to sell products or services. In contrast to advertisements and commercials, the mass media routinely supply public service messages that give valuable health-related information.

Labels and Directions

Federal law requires that many consumer product labels, including many kinds of food (see Chapter 5) and all medications, contain specific information.

When a drug is prescribed by a health care provider and dispensed by your pharmacist, a detailed information sheet describing the drug should be available information pertaining to the drug's chemical formu-

Consumer Protection Agencies and Organizations

Federal Agencies

Office of Consumer Affairs, Food and Drug Administration
U.S. Department of Health and Human Services
5600 Fishers Lane
Rockville, MD 20857
(301) 443-5006

Federal Trade Commission
Consumer Inquiries
Public Reference Branch
6th Street and Pennsylvania Avenue
Washington, D.C. 20580
(202) 326-2222

Fraud Division
Chief Postal Inspector
U.S. Postal Service
475 L'Enfant Plaza
Washington, D.C. 20260
(202) 268-4299

Consumer Information Center
Department SC
Pueblo, CO 81009
(719) 948-3334

U.S. Consumer Product Safety Commission Hotline
Washington, D.C.
(800) 638-CPSC

Consumer Organizations

Consumers Union of the U.S., Inc.
101 Truman Avenue
Yonkers, NY 10703
(914) 378-2000

The National Consumers' League
1522 K Street, N.W.
Suite 406
Washington, D.C. 20005
(202) 639-8140

Professional Organizations

American Medical Association
535 N. Dearborn
Chicago, IL 60610
(312) 464-5000

American Hospital Association
840 N. Lake Shore Dr.
Chicago, IL 60611
(312) 280-6000

American Pharmaceutical Association
Health Education Center Service
2215 Constitution Avenue, N.W.
Washington, D.C. 20037
(202) 628-4410

---

lation, its mode of action, and its contraindications can be obtained from this sheet (Figure 17-1). Generally your pharmacist will provide you with this information only when you request it.

Many doctors and health care agencies provide consumers with detailed directions about their health problem. As a patient, you should study these directions and follow them closely.

Folklore

Because it is often passed down from generation to generation, folklore about health is the primary source of health-related information for some people.

The truthfulness of health-related information obtained from family members, neighbors, and co-workers is difficult to evaluate. As a general rule, however, we would recommend caution concerning its scientific soundness. A blanket criticism is not warranted, however, since folk wisdom is on occasion grounded in scientific soundness. Also, the emotional support provided by the suppliers of this information could be the best medicine some people need.

Testimonials

People feel strongly about sharing information that has been beneficial to them. The recommendations made by other people concerning a particular practitioner or health-related product may at first appear to be nothing more than testimonials. Since they are frequently the basis for decision-making by others, we assign a small measure of importance to them as sources of health-related information. However, the exaggerated testimonials that accompany the sales pitches of the medical quack or the "satisfied" customers appearing on television commercials should never be interpreted as valid endorsements.

Mass Media Exposure

Health programming on cable television stations, lifestyle sections in newspapers, health care correspondents appearing on national network news shows, and a growing number of health-oriented magazines are four examples of health-related information in the mass media.

Although in general health-related information is presented well, it is presented with such quickness

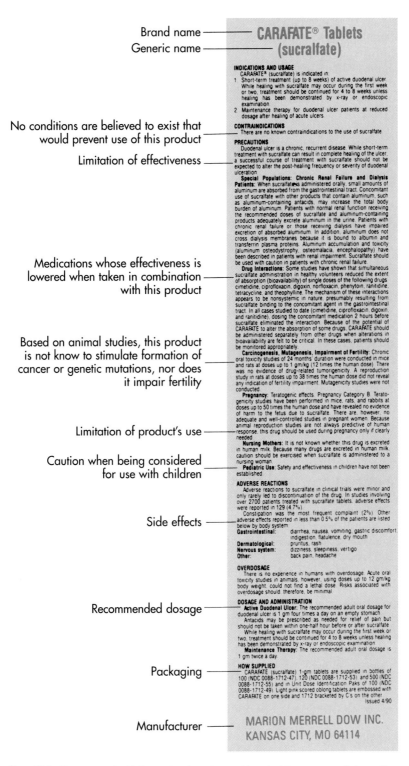

Brand name
Generic name

No conditions are believed to exist that would prevent use of this product

Limitation of effectiveness

Medications whose effectiveness is lowered when taken in combination with this product

Based on animal studies, this product is not know to stimulate formation of cancer or genetic mutations, nor does it impair fertility

Limitation of product's use

Caution when being considered for use with children

Side effects

Recommended dosage

Packaging

Manufacturer

Figure 17-1 Pharmaceutical information inserts provide valuable consumer information.

that it is distracting. By and large, however, the consumer who desires more complete coverage of a health-related topic can obtain it by combining media sources. For instance, a topic introduced with only a few seconds of coverage on a national network news program may be covered with somewhat greater depth on the cable news and later be the focus of a television documentary. An example of this multifocused approach to health-related information is the coverage given to AIDS, heart disease, and cancer.

Practitioners

The health care consumer also receives much information from individual health practitioners and their professional associations. In fact, the *patient education* role is so clearly seen by today's health care practitioner that to find one who does not exchange some information with a patient would be unusual. Also, pamphlets, audio and video tapes, and other teaching aids are routinely found in practitioners' offices. Education enhances patient **compliance** with health care directives, which is important to the practitioner and the consumer.

A major development in the area of practitioner-provided information and patient education has been the evolution of the hospital as an educational institution. Wellness centers, chemical dependence programs, sports medicine centers, and community-centered outreach programs are becoming more common. In addition to generating information regarding particular biomedical needs and generating revenues for the hospitals, these centers promote wellness through a variety of methods and materials.

Health Reference Publications

It is now believed that a substantial portion of all households own or subscribe to a health reference publication, such as the *The Wellness Book*,[3] the *Physicians' Desk Reference*,[4] or a newsletter such as *The Harvard Medical School Health Letter*, or *The Johns Hopkins Medical Letter: Health After 50*.

Personal computer programs and video cassettes featuring health-related information are important sources of information for some consumers. As long as consumers' demand for health reference material remains, materials will be developed to meet these demands.

Reference Libraries

Even though a large percentage of households possess health-related reference material and health care professionals are dispensing more and more information to the consumer, public and university libraries continue to be much-used sources of health-related information. Reference librarians are consulted, and audio-visual collections and printed materials can be checked out.

Consumer Advocacy Groups

A variety of nonprofit consumer advocacy groups patrol the health care marketplace, particularly in relation to services and products. These groups produce and send out information designed to aid the consumer in recognizing questionable services and products. Large, well-organized groups such as The National Consumers' League and Consumers' Union, and smaller groups at the state and local level, champion the right of the consumer to receive valid and reliable information about health care products and services.

Voluntary Health Agencies

Volunteerism and the traditional approach to health care and health promotion are virtually inseparable. Few other countries boast so many national voluntary organizations, with state and local affiliates, dedicated to the enhancement of health through research, service, and public education. The American Cancer Society, the American Red Cross, and the American Heart Association are all voluntary health agencies. Consumers can, in fact, anticipate finding a voluntary health agency for virtually every health problem.

Many voluntary organizations focus on the dissemination of information through many avenues, including the support of curriculum development in public schools, provision of speakers for conventions and meetings, and distribution of printed and visual materials. These organizations are among the most active and effective sources of consumer information.

Government Agencies

Government agencies are effective providers of information to the public. Through meetings and release of information to the media, agencies such as the Food and Drug Administration, Federal Trade Commission, United States Postal Service, and Environmental Protection Agency contribute to public awareness of health issues. Particularly in terms of labeling, advertising, and the distribution of information through the mail, government agencies also control the quality of information sent out to the buying public. The various divisions of the National Institutes of Health regularly release research findings and recommendations pertaining to the clinical practices, which in turn reach the consumer through clinical practitioners.

Despite their best intentions, federal health agencies are often less effective than what the public deserves. A variety of factors including inadequate staff, poor administration, and lobbying by special interest groups prevent these federal agencies from enforcing the consumer protection legislation that exists. As a result, the public is left with a sense of false confidence regarding the consumer protection provided by the federal government.

State government also provides the public with health-related information. State agencies are primary sources of information, particularly in the area of public health and environmental protection. In addition to these agencies, state funding of universities is an important contribution to the basic research that generates health-related information for the consumer. State universities also train educators and health professionals, who in turn help consumers.

Qualified Health Educators

Health educators can be found working in a variety of settings and providing their services to diverse groups of individuals. *Community health educators* are found working with virtually all of the agencies mentioned in this section; *patient educators* function in primary care settings; and *school health educators* are found at all educational levels. Increasingly, health educators are being employed in a wide range of wellness-based programs in community, hospital, corporate, and school settings.

Through a variety of approaches health educators attempt to influence the knowledge, attitudes, and practices of individuals in ways that will affect health in a positive way. For health educators in the community setting, expertise is directed toward empowering groups of people so that they can use resources to enhance their own health. For example, by teaching community members to write effective grant proposals, they can raise funds for application among various health concerns as they arise.

HEALTH CARE PROVIDERS

The types and sources of health information just discussed can contribute greatly to the decisions we make as informed consumers. An understanding of the many health-related services available can add to our growth as wise consumers. The choices we make about physicians, health services, and medical payment plans will reflect our commitment to remain healthy and our trust in specific persons who are trained in keeping us healthy.

Why We Consult Health Care Providers

Most of us seek care and advice from medical and health practitioners when we have a specific problem. A bad cold, a broken arm, or a newly discovered lump can make us realize that we need to consult health care professionals. Yet *diagnosis* and *treatment* are only two reasons why we might require the services of health care providers.

We might also encounter health practitioners in the context of *screening*. Screening is the examination of large numbers of people to discover particular diseases or health characteristics. Your earliest experience with screening may have been in elementary school, where physicians, nurses, audiologists, and dentists sometimes examine all children for normal growth and development patterns. As an adult, you might use the services of health care practitioners at a shopping center when you volunteer to be screened for hypertension or diabetes. Although screening should be considered much less precise than actual diagnosis, screening serves to identify people who should seek further medical examination.

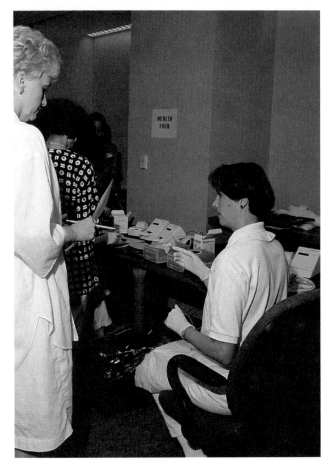

Screening at an office health fair.

Consultation is a fourth reason why knowledgeable consumers seek health care providers. A consultation is the use of two or more professionals to deliberate a person's specific health problem or condition. Consultations are especially helpful when a physician requires the opinion of a specialist. The use of an additional practitioner as a consultant can also help reassure patients who may have doubts about their own condition or about the abilities of their physician.

Prevention is a fifth reason why we might seek a health care provider. With the current emphasis on trying to stop problems before they begin, the use of health care providers for prevention is becoming more common. People want information about how to prevent needless risks and promote their health and are seeking such advice from physicians, nurses, dentists, exercise physiologists, health educators, and patient educators. The Health Action Guide on p. 426 gives guidelines to follow when choosing a physician.

compliance (kum **ply** ence) willingness to follow the directions provided by another person.

Health ACTION Guide

Choosing a Physician

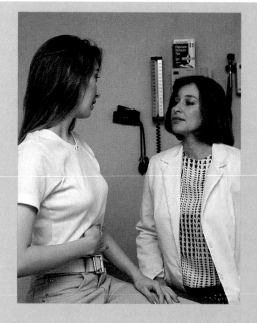

When choosing a physician, plan to obtain answers to the following questions *during* your initial visit:

▼ Obtain a description of the physician's medical background such as education, residencies, and specialty areas.

▼ How does the physician keep up with new developments in the medical profession? Does the physician attend seminars and conferences, take courses, read medical journals, write articles, participate in professional organizations, or teach at a medical school?

▼ What are the normal office hours? What should be done if help is needed outside of normal office hours?

▼ What is included in a comprehensive physical exam?

▼ How does the physician feel about second and third opinions?

▼ Which hospitals is the physician affiliated with in your area?

▼ With which specialists is the physician associated?

▼ What is the physician's fee schedule?

Ask yourself the following questions *after* your visit:

▼ Was I comfortable with the physician's age, sex, race, and national origin?

▼ Was I comfortable with the physician's demeanor? Did I find communication with the physician to be understandable and reassuring? Were all my questions answered?

▼ Did the physician seem interested in having me as a patient?

▼ Are the physician's training and practice specialty in an area most closely associated with my present needs and concerns?

▼ Does the physician have staff privileges at a hospital of my preference?

▼ Does the physician's fee-for-service policy in any way exclude or limit my ability to receive necessary services?

▼ Did the physician take a complete medical history as a part of my initial visit? Was prevention, health promotion, or wellness addressed by the physician at any point during my visit?

▼ Did I at any point during my visit sense that the physician was unusually reluctant or anxious to try new medical procedures or medications?

▼ When the physician is unavailable, are any colleagues on call for 24 hours? Did I feel that telephone calls from me would be welcomed and responded to in a reasonable period?

If you have answered yes to the majority of these questions, you have found a physician with whom you should feel comfortable. If you have been using the services of a particular physician but are becoming dissatisfied, how could you resolve this dissatisfaction? ▼

Another general reason why we consult health practitioners is in the broad area of *research*. We might seek the service of a medical research scientist when we have a critical question in a relatively unexplored area of knowledge. We also might require the help of a health care provider in interpreting the results from conflicting research reports. We might come into contact with health care practitioners for research reasons if we were to volunteer to be a subject in experiments related to medical care, drug therapy, exercise physiology, or health education.

Physicians and Their Training

In every city and many smaller communities, the local telephone directory will attest to the many types of physicians engaged in the practice of medicine. These health care providers hold the academic degree of Doctor of Medicine (MD) or Doctor of Osteopathy (DO).

At one time, **allopathy** and **osteopathic** medicine were clearly different health care professions in terms of their healing philosophies and modes of practice. Today, however, MDs and DOs receive similar educations and engage in very similar forms of practice. Both can function as **primary care physicians** or as board-certified specialists. The differences that exist are in terms of the osteopath's greater tendency to use manipulation in treating health problems. Additionally, DOs perceive themselves as being more holistically oriented than MDs.

The training of medical physicians and osteopathic physicians is a long process. Usually, 4 years of undergraduate preparation is required. There is heavy emphasis on the sciences—biology, chemistry, mathematics, anatomy, and physiology. Most undergraduate schools have preprofessional courses of study for students interested in medical or osteopathic schools.

Once accepted into professional schools, students generally spend 4 or more years in intensive training that includes advanced study in the preclinical medical sciences and clinical practice. Upon the completion of this phase of training, the students are awarded the MD or DO degree and then take the state medical license examination. Most newly licensed physicians complete an internship at a hospital. During this period interns gain experience in various clinical areas or begin specialization in areas that continue in residency programs. Residency programs vary in length from 3 to 4 years. At the conclusion, board-eligible or board-certified status is granted. The box on p. 429 describes several of the more familiar areas of specialization.

Nonallopathic Practitioners

In addition to medical physicians and osteopathic physicians, several forms of alternative health care exist within the large health care market. Included within this group is **chiropractic, acupuncture,** homeopathy, massage, **reflexology,** and **ayurveda.** Although long scoffed at by traditional medicine as being ineffective and unscientific, many persons use these forms of health care and feel strongly that they are as effective (or more effective) than allopathic and osteopathic medicine.

At the urging of many persons in both the medical community and alternative health care fields, the National Institutes of Health have agreed to fund the first study of the effectiveness of alternative health care procedures.[5,6] Although not much money is available for this study, NIH will undertake carefully controlled studies such as those used in traditional medical research. Perhaps through the use of double-blind formats and the careful selection of participants, a clearer picture of the true effectiveness of alternative health care approaches will appear.

Restricted Practice Health Care Providers

We receive much of our health care from medical physicians. However, most of us also use the services of various health care specialists who also have advanced graduate level training. These specialists hold doctoral degrees other than the MD or DO degrees. Although not medical physicians, they nevertheless have had extensive training and practice on a fee-for-service basis. Among these professionals are dentists, psychologists, podiatrists, and optometrists.

Dentists (Doctor of Dental Surgery, DDS) are trained to deal with a wide range of diseases and impairments of the teeth and oral cavity. Dentists undergo undergraduate predental programs that emphasize the natural sciences, followed by 4 additional years of graduate study in dental school and, with increasing frequency, an internship program. State licensure examinations are required. As with medical physicians, dentists can also specialize; fields range from *oral surgery* to **orthodontics** to **prosthodontics.** Dentists are also permitted to prescribe therapy programs (such as appliances for the treatment of temporomandibular joint dysfunction) and drugs that per-

allopathy (ah **lop** ah thee) system of medical practice in which specific remedies (often pharmaceutical agents) are used to produce effects different from those produced by a disease or injury.

osteopathy (os tee **op** ah thee) system of medical practice that combines allopathic principles with specific attention to postural mechanics of the body.

primary care physician the physician who sees a patient on a regular basis, rather than a specialist who sees the patient only for a specific condition or procedure.

chiropractic (ky row **prac** tick) manipulation of the vertebral column to relieve pressure and cure illness.

acupuncture (**ack** you punc shur) insertion of fine needles into the body to alter electroenergy fields and cure disease.

reflexology (re flex **ol** oh gee) massage applied to specific areas of the feet in order to treat illness and disease in other areas of the body.

ayurveda (ai yur **vey** da) traditional Indian medicine based on herbal remedies.

orthodontics (ore tho **don** ticks) dental specialty that focuses on the proper alignment of the teeth.

prosthodontics (pros tho **don** ticks) dental specialty that focuses on the construction and fitting of artificial appliances to replace missing teeth.

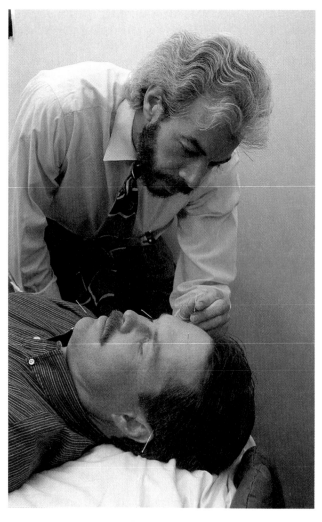

Acupuncture.

⭐ Dental Care

Tooth and gum disease can be prevented. With proper care, your teeth should last a lifetime. Every person should do the following:

★ **Brush and floss correctly every day.**

★ **Eat nutritious meals; avoid sweets between meals.**

★ **Visit a dentist regularly for checkups and cleaning.**

★ **Watch for symptoms that indicate problems (red, swollen, or bleeding gums; loose teeth; improper bite; chronic bad breath or bad taste).**

★ **Get treatment quickly if needed.**

Good dental health is more easily obtained than ever before, but it takes commitment! It's up to you!

tain to their practices (primarily analgesics and antibiotics).

Psychologists provide services that allow us to improve our understanding of behavior patterns or perceptions. Over 40 states have certification or licensing laws that prohibit unqualified persons from using the term *psychologist*. It is important for a consumer to examine the credentials of a psychologist. Legitimate psychologists have received advanced graduate training (often leading to a PhD or EdD degree) in clinical, counseling, industrial, or educational psychology. Furthermore, these practitioners will have passed state certification examinations and, in many states, will have met further requirements that allow them to offer health services to the public. Psychologists may have special interests and credentials from professional societies in individual, group, family, or marriage counseling. Some are certified as sex therapists.

Unlike *psychiatrists*, who are medical physicians, psychologists cannot prescribe or dispense drugs. They may refer to or consult with medical physicians about clients who might benefit from drug therapy.

Podiatrists are highly trained clinicians who practice podiatric medicine, or care of the feet (and ankles). Although not MDs or ODs, doctors of podiatric medicine (DPM) treat a wide variety of conditions related to the feet, including corns, bunions, warts, bone spurs, hammertoes, fractures, diabetes-related conditions, athletic injuries, and structural abnormalities. Podiatrists perform surgery, prescribe medications, and apply orthotics, splints, and corrective shoes for structural abnormalities of the feet.

Doctors of podiatric medicine follow an educational path similar to that taken by MDs and ODs, consisting of a 4-year undergraduate preprofessional curriculum, 4 additional years of study in a podiatric medical school, and an optional residency of 1 or 2 years. Board-certified areas of specialization include surgery, orthopedics, and podiatric sports medicine. Hospital affiliation generally requires board certification in a specialized area.

Optometrists are eye specialists who deal primarily with vision problems associated with *refractory errors*. They examine the eyes and prescribe glasses or contact lenses to correct visual disorders. Sometimes optometrists also attempt to correct certain ocular muscle imbalances with specific exercise regimens. Optometrists must complete undergraduate training and additional years of coursework at one of 16 accredited colleges of optometry in the United States or two Canadian colleges before taking a state licensing examination.[7]

Opticians are technicians who manufacture and fit eyeglasses or contact lenses. Although they are rarely licensed by a state agency, they perform the important function of grinding lenses to the precise prescription designated by an optometrist or ophthalmologist. To

Medical Specialties

The American Board of Medical Specialties is a nonprofit organization that represents 23 medical specialty boards.* Each board is composed of expert physicians already qualified in a particular field. These specialty boards evaluate physicians who wish to practice in a specific area of medicine. Some of the more common specialty areas consumers might encounter are listed below.

SPECIALTY	SCOPE OF PRACTICE
★ Allergy	Treatment of sensitivity disorders
★ Anesthesiology	Use of drugs to sedate or anesthetize
★ Cardiovascular surgery	Various forms of heart surgery
★ Dermatology	Skin diseases and disorders
★ Emergency medicine	Care of accident victims
★ Family practice	Broad-based family medical care
★ Geriatrics	Diseases and disorders of the elderly
★ Gynecology	Female reproductive health care
★ Internal medicine	Nonsurgical treatment of internal organ systems
★ Neurology	Diseases and disorders of the nervous system
★ Nephrology	Kidney diseases and disorders
★ Obstetrics	Prenatal care and child delivery
★ Oncology	Treatment of unusual growths and tumors
★ Ophthamology	Disorders of the eye
★ Orthopedic surgery	Surgery for structural disorders of the bones and joints
★ Otorhinolaryngology	Ear, nose, and throat problems
★ Pathology	Diagnosis of disease through the examination of body tissues
★ Pediatrics	Childhood health concerns
★ Psychiatry	Mental and emotional diseases or disorders
★ Radiology	Use of radiation to diagnose and treat diseases and injuries
★ Urological surgery	Surgery for urinary tract diseases and male reproductive dysfunctions

*Governed by these 23 medical boards are 85 practice specialties.

save money and time, many consumers take an optometrist's prescription for glasses or contact lenses to a large-volume retail store that deals exclusively with eyewear products.

Nurse Professionals

Nurses constitute a large group of health professionals who practice in a variety of settings. Frequently, the responsibilities of nurses vary according to their academic preparation. Registered nurses (RNs) are academically prepared at two levels: (1) the technical nurse, and (2) the professional nurse. The technical nurse is educated in a 2-year associate degree program. The professional nurse receives 4 years of education and earns a bachelor's degree. Both technical and professional nurses must successfully complete state licensing examinations before they can practice as RNs.

Many professional nurses continue their education

and earn master's and doctoral degrees in nursing or other health-related fields. Some professional nurses specialize in a clinical area (such as pediatrics, gerontology, public health, or school health) and become certified as *nurse practitioners.* Working under the supervision of physicians, nurse practitioners perform many of the diagnostic and treatment procedures performed by physicians. The ability of these highly trained nurses to function at this level provides communities with additional primary care providers, as well as freeing physicians to deal with more complex cases. Many college health centers employ nurse practitioners because of their ability to deliver high quality care at a smaller cost to the institution.

Licensed practical nurses (LPNs) are trained in hospital-based programs ranging from 12 to 18 months. Because of their brief training, LPNs' scope of practice is limited. Most LPN training programs are gradually being phased out.

Allied Health Care Professionals

Our primary health care providers are supported by a large group of *allied health care professionals,* who often take the responsibility for highly technical services and procedures. Such professionals include respiratory and inhalation therapists, radiological technologists, nuclear medicine technologists, pathology technicians, general medical technologists, operating room technicians, emergency medical technicians, registered nurse midwives, physical therapists, occupational therapists, dental technicians, physician assistants, and dental hygienists. Depending on the particular field, the training for these specialty support areas can take from 1 to 5 years of post–high school study. Programs include hospital-based training leading to a diploma through associate, bachelor's and master's degrees. Most allied health care professionals must also pass state or national licensing examinations.

SELF-CARE

The emergence of the **self-care movement** indicates that many of us are becoming more responsible for the maintenance of our health. We are developing the expertise to prevent or manage numerous types of illness, injuries, and conditions. We are learning to assess our health status and treat, monitor, and rehabilitate ourselves in a manner that was once thought possible only with the direct help of a physician or some other health care specialist.

The benefits of this movement are that self-care can (1) lower our health care costs, (2) be effective care for particular conditions, (3) free physicians and other health care specialists to spend time with other patients and (4) enhance our interest in health-related activities.

In what situation is self-care an appropriate alternative to professional care? We can identify three areas.

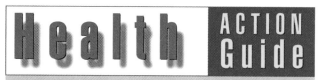

Home Tests

When using home tests, be sure to follow these simple guidelines:

▼ Check expiration date (chemicals lose potency, and results could be affected).
▼ Store products as directed (they can be affected by heat and cold).
▼ Read labels and package inserts carefully; follow directions exactly.
▼ Keep accurate test results.
▼ Follow directions for positive, negative, and unclear results.
▼ Use a stopwatch if precise timing is necessary.
▼ Ask your pharmacist or physician for information when questions arise.

If you have previously used home tests, did you use them correctly? Many untrained and inexperienced persons use these kits; are the directions complete enough? How confident are you about the results obtained from home testing? ▼

First, self-care may be appropriate for certain acute conditions that have familiar symptoms and are *self-limiting.* Common colds and flu, many home injuries, sore throats, and nonallergic insect bites are often easily managed with self-care.

A second area in which we might use self-care is *therapy.* For example, many people are now administering allergy shots and continuing physical therapy programs in their homes. Asthma, diabetes, and hypertension are also conditions that can be managed or monitored with self-care.

A third area in which self-care has appropriate application is *health promotion.* Weight loss programs, physical conditioning activities, and stress reduction programs are particularly well suited to self-care. In most communities a variety of organizations specialize in these areas of health promotion.

People interested in practicing more self-care must be skilled consumers. The self-care marketplace is growing very rapidly and is expected to be a multibillion dollar industry by the end of the decade. Equipment such as blood pressure–measuring instruments, stethoscopes, and diagnostic kits, as well as over-the-counter drugs, can represent significant investments. Clearly, your money, time, and willingness to develop expertise are important components in this growing area of health care consumerism.

Health ACTION Guide

Hospitals

Despite efforts in self-care and health promotion, most people will experience hospitalization at some time in their lives. Serious threatening illnesses and rarer diseases are best treated in larger research-oriented hospitals at major medical centers or regional teaching hospitals. Less serious illness or elective procedures can be accommodated in community hospitals. Regardless of the type of hospital, however, these characteristics should be looked for:[8]

▼ The hospital building should be neat, clean, and well maintained.

▼ There should be recreational relaxation areas for patients to use, including outside areas.
▼ The public areas of the hospital (lobbies, snackbars, parking structures, and business areas) should be comfortable and clean.
▼ Visiting hours should be liberal, and children should be allowed some access.
▼ Accommodations should be available for family and friends to stay overnight.
▼ Patients' meals should be carefully selected, attractively prepared, and efficiently served.
▼ Special meals should be provided when medically appropriate, and families should be assisted in postdischarge meal planning.
▼ Hospital rooms should be attractive, comfortable, and well situated for nursing services.
▼ Smoking by patients, staff, and visitors should be carefully controlled.

HEALTH CARE FACILITIES

Most of us have a general idea of what a hospital is. However, all hospitals are not alike. They usually fall into one of three categories—private, public, or voluntary hospitals. *Private hospitals* (or proprietary hospitals) function as profit-making hospitals. They are not supported by tax monies and usually accept only clients who can pay all of their expenses. Although there are some exceptions, these hospitals are generally smaller than tax-supported voluntary hospitals. Commonly owned by a group of business investors, a large hospital corporation, or a group of physicians, these hospitals sometimes limit their services to a few specific types of illnesses.

Public hospitals are supported primarily by tax dollars. They can be operated by government agencies at the state level (such as state mental hospitals) or at the federal level (such as the Veterans Administration Hospitals and various military service hospitals such as Walter Reed Army Hospital). Large county or city hospitals are frequently public hospitals. Routinely, these hospitals serve indigent segments of the population. They also function as *teaching hospitals*.

The most commonly recognized type of hospital is the *voluntary hospital*. Voluntary hospitals are maintained as nonprofit, public institutions. Often supported by religious orders, fraternal groups, or charitable organizations, these hospitals usually offer a wider range of comprehensive services than do private hospitals or clinics. Voluntary hospitals are supported by patient fees (covered by health insurance), Medicare reimbursement, and Medicaid and public assistance reimbursement.

In the last decade, voluntary hospitals have expanded their scope of services. Today it is not unusual to find **wellness centers,** stress centers, cardiac rehabilitation centers, chemical dependence programs, health education centers, and satellite centers for well-baby care and care for the homeless being operated by hospitals. The repercussions from this expanding concept of health care versus the financial losses of a declining patient population are not always easy to determine. Regardless, these new services enhance the health of those who have access to them.

Other health care facilities include *clinics* (both private and tax supported), *nursing homes* (most of which are private enterprises), and *rehabilitation centers.* Rehabilitation centers are often supported by charitable organizations devoted to the care of chronically ill or handicapped persons, orthopedically injured persons, or burn victims.

Within recent years a number of private, 24-hour drop-in medical emergency and surgical centers have emerged. These clinics have their own professional staffs of physicians, nurses, and allied health professionals. They provide direct competition with the larger hospital-based facilities. Some clinics specialize in women's health needs, including gynecological care, prenatal care, and childbirth services.

self-care movement trend toward individuals taking increased responsibility for prevention or management of certain health conditions.

wellness centers units within hospitals or clinics that provide a wide range of rehabilitation, disease prevention, and health enhancement programs.

TABLE 17-1	Average Daily Cost Per Patient in a Community Hospital (1993 dollars)
Year	**Amount**
1971	$295.93
1981	$451.15
1991	$797.27

Table 17-1 summarizes the increased cost of hospital care over the last two decades.

Patients' Institutional Rights

Regardless of the type of institution that you are a patient in, you have a variety of rights. These are, of course, intended to protect you from unnecessary harm and financial loss. The hospital too can expect your cooperation as a patient. Figure 17-2 explains these relationships more fully.

Rights: The Patient's and the Institution's

AS A PATIENT, YOU CAN EXPECT FROM THE INSTITUTION:

- To be treated with respect and dignity
- To be afforded privacy and confidentiality consistent with federal and state law, institutional policies, and the requirements of your insurance carrier
- To be provided services on request, so long as they are reasonable and consistent with appropriate care
- To be fully informed of the identity of the physicians and staff providing care
- To be kept fully updated as to your condition, including its management and your prognosis for recovery
- To be listened to regarding your concerns over the type and extent of care received

THE INSTITUTION CAN EXPECT YOU, AS A PATIENT:

- To keep all appointments
- To provide all background information pertinent to your condition
- To treat hospital personnel with respect
- To ask questions and seek clarification about matters pertaining to your condition
- To maintain the treatment indicated by your physician
- To provide information needed in providing the fullest insurance coverage and to raise questions concerning hospital charges

AS A PATIENT, YOU MAY AT ANY TIME:

- Refuse treatment
- Seek a second opinion
- Discharge yourself from the institution

Figure 17-2 Patients' institutional rights.

HEALTH-CARE COSTS AND REIMBURSEMENT

As depicted in Figure 17-3 on p. 433, there are many avenues for receiving health care. However, being able to afford quality health care is among the most important concerns of the American public. Today over 37 million Americans lack health insurance to pay health care costs, including over 10 million dependent children.[9] Furthermore, Americans are less optimistic today about their ability to have adequate health insurance coverage, find reasonably priced health care, and afford long-term home-bound or nursing home care than ever before.[10] Unfortunately, the word *crisis* is appropriate to use when talking about our ability to continue to afford high-quality health care today.

Central to our concern with health care today is its cost. As a nation, Americans are now spending over $1 trillion a year on health care, and by the year 2000 the amount is expected to exceed $1.5 trillion.[11] At today's rates, annual health care costs per person will approach $4000 by the year 1995 and $5500 by the year 2000.[11] When viewed on the basis of household expenditures for health care, Americans spent approximately $640 billion in 1990. Table 17-2 depicts the distribution of this money.[12] For the country as a whole, nearly 15% of our Gross National Product (GNP) is devoted to health-care costs.

In light of factors such as the high cost of modern medical technology, an emphasis on long life at all cost, the growing number of older persons with chronic conditions that require expensive extended care, and the AIDS epidemic, controlling the cost of medical care is among one of the most complex problems facing the nation. Nevertheless, well over 40 different plans have been advanced in response to this problem. These range from only modest changes to the current system to tax credit strategies and mandatory employment-based insurance to a federally controlled national health plan.[13] However, no single plan has yet caught the favor of the American public or their policymakers in Washington.

TABLE 17-2	Household Health-Care Expenditures
Commodity	**Amount (in billions)**
Hospitals	$256.0
Physicians	$125.7
Nursing homes	$ 53.1
Drugs/supplies	$ 54.6
Dental care	$ 34.0
Other	$120.0

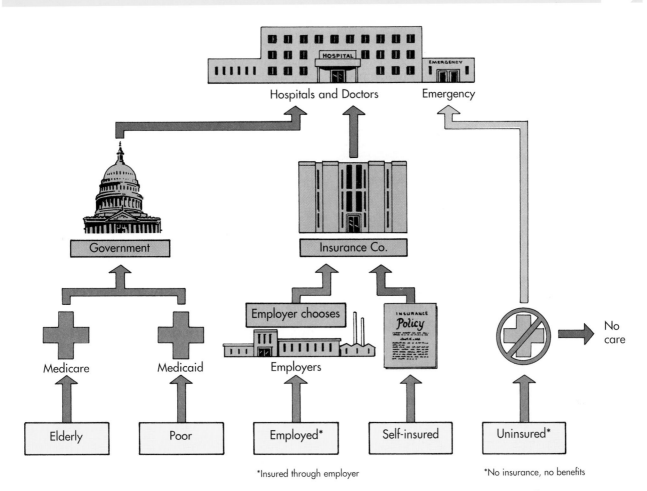

Figure 17-3 How you get medical coverage: the current system involves many layers of bureaucracy between people and their doctors.[14]

Health Insurance

Health insurance is a financial agreement between an insurance company and an individual or group for the payment of health costs. After paying a premium to an insurance company, the policyholder is covered for specific benefits. Each policy is different in terms of coverage for illnesses and injuries. Merely having an insurance policy does not mean that all of your health care expenses will be covered. Most health insurance policies require various forms of payments on the part of the policyholder, which include provisions for deductible amounts, fixed indemnity benefits, coinsurance, and exclusions. For the majority of Americans, participation in the health care system is possible if they have adequate health insurance.

A *deductible* amount is an established amount that the insuree must pay before the insurer reimburses for services. For example, if you have been billed for $500 worth of services, your policy might require you to pay $200 before the insurance company will pay the other $300. Usually, the lower the deductible amount is, the higher your premiums will be.

A policy with *fixed indemnity benefits* will pay only a specified amount for a particular procedure or service. If your policy pays only $1000 for an appendectomy and the actual cost of your appendectomy was $1500, then you owe the health care providers $500. A policy with full service benefits, which pays the entire cost of a particular procedure or service, may be worth the extra cost.

Policies that have *coinsurance* features require that you and the insurance company share the costs of certain covered services, usually on a percentage basis. One standard coinsurance plan requires that you pay 20% of the costs above a deductible amount, and the company pays the remaining 80%.

An *exclusion* refers to a service or expense that is not covered by your policy. Elective or cosmetic surgery procedures, unusual treatment protocols, prescription drugs, and certain kinds of consultations are common exclusions in many policies. Illness and injuries you already have at the time you purchase your policy (pre-existing conditions) often are excluded. Also, injuries incurred during high-risk activities (ice hockey, hang gliding, mountain climbing, intramural sports) might not be covered by a policy.

Health insurance can be obtained through *individual policies* or *group plans.* Group health insurance plans usually offer the widest range of coverage at the least

Health Insurance: Types of Coverage

When considering a health insurance policy, you should evaluate the following types of coverage.

Hospital. Hospital coverage refers to insurance that covers inpatient hospital expenses. With hospital expenses approaching $800 per day, you want to be certain that your policy provides for this expense.

Surgical. Surgical coverage provides for the fees surgeons charge for specific surgical care.

Regular medical. Regular medical covers physicians' fees for nonsurgical care. Often maximum benefits are specified for certain types of nonsurgical procedures.

Major medical. Major medical coverage is for unusually large, often unpredictable, medical expenses. Major medical coverage is designed to extend beyond a health insurance policy's regular medical coverage. Although major medical benefits have very high maximum benefit limits (often hundreds of thousands of dollars), these benefits are often paid on a coinsurance basis. Thus you may pay a portion of the medical expense.

Dental. Initial coverage provides for various types of dental care.

Disability. Disability insurance (also called *income protection insurance*) provides for income lost because of your inability to work after an illness or injury. ★

Health Insurance for College Students

The days when students could leave for college confident that their health needs would be met by the family health insurance plans held by their parents are nearly gone. Today many young adults 18 years of age and older need to provide their own health care coverage, regardless of whether they are students. Accordingly, colleges and universities are likely to offer health care insurance packages for students to purchase on an annual basis. The annual premium for a typical student health insurance program may range from $300 for a single student up to $1400 for a student with a spouse and dependent children. When considering your health insurance coverage, it is important to learn whether more affordable health insurance of equal or better coverage than that sold by your school could be purchased from an insurance agent. ★

expensive price and often are purchased by companies for their employees. Fortunately, no employee is refused entry into a group insurance program. However, when employees leave the company, they often lose their group health insurance coverage. Today as many major American companies downsize, tens of thousands of employees can lose this important group health insurance, virtually without warning.

Individual policies are purchased by one person (or a family) from an insurance company. These policies are often much more expensive than group plans and may provide much less coverage. Persons who do not have access to a group plan should still attempt to secure individual policies, since the financial burdens resulting from a major accident or illness that is not covered by some form of health insurance can be devastating. The Health Action Guide on p. 435 gives the consumer some questions to consider before purchasing a health insurance policy.

Health Maintenance Organizations

The emergence of *health maintenance organizations (HMOs)* during the past 20 years lends testimony to the fact that health care and preventive medicine can go hand in hand. HMOs are health care delivery plans under which health care providers agree to meet the covered medical needs of subscribers for a prepaid amount of money. For a fixed monthly fee, enrollees are given comprehensive health care with an emphasis on preventive health care. Enrollees receive their care from physicians, specialists, allied health professionals, and educators who are hired or contractually retained by the HMO.

One of the potential advantages offered by HMOs is *cost containment.* Since most of the medical services with an HMO are centralized, there is little duplication of facilities, equipment, or support staff. Central filing of records allows several HMO physicians to have access to a single client's record file. This saves time, administrative costs, and the overlapping of care. HMOs also routinely use health promotion activities to encourage clients to practice illness prevention.[15] All of these approaches can help lower health care costs.

Additional new approaches to reducing health costs involve the formation of *independent practice associations (IPAs)* and *preferred provider organizations (PPOs).* An IPA is a modified form of an HMO that uses a group of doctors who offer prepaid services out of their own offices and not in a central HMO facility. IPAs have been viewed as "HMOs without walls." A PPO is a group of private practitioners who sell their services at reduced rates to insurance companies. When policyholders choose a physician who is in that company's PPO, the insurance company will pay the entire physician's fee. When a policyholder selects a non-PPO physician, the insurance company will pay only a portion of that physician's fee.

Health ACTION Guide

Selecting Insurance

Before you purchase a health insurance policy, ask yourself the following questions. The more questions you can answer with a "yes," the better you should feel that the policy you select is right for you.

GENERAL QUESTIONS

▼ Do I really need an individual insurance policy?

▼ Am I already covered by a group insurance policy?

▼ Is the insurance company I'm considering rated favorably by *Best's Insurance Reports* or my state insurance department?

▼ Have I compared health insurance policies from at least two other companies?

▼ Does this company have a "return rate" of 50% or more?

▼ Can I afford this insurance policy?

▼ Do I understand the factors that might raise the cost of this policy?

SPECIFIC QUESTIONS

▼ Do I clearly understand which health conditions are covered and which are not?

▼ Do I clearly understand whether I have fixed indemnity benefits or full service benefits?

▼ Do I clearly understand the deductible amounts of this policy?

▼ Do I clearly understand when the major medical portion of this policy starts?

▼ Do I clearly understand all information in this policy that refers to exclusions and preexisting conditions?

▼ Do I clearly understand any disability provisions of this policy?

▼ Do I clearly understand all information concerning both cancellation and renewal of this policy?

Government Insurance Plans

Created in 1965 by amendments to the Social Security Act, Medicare and Medicaid represent governmental types of health insurance. Medicare provides health care reimbursements primarily for persons aged 65 years or older. Medicare is a *contributory* program— that is, through their working years, all employed citizens contribute a portion of their salaries (through social security taxes) to the Medicare fund. At present, that amount is 1.45% of the social security taxes (FICA) paid on annual earnings.[16] When they reach age 65 years, some of their health care expenses are covered by Medicare. Regardless of their age, persons who require kidney dialysis or transplant are covered by Medicare.

Medicare is actually composed of two parts. Medicare A is basically a hospital insurance program. Part A will pay for necessary hospital care (semiprivate room) after payment of the required deductible, for medically necessary inpatient care in a nursing home (skilled level care), and hospice care. In addition, it will pay 80% of the cost of approved durable medical equipment, such as walkers, and for all units of blood used by an inpatient, after the first three units.[17] Medicare B is a voluntary program (for which the subscriber must pay a monthly fee) that supplements Medicare A. Medicare B provides regular medical insurance that covers a broad range of physicians' fees and other health care services. Physicians who "accept assignment" from Medicare agree to charge their elderly patients only the amount that Medicare will cover. Those who do not accept assignment may charge an amount up to 115% of the Medicare amount. However, by doing so they will be asking their elderly patients not only to pay the 20% co-payment but an additional 15% as well. Consequently, many elderly will go only to physicians who accept assignment. Both Medicare plans are subject to yearly changes in coverages and administrative procedures.

One of the more recent attempts by Medicare at cost containment in the area of health care is the *prospective pricing system* established in 1984 by the federal government. Under this system, Medicare reimbursements to hospitals are based on 467 *diagnosis-related groups (DRGs)* rather than on the costs accrued by the hospitals. Each hospital stay is now assigned a DRG classification, and reimbursement to the hospital is based on that classification. This system encourages hospitals to deliver services at or below the DRG payment schedule.

Medicaid is a *noncontributory* program for citizens who are receiving other types of public welfare assistance. It is designed to provide both medical and hospital coverage. Unlike Medicare, Medicaid has no age

---

Medicare (med ih care) contributory governmental health insurance, primarily for persons 65 years of age or older.

Medicaid (Med ih cade) noncontributory governmental health insurance for persons receiving other types of public assistance.

Learning FROM ALL Cultures

Health Care in the United States and Canada

Approximately 14% of the United States population does not have access to health care. This amounts to approximately 37 million people, primarily among the poor.[18] A substantial number of people lacking medical coverage are people who work full time at very low-paying jobs without health-care benefits. This population may suffer more than the very poor or unemployed because they may not be poor enough to qualify for Medicaid.[19]

Usually people who need emergency or immediate care will not be turned away at a hospital. However, people without health coverage lack primary care—preventive measures like check-ups, screenings, and prenatal care. Because of this lack of preventive attention they eventually may need more extensive and costly care.[19]

Other countries, such as Canada, have addressed the issue of universal health care. Since 1972 Canadian residents have been guaranteed health insurance coverage through a system funded by the federal government and the ten provincial and two territorial governments. Of the total health care cost, 30% to 40% is paid by the federal government, about 25% comes from private sources, and the rest is contributed by the provinces, usually through taxes.[20]

Each individual is guaranteed health care in Canada, but the system is not socialized medicine. Physicians do not work for the government but are independent providers. Providers must, however, accept the provincial plan's reimbursement as total payment if a province is to continue to receive federal support.[20]

Would the Canadian system work in the United States? From where in the federal and state budgets would the funding come? Some argue that there are too many groups of people who would not benefit from a system like the Canadian one. Why would certain groups oppose such a system? ●

---

requirements and is administered cooperatively through federal and state agencies. Medicaid is particularly important to older adults, since it will cover nursing home care once eligibility is established.

Because of the bureaucracy currently surrounding these two governmental insurance programs, a number of private physicians and voluntary hospitals are reluctant to accept Medicaid and Medicare clients. A major concern now seems to be how the United States can provide proper health care for all of its citizens, including the aged, economically disadvantaged, and those whose life savings can be quickly depleted by a catastrophic illness.

MEDICARE SUPPLEMENT POLICIES (MEDIGAP)

Because Medicare A and Medicare B require deductibles and copayment to be made by patients before they will begin payment, insurance to cover these gaps in coverage has been developed. In the most basic "medigap" policies (policy version), often sold via television, reimbursement is made to the patient for the deductible and copayment portions of the approved charges, as determined by the DRG (Medicare A) and approved physician fee (Medicare B). More expensive and more comprehensive Medicare supplement policies (policy versions B through J) are also available that pay for hospital care and equipment not covered by Medicare A and for physician fees that ex-

ceed the approved amount of coverage for Medicare B. The difference in costs between the basic medigap policies and the more comprehensive policies that literally pay for everything that is not covered by Medicare is substantial.

EXTENDED CARE INSURANCE

With the aging of the population and the greater likelihood that nursing home care will be required (at about $32,000 per year), extended care policies have been developed and are being sold. When purchased at an early age (by mid-50s), these policies are much more affordable than if purchased when it is apparent that a spouse or family member will require institutional care. However, not all older adults will need extensive nursing home care, so an extended care policy could be an unnecessary expenditure.

National Health Care: A Solution?

In light of the extensive cost of modern health care services and the large number of people lacking health insurance, *national health care* coverage might be a solution. Forms of national health care coverage exist in Canada, England, and Sweden. The most vocal critics of America's lack of a comprehensive health care delivery system point out that, among highly developed countries, only the United States and South Africa lack such a system. In countries with a comprehensive sys-

Legislation for National Health Care

American health care is technically superior to any in the world but increasingly unavailable to the public. As costs spiral upward, millions of Americans go without health care insurance, and primary care physicians are in even shorter supply. Today Americans await the health care reforms that are currently being developed in Washington. The Clinton administration has promised that change will occur, while the task of formulating these reforms has been turned over to Hillary Rodham Clinton. Planning, approval, and implementation of reform are expected to be a slow process as various special interest groups jockey for position in the new health care delivery system and massive funding sources are established.

Although planning is far from finished, many of the following features are expected in the health care reform package:

★ Universal health care coverage for the unemployed through insurance paid for by workers, employers, and the government

★ One health care package per family, regardless of the number of family members employed

★ Benefits that cover a wide range of health care needs including preventive care, prescription drugs, emotional health services, and some dental care

★ Supportive services to make the system more accessible for those seeking care, including transportation, child care, and language services

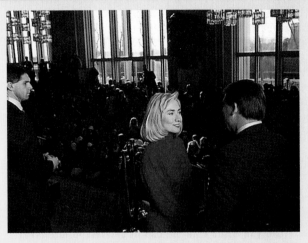

★ Organization of providers into service areas to make health care services competitively priced

★ Home care for older adults to decrease the need for institutional care

★ Emphasis on health maintenance organizations that allow consumers to choose their own providers

★ Increased use of nonphysician professionals and alternative health care providers

Perhaps within the next 3 to 5 years the delivery of health care services to the American public will show signs of reform. ★

tem such as those previously mentioned, citizens receive cradle-to-grave health care. This coverage is supported, in most cases, through taxation.

The box above is an overview of the plan advanced by the Clinton administration, which is under critical review.

HEALTH-RELATED PRODUCTS

As you might imagine, prescription and over-the-counter drugs constitute an important part of our discussion of health-related products.

Prescription Drugs

Caution: Federal law prohibits dispensing without prescription.

This FDA warning appears on the labels of approximately three fourths of all medications. Prescription drugs must be ordered for us by a licensed practitioner. Because these compounds are legally controlled and may require special skills in their administration, our access to these drugs is limited.

Although over 2500 compounds listed in the current edition of the *Physicians' Desk Reference* represent

the drugs that can be prescribed by a physician, only 200 drugs make up the bulk of the 827 million new prescriptions and 773 million refills ordered in 1992.[21] The most frequently prescribed drugs, by units dispensed, are Amoxil, Lanoxin, Zantac, Premarin, Xanax, and Dyazide. Working through physicians and pharmacists, pharmaceutical companies contribute to the improvement of health while generating sales in excess of $25.6 billion per year.[22] Health care dollars spent for prescription drugs account for 13% of the total health care costs accrued by Americans.

Research and Development of New Drugs

As a consumer of prescription drugs, you may be curious about the process by which drugs gain FDA approval for marketing. The rigor of this process may be why fewer than 15 to 20 new drugs are added to our national pharmacopeia each year.

On a continuous basis, the nation's pharmaceutical companies are exploring the molecular structure of various chemical compounds in an attempt to discover important new compounds with desired types and levels of biological activity. Once these new compounds are identified, extensive in-house research

Animals in Research

Despite the scientific community's position that drug research cannot be successfully undertaken without the use of animals, animal rights activists continue to protest the use of any animals for pharmaceutical and medical research. They contend that adjuncts such as epidemiological data bases and computer simulation models are sufficient to adequately determine the safety and effectiveness of new drugs. Because of the importance of animals to research, guidelines for the proper housing, feeding, handling, veterinary care, and disposal of animals used in research have been issued by several branches of the federal government, some state governments, and organizations such as the American Association for the Accreditation of Laboratory Animal Care (AAALAC).[23]

Do you agree with the use of animals in furthering pharmaceutical and medical research? ★

with computer simulations and animal testing is required to determine whether clinical trials with humans are warranted. Of the 125,000 or more compounds under study each year, only a few thousand receive such extensive preclinical evaluation. Even fewer of these are then taken to the FDA to begin the evaluation process necessary to gain approval for further research with humans. Once a drug is approved for clinical trials, the chemical companies can secure a patent, which prevents the drug from being manufactured by other companies for the next 17 years.

Over the course of approximately 7 years, a pharmaceutical company must supply the FDA with extensive information pertaining to (1) the biological source of the new compound, (2) the steps required to manufacture the compound, (3) animal studies conducted by the company, (4) proposed clinical studies, (5) credentials of the physicians who will be involved in the clinical studies, (6) prior research on the drug, and (7) patient consent. The company must also agree to inform the FDA of all pertinent information as it is generated.

Clinical studies with humans are performed during the last 3 to 4 years of the 7-year period. The $125 million price tag for bringing a new drug into the marketplace reflects this slow, careful process. If this 7-year process goes well, a pharmaceutical company will enjoy 10 years of protected retail sales.

Generic Versus Brand Name Drugs

When a new drug comes into the marketplace, it carries with it three names: its **chemical name,** its **generic name,** and its **brand name.** During the time the 17-year patent is in effect, no other drug with the same chemical formulation can be sold. When the patent expires, other companies can manufacture a drug of equivalent chemical composition and market it under the brand name drug's original generic name. Because extensive research and development are not necessary at this point, the production of generic drugs is far less costly than the initial development of the brand name drug. Nearly all states allow pharmacists to substitute generic drugs for brand name drugs, as long as the prescribing physician approves. However, some concern exists over whether certain generic drugs have the same levels of *bioavailability* as brand name drugs and whether data on effectiveness were reported honestly by generic drug manufacturers to the FDA.

When such generic drugs are discovered, they are immediately withdrawn from the market and reformulated. To date, very few generic drugs initially introduced into the marketplace have been taken off for reformulation. In each case in which this has occurred, the drug returned in an appropriately effective form. In a few cases, generic drugs have proven to be equally as effective as their brand name counterpart. For some patients, however, the particular dye used in the manufacturing of the capsule or coating caused discomfort and forced a return to the brand name product.

Over-the-Counter Drugs

When did you last take some form of medication? For many of you the answer might be "I took aspirin this morning." In making this decision, you engage in self-diagnosis, determine a course for your own treatment, self-administer your treatment, and free a physician to serve a person whose illness is more serious than yours. None of this would have been possible without readily available, inexpensive, and effective over-the-counter (OTC) drugs.

In comparison with the 2500 prescription drugs available, there are perhaps as many as 300,000 different OTC products, routinely classified into 26 different families (see the box on p. 441). Like prescription drugs, nonprescription drugs are regulated by the FDA. However, for OTC drugs the marketplace is a more powerful determinant of success. Table 17-3 compares common OTC pain relievers.

The regulation of OTC drugs is based upon a provision in a 1972 amendment to the 1938 Food, Drug, and Cosmetic Act. As a result of that action, OTC drugs were placed in three categories on the basis of the safety and effectiveness of their active ingredient(s).

Drugs assigned to category I are those in which active ingredients are deemed to be both safe and effective, and the product is honestly labeled. Category II products are either not safe and effective, or untruthfully labeled and are to be removed from shelves within 6 months. Category III is reserved for products for which there are insufficient data to determine safety and/or effectiveness. Category III drugs were

TABLE 17-3 **Common Over-the-Counter Pain Relievers: How They Stack Up**

Aspirin (Bayer, Bufferin)	Acetaminophen (Tylenol)	Ibuprofen (Advil, Nuprin)
How they work		
Suppresses the body's pain and inflammation promoting chemicals at site of pain or injury	Apparently blocks pain-promoting chemicals in brain; no antiinflammatory effect	Works similarly to aspirin
Additional benefits		
In small daily doses, aspirin's blood-thinning properties help reduce the likelihood of heart attack or stroke in those at risk	Easier on stomach than aspirin	Easier on stomach than aspirin
Relatively inexpensive	Virtually no side effects when used according to product guidelines	Requires lower dose to produce same painkilling effect as aspirin
Disadvantages		
Stomach irritation	May not work as effectively against swelling or arthritis-related pain as aspirin or ibuprofen	Does not offer heart protection benefits
Risks		
Possibility of gastrointestinal bleeding	Prolonged or intensive use may result in liver damage	High doses may lead to kidney damage

Whether or not prolonged use of any of these OTC pain relievers is good or bad for you is something you must decide with your physician. Your age, weight, family, and personal medical histories all play a role in determining how and at what dosage you will benefit from these products.

sold until 1981 when the FDA dropped this category entirely. Today, only category I OTC drugs that are safe, effective, and truthfully labeled are to be sold. The FDA's drug classification process also allows some OTC drugs to be made stronger and some prescription drugs to become nonprescription drugs by reducing their strength through reformulation.

The current labeling of OTC drugs also reflects the regulatory process described. The labels must clearly state the type and quantity of active ingredients, alcohol content, side effects, instructions for appropriate use, warnings against inappropriate use, and the risks of polydrug use. Unsubstantiated claims must be carefully avoided in advertisements for these products.

Cosmetics

Concern over the safety of cosmetics has existed for more than 50 years. Hyperallergic reactions, bacterial infections, and the presence of carcinogens and teratogens (agents that cause birth defects) remain at the center of this concern. Because cosmetics are not generally classified as drugs, their regulation is limited in terms of FDA involvement. Legislation is regularly proposed that would increase the ability of the FDA to better control this important segment of the personal care retail trade.

HEALTH CARE QUACKERY AND CONSUMER FRAUD

A person who earns money by marketing inaccurate health information, unreliable health care, or ineffective health products is called a fraud, quack, or charlatan. **Consumer fraud** flourished with the old-fashioned medicine shows of the late 1880s. During medicine shows, self-proclaimed "doctors" would sell their tonics and potions (primarily alcohol-based) from cov-

chemical name name used to describe the molecular structure of a drug.

generic name (je **nare** ick) common or nonproprietary name of a drug.

brand name specific patented name assigned to a drug by its manufacturer.

consumer fraud marketing of unreliable and ineffective services, products, or information under the guise of curing disease or improving health; quackery.

PERSONAL ASSESSMENT

Circle the selection that best describes your practice. Then total your points for an interpretation of your health consumer skills.

1 Never
2 Occasionally
3 Most of the time
4 All of the time

1. I read all warranties and then file them for safekeeping.   1 2 3 4
2. I read labels for information pertaining to the nutritional quality of food.   1 2 3 4
3. I practice comparative shopping and use unit pricing, when available.   1 2 3 4
4. I read health-related advertisements in a critical and careful manner.   1 2 3 4
5. I challenge all claims pertaining to secret cures or revolutionary new health devices.   1 2 3 4
6. I engage in appropriate medical self-care screening procedures.   1 2 3 4
7. I maintain a patient-provider relationship with a variety of health-care providers.   1 2 3 4
8. I inquire about the fees charged before using a health-care provider's services.   1 2 3 4
9. I maintain adequate health insurance coverage.   1 2 3 4
10. I consult reputable medical self-care books before seeing a physician.   1 2 3 4
11. I ask pertinent questions of health-care providers when I am uncertain about the information I have received.   1 2 3 4

12. I seek second opinions when the diagnosis of a condition or the recommended treatment seems questionable.   1 2 3 4
13. I follow directions pertaining to the use of prescription drugs, including continuing their use for the entire period prescribed.   1 2 3 4
14. I buy generic drugs when they are available.   1 2 3 4
15. I follow directions pertaining to the use of OTC drugs.   1 2 3 4
16. I maintain a well-supplied medicine cabinet.   1 2 3 4

YOUR TOTAL POINTS   _____

INTERPRETATION

16-24 points   A very poorly skilled health consumer
25-40 points   An inadequately skilled health consumer
41-56 points   An adequately skilled health consumer
57-64 points   A highly skilled health consumer

TO CARRY THIS FURTHER . . .

Could you ever have been the victim of consumer fraud? What will you need to do to be a skilled consumer?

Categories of Over-the-Counter (OTC) Drugs

★ Antacids

★ Antimicrobials

★ Sedatives and sleep aids

★ Analgesics

★ Cold remedies and antitussives

★ Antihistamines and allergy products

★ Mouthwashes

★ Topical analgesics

★ Antirheumatics

★ Hematinics

★ Vitamins and minerals

★ Antiperspirants

★ Laxatives

★ Dentrifices and dental products

★ Sunburn treatments and preventives

★ Contraceptive and vaginal products

★ Stimulants

★ Hemorrhoidals

★ Antidiarrheals

★ Dandruff and athlete's foot preparations

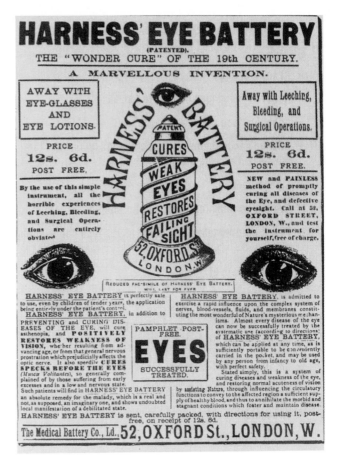

Health quackery as it appeared in the late 1800s.

ered wagons, often to gullible people who wanted cures for everything from gout to rheumatism.

Unfortunately, consumer fraud still flourishes. One need look no further than large city newspapers to see questionable advertisements for disease cures and weight loss products. Quacks have found in health and illness the perfect avenues to realize maximum gain with minimum effort.

When people are in poor health they may be afraid of dying. So powerful are their desires to live and be free of suffering that people are vulnerable to promises of health improvement and life extension. Even though many persons have great faith in their physicians, they also would like to have access to experimental treatments or products touted as being superior to currently available therapies. When tempted with the promise of real help, people are sometimes willing to set aside traditional medical care.

In another sense, many victims of consumer fraud participate in their own demise. Since the days of the medicine shows, the quack has recognized that many persons have a measure of gullibility, blind faith, impatience, superstition, ignorance, or hostility toward professional expertise. The fraud provides an answer for those who believe in miracle cures.

Regardless of the specific motivation that leads people into consumer fraud, the outcome is frequently the same. First, the consumer suffers financial loss. The services or products provided are grossly overpriced, and the consumers have little recourse to help them recover their money. Second, the consumers often feel disappointed, guilty, and angered by their own carelessness as consumers. Finally, consumer fraud may lead to unnecessary suffering. Far too frequently, premature deaths result from the faith that consumers place in the fraudulent products or services.[24]

Stocking Your Medicine Cabinet

A well-supplied medicine cabinet can be a valuable aid in maintaining a high level of health. How well supplied is yours?

SUPPLIES

★ Absorbent cotton

★ Adhesive bandages of assorted sizes

★ Adhesive tape

★ Dosage spoon (common household teaspoons are rarely the correct dosage size)

★ Elastic bandage

★ Eye cup for flushing objects out of the eye

★ Fever thermometer, including rectal type for a young child

★ First aid manual

★ Heating pad

★ Hot water bottle

★ Ice bag

★ Small blunt-end scissors

★ Sterile gauze in pads and a roll

★ Tweezers

★ Vaporizer or humidifier

NONPRESCRIPTION DRUG ITEMS

★ Analgesic—aspirin and/or acetaminophen. Both reduce fever and relieve pain; only aspirin can reduce inflammation.

★ Antacid

★ Antibacterial topical ointment

★ Antidiarrhetic

★ Antiseptic solution

★ Burn ointment

★ Calamine for poison ivy and other skin irritations

★ Cough syrup—nonsuppressant type

★ Decongestant

★ Emetic (to induce vomiting)—syrup of ipecac and activated charcoal to induce vomiting. Read the instructions on how to use these products.

★ Hydrocortisone creams for skin problems

★ Petroleum jelly as a lubricant

The medicine cabinet might also include antinausea medication if any family member is prone to motion sickness, a laxative, and some liniment. Seasonal items, such as insect repellants and sunscreens, round out the list. ★

HOW TO BECOME A SKILLED CONSUMER

After this discussion of health-influencing information, services, and products, you should be a wiser, more prepared consumer. However, information alone is not enough. We would like to offer six suggestions that may help you become a more skilled assertive consumer.

▼ *Prepare yourself for consumerism.* In addition to this personal health course, your university may offer a course on consumerism. Trade books on a variety of consumer topics are available in the library, as well as in bookstores. Consumer protection agencies can provide direction in selected areas. Governmental agencies may also provide assistance for your consumer choices.

▼ *Engage in comparative shopping.* In our free enterprise system, virtually every service or product can be duplicated on the open market. Very few one-of-a-kind items exist. Take the time to study your choices before purchasing a product or service.

▼ *Insist on formal contracts and dated receipts.* Under the consumer laws in most states, you have a limited period in which to void a contract. Formal documentation of your actions as a consumer will provide you with the maximum protection available.

▼ *Obtain written instructions and warranties.* Be certain of the appropriate use of any product you purchase. If you inappropriately use a product, you might void its warranty. Be familiar with what you can reasonably anticipate from the purchases you make. Also, be aware that a written warranty supersedes any verbal assurances a salesperson might make.

▼ *Put your complaints in writing.* There is no substitute for a carefully constructed record of your complaints. By having accurate records of the names and addresses of all persons and companies with whom you have done business, you will be able to document your actions as a consumer.

▼ *Press for resolution of your complaints.* As a consumer, you are entitled to effective products and services. If your consumer complaints are not resolved, legal recourse through the courts is available. You should not hesitate to assert your rights, not only for your own sake, but for consumers who might subsequently become victims.

Consumerism is an active relationship between you and a provider. If the provider is competent and honest and you are an informed and active consumer, both of you will profit from the relationship. However, if the provider is not competent or honest, you can protect yourself by following these six suggestions.

Summary

✔ Sources of health information include family, friends, commercials, labels, and information supplied by health professionals.

✔ Physicians can be either Doctors of Medicine (MD) or Doctors of Osteopathy (DO). Both receive similar training and engage in similar forms of practice.

✔ While alternative health care providers, including chiropractors, naturopaths, and acupuncturists, meet the health care needs of many people, systematic study of these forms of health care is only now underway.

✔ Restricted practice health care providers play important roles in meeting the holistic health needs of the public.

✔ Nursing at all levels, is a critical health care profession.

✔ Self-care is a viable approach to preventing illness and reducing the use of health care providers.

✔ Our growing inability to afford health care services has reached a crisis proportion in this country.

✔ Health insurance is critical in our ability to afford modern health care services.

✔ Health maintenance organizations (HMOs) provide an alternative way to receive health care services.

✔ Medicare and Medicaid are governmental plans for paying for health care services.

✔ National health care, in some fashion, seems likely to be implemented.

✔ The development of prescription medication is a long and expensive process.

✔ Critical health consumerism requires careful use of health-related information, products, and services.

Review Questions

1. Determine how you would test the accuracy of the health-related information you have received in your lifetime.

2. Identify and describe some sources of health-related information presented in this chapter. What factors should you consider when using these sources?

3. Point out the similarities between allopathic and osteopathic physicians. What is a nonallopathic health care practitioner? Give examples of each type of nonallopathic practitioner.

4. Describe the services that are provided by the following limited health care providers: dentists, psychologists, podiatrists, optometrists, and opticians. Identify several allied health care professionals.

5. In what ways is the trend toward self-care evident? What are some reasons for the popularity of this movement?

6. Identify and describe three general categories of hospitals. What new types of health care facilities are emerging in our society?

7. What is health insurance? Explain the following terms relating to health insurance: deductible amount, fixed indemnity benefits, full-service benefits, coinsurance, exclusion, and preexisting illnesses.

8. What is a health maintenance organization? How do HMO plans reduce the costs of health care? What are IPAs and PPOs?

9. What do the chemical name, brand name, and generic name of a prescription drug represent? OTC drugs are categorized according to what two factors?

10. What is health care quackery? What responsibilities have been given to the FDA? What can a consumer do to avoid consumer fraud?

Think About This . . .

✔ How do you rate yourself as an informed consumer of health information, services, and products?

✔ Are there any types of providers mentioned in this chapter whom you would not choose to consult? Explain your answer.

✔ To what extent and in what ways have you engaged in self-care?

✔ Many insurance companies exclude certain kinds of illness (such as AIDS) from coverage, and will not pay for the needed drugs. Who then should cover the cost?

Under what circumstances do you think that expensive medications should be prescribed for terminal patients?

✔ Is life insurance more important than health insurance for young adults? Explain your answer.

✔ Why do you think it is difficult to get people to seek help for preventive care although it is usually less expensive than treatment services?

✔ When you read a newspaper or magazine, do some advertisements seem questionable to you?

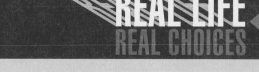

YOUR TURN

▼ Do you experience migraine headaches or some other chronic physical condition that causes you intense pain? If so, how do you deal with it, and what are the results?

▼ Have you ever sought alternative forms of treatment for a chronic painful condition, or do you know anyone who has? If so, what were the results?

▼ Ellen Gorman seems determined to explore alternative therapies for her migraine headaches. Based on what you have learned in this chapter, what are some cautions you can offer her? What questions

should she be asking about any practitioner she consults?

AND NOW, YOUR CHOICES . . .

▼ Would you consider using an alternative approach to treatment for a condition like Ellen's? Why or why not?

▼ If you did decide to seek alternative treatment, would you tell your regular physician? Why or why not? ▼

References

1. Sale of peroxy products halted, investigators' report, *FDA Consumer* 24(10):38, 1990.
2. Injunction actions, *FDA Consumer* 28(2):47, 1994.
3. Benson H, Stuart E: *The wellness book: guide to maintaining health and treating stress-related illness*, New York, 1992, Birch Lane Press (Carol Publishing Group).
4. *Physicians' desk reference*, ed 46, Oradel, NJ, 1993, Medical Economics.
5. Bryant J: NIH panel reviews "unconventional" medical practices, *The NIH Record* 44(14);1, 1992.
6. Nelson H: USA-NIH approach to unconventional therapies, *Lancet* 340(8811):106, 1992.
7. American Optometric Association, Office of the Executive Director, personal communication, May 10, 1994.
8. Inlander C: *Take this book to the hospital with you: a consumer guide to surviving your hospital stay*, New York, 1991, Pantheon Books.
9. Employee Benefit Research Institute, *USA Today*, p. 1B, March 11, 1991.
10. Carlson E: AARP submits health-care reform proposal to members for their review, *AARP Bulletin* 33(3):1, 1992.
11. Federal budget estimates for 1991-1996; Department of Health and Human Services estimate for 1991; Department of Commerce estimates, for 1991-1996, *USA Today*, p. 3B, May 6, 1991.
12. Levit K, Cowan C: Businesses, households, and governments: health care cost, 1990, *Health Care Financing Review* 13(2):83, 1991.
13. Aaron H: *Serious and unstable condition: financing America's health care*, Washington, 1991, Brookings Institute.
14. SAMHSA: Newsletter, Department of Health and Human Services, 1(4):3, 1993.
15. McKenzie JF, Pinger RR: *Introduction to community health*, New York, 1995, Harper Collins College Publishing.
16. U.S. Department of Health and Human Services, Social Security Administration: *Medicare*, SSA Publication No. 06-10043, May 1993.
17. Detlefs D, Myers R: *1993 Medicare: What you need to know about Medicare in simple, practical terms*, 1992, William M Mercer.
18. Ries P: Characteristics of persons with and without health care coverage: United States, 1989. *Advance Data from Vital and Health Statistics, No. 201*. Hyattsville, MD, 1991, National Center for Health Statistics, Centers for Disease Control.
19. Butler PA: *Too poor to be sick: access to medical care for the uninsured*, Washington, DC, 1988, American Public Health Association.
20. Fuchs BC, Skolovsky J: *CRS report for Congress: the Canadian health care system*, Washington, DC, 1990, Congressional Research Service, The Library of Congress.
21. Simonsen L: What are pharmacists dispensing most often? *Pharmacy Times* 59(4):29, 1993.
22. Annual Rx review: Nicotine patches lead Rx activity to new heights, *Drug Topics* 137(7):72, 1993.
23. *Using animals in intramural research: guidelines for investigators*, NIH Animal Care and Use Committee, NIH Training Center, US Government Printing Office, 1992-331-302.
24. Cornacchia HJ, Barrett S: *Consumer health: a guide to intelligent decisions*, ed 5, St Louis, 1993, Mosby.

Suggested Readings

Aaron H: *Serious and unstable condition: financing America's health care*, Washington, 1991, Brookings Institute.

A respected economist evaluates the present critical condition of the American health care system. An evaluation of various approaches to moderating these problems is provided. Presents strengths and weaknesses, as well as short-term and long-term problems for each approach.

Inlander C: *Take this book to the hospital with you: a consumer guide to surviving your hospital stay*, New York, 1991, Pantheon Books.

Because most of us will experience hospitalization, the author provides a checklist for evaluating the "patient friendliness" of hospitals. Provides additional hints for making hospital stays more pleasant.

Taylor RL: *Health fact, health fiction—getting through the media maze*, Dallas, 1990, Taylor Publishing.

A physician writes about the problem of health hype through the media. Too many people act on health information that is not credible. Encourages a sound approach for evaluation of health messages and health risks.

18

Environment

Influences from the World Around Us

Throughout this book you have read about areas of health over which you have significant control. For example, you select the foods you eat, how much alcohol you consume, and how you want to manage the stressors in your life. You make many of these kinds of decisions on a daily basis, often subconsciously.

The study of the environment and its impact on your health provides an interesting contrast to the daily controls you have on your own health. Perhaps because of the natural processes of life and death and the vital role the environment plays, we are inclined to think that we cannot make personal decisions concerning it. This is, however, changing.

In comparison with the 1980s when concerns about the environment focused on problems over which individuals had little direct responsibility or control (such as the ozone layer and nuclear accidents), the 1990s are characterized by a focus on the individual and the home. Environmentally related issues such as the disposal of municipal waste, the recycling of glass and aluminum, the venting of radon gas from basements, and the reduction of water use during periods of drought reflect the fact that individuals must act to support our environment.

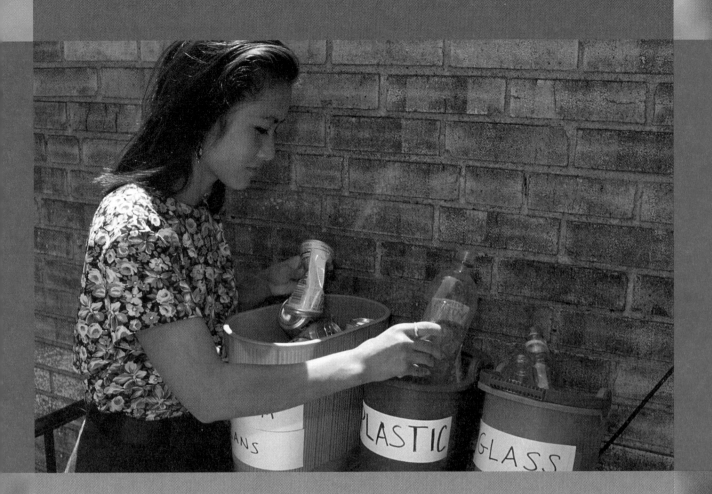

ENVIRONMENTAL HEALTH

The following objectives are covered in this chapter:

▽ Reduce human exposure to criteria air pollutants, as measured by an increase to at least 85% in the proportion of people who live in counties that have not exceeded any Environmental Protection Agency standard for air quality in the previous 12 months. (Baseline: 49.7% in 1988; p. 320.)

▽ Reduce human exposure to solid waste-related water, air, and soil contamination, as measured by a reduction in average pounds of municipal solid waste produced per person each day to no more than 3.6 pounds. (Baseline: 4.0 pounds in 1988; p. 325.)

▽ Expand to at least 35 the number of states in which at least 75% of local jurisdictions have adopted construction standards and techniques that minimize elevated indoor radon levels in those new building areas locally determined to have elevated radon levels. (Baseline: 1 state in 1989; p. 329.)

▽ Establish programs for recyclable materials and household hazardous waste in at least 75% of counties. (Baseline: approximately 850 programs in 41 states collected household toxic waste in 1987; extent of recycling collections unknown; p. 331.)

HEALTHY PEOPLE 2000 OBJECTIVES

REAL LIFE
REAL CHOICES
Poverty and Pollution: Partners in Crime?

▼ **Name:** David Cloudwalker
▼ **Age:** 23
▼ **Occupation:** Medical student

"Save the Earth!" "Fight Pollution!" "Clean Air NOW!"

Slowing his beat up VW bug to let a throng of student demonstrators cross the street, David Cloudwalker glances at the signs they carry and shakes his head. Four hundred years of abusing and exploiting the environment, and these people think all it takes to clean up the mess is signs and marches. How many of these kids, he wonders, know what it's like to pay every day of your life for the waste dump someone else has made of your native land?

David knows. A member of the Crow nation, he grew up with eight brothers and sisters in grinding poverty on the edge of an old mining town in Montana. Scarred hillsides and towering slagheaps stand in stark contrast to the craggy majesty of ancient mountains and the colorful profusion of native wildflowers. The clear cold stream where David's ancestors fished still gleams and sparkles . . . but with the rainbow hues of chemical waste from the nearby plastics plant. The vast blue bowl of western sky is streaked with black plumes from the factory's exhaust stacks, and the roar and crash of freight trains shatter the peaceful mountain night.

Like other families in Indian Hollow, the Cloudwalkers had no health insurance and little access to medical care. Sanitation facilities were crude and poorly maintained, and people always seemed to be passing the same disease-causing germs back and

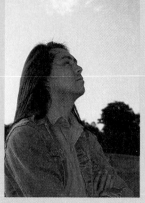

forth. David's father, a laborer at the plastics factory, died at the age of 36 of what the plant physician vaguely called "weak lungs." But George Cloudwalker never smoked, and as a young man he won every running competition at tribal gatherings. His weak lungs, David is sure, were the result of long-term exposure to the choking filth of the factory air. Two of David's brothers have worked at the plant since high school, and they always seem to be coughing or wiping watery eyes. And now a new generation of kids is coughing, sneezing, and getting gastrointestinal "bugs."

The lands of David's ancestors have been invaded not only by technology but also by tourists. The once abandoned mining town has been restored to attract summer visitors. The old brick and frame storefronts of the main street now display pricey western and Native American clothing, jewelry, and souvenirs. Costly cars with out of state license plates line the dusty streets, and synthetic country music thunders from speakers on the pavilion of a trendy line-dance spot.

David doesn't long to be a painted warrior or a daring buffalo hunter. He's working his way through one of the top medical schools in the country, and his goal is to become a neurosurgeon. But he's proud of his heritage, and he's both sad and angry about the heedless exploitation of our country's vast natural riches.

As you study this chapter, think about David's experiences as a Native American dealing with environmental damage, and prepare yourself to answer the questions in **Your Turn** at the end of the chapter. ▼

TRANSITION TO A POSTINDUSTRIAL SOCIETY

Before the industrial revolution our environmental resources supported the physical well-being of most people. The air was crisp, the water was clean, and the land was fertile. When forms of pollution occurred, they were the results of natural events, such as floods, dust storms, forest fires, and volcanoes. Agrarian living was the rule in this decentralized society. When the industrial revolution occurred at the turn of the century, many people moved to the large cities where fac-

tory labor was needed. Population growth in urban areas increased significantly faster than did growth in rural communities.

These major shifts produced problems for the health of the country. Segments of our population were subjected to overcrowding, poor sanitation and waste disposal, industrial waste, and environmental pollutants of various kinds. Over time it became clear that life in the ubran centers was more precarious than that in rural areas. A few people returned to rural areas, but the majority were economically unable to move. They remained in large cities, close to the in-

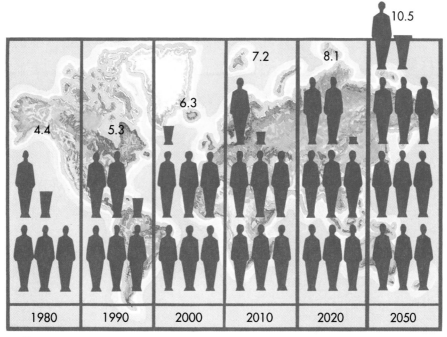

Figure 18-1 At its current rate of growth, the world's population will reach 10 billion approximately 25 years sooner than predicted only a decade ago.

dustrial centers that promised a "better tomorrow."

From an environmental point of view, this better day has not arrived. Our environment has deteriorated: our air is polluted, our fresh water is scarce, and our land is filled with toxic chemicals. Although our society is rapidly moving toward the high technology of postindustrialism, our natural resources are dwindling to the point where even our own technologies may not be able to reduce the negative impact on our health.

WORLD POPULATION GROWTH

Population growth affects the environment beyond our own homes and communities to include the entire planet.

Each year the population of the world grows by 90 million people. By the middle of the next century there could be 50% more people than there are today (Figure 18-1). By the year 2060 it is projected that 10.8 billion persons will be alive. By the year 2000 more than half of the developing countries in the world may not be able to feed their populations from foods grown on their own lands.[1] As seen in Somalia, the consequence of overpopulation, combined with nonenvironmental factors such as limited agriculture and governmental

instability, can lead to human suffering of the highest magnitude. However, as the earth's population increases by 1 million persons every 4 years, we struggle to make family planning available to everyone, to encourage later marriage and childbearing, to encourage breastfeeding for not only the health of infants but also to lengthen the interval between pregnancies, and to improve the status and well-being of women so that they have new roles for themselves and their families. Failing to control population growth, crowding, water pollution and scarcity, hazardous waste accumulation, and air pollution will move us closer yet to ecological disaster.

AIR POLLUTION

If you think that air pollution is a modern concern reflecting technology that has gone astray, keep in mind that our air is routinely polluted by nature. Sea salt, soil particles, ash, dust, soot, mcirobes, assorted trace elements, and plant pollens are consistently found in the air we breathe.

Pollution caused in part by humans also has a long history. From the fires that filled our ancestors' caves with choking smoke, through the "killer fogs" of nineteenth century London, to the dust storms of the Great

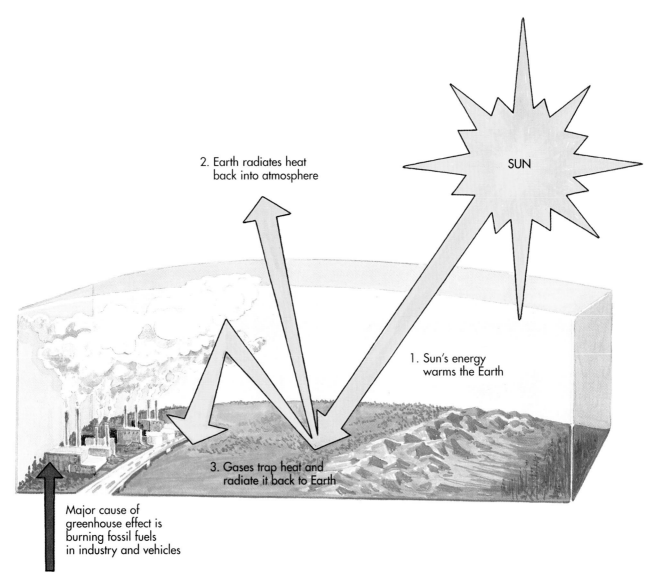

2. Earth radiates heat
back into atmosphere

SUN

1. Sun's energy
warms the Earth

3. Gases trap heat and
radiate it back to Earth

Major cause of
greenhouse effect is
burning fossil fuels
in industry and vehicles

Figure 18-2 The greenhouse effect.

Depression, humans have contributed to air pollution. Only since World War II, however, has air pollution become a widely recognized concern in North America.

Sources of Air Pollution

The sources of our modern air pollutants are familiar to you. A leading source is the internal combustion engine. Automobiles, trucks, and buses contribute a variety of materials to the air, including carbon monoxide and hydrocarbons. Industrial processes, domestic heating, refuse burning, and use of pesticides and herbicides also contribute to our air pollution problem. In recent years the massive deforestation of the tropical rain forest in the Amazon River basin of South America has contributed significant amounts of gaseous and particulate pollutants to the air.

GASEOUS POLLUTANTS

The pollutants dispersed into the air by the sources just identified are generally in the form of gases, including carbon dioxide and carbon monoxide. Carbon dioxide is the natural byproduct of combustion and is produced whenever fuels are burned. Electricity production, car and truck emissions, and industry are the principal producers of carbon dioxide. According to many scientisits, increasing levels of carbon dioxide may result in a **greenhouse effect.** A greenhouse effect would cause the earth's surface temperature to increase. An increase of only a few degrees Fahrenheit could produce significant increases in violent storms, unbearably hot summer days, and prolonged droughts.[3] Figure 18-2 depicts the development of the greenhouse effect. Table 18-1 shows the worldwide sources of carbon dioxide. At the time of this writing

Scripps Institute of Oceanography is proposing the use of sound wave transmission to determine the extent to which the oceans have warmed.[3]

Carbon monoxide, the colorless and odorless gas produced when fuels are burned incompletely, has already been discussed in conjunction with cardiovascular disease (see Chapter 10). Also occurring in gaseous form are methane, from decaying vegetation; the terpenes, produced by trees; and benzene and benzopyrene, produced by incomplete combustion of many types of hydrocarbons, which may cause cancer when taken into the respiratory system.[4]

Nitrogen and sulfur compounds are pollutants produced by a variety of industrial processes, including the burning of high sulfur content fuels, especially coal (Figure 18-3). When nitrogen and sulfur oxides combine with moisture in the atmosphere, they are converted to nitric and sulfuric acid. The resulting **acid rain,** acid snow, and acid fog are responsible for the destruction of aquatic life and vegatation in the eastern United States and Canada.[5]

Smog is another familiar type of air pollution. In urban areas located in cooler climates (or other cities during the winter months), sulfur oxides and particu-

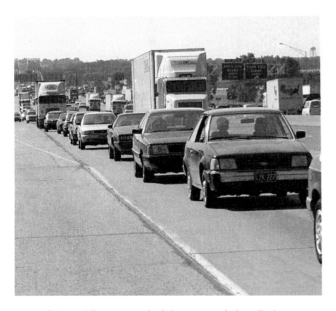

Automobiles are a principle source of air pollution.

TABLE 18-1 Worldwide Sources of Carbon Dioxide	
USA	23%
USSR	19%
Western Europe	15%
China	10%
Eastern Europe	7%
Latin America	6%
Japan	5%
Others	5%
Middle East	4%
Africa	3%
Canada	2%

⭐ **Gulf War Syndrome**

In January 1991 over 700,000 American military personnel were involved in the Persian Gulf War under the operational title of Desert Storm. Since their return to the United States, veterans have reported a variety of physical ailments that have become known as the Gulf War Syndrome (GWS). Today, over 20,000 people have been identified with symptoms of GWS and 1000 new victims join the list each month. Among the symptoms which the veterans have experienced are skin rashes, shortness of breath, chest pain, insomnia, poor thinking abilities, fatigue, and intermittent diarrhea. Somewhat less frequently reported are nightmares, hair loss, night sweats, and coldlike symptoms.

As the number of GWS victims increased during the period 1991 to 1993, demands for a serious scientific investigation of this mysterious condition increased. Early epidemiological evidence determined that there could be several causative factors. Among these were exposure to toxic compounds, as well as smoke from oil well fires, diesel fumes, pesticides, toxic plants, depleted uranium (from unused shells), direct contact with captured enemy soldiers, and chemical or biological weapons. The Pentagon, however, steadfastly denies that chemical and biological weapons were ever employed in the Gulf War.

At the time of this writing, early evaluations of a random sample of veterans failed to produce enough consistency in symptoms for a panel of medical and environmental health experts to support the existence of a true syndrome.[6] Rather, health experts recommend that the Department of Defense gather further data to help define the illness and determine its probable cause. ★

greenhouse effect warming of the earth's surface that is produced when solar heat becomes trapped by layers of carbon dioxide and other gases.

acid rain rain that has a lower pH (more acidic) than that normally associated with rain.

smog air pollution made up of a combination of smoke, photochemical compounds, and fog.

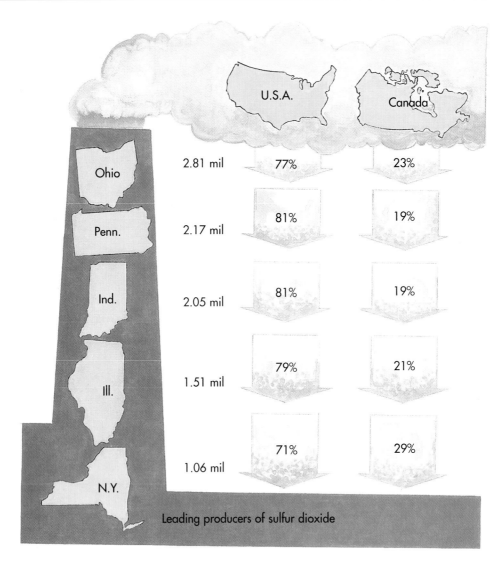

Figure 18-3 States that are the leading producers of sulfur dioxide. This results in the distribution of acid rain, snow, and fog to the Eastern United States and Canada.

late matter (from heating systems) combine with moisture to form a grayish haze, or smog. This gray-air smog contributes to respiratory problems that are common in these areas during the winter months. In warmer areas (or during the summer months in other areas), brown-air smog develops when hydrocarbons and particulate matter from automobile exhaust interact in the presence of sunlight.[5] This photochemical smog produces ozone. Ozone is highly reactive to the human respiratory system, plants, and materials such as rubber.

Obviously the elderly, smokers, and people with respiratory conditions should be cautious. Of course, maintaining a high level of respiratory system health is to the advantage of everyone, but particularly to people who must live in or near smog-prone areas.

An environmental concern currently being studied is the destruction of the ultraviolet light–absorbing **ozone layer.**[7] Nitrous oxides and materials containing **chlorofluorocarbons (CFCs)** can destroy this protective ozone layer within the stratosphere (Figure 18-4). Nitrous oxides come from the burning of fossil fuels like coal and gasoline. CFCs are used in air conditioners, many-fast food containers, insulation materials, and solvents. Today, an alternative group of compounds, the hydrofluorocarbons (HFCs) are replacing CFCs with significantly less potential for harming the ozone layer.

Although changes in the ozone layer have been recognized for over a decade, the progress of deterioration has not advanced as rapidly as once projected. The holes in the layer that appear seasonally over the

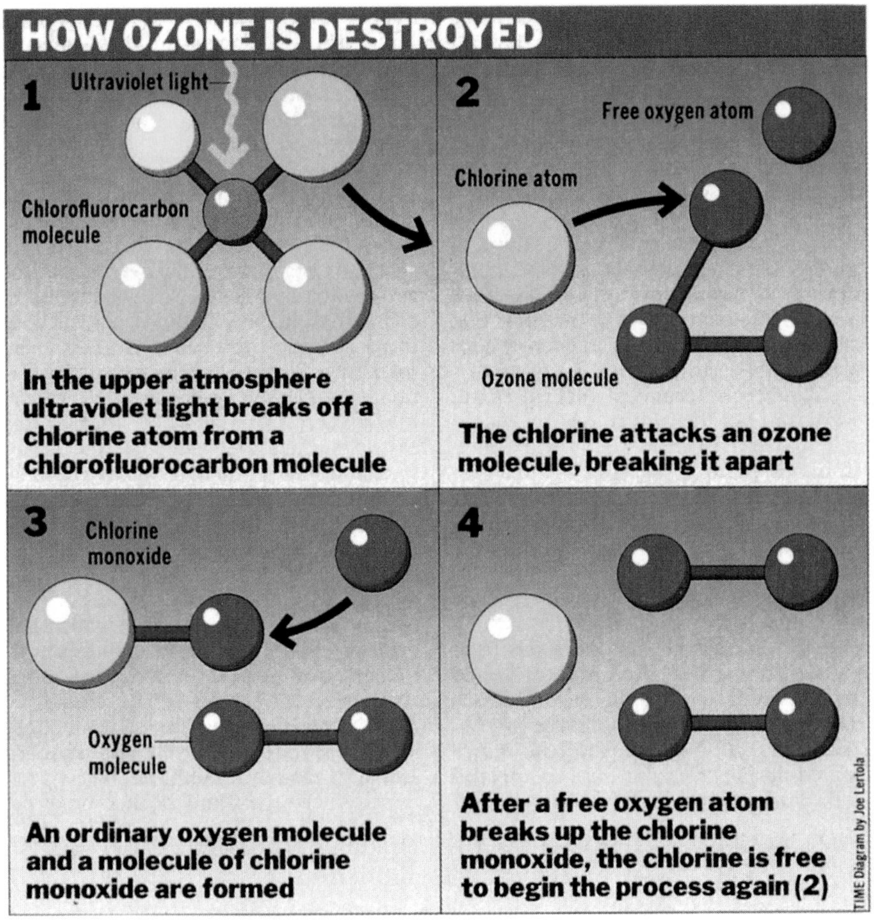

HOW OZONE IS DESTROYED

1

Ultraviolet light

Chlorofluorocarbon molecule

In the upper atmosphere ultraviolet light breaks off a chlorine atom from a chlorofluorocarbon molecule

2

Free oxygen atom

Chlorine atom

Ozone molecule

The chlorine attacks an ozone molecule, breaking it apart

3

Chlorine monoxide

Oxygen molecule

An ordinary oxygen molecule and a molecule of chlorine monoxide are formed

4

After a free oxygen atom breaks up the chlorine monoxide, the chlorine is free to begin the process again (2)

TIME Diagram by Joe Lertola

Figure 18-4 Process in which ozone is destroyed.

Antarctic and Arctic are, however, larger than in the early 1980s. Despite the progress in reducing CFC use in this country, continued use in other areas of the world prevents complete stabilization of the layer. Consequently, health dangers, such as skin cancer, cataracts, snow blindness, and premature wrinkling of skin, will continue.

PARTICULATE POLLUTANTS

There are many *particulate pollutants*, including both naturally occurring materials and particles derived from industrial processes, mining, and agriculture. Inhalation of particulate matter can cause potentially fatal respiratory diseases, including *silicosis* from quartz dust, *asbestosis* from asbestos fibers, and *byssinosis* from cotton fibers. Because of its widespread

⭐ Environmental Terrorism

In terms of air pollution, no single episode of contamination has ever surpassed that of the oil well fires in Kuwait. The 727 wells set on fire by retreating Iraqi troops in January 1991 burned 5,000,000 barrels of crude oil per day. The oil was converted into thick oily pollutants and noxious gases that were released into the atmosphere. The last of these fires was not extinguished until November 1991. Today children and adults with allergies, bronchial asthma, and pneumonia are commonly seen in Kuwaiti hospitals. Long-term influences may include lung cancer. ⭐

ozone layer (**oh** zone) layer of triatomic oxygen that surrounds the Earth and filters much of the sun's radiation before it can reach the Earth's surface.

chlorofluorocarbons (CFCs) (klor oh **floor** oh car bons) gaseous chemical compounds that contain chlorine and fluorine.

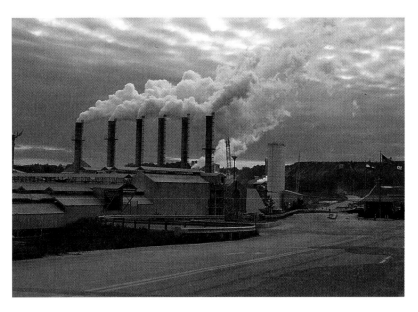

Industry contributes to air pollution.

presence, asbestos is a particular concern. In 1989 the *EPA* ordered asbestos use to be stopped by the year 1997. If you work or live in a building with asbestos-wrapped pipes, inquire as to when the asbestos will be removed.

Trace mineral elements, including lead, nickel, iron, zinc, copper, and magnesium, are also among the particles polluting the air. Chronic **lead toxicity** is among the most serious health problems associated with this form of air pollution. Legislation requiring the use of nonleaded gasoline was an important step toward reducing the levels of lead in the air. Those persons who must live or work in areas that have higher levels of lead in the air (or whose drinking water comes through lead pipes) may sustain damage to hemoglobin, their gastrointestinal tracts, or their central nervous systems. Lead toxicity is disproportionately seen in young minority children of low-income families, principally because of the lead-based paints found in older houses, heavy motor vehicle traffic on city streets, and the use of lead soldering in older plumbing systems. For these children, lower IQs, attention disorders, and long-term learning disabilities may result.

Temperature Inversions

On a normal sunny day, radiant energy from the sun warms the ground and the air immediately above it. As this warmed air rises, it carries pollutants upward and disperses them into a larger, cooler air mass above. Cool air sinking to replace the rising warmed air minimizes the concentration of pollutants.

On those occasions when high pressure settles over an area, warm air can be trapped immediately above the ground. Unable to rise, this trapped, warm, pol-luted air layer stagnates and produces a potentially health-threatening *subsidence inversion.*[5] (This is the inversion layer that meterologists talk about on the evening news.) In 1969, a subsidence inversion formed over much the eastern United States, resulting in respiratory distress and deaths among people with respiratory disease.

A second form of thermal inversion, *radiation inversion,* is frequently seen during winter.[5] At this time of year late afternoon cooling of the ground causes a layer of cool air to develop under a higher, warmer layer of air. With the inability of the cool layer of air to rise, pollutants begin to accumulate near the ground and remain there until the next morning. Warming of the ground later in the morning restores the heating of the lower level air and reestablishes the normal dispersal of pollutants.

Indoor Air Pollution

Not all air pollution occurs outside. Concern is growing over the health risks associated with indoor air pollution. Toxic materials including cigarette smoke (see Chapter 9), asbestos, radon, formaldehyde, vinyl chloride, and cooking gases can be found in buildings ranging from houses and apartments to huge office complexes and manufacturing plants. Science majors know that the odors that abound near their chemistry laboratories represent exposure to indoor air pollution.

Of all of the indoor air pollutants, none is of greater concern than cigarette smoke. In December 1992 the Environmental Protection Agency identified environmental tobacco smoke to be a Group A (known human) carcinogen.[8] It now is believed that 3000 lung cancer deaths occur annually due to this pollutant.

Health ACTION Guide

Preventing Indoor Air Pollution

To minimize the level of indoor pollution in your home, follow these simple steps. How easy or difficult would it be to improve your current level of prevention?

▼ Hang dry-cleaned clothing outside to air out before hanging it in the closet.
▼ Clean humidifiers, and replace belts on a regular basis.
▼ Limit use of aerosol personal care products to the bare minimum.

▼ Store fuel for mowers, snow blowers, trimmers, and other gasoline powered tools in an approved container in a well-ventilated area.
▼ Do not run the engine of a car in an attached garage or closed carport.
▼ Properly close containers of household cleaning products that are capable of emitting toxic fumes.
▼ Ventilate rooms in which new carpet and drapes have been installed as often as possible.
▼ Have fireplaces cleaned and inspected regularly.
▼ Eliminate smoking of cigarettes within the home.
▼ Discard unused paint, hobby supplies, herbicides, and pesticides on a regular basis.
▼ Inspect gas appliances for proper ventilation.
▼ Use products that are as free as possible from asbestos and formaldehyde when remodeling.

Between 150,000 and 300,000 illnesses in infants and young children occur annually as a result of exposure to environmental tobacco smoke.[8]

Environmental tobacco smoke joins formaldehyde (from building material), vinyl chloride (from PVC plumbing), and other pollutants (including radon from natural radiation sources and asbestos from insulation) to form the basis of the sick building syndrome.[9] For people with respiratory illnesses and immune system hypersensitivities, as well as the elderly, home or work sites could be less healthy than traditionally thought.

Health Implications

Because of the complex nature of many health problems, it is difficult to clearly assess the impact of air pollution on health. Age, sex, genetic predispositions, occupation, residency, and personal health practices complicate this assessment. Nevertheless, air pollution may severely affect health problems for elderly persons, persons who smoke or have respiratory conditions such as asthma, and persons who must work in polluted air.

In an attempt to improve air quality in the decades ahead and thus minimize health problems, legislation passed in 1991 established objectives for the future. Specific standards and timeliness to achieve them by the year 2020 were detailed for utilities, vehicles, municipalities, fuels, and industry.

WATER POLLUTION

Although water is the most abundant chemical compound on the earth's surface, we are finding it increasingly difficult to maintain a plentiful and usable sup-

TABLE 18-2 **Home Water Use**	
Use	**Gallons**
Washing car	100
Taking a bath	36
Washing clothes	35 to 60
Washing dishes	10 to 30
Brushing teeth	10 to 20
Shaving	10 to 20
Watering lawn	8/min
Taking a shower	7/min
Flushing toilet	5 to 7
Leaky faucet	2/day

ply. Pollution is depriving us of the water we need to meet the needs of a typical household, as shown in Table 18-2.

Yesterday's Pollution Problem

Like air pollution, water pollution is not solely a phenomenon of twentieth century overpopulation or unchecked technology. Nature has, in fact, routinely polluted our surface and ground water with minerals leached from the soil, acids produced by decaying vegetation, and the decay of animal products. Also,

---

lead toxicity (tok **sis** ih tee) blood lead level above 25 micrograms/deciliter. (If adopted, the new standard will be 10 micrograms/deciliter).

people have polluted their own water supplies. Waterborne contaminants that resulted in outbreaks of dysentery, typhoid fever, cholera, and infectious hepatitis can be traced to poor sanitation practices in centuries past. As recently as one generation ago, people living in rural areas occasionally found that their feed lots, chicken coops, and septic tank systems polluted their water supplies.

Today's Pollution Problem

In addition to the natural sources of water pollution already described, today's water sources are often damaged by pollutants derived from agricultural, urban, and industrial sources. Most of these pollutants are either biological or chemical products, and many can be either removed from the water or brought within acceptable safety limits. For some pollutants, however, management technology has been only partially successful or is still being developed.

Sources of Water Pollution

Water pollution is not the result of only one type of pollutant. In fact, many sources of water pollution exist.

PATHOGENS

Pathogenic agents, in the form of bacteria, viruses, and protozoa, enter the water supply through human and animal wastes. Communities with sewage treatment systems designed around a combined sanitary/storm system can, during heavy rain or snow melt, allow untreated sewage to rush through the processing plant. For example, following a heavy downpour, New York City's combined storm-sanitary system will allow 84 billion gallons of waste water (sewage, precipitation, and industrial waste) into the Hudson River.[10] In addition, pathogenic organisms can enter the water supply when sewage is flushed from boats. Pathogenic agents are also introduced into the water supply from animal wastes at feed lots and at meat processing facilities. Pet dropping have also been found contaminating water supplies.

Sewage treatment plants and public health laboratories routinely test for the presence of pathogenic agents. The presence of **coliform bacteria** indicates human or animal feces.

BIOLOGICAL IMBALANCES

Aquatic plants tend to thrive in water rich in nitrates and phosphates. This overabundance leads to **eutrophication,** which can render a stream, pond, or lake unusable.[11]

During hot, dry summers aquatic plants die in large numbers. Since the decay of vegetation requires aerobic bacterial action, the *biochemical oxygen demand* will be high.[2] To satisfy the biochemical oxygen demand, much of the water's oxygen is used. When such a condition exits, fish may be killed in great numbers.

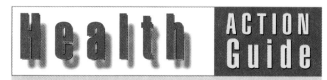

Drinking Water

When traveling outside of the United States, you should be aware that water supplies in more than 100 countries are considered unsafe. You can avoid waterborne illnesses by following these guidelines:

▼ Drink bottled water (but be careful of locally bottled water; it can also be unsafe).
▼ Boil water.
▼ Use iodine or water-purification tablets.
▼ Avoid using ice.
▼ Do not use tap water when brushing teeth.
▼ Avoid vegetables and fruits washed in unclean water.

To take the above advice further, before traveling be certain that all your immunizations are current, and request medication for diarrhea from your physician. ▼

Putrefaction of the dead fish not only further pollutes the water, but also fouls the air.

Contamination of water by nitrates and phosphates can occur in a number of unintentional ways. In rural areas runoff from fields carries fertilizers into the water supply. Animal wastes contribute nitrogen and phosphorus to the water supply. Some detergents used in homes and industries contain phosphates that can pass undegraded through all but the most extensive sewage treatment process.

TOXIC SUBSTANCES

Of the pollutants found in today's water supply, perhaps none are of greater concern than toxic chemical substances. These chemical toxins, including metals as well as hydrocarbons, are dangerous because they have the ability to enter the food chain. When they do so, their concentration per unit of weight increases with each life form in the chain. This increase is called *biological magnification*. By the time humans consume the fish that have fed on the contaminated lower forms of aquatic life, the toxic chemicals have been concentrated to dangerous levels.[2]

Among the important toxic substances is *mercury*, in the form of methyl mercury. Derived from industrial wastes, methyl mercury is ingested and concentrated by shellfish and other fish. When humans eat these fish regularly, mercury levels increase to the point that hemoglobin and central nervous system function can be

Health ACTION Guide

Tips for Cooking Fish

For those who enjoy eating fish, experts recommend the following steps to minimize the risk of overexposure to the toxic chemicals concentrated in the tissue of fish;

▼ Fillet fish; throw away skin and guts as well as fatty areas which are usually brownish.
▼ Do not always eat the same kind of fish, or even different kinds of fish from the same pond, lake, or stream.
▼ Eat smaller fish rather than the larger fish of the same variety.
▼ Select fish varieties that live nearer the surface.
▼ Grill or broil fish to cut down on fat retention.
▼ If you fish, be aware of local restrictions about contamination of fish.

Eating fish can be very nutritious, but exercise caution regarding the amount and types of fish eaten. ▼

rounding water supply. Tests are now being conducted at these dump sites to determine the extent of contamination of the underground water supply. Studies on persons who have been exposed to high levels of PCBs in drinking water are being conducted. More is being learned concerning long-term exposure to these hydrocarbons. In laboratory animals, PCBs produce liver and kidney damage, gastric and reproductive disorders, skin lesions, and tumors.[2] Most recently a report indicates that PCBs have been found in women with breast cancer.[12] The U.S. **Environmental Protection Agency (EPA)** ordered that all PCBs in electrical transformers be removed by 1990.

MISCELLANEOUS SOURCES

Three additional types of pollution that affect our water are important, although their impact on human health is not fully understood. The pollution from these sources is detrimental to aquatic life, alters the esthetic value of our waterways, and reduces recreational use of our rivers, lakes, and shores.

Oil spills include not only the major spills resulting from tanker accidents, but also spills that occur on inland waters and those that result from the seeping of crude oil from the ground. Any kind of oil spill can foul our water. Fish, aquatic plants, sea birds, and

seriously altered. Death from mercury poisoning is well documented.

A variety of other metals have also been found in North American rivers and lakes. Arsenic, cadmium, copper, lead, and silver are all capable of entering the food chain. In many cases, only very low levels of these metals need to be ingested before changes in health become evident.

Of the wide variety of agricultural products currently used on American and Canadian farms, **pesticides** are among the most toxic. Containing more than 1800 different chemical compounds, pesticides deliver a diverse array of chemicals to our water supplies.

Most serious of the toxic chemicals found in our water are the *chlorinated hydrocarbons,* including dichlorodiphenyltrichloroethane (DDT), chlordane, and chlordecone (Kepone). The **mutagenic, carcinogenic,** and **teratogenic** effects of these hydrocarbon products need further scientific exploration.

Polychlorinated biphenyls (PCBs) are a second group of hydrocarbons causing a great deal of concern because of their presence in the water supply.[2] PCBs are, on the basis of their chemical structure, very stable, heat-resistant compounds that have been used extensively in transformers and electrical capacitors. In many areas of the country discarded electrical equipment has broken open and released PCBs into the sur-

coliform bacteria (**co** lih form back **teer** ee uh) intestinal tract bacteria, presence in a water supply suggests contamination by human or animal waste.

eutrophication (yo trofe ih **kay** shun) enrichment of a body of water with nutrients, which causes overabundant growth of plants.

putrefaction (pyoo tre **fak** shun) decomposition of organic matter.

pesticide (**pes** tih side) agent used to destroy pests.

mutagenic (myoo ta **jen** ick) capable of promoting genetic alterations in cells.

carcinogenic (kar sin oh **jen** ick) related to the production of cancerous changes; property of environmental agents, including drugs, that may stimulate the development of cancerous changes within cells.

teratogenic (ter ah toe **jen** ick) capable of promoting birth defects.

Environmental Protection Agency (EPA) federal agency charged with the protection of natural resources and the quality of the environment.

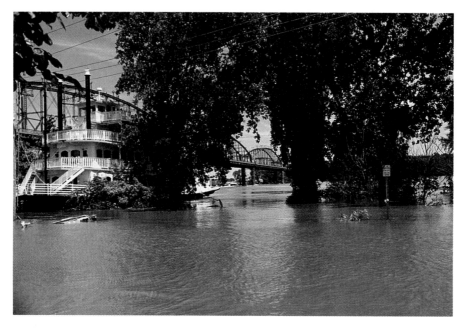

Flooding along the Missouri River in 1993. This riverboat attraction was alongside a road and picnic area.

beaches can be damaged by both surface oil film and tar masses that float below the surface or roll along the ocean bottom.

The costly vacuuming of oil, the use of detergents to break up oil slicks, and, eventually, the consumption of oil by bacteria can perhaps return polluted water to a more normal state.

Power plants that use water from lakes and rivers to cool their stream turbines cause *thermal pollution.* When this heated water is returned to its source, temperatures in the water may rise significantly. As temperatures increase, the oxygen-carrying capacity of the water decreases and the balance of aquatic life forms is altered. In water that is raised only 10° C (18° F), entire species of fish can disappear and aquatic plants can proliferate out of control.[13]

Sediments in the form of sand, clay, and other soil constituents regularly reach waterway channels. Rivers, lakes, reservoirs, and oceans serve as settling basins for these sediments. As land is cleared for agriculture and commercial development, the effects of sedimentation grow. Water that is polluted by these sediments is deprived of sunlight. Thus plant life is reduced and the water channels eventually become filled as the materials settle. If cleared land areas cannot be returned to vegetative cover, then dredging may be required to keep the waterway usable, although this is an expensive and relatively ineffective response.

Today a trip to the beach is often an adventure in water pollution. Besides oil, a wide variety of objects can be seen in the water as it washes the sand. Plastic, foam, glass, cigarette butts, paper, metal cans, and medical wastes are most frequently seen. When volunteers cleaned selected beaches during 1989, the coastal states of Florida, Texas, and California reported picking up 400,000, 316,000, and over 207,000 pounds of debris, respectively!*

Chlorine, one of the most extensively used chemicals in industry, is now recognized as a prevalent pollutant of the country's water supply, particularly for the Great Lakes. Experts believe that elevated levels of chlorine could result in a variety of health problems in humans, including memory problems, stunted growth, and even some forms of cancer. For many animals such as eagles, mink, lake trout, and turtles, chlorine seems to be closely related to changes in reproductive processes.

When implemented, 1994 amendments to the Clear Water Act will force significant changes in the plastics, organic chemicals, pulp and paper, and wastewater management industries, since they will be required to replace chlorine with an acceptable substitute. Many of these industries contend that they do not have an acceptable substitute and, thus, the elimination of chlorine will result in job losses. Fortunately, municipal water supply purification is not a significant contributor to the chlorine problem.

Effects on Wetlands

The progressive loss of *wetlands* due to drainage and the dumping of debris is of great concern. With the loss of wetlands, the natural habitat for countless

---

*As reported by the Center for Marine Conservation.

species of fish, shellfish, birds, and marine mammals is lost. By the end of this century, over half of the country's wetlands will have vanished.[14] On a more positive note, concerted efforts to reestablish wetlands are occurring in some areas of the country, such as California. Unfortunately, at the same time, continued loss occurs in other areas.

Effects on Health

When our water becomes polluted, its quality falls below acceptable standards for its intended use, and some aspects of our health will be negatively influenced. Polluted water is associated with disease and illness, but it also distresses us emotionally, limits our social activities, and challenges us intellectually and spiritually to be more active stewards of our environment.

This became extremely evident during the Great Flood of 1993 in which thousands of people living and working along the Mississippi and Missouri rivers and their tributaries faced the pollution carried by flood water. With water equal in volume to another Great Lake, entire communities were completely covered. Untreated sewage, oil and gasoline, animal carcasses, pesticides, and every conceivable form of debris possible (including caskets!) were carried along by the flood waters. Cleanup efforts as well as the restoration of homes and livelihoods will continue for a long time to come.

LAND POLLUTION

Since we live, work, and play on land, it may be difficult to believe that land constitutes only about 30% of the earth's surface. The rest is, of course, water. When we consider the rivers, streams, marshes, and lakes found on our land surfaces, our land surface seems even smaller. Uninhabitable land areas, such as swamps, deserts, and mountain ranges, further reduce the available land on which we humans can live. Our land is a precious commodity—one that we have taken for granted.

The effects of our growing population on our limited land resources are becoming more evident. However, the greatest impact on our land comes from the products our society discards: solid waste products and chemical waste products.

Solid Waste

The trash that is collected from our homes is composed of a wide variety of familiar materials. Each year, Americans dispose of paper, newspaper, cardboard, clothing, yard waste, wood pallets, food waste, cafeteria waste, glass, metal, disposable tableware, plastics, and an endless variety of other *municipal solid wastes (MSW)*. Each individual American produces over 4.3 pounds of MSW each year.[15] Collectively, we will produce 200 million tons of solid waste by 1995.

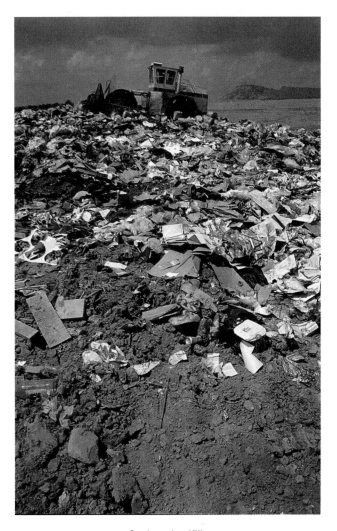

Sanitary landfill.

Although important, MSW makes up only a small amount of the solid wastes discarded in this country. Agricultural, mining, and industrial wastes contribute much more to our solid waste problems.

Regardless of the source, solid wastes require some form of disposal. Traditionally, these forms have been taken[16]:

▼ *Open dumping.* Solid waste is compacted and dumped on a dump site. Open dumps are discouraged or illegal in many urban areas.

▼ *Sanitary landfill.* Solid waste is compacted and buried in huge open pits. Each day, a layer of soil is pushed over the most recently dumped material to encourage decomposition, reduce unpleasant odors, and contain the material to keep it from being scattered.

▼ *Incineration.* Solid waste can be incinerated. A variety of types of incinerators exist, including cement kilns, boilers and furnaces, and commercial incinerators. Figure 18-5 depicts the sites of working and proposed incinerators within the United States.

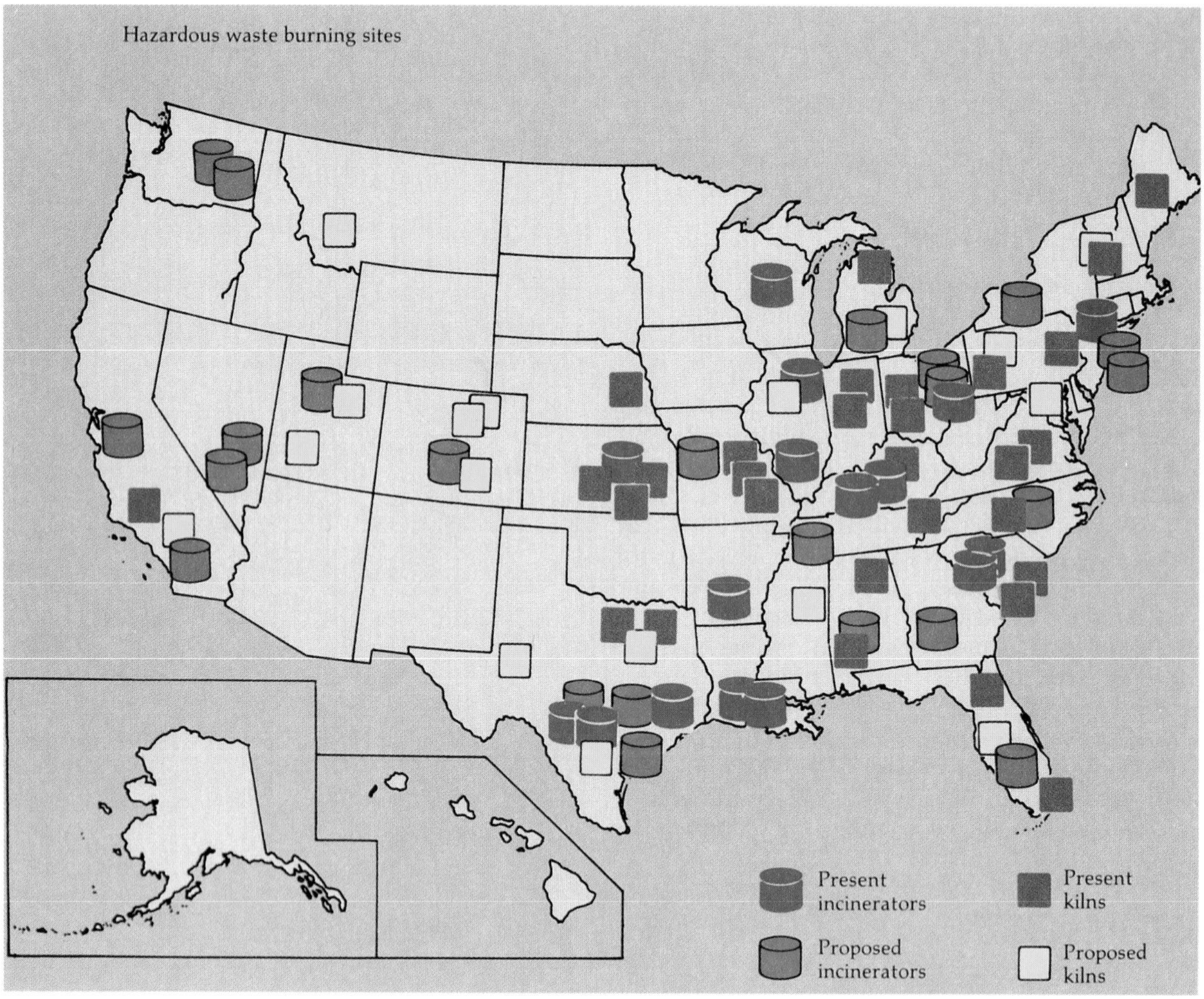

Figure 18-5 Present and proposed sites for the burning of hazardous waste.

▼ *Ocean dumping.* When near enough to the ocean, solid waste can also be collected, loaded into barges, and taken to offshore dump sites.

Our ability to solve our solid waste disposal problems may depend on **recycling,** or the ability to convert many of our disposable items into reusable materials. It has been difficult to convince manufacturers and the public that many of our solid waste products should be recycled. Efforts to recycle glass, aluminum, paper, and plastic have not been fully adopted by society. Cost of recycling and a lack of markets for reclaimed materials often discourage municipalities and industries from practicing more recycling. Lack of time and interest, failure to understand how to recycle, messiness, and the lack of curbside pickup are also frequently mentioned as reasons for not recycling in the home.

Chemical Waste

According to many environmental consumer group leaders, the quality of our lives is deteriorating, in part because of the unsafe disposal of hazardous chemicals from industrial and agricultural sources. In 1988 alone, according to the EPA, 4.57 billion tons of potentially toxic chemicals were released into the air, water, land, sewers, and into toxic waste dump sites. Currently, it is estimated that there are as many as 31,500 toxic waste dump sites sprinkled across the country.[2] Because it costs much more money to detoxify, recycle, and reuse toxic chemical products than to dump them, too many chemical companies have been more than willing to secretly and unlawfully bury their chemical wastes.

Because of the widespread dumping of toxic waste, the EPA, through the use of monies from its $12 billion

★ The Nature Conservancy

Beyond adopting practices that contribute to the health of the environment, is there a way that you can *join* in making a significant contribution to environmental stewardship? The answer is *yes!* One specific approach is through membership in The Nature Conservancy.

The Nature Conservancy is a national organization that obtains land through donation and bequests. It also purchases land and protects it in well-managed preserves. By the end of 1993, in this country and abroad, The Nature Conservancy had protected a total area of land larger than the size of the state of Michigan. Thousands of members further contribute by participating in a variety of activities designed to assist in the management of land. This includes clean-up projects, informative nature study tours, and publication of its popular magazine, The Nature Conservancy.

From rain forest to prairie, The Nature Conservancy is building a natural legacy for generations to come. ★

★ Prevention Versus Control: the Three *R*s

As consumers and environmentally concerned citizens, we need to do more than control the disposal of solid waste so that it does not adversely influence our health and the health of our environment. We must prevent this waste from occurring in increasing quantities. To accomplish this goal, a commitment to reduce, reuse, and recycle must be made.

The first step in dealing with the problem of solid waste disposal is to find ways to *reduce* the use of materials that eventually pollute our environment. A concerned public willing to make do with less, such as the amount of packaging material used with small consumer products, is a positive step. As concerned citizens, we must all learn to *reuse* as much as possible. Glass milk bottles that can be used again by the dairy, as well as cloth diapers rather than the nondegradable disposable diapers are examples of reuse at its best.

Finally, we must *recycle* as much material as possible. Recent experience has taught us that Americans will recycle when a system for collecting material is in place. However, recycling will go only as far as the demand and a market for recycled materials exists.

When combined, the three *R*s of reduction, reuse, and recycling could significantly reduce our need to engage in the more expensive disposal of toxic wastes. ★

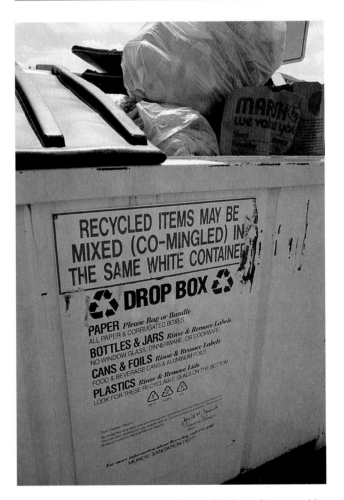

Recycling offers a way to convert disposable items into reusable ones.

Superfund, is supporting the cleanup of approximately 1200 toxic waste disposal sites in various parts of the country.[2]

To date, Superfund money has been difficult to use effectively. Currently only 80 officially completed sites have been returned to the standard of cleanliness required by the law. That is, if a water well were drilled in the middle of the site, water from that well would be pure enough for drinking. An additional 350 sites are in the process of being cleaned, and assessments have been made at more than 435 additional sites. Unfortunately, most of the fund's money has already been expended, largely in fighting lawsuits brought by the firms accused of polluting the land and under court order to pay for the required cleanup.[2]

Pesticides

Since Rachel Carson wrote her now-classic book *Silent Spring* in 1962, the public has been aware of the potential dangers associated with the use of some pesticides.

recycling (re **sike** ling) the ability to convert disposable items into reusable materials.

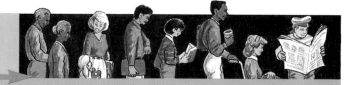

Learning FROM ALL Cultures

The Green Plan

In December 1990, Canada introduced an environmental plan for the 1990s to improve and protect the environment. The Green Plan was designed to create and implement programs to protect and clean up Canada's land, air, water, and resources and to curb waste and use of energy. The Plan called for an increase of 50% in spending on the environment over the next 6 years and for more funding for environmental groups not associated with the government.[17]

One particular area of concern included in the Green Plan is the ecosystems of the Arctic region. Forty percent of Canadian land is in the far North, therefore Canada has a history of involvement in Arctic issues. Most of the contaminants present in the Arctic region come from southern areas, but these pollutants are deposited in Arctic lakes. These toxins ulti-

mately affect the food chain. Scientists suspect that air toxins recirculate in the atmosphere, and when they get to the Arctic, the temperature is too cold for the toxins to pass off as vapor somewhere else. As a result, the Arctic could become the depository for pollutants. A goal of the Green Plan is to study the problem of contaminants in the Arctic and find solutions to the ongoing accumulation of toxins. Canada is also committed through the Plan to clean up hazardous waste sites in the far North.[17]

Pollution of the Arctic region is only one of many environmental concerns of the Green Plan. Considering the sparse population in the region and the harsh environment, should the cleanup and protection of the area be of great importance? ●

Although Carson's primary concern was with the pesticide DDT, a number of other hazardous pesticides have since been removed from the marketplace. Tighter controls established by the EPA have restricted the availability of other less hazardous pesticides. Clearly, farmers need to use effective poisons to save their crops from insect destruction. However, equal concern seems to be focused now on the effects of pesticides on water supplies, soil quality, animals, other insects, and humans. Harmful agents such as pesticides can enter an **ecosystem** and affect the entire food chain.

The world's worst industrial accident took place at a pesticide plant in Bhopal, India. In December 1984, the Union Carbide India Limited pesticide plant accidentally emitted over 16 tons of the chemical methyl isocyanate vapor into the air of neighborhoods adjacent to the plant. Within a few days, approximately 2500 people died and between 80,000 and 90,000 others were injured—many with lung damage, eye injuries, and liver and kidney disorders. This tragedy reminds us of the precarious relationship between our expanding technology and our immediate environment.

Herbicides

Herbicides also contribute to the growing problem of water and soil pollution, and to the contamination of the food chain. These weed-killing chemicals are sprayed on plants and incorporated into the soil with

plowing, but are not totally taken up by the plant tissues they are intended to kill. The extent to which pesticides and herbicides causes illnesses in humans is not fully known though the potential is there.

RADIATION

We live in the nuclear age and have since the end of World War II. Today the hopes for nuclear energy primarily lie in its enormous potential to reduce our dependence on fossil fuels as energy sources. Also, nuclear energy can (and already does) improve our industrial and medical technology, as evidenced by an expanding use of radioactive materials in the diagnosis and treatment of various health disorders.

The two greatest concerns over nuclear energy are (1) the negative health effects that come from day-to-day exposure to radiation and (2) the potential for a nuclear accident of regional or global consequences. Fission produces not only great energy but also **ionizing radiation** in the form of radioactive particles. We are exposed to various forms of ionizing radiation daily through natural radiation, including ultraviolet radiation from the sun and natural radioactive mineral deposits, and synthetic radiation, including waste from nuclear reactors, industrial products, and x-ray examinations. Most of the exposures we get on a daily basis produce negligible health risks. Although it is clear that no kind of radiation exposure is good for you, safe levels of exposure are difficult to determine.

TABLE 18-3 Selecting Sunglasses

Type	Some Benefits
By designation	
Cosmetic	Blocks at least 70% of UVB and 20% of UVA and less than 60% of visible light; designed for activities in nonintense light
General purpose	Blocks at least 95% of UVB, at least 60% of UVA, and from 60% to 92% of visible light; designed for activities in sunny places
Special purpose	Blocks at least 99% of UVB, at least 60% of UVA, and at least 97% of visible light; designed for use in very bright conditions, such as beaches and ski slopes
Polarized	Minimizes glare; good when driving or when near water or snow
Wraparound	Close fit offers greater protection against UV rays
By color	
Pink/Vermillion	Allows accurate perception in low-light conditions; allows moderate light in bright sunlight; popular with bike racers and skiers
Gray/Green	Only minimal distortion no matter how dark the lenses; good for everyday use
Brown/Amber	Blocks blue light, contrast is sharpened, reduces eyestrain; popular with skiers and boaters
Yellow	Good depth perception and contrast in low-light conditions; cuts through haze on foggy days
Mirror	Provides added protection against bright sunlight; reflective coating reduces glare; but check label to be sure of protection from UV radiation

Health Effects of Radiation Exposure

The health effects of radiation exposure depend on many factors, including the duration, type, dose of exposure, and individual sensitivity. Clearly, heavy exposure (as in a major nuclear accident) can produce **radiation sickness** or immediate death. Lesser exposure can be quite harmful as well. Particular concern is focused on the effects of radiation on egg and sperm production, embryonic development, and dangerous or irreversible changes to the eyes and skin. Cancer, particularly of the blood-forming tissue, is also a concern. From a health perspective, the message is clear. Avoid any unnecessary exposure to radioactive materials. Make it a point to question the value of diagnostic x-ray examinations, especially routine dental and chest x-ray studies and mammograms. Routine x-ray studies have been discouraged by numerous professional societies and consumer groups. Recent studies suggest that the risk is minimal for most persons.[18] Furthermore, if your skin is fair, you should limit your exposure to solar radiation. (See Chapter 11 for additional information on skin cancer.)

Selecting Sunglasses

For maximum visual health, the human eye needs protection from both forms of ultraviolet light: *UVA* (longer, weaker rays) and *UVB* (shorter, stronger rays) that are particularly harmful to the cornea. All nonprescription sunglasses must be accompanied by a tag when sold that details the type of protection from ultraviolet light that is provided. This information should be read carefully to determine how the sunglasses are to be used. In addition, since the color of the lens is often important to consumers, information about lens color should also be considered in the selection process (Table 18-3).

Electromagnetic Radiation

What do water bed heaters, electric razors, electric blankets, high-tension electrical transmission lines, and cellular telephone have in common? The answer is electromagnetic fields or electromagnetic waves, even more specifically, electromagnetic fields that come in close proximity to the body or pass very near your home, as in the case of transmission lines.

In recent years concern has been voiced as to whether the electromagnetic fields generated by these

ecosystem (ee koe sis tem) an ecological unit made up of both animal and plant life that interact to produce a stable system.

ionizing radiation (eye oh nye zing ray dee **ay** shun) form of radiation capable of releasing electrons from atoms.

radiation sickness illness characterized by fatigue, nausea, weight loss, fever, bleeding from mouth and gums, hair loss, and immune deficiencies, resulting from overexposure to ionizing radiation.

The crew of the MV Greenpeace detecting nuclear waste as it is dumped into the Sea of Japan.

familiar devices could cause cancer. Research using laboratory animals and epidemiological studies comparing people using these devices with those who do not have been far from conclusive. There is, however, a gradually growing belief that this form of radiation is to some degree capable of exerting a carcinogenic effect on human tissues. Therefore, until more research has been done, their use should be restricted by the consumers who own them. For example, heaters for water beds could be turned on early to allow the bed to warm and then turned off once in the bed, cellular telephone calls should be kept short, and a morning shave should not last more than a few minutes.

Nuclear Reactor Accidents and Waste Disposal

To generate the nuclear energy to produce electrical energy, more than 100 nuclear power plants have been constructed in North America. Built mostly by utility companies, these nuclear power plants were designed to produce electrical energy in an efficient, economical, and safe manner. Much public criticism has been directed at these power plants, claiming that their safety and efficiency have not been documented.

In July 1990 the U.S. Government revealed that during the late 1940s, tremendous amounts of radioactive materials were released from the reactors at the Hanford Nuclear Reservation in eastern Washington state. This was the first time the government publicly admitted that radiation releases could have caused human health problems such as cancers and birth defects. These releases were not reactor accidents; they were early forms of nuclear waste disposal.

The safe disposal of nuclear waste is a major problem that also has not been fully solved. The by-products of nuclear fission remain radioactive for many years. Although the current method for disposing of these wastes is to bury them, the question of eventual leakage into our environment is a valid one.

Since the Gulf War in early 1991, interest in building additional nuclear reactors has been renewed. To date, however, no new facilities have been proposed. Should construction of new nuclear power stations be undertaken, it is likely that questions about costs, environmental pollution, safety, and plant security would be important issues voiced by those who oppose the expanded use of nuclear energy.

Proponents of nuclear power maintain their stance that not one person in the United States has died as the result of a power plant accident. They point to a spotless safety record and reiterate that our fossil fuel supply is limited. Supporters of the nuclear industry feel that a public commitment to establishing more nuclear reactors is important for the future of our country. Currently, nearly 20% of our electrical energy is generated by nuclear power.

Concern over the safety of nuclear power plants was heightened in this country and around the world when on April 26, 1986, a **meltdown** occurred at the Chernobyl nuclear power plant in the Soviet Union. Human error was responsible for creating a situation in which excessive heat was allowed to build up in the core of the nuclear reactor. The resultant explosion killed two people, hospitalized hundreds, and exposed hundreds of thousands of people to nuclear ra-

meltdown the overheating and eventual melting of the uranium fuel rods in the core of a nuclear reactor.

Estimate Your Exposure to Radiation

Calculate your average annual exposure to radiation by filling in the blank spaces in the column on the right.

Radiation Source	Estimated Annual Dose (In Millirems)	

Natural Radiation

Cosmic rays from space At sea level	40	(U.S. average)
Add 1 m rem for each 100 feet you live above sea level		(Your risk)
Radiation in rocks and soil (ranges from 30-200)	55	(U.S. average)
Radiation from air, water, and food (ranges from 200-400)	25	(U.S. average)

Radiation From Human Activities

Medical and dental x-rays and treatments	80	(U.S. average)
Working or living in a stone or brick building (add 40 for each, if applicable)		(Your risk)
Smoking one pack of cigarettes per day (add 40 mrem)		(Your risk)
Nuclear weapons fallout	4	(U.S. average)
Air travel: add 2 m rem a year for each 1500 miles flown		(Your risk)
TV or computer screens—add 4 mrem/year for each 2 hours of exposure per day		(Your risk)
Occupational exposure (depends on occupation)	0.8	(U.S. average)
Living next to a nuclear power plant (boiling water reactor, add 76 m rem; pressurized water reactor, add 4 mrem)		(Your risk)
Living within 5 miles of a nuclear power plant (add 0.6 mrem)		(Your risk)
Normal operation of nuclear power plants, fuel processing, and research facilities	0.1	(U.S. average)
Miscellaneous—industrial wastes, smoke detectors, certain watch dials	2	(U.S. average)
YOUR TOTAL POINTS		

INTERPRETATION

The average annual exposure per person in the United States is 230 m rem. Of this, 130 m rem comes from natural radiation, and 100 m rem comes from human activities. Your exposure may be considerably higher than this depending on your place of residence, water supply, medical tests and treatments, occupation, and specific health behaviors, including smoking and exposure to sun.

TO CARRY THIS FURTHER

Having completed this assessment, were you surprised at the level of your annual exposure to radiation? How could you reduce your level of risk? What would you project for your future level of risk?

PERSONAL ASSESSMENT

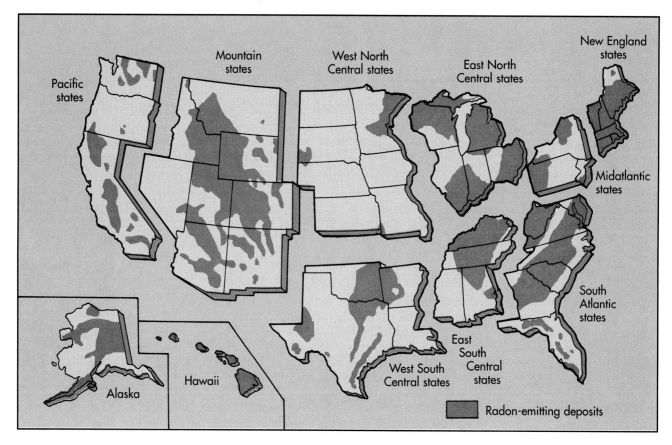

Figure 18-6 Mineral deposits in the United States that emit radon.

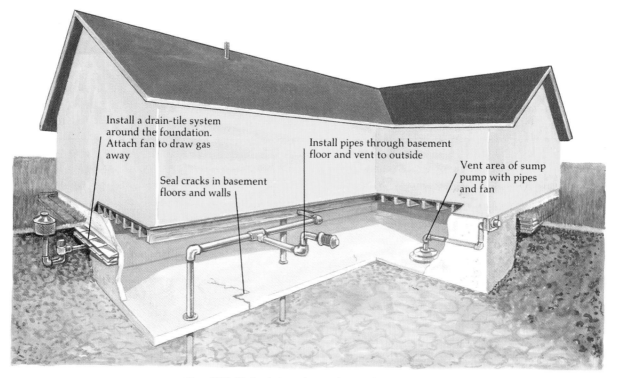

Figure 18-7 Methods to reduce radon gas levels in your home.

diation. As a result of the Chernobyl accident, the Russian government must resettle 200,000 persons at an estimated cost of $26 billion. Furthermore, a leading Soviet scientist has estimated that 10,000 miners and soldiers died as a result of exposure to radiation received during cleanup operations after the accident.

Radon Gas

Perhaps the form of radiation exposure that strikes closest to home is **radon gas.** Released from underlying rock formations and stone building materials, this radioactive gas enters buildings through a variety of routes (the water supply, block walls, slab joints, drains, even cracks in the floor) and is then found in unacceptably high levels. Because radon gas can concentrate when air is stagnant, energy-efficient airtight homes, schoolrooms, and buildings are most affected.[19] Tests conducted on homes in various areas of the country (Figure 18-6 shows areas high in radon) suggest that 20% of all homes have higher than normal levels and 10% have dangerously high levels. The importance of this lies in the relationship of radon exposure to the development of lung cancer. Current research indicates that radon exposure may increase the risk of developing lung cancer by 30% to 80%, depending on the level of exposure.[20]

Those who are concerned about the level of radon gas in their homes can purchase test kits (manufactured by some 200 companies at a cost of $10 to $50) or have their homes tested by radon testing laboratories. Consumers are, of course, cautioned that not all test kits are equally sensitive and that few states license radon testing companies. The repair of homes with high radon levels can be expensive, with some costing as much as $30,000. One form of repair, the installation of a home ventilation system, may cost from $300 to $500 (Figure 18-7).

NOISE POLLUTION

In much the same fashion that a weed is an unwanted plant and can ruin a lawn, noise is an unwanted sound that can be detrimental to our overall health. Or in some cases, a sound that is desirable such as music can function like a true noise because of the intensity of the presentation. Regardless, today's world is characterized by sounds whose loudness and unrelenting presence are dangerous to our health. This intense sound can reduce our hearing acuity, disrupt our emotional tranquility, infringe on our social interactiveness, and interrupt our concentration.

Noise-induced Hearing Loss

Sound, or a wave of compressed air molecules moving in response to a pressure gradient, is characterized by two qualities—*frequency* and *intensity.* High intensity is primarily responsible for the loss of **auditory acuity** experienced by many persons living in noise-polluted environments. Intensity of sound exceeding 80 to 85 *decibels* (1200 to 4800 cycles per second frequency range) can cause hearing damage. The box on p. 486 shows sound intensity associated with several common environmental sound sources.

The interpretation of a sound (hearing) is a sophisticated and sensitive physiological process involving the progressive conversion of acoustical energy to mechanical energy, then to hydraulic energy, and, finally, to electrochemical energy. Electrochemical energy is subsequently transmitted by the acoustic nerve to the brain for interpretation. The destructive influence of exposure to sounds of high intensity lies in the destruction of special *hair cells* in the *cochlea* that are responsible for converting hydraulic energy into electrochemical energy. Loud music, jet engine noise, vehicular traffic, and a wide range of industrial noises can collapse these sensitive cells. Ironically, the cells that are damaged are those responsible for hearing the high-frequency sounds associated with normal conversation. Thus the environmental sources of noise rob you of your ability to hear sound of a far greater *value—the sound of the unamplified* human voice.

The damage just described is initially reversible. However, with continued exposure, the changes in the sensitive cells of the inner ear become permanent. Because the hearing loss inflicted by intense environmental sound is so serious, **audiologists** are now stating that most persons older than 15 years are no longer capable of having *maximum auditory acuity.*

Noise as a Stressor

In addition to the damaging effects of noise on auditory acuity, the role of noise as a stressor has long been recognized. Indeed, the absence of noise (silence) and prolonged noise are both proven techniques to break the will of prisoners during war. Recently, however, attention has shifted to the role of noise in terms of the stress response, presented in Chapter 3. In people stressed by unrelenting noise, the elevated epinephrine levels contribute to hypertension and other stress-related health problems.

---

radon gas (**ray** don) a naturally occurring radioactive gas produced by the decay of uranium.

auditory acuity clarity or sharpness at which a particular sound can be heard.

audiologists (aw dee **ol** oh jists) health care professionals trained to assess auditory function.

Noise Pollution and Its Effects on Hearing

The loudness of sounds is measured in decibels (dB). Sound intensity is determined logarithmically, not arithmetically. Each increase of 10 dB produces a tenfold increase in sound intensity. Thus 30 dB has 10 times the intensity of 20 dB, 40 dB has 100 times the intensity of 20 dB, and 110 dB sounds 10 times as loud as 100 dB. Hearing damage depends on the dB level and the length of exposure. Presented below are dB ranges, common sources, and effects on hearing.

Decibel	Common sources	Effect on hearing
0	Lowest sound audible to human ear	
30	Quiet library, soft whisper	
40	Quiet office, study lounge, bedroom away from traffic	
50	Light traffic at a distance, refrigerator, quiet conversation, gentle breeze	
60	Air conditoner at 20 feet, normal conversation, sewing machine	
70	Busy traffic, noisy office or cafeteria	Annoying, and may start to affect hearing if constant
80	Heavy city traffic, alarm clock at 2 feet, typical factory	Start to affect hearing if exposed more than 8 hours
90	Truck traffic, noisy home appliances, shop tools, lawn mower	Temporary hearing loss can occur in less than 8 hours
100	Chain saw, pneumatic drill (jackhammer), loud motorcycle or farm equipment	Unprotected exposure for 2 hours can produce serious damage to hearing
120	Rock band concert in front of speakers, sandblasting, loud thunderclap	Immediate danger threat
140	Shotgun blast, jet plane from 50 feet	Immediate pain threat; any length of exposure is dangerous
180	Rocket pad area during launch (without ear protection)	Immediate, irreversible, and inevitable hearing loss

Health ACTION Guide

Reducing Noise Pollution

Beyond giving your political support to legislation and enforcement policies designed to reduce environmental noise pollution, what can you do to lessen the degree of noise pollution in your life? The following suggestions are only a few of the recommended approaches:

▼ Limit your exposure to highly amplified music. The damage from occasional exposure to sound intensity between 110 and 120 decibels can be reversible. Daily exposure, however, will result in permanent hearing loss.

▼ Reduce the volume on your portable headsets. When others can hear the music coming through your headset while you are wearing it, you should probably turn down the volume.

▼ Wear ear plugs (wax or soft plastic) and sound-absorbing ear muffs when using firearms or operating loud machinery.

▼ Maintain your automobile, motorcycle, or lawn mower exhaust systems in good working order.

▼ Furnish your room, apartment, home, and office with sound-absorbing materials. Drapes, carpeting, and cork wall tiles are excellent for reducing both interior and exterior noises.

▼ Establish noise reduction as a criterion in selecting a site for your residence. An apartment complex near a freeway or airport or property near an interstate highway may prove to be less than desirable.

Since you are a person with a lifetime of hearing ahead, noise pollution reduction deserves your participation and your support. ▼

Organizations Related to Environmental Concerns

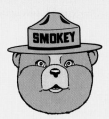

FEDERAL DEPARTMENTS, AGENCIES, AND OFFICES

★ Environmental Protection Agency, 401 M St. S.W., Washington, DC 20460; (202) 382-2090

★ Council of Environmental Quality, 722 Jackson Pl. N.W., Washington, DC 20503; (202) 395-5750

★ Department of Energy, Forrestal Bldg., 1000 Independence Ave. S.W., Washington, DC 20585; (202) 586-6210

★ Department of Interior, Interior Bldg., 1849 C St. N.W., Washington, DC 20240; (202) 208-3100

★ National Oceanic and Atmospheric Administration, Rockville, MD 20852; (301) 443-8910

★ United States Fish and Wildlife Service, 1849 C Street, N.W., Washington, DC 20240; (202) 208-5634

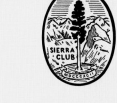

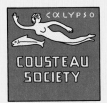

NATIONAL ORGANIZATIONS

★ National Wildlife Federation, 1400 16th St. N.W., Washington, DC 20036; (202) 797-6800 and (800) 432-6564

★ Sierra Club, 730 Polk St., San Francisco, CA 94109; (415) 776-2211

★ Cousteau Society, Inc., 870 Greenbriar Circle, Suite 402, Chesapeake, VA 23320 (804) 523-9335

★ Greenpeace USA, 1436 U Street, N.W., Washington, DC 20009; (202) 462-1177

★ The Wilderness Society, 900 17th Street, N.W., Washington, DC 20006; (202) 833-2300

CANADIAN ORGANIZATIONS

★ Environment Canada, Ottawa, Ontario K1A OH3; (819) 997-1441

THE WILDERNESS SOCIETY

Are You Helping the Environment?

PERSONAL ASSESSMENT

How many ways can you help the environment? Give yourself two points for each of the following that you do on a regular basis, one point for each that you do occasionally, and a zero for those that you do not do. Total your points and compare your score with those that follow the assessment.

_____ 1. Promptly repair leaky faucets.

_____ 2. Use the microwave as often as possible rather than the stove or the oven.

_____ 3. Buy brands that come in minimal amounts of packaging.

_____ 4. Do not run excess water while washing dishes.

_____ 5. Use paper bags rather than plastic.

_____ 6. Use sponges or dishcloths for spills rather than paper towels.

_____ 7. Recycle newspapers rather than throw them out.

_____ 8. Snip six-pack rings.

_____ 9. Walk or bicycle rather than drive.

_____ 10. Purchase products in the larger sizes.

_____ 11. Preheat your oven for the minimal amount of time necessary.

_____ 12. Turn off water while brushing your teeth.

_____ 13. Do not use a trash compactor.

_____ 14. Serve fresh fruits and vegetables rather than processed foods.

_____ 15. Pull weeds by hand rather than spraying.

_____ 16. Carpool to work.

_____ 17. Limit garbage disposal use as much as possible.

_____ 18. Use canvas or cloth bags for shopping.

_____ 19. Sweep driveways and sidewalks rather than use a hose.

_____ 20. Recycle bottles and jars.

_____ 21. Pick up litter when you see it.

_____ 22. Make note pads out of used office stationery and paper.

_____ 23. Wear clothing that is right for the weather.

_____ 24. Use rechargeable batteries.

_____ 25. Clean the lint screen in the dryer after each load.

_____ 26. Put trash in only one bag (or the fewest needed).

_____ 27. Use refillable containers for household products (such as liquid hand soap).

_____ 28. Keep the water heater at the lowest level needed.

_____ 29. Open blinds and curtains during daylight periods during winter months.

_____ 30. Close blinds and curtains during periods of bright sunshine during summer months.

_____ 31. Turn off lights when you leave a room.

_____ 32. Take quick showers rather than leisurely baths.

_____ 33. Turn off stereos, radios, and televisions when leaving the house.

_____ 34. Turn off the water when washing the car and use a bucket when possible.

_____ 35. Place a brick or a plastic bottle of water inside the toilet storage tank.

_____ 36. Buy laundry detergents that are phosphate-free when there are other options available.

_____ 37. Drink "ice water" from the refrigerator rather than run tap water to get it cooler.

_____ 38. Run the dishwasher only when full.

_____ 39. Use hairspray in nonaerosol bottles.

_____ 40. Clean and change filters on the furnace and air conditioner on a regular basis.

_____ 41. Keep a reusable mug or cup at home or the office.

_____ 42. Purchase clothing that can be washed rather than only dry cleaned.

_____ 43. Wash clothing only when dirty.

_____ 44. Close the refrigerator door promptly.

_____ 45. Keep the car properly tuned.

_____ 46. Collect rain water for use in plants and gardens.

_____ 47. Donate outgrown clothing to nonprofit organizations.

_____ 48. Participate in organized clean-up days when they are held in your community.

_____ 49. Replace conventional shower head with a water-conserving model.

_____ 50. Write elected officials to support environmental legislation.

_____ YOUR TOTAL POINTS

INTERPRETATION

90-100 points: Your conservation efforts are in the superior range. Keep up the excellent work!

80-89 points: You are clearly above average and should also be congratulated!

70-79 points: Although your score is average, your efforts at conserving the environment are important contributions to the total effort. Keep up the good work and look for additional ways to conserve.

60-69 points: Your score is passing but below average. Try to find more ways to help the environment. You have room for improvement.

59 and below: Time has not run out! You can still earn a passing grade but you need to follow the suggestions in this assessment and chapter to help the environment.

TO CARRY THIS FURTHER

Share these suggestions, or any others that you find useful, with family, friends, classmates, and other associates as a means of further helping our environment.

PERSONAL ASSESSMENT

Your Role in Creating a Sustainable Environment

As we search for solutions to complex environmental problems, we may have to make some difficult decisions. For example, will Third World populations be forced to use contraception or sterilization? Will we attempt to feed the world's hungry people? Will we continue to protect endangered species of plants and animals? Will we strive more forcefully for nuclear disarmament? Can we commit ourselves to cleaning up all of our toxic waste sites? Answers to these complex questions about *stewardship* will probably be based not only on our knowledge, but also on our moral predispositions.

Answers to these sorts of complex questions can come from recognizing the value of a *sustainable environment.* This environment will be developed only when individuals and groups are willing to[2]:

★ Evaluate their environment

★ Become environmentally educated

★ Choose a simpler, less consumption-oriented lifestyle

★ Recognize the limitations of technology in solving problems

★ Become involved in environmental protection activities

★ Work with people on all sides of environmental issues

These suggestions might sound abstract for a person confronted with a local environmental problem. However, each of these steps can be applied to a local situation with only limited modifications. The PCB soil contamination in Indiana, the nerve gas weapons storage in Kentucky, the toxic waste site cleanup in Missouri, and the transportation of nuclear waste materials in California and other states represent local issues to which these steps can be applied. Are you committed enough to a sustainable environment to practice these steps? ★

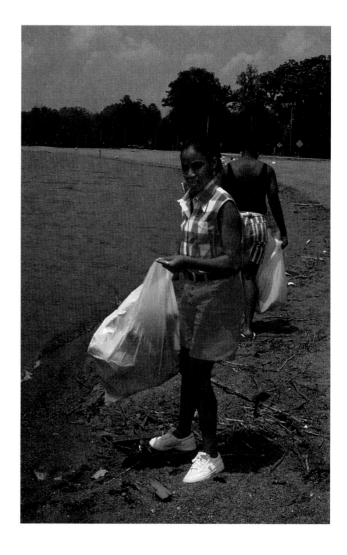

IN SEARCH OF BALANCE

How often have you heard people yearn for a return to the "good old days"? They reminisce about times when people moved more slowly, cared more for their neighbors, and appreciated their natural resources. After listening to these nostalgic impressions, you could believe that our society was once almost idyllic—with little or no pollution, population concerns, or threats of nuclear accidents?

Certainly it is nice to dream, but it is doubtful that our advancing technology and exploding worldwide population will permit us to find such an ideal world. Instead, we need to focus on finding the appropriate balance between technological growth and environmental deterioration. Perhaps some of the organizations listed on p. 469 can help us in our efforts.

We must learn to think beyond the present. Each decision we make for the future should be considered in light of its influence on our environmental systems. If our future decisions are based solely on financial gain or personal convenience, we will be committing a monumental disservice to our children and future generations.

Summary

- ✔ World population is increasing at an alarming rate and with adverse effects on the environment.
- ✔ Worldwide increases in carbon dioxide production could result in a greenhouse effect, leading to climatic warming.
- ✔ Acid rain, acid fog, acid snow, as well as smog, result from the release of gaseous and particulate pollutants into the air.
- ✔ Deterioration of the ozone layer could result in exposure to high levels of ultraviolet radiation and serious health problems.
- ✔ Particular pollutants, including lead, can produce serious health problems.
- ✔ Temperature inversions increase the seriousness of air pollution.
- ✔ Indoor air pollution is now recognized as a serious affront to health.

- ✔ Water pollution results from a variety of causative agents, including toxic chemicals and human/animal wastes.
- ✔ Municipal solid wastes are a small but important component of all solid waste.
- ✔ Solid wastes are traditionally buried, dumped, or incinerated.
- ✔ Reduction, reuse, and recycling are important aspects of the prevention of environmental pollution.
- ✔ Radiation, including radon, ultraviolet, and ionizing radiation from nuclear power plants, could result in serious health problems.
- ✔ Noise pollution can lead to hearing loss, particularly within the human voice range.

Review Questions

1. In what direction is world population changing? What could be the consequences of this change on the environment? How can the rate of this change be moderated?

2. What is the greenhouse effect? How does deforestation influence this process? What is the anticipated consequence of the greenhouse effect?

3. How are acid rain, acid fog, and acid snow produced? What and where is the damage attributed to them?

4. What is causing the deterioration of the ozone layer? What step has been taken to slow this process? What are the consequences of ozone layer deterioration?

5. What are the major particulate pollutants in our air? What is the principal risk associated with lead as a pollutant? What specific diseases are associated with particular material in our air?

6. How are gray-air smog and brown-air smog formed? When and where is one form more likely to be seen than the other?

7. What air pollutant has recently been classified as a Type A carcinogen? What other pollutants contribute to indoor air pollution?

8. What toxic chemicals are most often the sources of water pollution? What is the consequence of having too little oxygen dissolved in water? What is thermal pollution?

9. What are several forms of municipal solid waste? How much municipal solid waste does the typical person produce per day? How much do Americans produce in a year?

10. How are solid wastes most often disposed of? Why are these techniques less than fully acceptable?

11. What are the three *Rs* of better solid waste prevention?

12. What are the principal sources of radiation that are of concern today? Which are natural sources of radiation, and which are the result of human intervention? What familiar appliances may be sources of electromagnetic fields?

13. How does noise pollution result in hearing loss? What are the most common sources of noise pollution?

Think about This . . .

✔ To what extent do your driving habits contribute to air pollution?

✔ In what ways do your recreational activities contribute to water pollution?

✔ If land were very affordable, would you build a new house on land reclaimed from a toxic waste dump site?

✔ How close to a nuclear power plant would you feel comfortable living?

✔ Is your home protected from the possibility of radon gas?

✔ The environmental focus of the 1990s has shifted from global concerns such as the ozone layer, deforestation, and world population to local concerns such as recycling and indoor air pollution. Will it now be possible to "think globally while acting locally"?

✔ Would you be willing to spend more for a light bulb designed to last 20,000 hours, use little energy, and last several years rather than a much less expensive incandescent bulb to reduce energy costs?

REAL LIFE
REAL CHOICES

YOUR TURN

▼ What are the major sources of air and water pollution in the environment today?

▼ What are the sources of environmental pollution in David Cloudwalker's home town?

▼ Do you think environmental damage falls more heavily on poor people and/or minorities? Why or why not?

AND NOW, YOUR CHOICES

▼ If you had grown up in circumstances similar to David's, how would you react to student "clean air" demonstrators on your campus?

▼ If you were one of the demonstrators on David's campus, how would you respond to his observation that signs and marches won't clean up the mess in our environment? ▼

References

1. Greenhouse gas giants, *USA Today,* June 3, 1992 (based on data supplied by the World Resource Institute).
2. Miller GT: *Living in the environment,* ed 7, Belmont, Calif, 1992, Wadsworth Publishing.
3. Goodavage M, Sanchez S: Testing for global warming, *USA Today,* May 13, 1994, 10A.
4. Arms K: *Environmental science,* ed 2, Fort Worth, 1994, Saunders College Publishers.
5. Chiras D: *Environmental science: action for a sustainable future,* ed 3, Redwood City, Calif, 1991, Benjamin/Cummings.
6. Milner BI, Axelrod BN, Sillanpas M: Is there a Gulf War syndrome? *JAMA* 271(9):661, 1994 (letter).
7. Kerr JB, McElroy CT: Evidence for large upward trends of ultraviolet-B radiation linked to ozone depletion, *Science* 262:1032-1034, 1993.
8. *Respiratory health effects of passive smoking: lung cancer and other diseases,* Office of Health and Environment, Office of Research and Development, U.S. Environmental Protection Agency, EPA/600/6-90/006F) December 1992.
9. Menzie R, et al: The effect of varying levels of outdoor-air supply on the symptoms of sick building syndrome, *N Engl J Med* 328(12): 821-827, 1993.
10. Urban sewage overflow, *USA Today,* April 29, 1992, 7A (based on data supplied by Natural Resources Defense Council, Center for Marine Conservation).
11. Cunningham W, Saigo B: *Environmental science: a global concern,* ed 2, Dubuque, Ia, 1992, William C Brown.
12. Falck F, et al: Pesticides and polychlorinated biphenyl residues in human breatr lipids and their relationship to breast cancer, *Arch Environ Health* 47(2):143-146, 1992.
13. Chiras D: *Environmental science: a framework for decision making,* ed 2, Menlo Park, Calif, 1988, Benjamin-Cummings Publishing.
14. Cunningham WP: *Understanding our environment,* Dubuque, Ia, 1994, William C Brown.
15. Franklin W, Franklin M: Putting the crusade into perspective: recycling and waste generation both are on the rise, *EPA Journal* 18(3):7, 1992.
16. Rathje W: Rubbish, *The Atlantic* 264(6):99, 1989.
17. Hansen P: Canada's green plan, *Canada Today/d'aujour'dhui* 22(1):3, 1991.
18. Boice J et al: Diagnostic x-ray procedures and risk of leukemia, lymphoma, and multiple myeloma, *JAMA* 265(10):1290, 1991.
19. Kerr R: Indoor radon: the deadliest pollutant, *Science* 246:606, 1988.
20. Pershagen G, et al: Residential radon exposure and lung cancer in Sweden, *N Engl J Med* 330(3):159-164, 1994.

Suggested Readings

50 simple things you can do to save the earth, 50 simple things kids can do to save the earth, and *The student environmental action guide,* The Earth Works, Berkeley, Calif, 1992, The Earth Works Group.

A collection of three of the most practical and comprehensive books written on how we can become stewards of the environment. Each book is intended for a specific group (adults, children, and college students) and offers advice in the context of each group's experiences and environment.

Fisher DE: *Fire and ice—the greenhouse effect, ozone, depletion, and nuclear winter,* New York, 1990, Harper & Row.

An interesting look at a number of environmental problems facing the world today. Proposed solutions are offered; also contains an appendix listing many citizen environmental groups.

French HF: *Clearing the air—a global agenda,* Washington, DC, 1990, The Worldwatch Institute.

One in a series of published papers by the Worldwatch Institute, a nonprofit research institute focusing on global problems. Reviews the health threats of air pollution, ways to reduce harmful air emissions, and the agenda, for clean air.

Pedersen A: *The kid's environment book: what's awry and why,* Santa Fe, NM, 1992, John Muir Publishing.

Explains serious environmental problems to children without scaring them. Intended for children 8 years of age and older.

Smith AA: *Campus ecology: a guide to assessing environmental quality and creating strategies for change,* Los Angeles, 1993, Living Planet Press.

A guidebook for campus groups identifying environmental concerns found on the college campus and suggesting approaches to resolving these concerns. Numerous case studies are included.

19

Violence and Safety

Coping in Today's Society

As recently as 15 years ago, the suspicious disappearance of a school-age child or the death of a bystander during a drive-by shooting was virtually unheard of. In the mid-1990s, violent crimes are committed so frequently in the United States that they rarely make front page headlines. However, in June 1994 the brutal deaths of Nicole Brown Simpson (former wife of football Hall of Famer O.J. Simpson) and her friend put one form of violence—domestic violence—back on the front page.[1]

Domestic violence directed at women and children seems to be increasing, and many persons fear being a random victim of a homicide, robbery, or carjacking. Law enforcement officials contend that gang activities and hard core drug involvement are major factors that have increased violent behavior in our society.

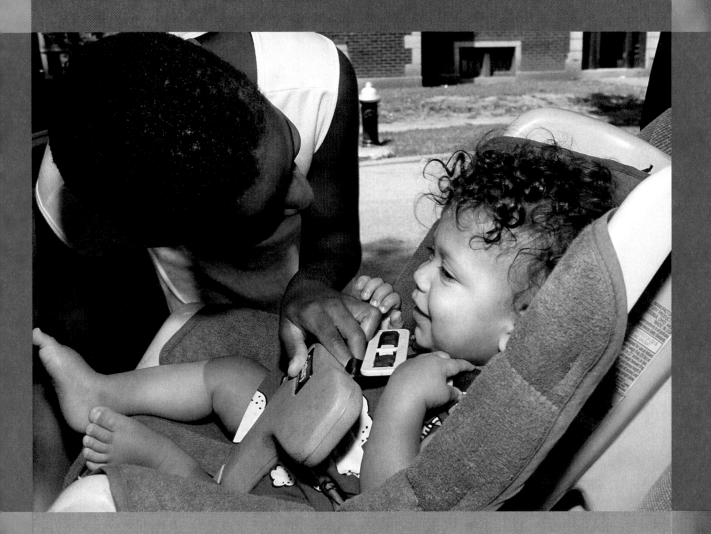

VIOLENCE AND SAFETY: COPING IN TODAY'S SOCIETY

The following objectives are covered in this chapter:

▽ Reduce homicides to no more than 7.2 per 100,000 people. (Age-adjusted baseline: 8.5 per 100,000 in 1987; p. 278.)

▽ Reduce physical abuse directed at women by male partners to no more than 27 per 1000 couples. (Baseline: 30 per 1000 in 1985; p. 233.)

▽ Reduce assault injuries among people age 12 and older to no more than 10 per 1000 people. (Baseline 11.1 per 1000 in 1986; p. 233.)

▽ Reverse to less than 25.2 per 1000 children the rising incidence of maltreatment of children younger than age 18. (Baseline: 25.2 per 1000 in 1986; p. 232.)

▽ Reduce rape and attempted rape of women age 12 and older to no more than 108 per 100,000 women. (Baseline: 120 per 100,000 in 1986; p. 234.)

REAL LIFE
REAL CHOICES
Date Rape: Shattered Trust

▼ **Names:** Debra Hemsath and Ron Mayer
▼ **Ages:** 19 and 20
▼ **Occupations:** College students

"I kept saying no, but he didn't stop. Even when I started screaming, he just wouldn't stop. It's not like I don't want him to touch me—maybe I let things go too far—but I wasn't ready for sex yet, and I told him so." Trembling violently, her hands covered her face, gulping back tears, Debra Hemsath is recounting to a counselor in the student health center how an enjoyable evening with the man she'd been dating for 3 weeks turned into an emotional nightmare.

"We'd both had a lot of beers—way more than we'd had on other dates. I wasn't the only one who was in the mood—she was getting pretty hot and heavy herself. I mean, it wasn't like this was our first date, or some one-night stand. I really liked her, and she knew it." Baffled, frustrated, alternating between anger and guilt, Ron Mayer is trying to explain to his closest friend how a pleasant interlude in his apartment turned into an accusation of date rape from a woman about whom he was beginning to feel pretty serious.

Between the enjoyable moments in Ron's dimly lit apartment and Debra's shattering accusation of rape there might lie a hundred misunderstandings, missed cues, false assumptions, and misinterpretations. Add in the emotional baggage each of them brought to the situation (family attitudes about sex, previous experiences in intimate relationships) plus Debra and Ron's affection for and attraction to each other, and the stage is set for the kind of collision that took place between these two students.

As you study this chapter, think about the factors that contributed to Debra and Ron's situation, and prepare yourself to answer the questions in **Your Turn** at the end of the chapter. ▼

Although violence may seem to be focused in urban areas, no community is completely safe. Even people who live in small towns and rural areas now must lock their doors and remain vigilant about protecting their safety. Crime on the college campus is on the rise,[2] and much of the campus violence is a direct result of alcohol use.

For some students the content in this chapter may be the most important information in this textbook. Becoming a victim of violent behavior or sustaining an unintentional injury can harm your health as much (or more) than any unhealthy behavior. The goal of this chapter is to help you understand the scope of violence in our society and learn what you can do to prevent yourself from becoming a victim.

INTENTIONAL INJURIES

Intentional injuries are injuries that are committed on purpose. With the exception of suicide (which is self-directed), intentional injuries reflect violence committed by one person acting against another person. Categories of intentional injuries include homicide, robbery, rape, suicide, assault, child abuse, spouse abuse, and elderly abuse (see Chapter 20). Each year in the United States intentional injuries cause about 50,000 deaths and another 2 million nonfatal injuries.[3]

The U.S. Department of Justice reported 6.4 million violent crimes (excluding homicide) were committed in 1991.[4] Stated in another way, there were 31 violent crimes for every 1000 persons age 12 and older. Although this rate of violent crime may sound high, it is lower than the record of 35 crimes per 1000 persons in 1981. Let's look at some of these violent crimes in more detail.

Homicide

Homicide (or murder) is the intentional killing of one person by another. In 1993 a total of about 24,500 people were murdered in the United States. This figure reflects an increase of about 3% over the 1992 total of 23,760.[5] Sadly, the United States leads the industrialized world in homicide rates. Lowering the homicide rate is one of the key violence-related Healthy People 2000 objectives.

It is not surprising that Americans are especially fearful of the possibility of being murdered. Television news programs seem to report murders daily. There are some clear trends when it comes to the persons involved in homicides. The most vulnerable group of homicide victims are African-Americans, especially young African-American males. Homicide is the leading cause of death for African-American males ages 15 to 44. African-American males have a 1 in 21 lifetime chance of becoming a victim of homicide.[6]

Another clear trend related to homicide is the extent to which illegal drug activity is related to homicide. A variety of research studies from large cities indicate

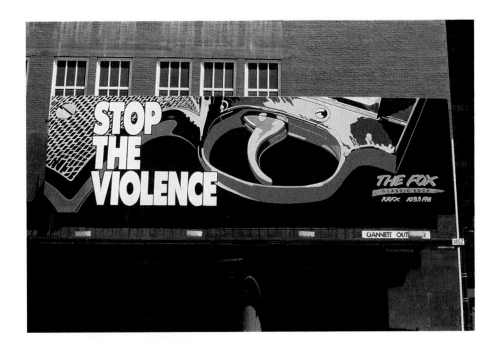

that from 25% to 50% of all homicides are drug related.[7] Most of these murders are related to activities involved in drug trafficking, including disputed drug transactions. Additionally, high percentages of both homicide assailants and victims have drugs in their systems at the time of the homicide.[7]

Finally, another clear trend is that handguns are the weapon of choice for homicides. In 1992 handguns were used in over half (13,200 murders) of the homicides in the United States.[8] This is not surprising, because handgun use among most categories of violent crime reached record levels in 1992. In 1992, 13% of all violent crimes were committed with offenders using handguns.[8] The proliferation of handguns and their use in violent crimes led to the recent passage of the so-called Brady Bill (see box on p. 480).

Domestic Violence

Family life in the 1990s is a far cry from that portrayed in the popular 1950s and 1960s television shows like the *Donna Reed Show, Father Knows Best,* and *Ozzie and Harriet.* The composition of families has changed considerably. In the 1950s, a common family pattern was children being raised by two parents. Generally the father was the income earner and the mother stayed at home and managed the growing family.

Today family patterns are much more complex. Children are more frequently being raised in blended families or in families headed by single parents. In fact, since 1970 single-parent households have increased 100%, from 4 to 8 million homes.[9] A much higher percentage of women are employed outside the home. Because of pressing family economic concerns, many children take care of themselves during after-school hours. Sociologists indicate that families, and the individuals in those families, are under more stress than ever.

Add to this precarious nature of the American family, the additional factors of increased societal drug use, increased presence of handguns, and increased crime and violence. What emerges is no surprise—increased domestic violence.

PARTNER ABUSE

Partner abuse refers to violence committed against a domestic partner. Most frequently the victims are women, and a significant percentage of these women are spouses or former spouses of the assailant. Figures from the U.S. Department of Justice[11] are frightening and make it difficult to believe that the U.S. can achieve its Healthy People 2000 objective in this area. More than 2.5 million women are victims of some form of violence every year. Nearly two in three female victims of violent crimes are related to or know their attacker. About three out of four female victims resist the actions of their offenders either physically or verbally.

---

intentional injuries injuries that are purposefully committed by a person.

homicide (**hom** ih side) the intentional killing of one person by another person.

partner abuse violence committed against a domestic partner.

The Brady Bill

On November 31, 1993, President Bill Clinton signed into law the most sweeping handgun-control bill since 1968 (when Congress banned mail-order purchases of rifles, shotguns, handguns, and ammunition shortly after the assassinations of Robert Kennedy and Dr. Martin Luther King, Jr.). This bill was named after James Brady, the former White House press secretary who was seriously wounded in the 1981 assassination attempt on President Ronald Reagan.[10]

The signing of the Brady Bill into law was the culmination of a 7-year crusade by Mr. Brady and his wife, Sarah. This gun control bill was endorsed by virtually every major law-enforcement organization in the country. The Brady Bill was opposed by the National Rifle Organization, which was convinced that the bill endangered the constitutional right to bear arms and would not deter violent crime to any significant degree.

The bill requires a 5-day waiting period and a background check on handgun buyers. The purpose of the background check is to prevent persons with certain criminal records from purchasing handguns from licensed dealers. At the time of this writing, it is too early to determine the effect that the Brady Bill has had on handgun purchases and violent crime.[10] ★

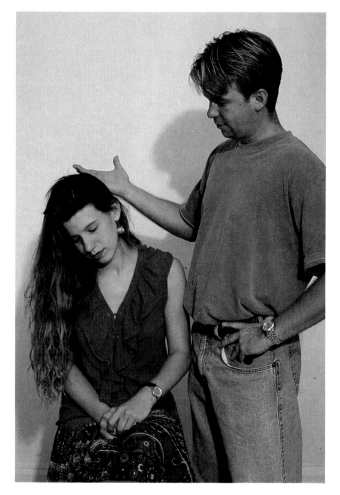

Emotional abuse can lead to physical abuse.

The most vulnerable female victims are African-American and Hispanic, live in large cities, are young and unmarried, and are from lower socioeconomic groups.[11] However, these trends do not mean that only women from these classifications are vulnerable to violent behavior. Women across all economic, racial, and age categories are potential victims. For example, in the aftermath of the tragic murder of Nicole Brown Simpson in June 1994, a picture emerged of an affluent woman who had been seriously injured by violent behavior.

One of the real difficulties related to domestic violence is the vast underreporting of violent acts to law enforcement authorities. It is estimated by the U.S. Department of Justice that about half of the victims of domestic violence do not report the crime to police. All too many victims view their violent situations as private or personal matters and not actual crimes. Despite painful injuries, too many victims view the offenses against them as minor.[11]

Of course, it is easy to criticize the victims of domestic violence for not reporting the crimes committed against them. However, this may be unfair. Why do women stay in these relationships? Many women who are injured may fear being killed if they report the crime. Women may also fear for the safety of their children. Women who receive economic support from an abuser may fear being left with no financial assistance.

However, help is available for victims of partner abuse. Most communities have family support or domestic violence hotlines that abused persons can call for help. Communities are establishing shelters where abused women and their children can seek safety while their cases are being handled by the police or court officials. If you are being abused or know of someone who is the victim of domestic violence, do not hesitate to use the services of these local hotlines or shelters. Also, check the resources listed in the Health Reference Guide at the back of this text.

CHILD ABUSE

The maltreatment of children under the age of 18 is indicated in one of the Healthy People 2000 objectives. Like many cases of partner abuse, **child abuse** tends to be a silent crime. It is estimated that about a million children are victims of child abuse and neglect each year.[12] Of course, some children are victims of repeated crimes, and since many victims do not report their crimes, the actual incidence of child abuse crimes is difficult to determine.

Children are abused in various ways.[13] Physical abuse reflects physical injury, such as bruises, burns, abrasions, cuts, wounds, and fractures of the bones and skull. Sexual abuse includes acts that lead to sexual gratification of the abuser. Examples include fondling, touching, and various acts involved in rape, sodomy, and incest. Child neglect is also a form of child abuse and includes an extreme failure to provide children with adequate clothing, food, shelter, and medical attention. A strong case can also be made for psychological abuse as a form of child abuse. Certainly, children are scarred by family members and others who routinely damage the psychological development of children. Unfortunately, this form of abuse is especially difficult to identify and measure.

The most frequent form of child abuse is neglect.[13] The incidence of child neglect is approximately three times the incidence of physical abuse and about seven times the incidence of child sexual abuse. Each form of abuse can have both devastating short-term and long-term consequences for the child.

Research studies in the various areas of child abuse reveal some interesting trends. It has become well established that abused children are much more likely than nonabused children to grow up to be child abusers themselves. It is also now understood that abused children are more likely to suffer from poor educational performance, increased health problems, and low levels of overall achievement. Recently, research also points out that abused children are significantly more likely than nonabused children to become involved in adult crime and violent criminal behavior.[13]

It is beyond the scope of this book to discuss, in detail, how to reduce child abuse. However, the violence directed against children can likely be lessened through a combination of early identification measures and violence prevention programs. Teachers, friends, relatives, social workers, counselors, psychologists, police, and the court system must not hesitate to intervene early in cases of suspected child abuse. The later the intervention, the more likely that the abuse will have worsened. Once abuse has occurred, it is likely to happen again.

Violence prevention programs can help parents and caregivers learn how to resolve conflicts, improve communication, cope with anger, improve parenting skills, and challenge the view of violence as entertainment.[14] In programs such as these, it may be possible to stop violence before it begins to damage the lives of young children. Figure 19-1 provides simple alternatives parents can choose to avoid hitting a child.[15]

Gangs and Youth Violence

In the last 15 years gangs and gang activities have been increasingly responsible for escalating violence and criminal activity. Before that time, gangs used fists, tire

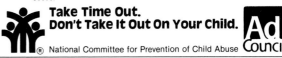

12 alternatives to lashing out at your child.

The next time everyday pressures build up to the point where you feel like lashing out — STOP! And try any of these simple alternatives.

You'll feel better . . . and so will your child.

1. Take a deep breath. And another. Then remember <u>you</u> are the adult . . .

2. Close your eyes and imagine you're hearing what your child is about to hear.

3. Press your lips together and count to 10. Or better yet, to 20.

4. Put your child in a time-out chair. (Remember the rule: one time-out minute for each year of age.)

5. Put yourself in a time-out chair. Think about why you are angry: is it your child, or is your child simply a convenient target for your anger?

6. Phone a friend.

7. If someone can watch the children, go outside and take a walk.

8. Take a hot bath or splash cold water on your face.

9. Hug a pillow.

10. Turn on some music. Maybe even sing along.

11. Pick up a pencil and write down as many helpful words as you can think of. Save the list.

12. Write for parenting information: Parenting, Box 2866, Chicago, IL 60690.

Take Time Out.
Don't Take It Out On Your Child.

National Committee for Prevention of Child Abuse

Ad Council

Figure 19-1 Alternatives to use to avoid hitting your child.[15]

irons, and, occasionally, cheap handguns ("Saturday night specials") as tools of enforcement. Now, gang members do not hesitate to use AK-47s (semiautomatic military assault weapons) that have the potential to kill large groups of people in a few seconds.

Most, but not all, gangs arise from big city environments where many disenfranchised, economically disadvantaged young persons live. Convinced that society has no significant role for them, gang members can receive support from an association of peers that has well-defined lines of authority. Rituals and membership initiation rites play important parts in gang socialization. Gangs often control particular territories

child abuse harm that is committed against a child; usually referring to physical abuse, sexual abuse, or child neglect.

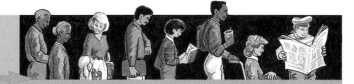

Learning FROM ALL Cultures

The Caning of Michael Fay

Can legally approved punishment be so harsh that it crosses the line and becomes an act of violence directed toward a prisoner? This was very much the question on the minds of Americans when an 18-year old American youth, Michael Fay, living in Singapore, was caned on the buttocks with a water-soaked rattan staff for alleged acts of vandalism.[18] Fay's caning was delivered in a Singapore prison by a martial arts expert, attended by a physician, and described by observers as being painful to the point of producing unconsciousness. Lifelong scars will remind Fay of his fate long after his interest in youthful pranks has passed.

Surrounding this incident is the question of whether another country should administer punishment that would be considered extreme by the customs (and laws) of our own. Those favoring the extreme nature of this punishment justify its intensity by suggesting that the low juvenile crime rate in Singa-

pore, when compared with our own crime rate, is the result of important lessons learned through pain. For them, Singapore's approach to controlling vandalism "works."

In contrast, people opposed to the rattan caning point out that the paint sprayed on cars in Singapore was easily removed, and therefore Fay's punishment was too violent. Many further believe that Americans should be punished in ways consistent with American law and custom, regardless of the country or culture in which the crime occurred.

In light of the diverse reactions to this incident, what is your opinion? Was caning an appropriate punishment, or an act of violence which was far too severe for the crime committed? Was quick, professionally inflicted pain less violent than a long period of incarceration? Do you think that a less violent physical punishment would be beneficial in reducing crime in the U.S.? ●

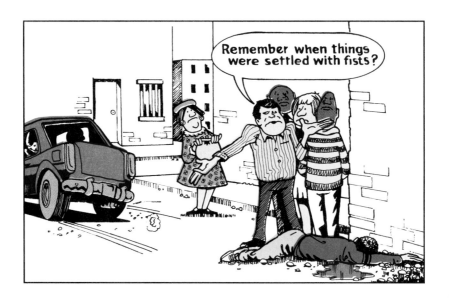

within a city.[16] Frequently, gangs are involved in criminal activities, the most common of which are illicit drug trafficking and robberies. In the mid-1990s, gang-related murders and drive-by shootings into groups of people are contributing to the rising death toll among young people.

It is not only older teenage males and young adults who are members of today's gangs. Increasingly, law

enforcement officials see younger persons (ages 12, 13, and 14) joining gangs. Some gangs have recently included young females as members and some cities report a growing number of all-female gangs. Some female gangs are reported to be every bit as ruthless as the male gangs.[17]

Youth violence is also spreading from the inner cities to the suburbs. Public health officials as well as

Health

Preventing a Carjacking

In the last 5 years a new form of violence has reached the streets of America. This crime is popularly called **carjacking.** Unlike auto theft, in which a car thief attempts to steal an unattended parked car, carjacking involves a thief's attempt to steal a car with a driver still behind the wheel.

Most carjacking attempts begin when a car is stopped at an intersection, usually at a traffic light. A carjacker will approach the driver and force him or her to give up the car. Resisting an armed carjacker can be extremely dangerous. Law enforcement officials offer the following tips to prevent carjacking[20]:

▼ Drive only on well-lit and well-traveled streets, if possible.

▼ Always keep your doors locked when driving your car.

▼ Observe traffic that may be following you. If you think that something suspicious is happening, try to locate a police officer or a busy, populated area to seek help.

▼ If someone approaches your car and you cannot safely drive away, roll the window down only slightly and leave the car running and in gear. If the situation turns bad, use your wits and quickly flee the scene, either in the car or on foot. *Remember: your life is worth more than your car.*

▼ If another car taps the rear bumper of your car (a common carjacking maneuver to get you to exit your car) and you feel uncomfortable about getting out of your car, tell the other driver that you are driving to the police station to complete the accident report. ▼

---

law enforcement personnel claim that youth violence is growing in epidemic proportions. Attorney General Janet Reno[19] has stated that youth violence is "the greatest single crime problem in America today."

Attempting to control gang and youth violence is particularly expensive for communities. When you consider that for every gang-related homicide there are about 100 nonfatal gang-related intentional injuries, it becomes obvious that gang violence is an expensive health care proposition. Furthermore, gang and youth violence takes an enormous financial and human toll on law enforcement, judicial, and corrections departments. Reducing gang and youth violence will be a daunting task for the nation as it approaches the year 2000.

Gun Violence

The tragic impact of gun violence has already been touched upon in a few sections of this chapter. Guns are being used more than ever in our society. In 1992 persons armed with handguns committed a record 931,000 violent crimes.[8] More than 60% of the homicides and 55% of the suicides committed each year in the U.S. involve the use of guns. As previously mentioned, gun violence is a leading killer of teenagers and young men, especially African-American males, and the use of semiautomatic assault weapons by individuals and gang members is increasing. Accidental deaths of toddlers and young children from loaded handguns is another dimension of the violence attributable to guns in our society.

The proliferation of firearm use has prompted major discussions concerning the enactment of gun con-

trol laws. For years, gun control activists have been in direct battle with the National Rifle Association (NRA) and its congressional supporters. Gun control activists want fewer guns manufactured and greater controls over the sale and possession of handguns. Gun supporters believe that such controls are not necessary and that people (the criminals) are responsible for gun deaths, not simply the guns. This debate will certainly continue.

Bias and Hate Crimes

One sad aspect of any society is how some segments of the majority treat certain people in the minority. Nowhere is this more violently pronounced than in **bias and hate crimes.** These crimes are directed at persons or groups of persons solely because of a racial, ethnic, religious, or other difference attributed to the victims. Victims are often verbally and physically attacked, their houses are spray painted with various slurs, and many are forced to move from one neighborhood or community to another.

---

carjacking a crime that involves a thief's attempt to steal a car while the owner is behind the wheel; carjackings are usually random, unpredictable, and frequently involve handguns.

bias and hate crimes criminal acts directed at a person or group solely because of a specific characteristic such as race, religion, ethnic background, or political belief.

Typically, the offenders in bias or hate crimes are fringe elements of the larger society who believe that the mere presence of someone with a racial, ethnic, or religious difference is inherently bad for the community, state, or country. Examples of groups commonly known to commit bias and hate crimes in the U.S. are white supremacists, skinheads, and the Ku Klux Klan. Increasingly, state and federal laws have been enacted to make bias and hate crimes serious offenses.

With a small but growing presence of neo-Nazi groups in Europe and clear evidence of so-called ethnic cleansing taking place in Bosnia, Serbia, Croatia and the former Soviet Union, bias and hate crimes are a worldwide problem. It is hoped that the recent push on college campuses to promote multicultural education, as well as the celebration of diversity, will make today's generation of college graduates well aware of the importance of tolerance and inclusion, rather than bigotry and exclusion.

Stalking

In recent years the crime of stalking has received considerable attention. **Stalking** refers to an assailant's planned efforts at pursuing an intended victim. Most stalkers are males. (One notable exception is the convicted female stalker of talk show host David Letterman.) Many of these stalkers are excessively possessive or jealous and pursue persons with whom they have had a former relationship. Some stalkers pursue people with whom they have had only an imaginary relationship.

Some stalkers have served time in prison and have waited for years to "get back" at their victims. In some cases stalkers go to great lengths to locate their intended victims and frequently know their daily whereabouts. Although not all stalkers plan to batter or kill their victims, their presence and potential for violence are enough to create an extremely frightening environment for the intended victim and the family.

Fortunately, since 1990 virtually all states have enacted or tightened their laws related to stalking and have created stiff penalties for those who do stalk. In many areas the criminal justice system is proactive in letting possible victims of stalking know, for example, when a particular prison inmate is going to be released. In other areas citizens are banding together to provide support and protection for persons who may be victims of stalkers.

If you think you are someone you know is being stalked, contact the police (or a local crisis intervention hotline number) to report your case and use their guidance. You can sense that you are a potential stalking victim either through the circumstances of a past relationship, or through the unusual behavior of someone who seems to be irrationally jealous of you or overly obsessed with you. Report a person who continues to pester you with phone calls, written notes or

Polly Klaas

Every parent's worst nightmare was played out in real life in the small town of Petaluma, California, in late 1993. On October 1 during a slumber party at her house, 12-year-old Polly Klaas was kidnapped by a knife-wielding man. For the next 2 months an unprecedented effort was undertaken to find this missing child. The Polly Klaas Foundation was immediately established and quickly raised half a million dollars to publicize her abduction. Over 1000 volunteers worked 12-hour shifts in hopes of finding Polly.[21]

In early December police arrested Richard Allen Davis, a twice-convicted kidnapper, and charged him with the abduction and murder of Polly. Four days after his arrest, Davis led police to Polly's body. With news coverage on national television networks, an entire nation began to mourn the death of Polly Klaas. The remaining money in the Polly Klaas Foundation was expected to be used to help find other missing children.[21]

The Polly Klaas case reflects random violence of the most heinous kind. Unfortunately her case was not an isolated one. In late 1993 10-year-old Cassidy Senter and 9-year-old Angie Housman were also kidnapped and killed in suburban St. Louis. The coverage of their cases on nationally televised news programs served to remind us that all children are vulnerable to random violence. ★

letters, or unwanted gifts. Report people who make persistent efforts to be with you after you have told them you do not want to see them. Until the situation is resolved, be alert for potentially threatening situations and keep in close touch with friends.

SEXUAL VICTIMIZATION

Ideally, sexual intimacy is a mutual, enjoyable form of communication between two people. Far too often, however, relationships are approached in an aggressive, hostile manner. These sexual aggressors always have a victim—someone who is physically or psychologically traumatized. *Sexual victimization* occurs in many forms and in a variety of settings. In this section we briefly look at sexual victimization as it occurs in rape and sexual assault, sexual abuse of children, sexual harassment, and the commercialization of sex.

Rape and Sexual Assault

As violence in our society increases, the incidence of *rape* and *sexual assault* correspondingly rises. The victims of these crimes fall into no single category. Victims of rape and sexual assault include young and old, male and female. Victims include the mentally retarded, prisoners, hospital patients, and college stu-

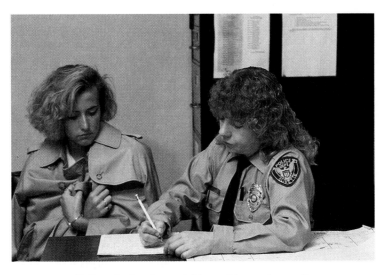

Self-protection is crucial to avoid sexual assault.

dents. We all are potential victims, and self-protection is critical. (See the Health Action Guide on rape prevention and the box on p. 486 for help for the rape victim.)

MYTHS ABOUT RAPE

Despite the fact that we are potential victims, many of us do not fully understand how vulnerable we are. Rape in particular has associated with it a number of myths (false assumptions). Among these are:

▼ *Women are raped by strangers.* In approximately half of all reported rapes the victim had some prior acquaintance with the rapist. Increasingly, women are being raped by husbands, dating partners, and relatives.

▼ *Rapes almost always occur in dark alleys or deserted places.* The opposite is true. Most rapes occur in or very near the victim's residence.

▼ *Rapists are easily identified by their demeanor or psychological profile.* Most experts indicate that rapists generally do not differ significantly from their non-rapist counterparts.

▼ *Incidence of rape is overreported.* Estimates are that only one in five rapes is reported.

▼ *Rape happens only to people in low socioeconomic classes.* Rape cuts across all socioeconomic classes. Each person, male or female, young or old, is a potential victim.

▼ *There is a standard way to escape from a potential rape situation.* Each rape situation is different. No one method to avoid rape can work in every potential rape situation. Because of this, we encourage personal health classes to invite speakers from a local rape prevention services bureau to discuss approaches to rape prevention.

Sometimes a personal assault begins as a physical assault that may turn into a rape situation. Rape is generally considered a crime of sexual aggression in which the victim is forced to have sexual intercourse. Current thought concerning rape characterizes this behavior as a violent act that happens to be carried out through sexual contact.

ACQUAINTANCE AND DATE RAPE

In recent years closer attention has been paid to the sexual victimization that occurs during relationships. *Acquaintance rape* refers to forced sexual intercourse between individuals who know each other. *Date rape* is a form of acquaintance rape that involves forced sexual intercourse by a dating partner. Studies on a number of campuses suggest that about 20% of college women reported having experienced date rape. An even higher percentage of women report being kissed and touched against their will. Frequently alcohol is a major contributing factor in these rape situations. (See Chapter 8 concerning alcohol's role in campus crime.) Some men have reported being psychologically coerced into intercourse by their female dating partners. In many cases, the aggressive partner will display certain behaviors that can be categorized (see the box on p. 486).

Psychologists believe that aside from the physical harm of date rape, a greater amount of emotional damage may occur. Such damage stems from the concept

stalking (stawk ing) a crime involving an assailant's planned efforts to pursue an intended victim.

Health **ACTION Guide**

Rape Prevention Guidelines

To prevent rape from occurring:

▼ Never forget that you could be a candidate for personal assault.

▼ Use approved campus security or escort services, especially at night.

▼ Think carefully about your patterns of movement to and from class or work. Alter your routes frequently.

▼ Walk briskly with a sense of purpose. Try not to walk alone at night.

▼ Dress so that the clothes you wear do not unnecessarily restrict your movement or make you more vulnerable.

▼ Always be aware of your surroundings. Look over your shoulder occasionally. Know where you are so that you won't get lost.

▼ Avoid getting into a car if you do not know the driver well.

▼ If you think you are being followed, look for a safe retreat. This might be a store, a fire or police station, or a group of people.

▼ Be especially cautious of first dates, blind dates, or people you meet at a party or bar who push to be alone with you.

▼ Let trusted friends know where you are and when you plan to return.

▼ Keep your car in good working order. Think beforehand how you would handle the situation should your car break down.

▼ Limit, and even avoid, alcohol to minimize the risk of rape.

▼ Trust your best instincts if you are assaulted. Each situation is different. Do what you can to protect your life.

Date Rape

To avoid date rape, be cautious of the following behaviors:

★ **Disrespectful attitude toward you and others**

★ **Lack of concern for your feelings**

★ **Violence and hostility**

★ **Obsessive jealousy**

★ **Extreme competitiveness**

★ **A desire to dominate**

★ **Unnecessary physical roughness**

of broken trust. Date rape victims feel particularly violated because the perpetrator was not a stranger. It was someone they initially trusted, at least to some degree. Once that trust is broken, developing new relationships with other people becomes much more difficult for the date rape victim.

Nearly all victims of date rape seem to suffer from *posttraumatic stress syndrome*. They can suffer from anxiety, sleeplessness, eating disorders, and nightmares. Guilt concerning their own behaviors, self-esteem, and judgment of other people can be overwhelming and the individual may require professional counseling. Because of the seriousness of these consequences, all students should be aware of the existence of date rape.

Sexual Abuse of Children

One of the most tragic forms of sexual victimization is the sexual abuse of children. Children are especially vulnerable to sexual abuse because of their dependent relationships with parents, relatives, and caregivers (such as babysitters, teachers, and neighbors). Often, children are unable to readily understand the difference between appropriate and inappropriate physical contact. Abuse may range from blatant physical manipulation, including fondling, to oral sex, sodomy, and intercourse.

Because of the subordinate role of children in relationships involving adults, sexually abusive practices often go unreported. Sexual abuse can leave emotional scars that make it difficult to establish meaningful relationships later in life. For this reason, it is especially important for people to pay close attention to any information shared by children that could indicate a potentially abusive situation. Most states require that information concerning child abuse must be reported to law enforcement officials.

Sexual Harassment

Sexual harassment consists of "unwanted attention of a sexual nature that creates embarrassment or stress."[22] Examples of sexual harassment include unwanted physical contact, excessive pressure for dates, sexually explicit humor, sexual innuendos or remarks, job advancement based on sexual favors, and overt sexual assault. Unlike more overt forms of sexual victimization, sexual harassment may be applied in a subtle manner and can, in some cases, go unnoticed by coworkers and fellow students. Nevertheless, sexual ha-

Health ACTION Guide

Help for the Rape Victim

If you have been raped, seek help as soon as possible. The following procedures may be helpful.

▼ *Call the police immediately to report the assault.* Police can take you to the hospital and start gathering information that may help them apprehend the rapist. Fortunately, many police departments now use specially trained officers (many of whom are female) to work closely with rape victims during all stages of the investigation.

▼ If you would rather not contact the police immedi-

ately, *call a local rape crisis center.* Operated generally on a 24-hour hotline basis, these centers have trained counselors to help you evaluate your options, contact the police, escort you to the hospital, and provide aftercare counseling.

▼ *Do not alter any potential evidence related to the rape.* Do not change your clothes, douche, take a bath, or rearrange the scene of the crime. Wait until all the evidence has been gathered.

▼ *Report all bruises, cuts, and scratches, even if they seem insignificant.* Report any information about the attack as completely and accurately as possible.

▼ *You will probably be given a thorough pelvic examination.* You may have to ask for STD tests and pregnancy tests.

▼ Although it is unusual for a rape victim's name to appear in the media, you might *request that the police withhold your name* as long as is legally possible.

Health ACTION Guide

Avoiding Date Rape

The following are some ways for both men and women to avoid a date rape situation:

MEN

▼ *Know your sexual desires and limits.* Communicate them clearly. Be aware of social pressures. It's OK not to score.

▼ *Being turned down when you ask for sex is not a rejection of you personally.* Women who say "no" to sex are not rejecting the person; they are expressing their desire not to participate in a single act. Your desires may be beyond control, but your actions *are* within your control.

▼ *Accept the woman's decision.* "No" means "no". Don't read other meanings into the answer. Don't continue after you are told "no!"

▼ *Don't assume that just because a woman dresses in a sexy manner and flirts that she wants to have sexual intercourse.*

▼ *Don't assume that previous permission for sexual contact applies to the current situation.*

▼ *Avoid excessive use of alcohol and drugs.* Alcohol and drugs interfere with clear thinking and effective communication.

WOMEN

▼ *Know your sexual desires and limits.* Believe in your right to set those limits. If you are not sure, STOP and talk about it.

▼ *Communicate your limits clearly.* If someone starts to offend you, tell him so firmly and immediately. Polite approaches may be misunderstood or ignored. Say "no" when you mean "no."

▼ *Be assertive.* Often men interpret passivity as permission. Be direct and firm with someone who is sexually pressuring you.

▼ *Be aware that your nonverbal actions send a message.* If you dress in a sexy manner and flirt, some men may assume you want to have sex. This does not make your dress or behavior wrong, but it is important to be aware of a possible misunderstanding.

▼ *Pay attention to what is happening around you.* Watch the nonverbal clues. Do not put yourself into vulnerable situations.

▼ *Trust your intuitions.* If you feel you are being pressured into unwanted sex, you probably are.

▼ *Avoid excessive use of alcohol and drugs.* Alcohol and drugs interfere with clear thinking and effective communication.

rassment produces stress that cannot be resolved until the harasser is identified and forced to stop. Both males and females can be victims of sexual harassment.

Sexual harassment can occur in many settings, including employment and academic settings. On the college campus, harassment may be primarily in terms of sex for grades. When this occurs, it is important that the student think carefully about the situation and document the specific times, events, and places where the harassment took place. Consult your college's policy concerning harassment. Next, you could report these events to the appropriate administrative officer (perhaps the Affirmative Action Officer, Dean of Academic Affairs, or Dean of Students). You may also want to discuss the situation with a staff member of the university counseling center.

If harassment occurs in the work environment, the victim should document the occurrences and report them to the appropriate management or personnel official. Reporting procedures will vary from setting to setting. Sexual harassment is a form of illegal sex discrimination and violates Title VII of the Civil Rights Act of 1964.

In 1986 the U.S. Supreme Court ruled that the creation of a "hostile environment" in a work setting was sufficient evidence to support the claim of sexual harassment. This action served as an impetus for many women to step forward with sexual harassment allegations. The number of complaints filed with state agencies and the Equal Employment Opportunity Commission increased from 5694 cases in 1990 to over 10,900 in 1993.[23]

Not surprisingly, this soaring number of complaints has served as a wake-up call for employers. From university settings to factory production lines to corporate board rooms, employers are scrambling to make certain that employees are fully aware of actions that could lead to a sexual harassment lawsuit. Sexual harassment workshops and educational seminars on harassment are now common and serve to educate both men and women about this complex problem.

Violence and the Commercialization of Sex

Thus far, Chapter 19 has focused on the prevalence of violence in our society. Violence in the form of homicides, gang warfare, and partner abuse continues to be a growing problem. Whenever we pick up a news magazine or watch the television news, we can see graphic evidence of the results of violent acts. The remnants of drive-by shootings, wounded store clerks, and murder victims covered by white sheets leave us with images we would like to forget. However, these violent acts which we see reported daily in the media tend to be ones that are nonsexual in nature.

Unforunately, violence also is committed in the sexual arena. Child sexual abuse, rape, and violence against women represent acts that leave lasting scars on their vicims...scars most of us never see.

It is beyond the scope of this book to explore whether sexual violence can be related to society's exploitation or commercialization of sex. However, sexually related products and messages are intentionally placed before the public to try to sway consumer decisions. Do you believe that there could be a connection between commerical products such as violent pornography in films and magazines, and violence against women? Does prostitution directly lead to violence? Do sexually-explicit "900" phone numbers cause an increase in violent acts? Can the sexual messages in beer commericals lead to acquaintance rape? What do you think?

UNINTENTIONAL INJURIES

Unintentional injuries are injuries that have occurred without anyone intending that any harm be done. Common examples include injuries resulting from car crashes, falls, fires, drownings, firearm accidents, recreational accidents, and residential accidents. Each year unintentional injuries account for over 150,000 deaths and millions of nonfatal injuries.

Unintentional injuries are very expensive for our society, both from a financial standpoint and from a personal and family standpoint. Fortunately, to a large extent it is possible to avoid becoming a victim of unintentional injuries. By carefully considering the tips presented in the safety categories that follow, you will be protecting yourself from many preventable injuries.

Since this section of Chapter 19 focuses on a selected number of safety categories, we encourage readers to consider some additional related activities. For further information in the area of safety, consult a safety textbook (one of which is listed in the references for this chapter).[24] To review important points in the area of first aid skills, consult Appendix 2 in this text. Finally, we encourage you to take a first aid course from the American Red Cross. Red Cross first aid courses incorporate a significant amount of safety prevention information along with the teaching of specific first aid skills.

Personal Safety

Self-protection and the prevention of sexual assault are viable health issues that can threaten each of us—male or female. As violence in our society increases, the incidence of physical injury, sexual assault, and rape correspondingly rises. The recommendations that we present are intended to encourage you to think critically about how you can prevent personal assaults from happening to you.

▼ Never assume that you are an unlikely candidate for personal assault.

▼ Think carefully about your patterns of movement to and from class or work. Alter your routes frequently.

▼ Walk briskly, with a sense of purpose. Try not to walk alone at night.

▼ Dress so that clothes you wear do not unnecessarily restrict your movement or make you more vulnerable.

▼ Always be aware of your surroundings. Look over your shoulder occasionally. Know where you are so that you won't get lost.

▼ If you think you are being followed, look for a safe retreat. This might be a store, fire or police station, or a group of people.

▼ Be especially cautious of first dates, blind dates, or people you meet at a party or bar who push to be alone with you.

▼ Let trusted friends know where you are and when you plan to return.

▼ Keep your car in good working order. Think beforehand how you would handle the situation should your car break down.

▼ Trust your best instincts if you are assaulted. Each situation is different. Do what you can to protect your life.

Residential Safety

Many serious accidents and personal assaults occur in dorm rooms, apartments, and houses. As a responsible adult, you should make every reasonable effort to prevent these tragedies from happening. One good idea is to discuss some of the following points with your roommates (or housemates) and see what cooperative strategies you can implement:

▼ Fireproof your residence. Are all electrical appliances and heating and cooling systems in safe working order? Are flammable materials safely stored?

▼ Prepare a fire escape plan. Install smoke or heat detectors.

▼ Do not give personal information over the phone to a stranger.

▼ Use initials for first names on mailboxes and in phone books.

▼ Install a peephole and deadbolt locks on outside doors.

▼ Within reason, avoid living in first floor apartments. Change locks when moving to a new apartment or home.

▼ Put locks on all windows.

▼ Require repairmen or deliverymen to show valid identification.

▼ Do not use an elevator if it is occupied by someone who makes you feel uneasy.

▼ Be cautious around garages, laundry rooms, and driveways (especially at night). Use lighting for prevention of assault.

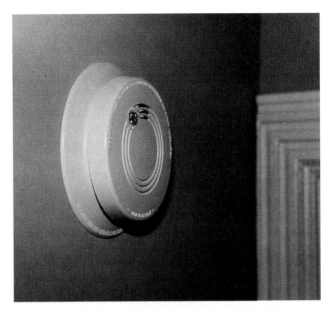

Smoke detectors are effective in saving lives, but they cannot be used properly without fresh batteries.

Recreational Safety

The thrills we get from risk taking are an essential part of our recreational endeavors. Sometimes we can get into serious accidents because we fail to consider important recreational safety information. Do some of the following recommendations apply to you?

▼ Seek appropriate instruction for your intended activity. Few skill activities are as easy as they look.

▼ Always wear your automobile seat belt.

▼ Make certain that your equipment is in excellent working order.

▼ Involve yourself gradually in an activity before attempting more complicated, dangerous skills.

▼ Enroll in a Red Cross first aid course to enable you to cope with unexpected injuries.

▼ Remember that alcohol use greatly increases the likelihood that people will get hurt.

▼ Protect your eyes from serious injury.

▼ Learn to swim. Drowning occurs most frequently to people who never intended to be in the water.

▼ Obey the laws related to your recreational pursuits. Many laws are directly related to the safety of the participants.

▼ Be aware of weather conditions. Many outdoor activities turn to tragedy with sudden shifts in the weather. Always prepare yourself for the worst possible weather.

unintentional injuries injuries that have occurred without anyone intending that harm be done.

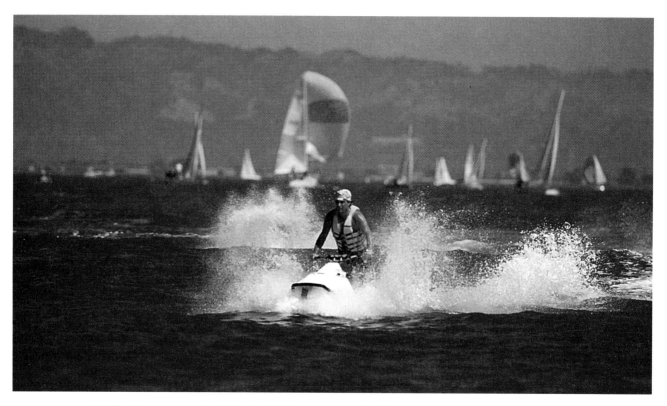

Jet skiing is a very popular but potentially dangerous activity. What safety precautions should this person follow?

Firearm Safety

Each year about 13,000 Americans are murdered with guns and another 2000 die in gun-related accidents. Most of the murders are committed with handguns. (Shotguns and rifles tend to be more cumbersome than handguns and thus are not as frequently used in murders, accidents, or suicides.) Over half of all murders result from quarrels and arguments between acquaintances or relatives. With many homeowners arming themselves with handguns for protection against intruders, it is not surprising that over half of all gun accidents occur in the home. Children are frequently involved in gun accidents, often after they discover a gun they think is unloaded. Handgun owners are reminded to adhere to the following safety reminders:

▼ Make certain that you follow the gun possession laws in your state. Special permits may be required to carry a handgun.
▼ Make certain that your gun is in good mechanical order.
▼ If you are a novice, enroll in a gun safety course.
▼ Consider every gun to be a loaded gun, even if someone tells you it is unloaded.
▼ Never point a gun at an unintended target.
▼ Keep your finger off the trigger until you are ready to shoot.

▼ When moving with a handgun, keep the barrel pointed down.
▼ Load and unload your gun carefully.
▼ Store your gun and ammunition safely in a locked container. Use a trigger lock on your gun when not in use.
▼ Take target practice only at approved ranges.
▼ Never "play" with guns at parties. Never handle a gun when intoxicated.
▼ Educate children about gun safety and the potential dangers of gun use. Children must never believe that a gun is a toy.

Motor Vehicle Safety

The greatest number of accidental deaths in America take place on highways and streets. When you are a young person, the way that you are most likely to die is from a motor vehicle accident. According to Bever,[24] the following is a description of a prime candidate for such a death:

. . . a male, 15 to 24 years of age, driving on a two-lane, rural road between the hours of 10 PM and 2 AM on a Saturday night. If he has been drinking and is driving a subcompact car or motorcycle, the likelihood that he and his passengers will have a fatal accident is even more pronounced.

Disabling injuries also result from motor vehicle accidents. With nearly 2 million such injuries each year, concern for the prevention of motor vehicle accidents should be important for all college students, regardless of age. With this thought in mind, we offer some important safety tips for motor vehicle operators:

▼ Make certain that you are familiar with the traffic laws in your state.
▼ Do not operate an automobile or motorcycle unless it is in good mechanical order. Regularly inspect your brakes, lights, and exhaust system.
▼ Do not exceed the speed limit. Observe all traffic signs.
▼ Always wear safety belts, even on short trips. Require your passengers to buckle up. Always keep small children in child restraints.
▼ Never drink and drive. Avoid horseplay inside a car.
▼ Be certain that you can hear the traffic outside your car. Keep the car's music system at a reasonable decibel level.

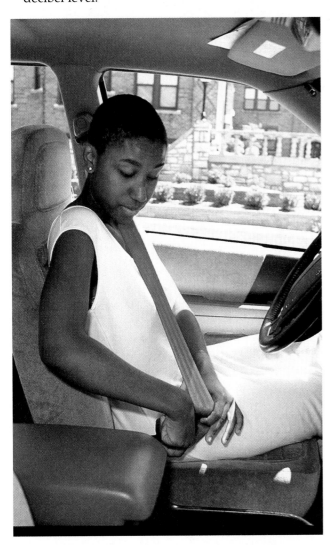

Always wear your seat belt, even on short trips.

▼ Give pedestrians the right-of-way.
▼ Drive defensively at all times. Do not challenge other drivers. Refrain from drag racing.
▼ Look carefully before changing lanes.
▼ Be especially careful at intersections and railroad crossings.
▼ Carry a well-maintained first aid kit that includes flares or other signal devices.
▼ Alter your driving behaviors during bad weather.

Home Accident Prevention for Children and the Elderly

Approximately one person in ten is injured each year in a home accident. Children and the elderly spend significantly more hours each day in a home setting than do young adults and midlife persons. It is especially important that accident prevention be given primary consideration for these groups. Here are some important tips to remember. Can you think of others? (See Figure 19-2.)

FOR BOTH GROUPS

▼ Be certain that you have adequate insurance protection.
▼ Install smoke detectors appropriately.
▼ Keep stairways clear of toys or debris. Install railings.
▼ Maintain electrical and heating equipment.
▼ Make certain that inhabitants know how to get emergency help.

FOR CHILDREN

▼ Know all the ways to protect from accidental poisoning.
▼ Use toys that are appropriate for the age of the child.
▼ Never leave young children unattended, especially infants.
▼ Keep any hazardous items (guns, poisons, etc.) locked up.
▼ Keep small children away from kitchen stoves.

FOR ELDERLY

▼ Protect from falls. (Consider rugs, floors, and stairs.)
▼ Install safety equipment in the bathroom (rails, slip-resistant surfaces).
▼ Be certain that elderly persons have a good understanding of the medications they may be taking. Know the side effects.
▼ Encourage elderly persons to seek assistance when it comes to home repairs.
▼ Make certain that all door locks, lights, and safety equipment are in good working order.

Refer to the next chapter for additional information related to the protection of older adults.

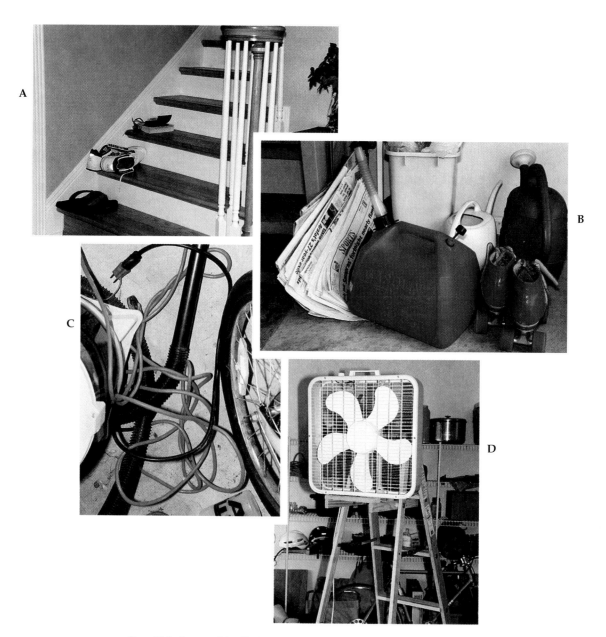

Figure 19-2 Can you identify the potential hazards in each of these scenes?

Answers for Figure 19-2: A, Cluttered stairs can lead to falls. **B,** Improper storage of a gasoline receptacle. **C** and **D,** Improper use of electric wires, extension cords, and an appliance.

Personal Safety Index

PERSONAL ASSESSMENT

This quiz will help you measure how well you manage your personal safety. For each item below, circle the number that reflects the frequency with which you do the safety activity. Then, add up your individual scores and check the interpretation at the end.

3 I regularly do this
2 I sometimes do this
1 I rarely do this

1. I am aware of my surroundings and do not get lost. 3 2 1
2. I avoid locations in which my personal safety could be compromised. 3 2 1
3. I intentionally vary my daily routine, such as walking patterns to and from class, parking places, jogging or biking routes, etc., so that my whereabouts are not always predictable. 3 2 1
4. I walk across campus at night with other people. 3 2 1
5. I am careful about disclosing personal information (address, phone number, social security number, my daily schedule, etc.) to people I do not know. 3 2 1
6. I carefully monitor my alcohol intake at parties. 3 2 1
7. I watch carefully for dangerous weather conditions and know how to respond if necessary. 3 2 1
8. I do not keep a loaded gun in my home. 3 2 1
9. I know how I would handle myself if I were to be assaulted. 3 2 1
10. I maintain adequate insurance for my health and my property. 3 2 1
11. I keep emergency information numbers near my phone. 3 2 1

12. I keep my first aid skills up-to-date. 3 2 1
13. I use dead bolt locks on the doors of my home. 3 2 1
14. I use the safety locks on the windows at home. 3 2 1
15. I check the batteries used in my home smoke detector. 3 2 1
16. I use adequate lighting in areas around my home and garage. 3 2 1
17. I have the electrical, heating, and cooling equipment in my home inspected regularly for safety and efficiency. 3 2 1
18. I use my car seat belt. 3 2 1
19. I drive my car safely and defensively. 3 2 1
20. I keep my car in good mechanical order. 3 2 1
21. I keep my car doors locked. 3 2 1
22. I have a plan of action if my car should break down while I am driving it. 3 2 1
23. I use appropriate safety equipment, such as flotation devices, helmets, elbow pads, etc., in my recreational activities. 3 2 1
24. I can swim well enough to save myself in most situations. 3 2 1
25. I use suggestions for personal safety each day. 3 2 1

TOTAL POINTS _____

INTERPRETATION:

Your total	may mean that:
70-75 points	You appear to carefully protect your personal safety.
65-69 points	You adequately protect many aspects of your personal safety.
60-64 points	You should consider improving some of your safety-related behaviors.
below 60 points	You must consider improving some of your safety-related behaviors.

TO CARRY THIS FURTHER

Although no one can be completely safe from personal injury or possible random violence, there are ways to minimize the risks to your safety. Scoring high on this assessment will not guarantee your safety, but your likelihood for injury should remain relatively low. Scoring low on this assessment should encourage you to consider ways to make your life more safe. Refer to Chapter 19 and this assessment to provide you with useful suggestions to enhance your personal safety. Which safety tips will you use today?

CAMPUS SAFETY AND VIOLENCE PREVENTION

This chapter will end on a positive note. Although many of the topics in this chapter are quite unsettling, students and faculty must continue to function adequately in the campus environment despite potential threats to our health. The first step in being able to function adequately is knowing about these potential threats. You have read about these threats in this chapter. Now you must think about how this information applies to your campus situation.

The campus environment is no longer immune to many of the social ills that plague our society. At one time the university campus was thought to be a safe haven from the "real world." Now there is plenty of evidence to indicate that significant intentional injuries and unintentional injuries can happen to anyone at any time on the college campus.

For this reason you must make it a habit to think constructively about protecting your safety. In addition to the personal safety tips presented earlier in this chapter, remember to use the safety assistance resources available on your campus. One of these might be your use of university-approved escort services, especially in the evenings as you move from one campus location to another. Another resource is the campus security department (campus police). Typically, campus police have a 24-hour emergency phone number. If you think you need help, do not hesitate to call this number. Campus security departments frequently offer short seminars on safety topics to student organizations or residence halls groups. Your counseling center on campus might also offer programs on rape prevention and personal protection.

If you are motivated to make your campus environment safer, you might wish to contact two organizations that specifically focus on campus crime.[2] The first is Safe Campuses Now, a nonprofit student group that tracks legislation, provides educational seminars, and monitors community incidents involving students. For information about Safe Campuses Now, including how to start a chapter on your campus, call (706) 354-1115. Another nonprofit organization, Security on Campus, Inc., aims at preventing campus violence and crime, but also helps victims enforce their legal rights. This group can be reached at (215) 768-9330. We encourage you to play an active role in making your campus a safer place to live. Good luck.

As We Go to Press...

As this text went to press the long-debated $30 billion Federal Crime Bill finally passed through the U.S. Congress in late August 1994. Touted as the most sweeping crime package in the history of the country, this bill provided $13.5 billion for law enforcement, $9.9 billion for prisons, and $6.9 for crime prevention. Key provisions in the bill called for up to 100,000 new police officers, a variety of crime prevention activities, stronger penalties for spouse abusers, and a ban on 19 kinds of assault-style firearms. What impact do you think this bill could have on crime?

Summary

- ✔ Everyone is a potential victim of violent crime.
- ✔ Each year in the United States intentional injuries cause about 50,000 deaths and another 2 million nonfatal injuries.
- ✔ Homicide is the leading cause of death for young African-American males. Handguns are the weapons of choice for homicides.
- ✔ Because of factors related to family structure, increased drug use and crime, and the inability of people to resolve conflicts peacefully, domestic violence is on the rise.
- ✔ Forms of child abuse include physical abuse, sexual abuse, and child neglect. Child neglect is the most common form.
- ✔ Youth violence is skyrocketing and much of the violence is related to gang activities.
- ✔ Bias and hate crimes, as well as the crime of stalking, are increasingly recognized as serious violent acts.
- ✔ Rape and sexual assault, acquaintance rape, date rape, and sexual harassment represent forms of sexual victimization in which victims often are both physically and psychologically traumatized.
- ✔ Unintentional injuries are injuries that occur without anyone intending that harm be done. The numbers of fatal and nonfatal unintentional injuries are exceedingly high.

Review Questions

1. Identify some of the categories of intentional injuries. How many persons are affected each year by intentional injuries?

2. What are some of the most important facts concerning homicide in the United States? How are the majority of homicides committed?

3. Identify changes in the traditional family structure that may be related to increased family stress and domestic violence. What additional factors also may be related to increased domestic violence?

4. What reasons might exist that explain why so many women do not report domestic violence?

5. Aside from the immediate consequences of child abuse, what additional problems do many abused children face in the future?

6. Explain why gangs and gang activities have increased tremendously over the last 15 years. What impact do gangs have on a community?

7. List some examples of groups that are known to have committed bias or hate crimes.

8. Identify some general characteristics of a typical stalker.

9. Explain some of the myths associated with rape. How can date rape be prevented?

10. Identify some examples of behaviors that could be considered sexual harassment. Why are employers especially concerned about educating their employees about sexual harassment?

11. Identify some common examples of unintentional injuries. Point out three safety tips from each of the safety areas listed at the end of this chapter.

Think about This . . .

✔ To what extent are you concerned about your personal safety? Are you comfortable with your level of concern? Or do you think you should be more or less concerned?

✔ According to published reports, after the tragic deaths of Nichole Brown Simpson and her friend, Ronald Goldman, phone calls to domestic violence hotlines increased tremendously. What were some of your feelings about domestic violence as you watched the news coverage of this story?

✔ Has there been any gun violence at your college? Are you aware of any students carrying guns or other concealed weapons on your campus?

✔ Do you know of educational programs on your campus that have dealt with rape prevention or sexual harassment? Where can you go on your campus to seek help for crises related to these issues?

✔ Is there a particular place on your campus where you believe that your personal safety is threatened? If so, how do you cope with this threat?

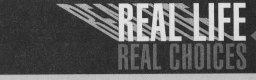

YOUR TURN

▼ According to current thinking, is rape (1) a crime motivated by sexual desire or (2) a crime of violence that is carried out through sexual conduct?

▼ In some cases men have accused women of date rape. Whether you are male or female, do you believe this could be a valid claim? Why or why not?

▼ Have you ever been involved in a date rape situation, as either the aggressor or the victim? If so, how did you deal with the situation at the time? Afterward? What behaviors on (1) your part and (2) your partner's part do you think contributed to the situation?

AND NOW, YOUR CHOICES

▼ Given what you know about rape in general and date rape in particular, what steps can you take to protect yourself from becoming involved in a situation like Debra and Ron's?

▼ If Ron or Debra were your friend, how do you think you could be most helpful to him or her in dealing with this experience? ▼

References

1. Turque B, Murr A et al: He could run . . . but he couldn't hide, *Newsweek*, June 27, 1994, p. 16.

2. Cohen G: Campus crime: a false sense of security, *U. Magazine*, May 1994, p. 18.

3. Bureau of Justice Statistics: *Injuries from crime: special report*, US Department of Justice, Washington, DC, 1989, US Government Printing Office.

4. Bureau of Justice Statistics: *Sourcebook of criminal justice statistics—1992*, US Department of Justice, Washington, DC, 1993, US Government Printing Office.

5. Marshall S: Killings rise 3%, despite overall drop in crime rate, *USA Today*, May 2, 1994, p. 3A.

6. Swanson JM, Albrecht M: *Community health nursing: promoting the health of aggregates*, Philadelphia, 1993, WB Saunders.

7. Bureau of Justice Statistics: *Drugs, crime, and the justice system: a national report*, US Department of Justice, Washington, DC, December, 1992, US Government Printing Office.

8. Bureau of Justice Statistics: *Guns and crime: handgun victimization, firearm self-defense, and firearm theft*, US Department of Justice, Washington, DC, April 1994, US Government Printing Office.

9. US Bureau of the Census: *Statistical abstract of the United States: 1993*, ed 113, Washington, DC, 1993, US Government Printing Office.

10. Hunt T: Brady Bill becomes law, *The Muncie Star*, December 1, 1993, p. 1.

11. Bachman R: *Violence against women: a national crime victimization survey report*, US Department of Justice, Washington, DC, January 1994, US Government Printing Office.

12. DeWitt CB: From the director, *Research in Brief*, National Institute of Justice, US Department of Justice, Washington DC, October 1992, US Government Printing Office.

13. Widom CS: The cycle of violence, *Research in Brief*, National Institute of Justice, US Department of Justice, Washington, DC October 1992, US Government Printing Office.

14. Prothrow-Smith D: Stop violence before it begins, *USA Today*, February 24, 1994, p. 11A.

15. National Committee for Prevention of Child Abuse: *12 alternatives to whacking your kid*, Chicago, undated pamphlet.

16. Covey HC, Menard S, Franzese RJ: *Juvenile gangs*, Springfield, Ill, 1992, Charles C Thomas.

17. Leslie C et al: Girls will be girls, *Newsweek*, August 2, 1993, p. 44.

18. Walsh J: The whipping boy, *Time*, May 2, 1994.

19. Kantrowitz B: Wild in the streets, *Newsweek*, August 2, 1993, p. 40.

20. Maynard G. The start of a trend: second carjacking attempt reported, *The Muncie Star*, October 21, 1993, p. 1.

21. Beck M et al: The sad case of Polly Klaas, *Newsweek*, December 13, 1993, p. 39.

22. Haas K, Haas A: *Understanding sexuality*, ed 3, St Louis, 1993, Mosby.

23. Ingrassia M: Sexual correctness: abused and confused, *Newsweek*, October 25, 1993, p. 57.

24. Bever DL: *Safety: a personal focus*, ed 3, St Louis, 1992, Mosby.

Suggested Readings

American Red Cross: *Responding to emergencies*, St. Louis, 1994, Mosby Lifeline.

    A comprehensive guide for handling first aid emergencies and a workbook used by many colleges and universities in their introductory first aid courses. Well illustrated and easy to follow; a considerable amount of safety and prevention information is included.

Petrocelli W, Repa K: *Sexual harassment on the job: what it is and how to stop it*, Berkeley, Calif, 1992, Nolo Press.

    A guide to identifying, handling, and preventing instances of sexual harassment for both women and managers. A major focus is on the legal issues involving harassment, including resource lists and various state laws.

Scott K: *Sexual assault: will I ever feel okay again?* Minneapolis, 1993, Bethany House Publishers.

    A survivor of rape tells about what it takes to rebound from the pain, fear, and shame. A good resource for victims, or those who know or work with victims.

UNIT SIX

Throughout Unit 6 we have explored the health-related issues of consumerism, the environment, and violence and safety. Now we relate these topics to the important developmental tasks of identity, independence, responsibility, social skills, and intimacy.

Forming an Initial Adult Identity

Whether we are able to admit it or not, we all want to find out "who we are." To develop the confidence to face the world and to contribute to its improvement require that we come to grips with personal strengths and limitations. Although it may be valuable to be able to understand and analyze others, it is much more significant that we discover, develop, and define our own identity. Examining attitudes and behaviors about health consumerism, the environment, and violence can help us learn about ourselves.

In the area of self-care, we can examine how we value and manage health; we learn about ourselves as we consider how we take care of ourselves when we are ill. Are you a person who must always visit a doctor when ill, or are you able to cope reasonably well with self-limiting conditions? Are you a skilled consumer in purchasing prescriptions or over-the-counter medications? Honest answers to these kinds of questions will help you understand your unique identity.

Establishing Independence

Gaining a sense of independence can be a refreshing, exciting experience for most young adults. Relocation, employment, and new friendships will propel you into consumer involvement on a scale greater than that required while at home or in college.

Besides choosing new health care providers, you will independently obtain the insurance needed to pay for these services. Health insurance and disability insurance are critical investments you must make.

Independence often brings with it new acquaintances who may attempt to push you into areas of consumerism for which you have no real need. Start preparing yourself now to live and work among people who will try to influence your consumer perspectives.

Assuming Responsibility

There is no area of responsibility more immediate than the responsibility you assume for your own safety. As violence in our society, including on campuses, escalates, you must be increasingly responsible for your actions and your responses to the actions of others. Make a concerted effort to understand the environmental cues associated with personal safety and plan ahead in dealing with threatening situations.

Developing Social Skills

Regardless of whether we are involved in decisions related to our environment or our consumer choices, we frequently make these decisions with other individuals, companies, or agencies. Our social skills help us convey our needs, interpret directions, and voice concerns. Effective speaking, listening, writing, reading, and cooperative working with others are the tools we need to refine as we work to improve our health or the health of others.

Sometimes in the areas of consumerism, environment, and safety, the social interactions we have with others may not always be pleasant. For example, voicing a complaint about a health-related product may require a face-to-face confrontation with a store manager. Speaking up at a public debate on a local environmental issue might be intimidating. Poise, tact, and a degree of assertiveness may be beneficial in both of these situations. Fortunately, these social skills can be developed and sharpened with practice.

Developing Intimacy

The development of intimacy suggests a certain quality in (or about) the environment in which interactions take place. Your physical environment should contribute to a safe, esthetic, and supportive backdrop to life. In the absence of such an environment, intimacy as well as safety can be compromised by a variety of concerns. The environment in which you pursue intimacy must be safe from acts of violence. Victimization of a person by a partner, including harassment and rape, is the antithesis of all that is implied in intimacy.

Part of intimacy is openness and honesty. These qualities must also be present in the intimate relationships that we have with health care providers and others whom we trust to deliver products, services, and information required for lifelong health.

UNIT SEVEN

This last unit examines two topics that many traditional age students initially prefer not to study: aging and death. These topics seem to run counter to a culture that idolizes youth, vitality, and health. Understandably, however, the content of Unit 7 is closely related to each of the five dimensions of health.

● Physical Dimension of Health

The inevitability of aging and death is beyond question. Unless we die suddenly at an early age, most of us will go through years of relatively good physical health before we reach a period of gradual decline. Eventually we will experience an extended period of failing health. Our deaths will probably result from a chronic health condition that our bodies cannot successfully overcome.

The above scenario is somewhat depressing because it has packed 50 to 60 years of physical change into one short paragraph. Overall, the physical changes described are those of decline, but this one-sided view neglects the fact that many persons today enjoy their highest levels of physical health late in life. As a part of a larger societal movement toward exercise, weight management, smoking cessation, and moderation in alcohol use, today's older adults often indicate that they are physically healthier than they were just a few years ago. This is an optimistic sign for young and old alike.

◆ Emotional Dimension of Health

The events associated with aging and death often influence the emotional dimension of health. The independence of grown children and the move to retirement can tax emotional health. Even the lack of change in life experience can influence how an aging person feels. For some persons, a life that continues unchanged will be seen as positive and stable, whereas for others it will produce stress or changes in mood, outlook, and self-perception. Another powerful stressor to the emotional dimension of an older person's health is the death of a spouse or close friend; this event reminds aging people that their lives are limited, and a major challenge to their emotional stability often takes place.

■ Social Dimension of Health

Three significant challenges to the social dimension of health for older persons are the independence of their children, the death of a spouse or close friend, and the changes in the neighborhood or town in which they live. When these events occur, many familiar, comfortable social relationships can be strongly influenced. Older persons may not have the interest and skill to replace these social contacts. You can do your best to fill the void created by these personal and social changes.

▲ Intellectual Dimension of Health

Intellectual activity is valuable to the overall health of older individuals. Contrary to popular belief, many older persons do not experience a major loss in their intellectual capacities. Fortunately, those who continue intellectual activity also tend to continue physical activity and social involvement and thus maintain their health resources.

● Spiritual Dimension of Health

The maturing of the spiritual dimension of health centers on an inward search that is evident in the form of overt behaviors. You can support an older person's need for introspection by recognizing his or her desire to participate in religious services, visit an art gallery, or attend a musical concert. You can be genuinely interested in an older adult's recollections of past experiences. Your willingness to discuss such topics as dying and death can also help an older person in the inward search for life's meaning.

Growing Older

Balancing Your Future With Your Past

20

The Maturing Adult

Moving Through Transitions

hat does it mean to be growing, developing, and aging? It probably depends on your perspective. For traditional age college students, growing and developing are usually positive experiences. They reflect a movement in the direction of future resources, recognition, and opportunity. Aging, in contrast, is perceived more negatively. Aging reflects a movement away from the very accomplishments and abilities toward which young people strive.

For college students who are in *midlife* (between 45 and 65 years of age) or are elderly (older than 65 years), all three terms might be equally positive. Growing and developing imply a potential for improvement, whereas aging reflects maturation, valuable insights, and sharpened skills.

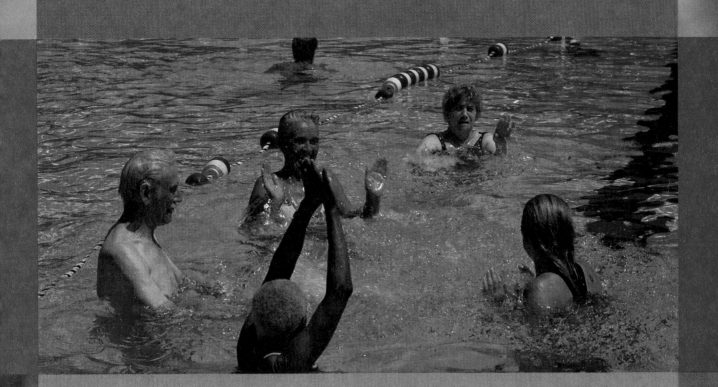

THE MATURING ADULT

The following objectives are covered in this chapter:

▼ Reduce to no more than 90 per 1000 people the proportion of all people age 65 and older who have difficulty in performing two or more personal care activities, thereby preserving independence. (Baseline: 111 per 1000 in 1984-85; p. 587.)

▼ Reduce to no more than 22% the proportion of people age 65 and older who engage in no leisure time physical activity. (Baseline: 43% in 1985; p. 589.)

▼ Increase years of healthy life to at least 65 years. (Baseline: An estimated 62 years in 1980; p. 588). Note: "Years of healthy life" is a summary calculation based on age of death, years of sickness, and years of disability.

REAL LIFE
REAL CHOICES

Growing Older: Over the Hill or Top of the Mountain?

▼ **Name:** Josh Washington
▼ **Age:** 22
▼ **Occupation:** Premed graduate and future medical student

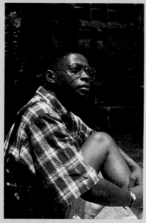

"Play ball!"

As these words are heard across the playing field, cousins and relatives all join in to enjoy a friendly game of softball at the twelfth annual Washington family reunion. Approaching his clan, Josh Washington is immediately surrounded by a happy, laughing throng, amidst all the shouting, hugging, kissing, and even a few tears.

Just past the chattering knot of relatives, Josh catches sight of his two grandmothers. Excusing himself, he moves toward the two older women. "Nana . . . Grandmother . ." On one side Josh is enfolded in the swift, strong embrace of Nana Keller, his mother's mother, while on the other side he feels the frail clutch of Grandmother Washington's birdlike hand. Smiling, he accepts their hugs, then stands back, still holding their hands, watching and listening. On this beautiful summer day, Josh is suddenly struck for the first time by the real meaning of aging and wonders what might explain the striking differences between his grandmothers.

They're both in their late 60s, both intelligent, well educated, and in comfortable circumstances. That, Josh thinks, is where any resemblance ends. Widowed 3 years ago after more than 40 good years of marriage, Nana Keller still teaches nutrition at the community college, gardens enthusiastically, is active in community projects, and plans to spend part of this summer at a university-sponsored health and nutrition meeting in the Middle East. Last winter, 3 weeks after spraining her ankle in a fall, she tossed her crutches aside and walked to her doctor's office to tell him she was fully recovered.

She's so intense, so involved, so . . . *alive,* Josh thinks, marveling as he always does at Nana Keller's unquenchable zest for life. How, he wonders, can Grandmother Washington be the same age, and yet so different? He studies his father's mother. For as long as Josh can remember, she's looked frail, timid, delicate, and, well, *old.* Although apparently in reasonable health, she always seems to have an ache or pain to prevent her from being active. She dislikes being outdoors (the sun, the wind, the sand, the insects) and is uncomfortable in many public places (germs, noise, dirt). A promising concert violinist before her marriage, she gave up her career to be a housewife and mother. She never mentions what must have been a painful sacrifice, but Josh, to whom she has imparted her passion for music, has seen the expression on her face when she leafs through old sheet music. A widow for more than 20 years with a comfortable income, she doesn't travel, rarely goes out except for her weekly afternoon of bridge and church on Sunday, and is increasingly isolating herself in the dim, silent brick house where Josh's father and his aunt grew up.

As you study this chapter, think about the similarities and differences between Josh's two grandmothers, and prepare yourself to answer the questions in **Your Turn** at the end of the chapter. ▼

In this chapter, growing, developing, and aging are considered in terms of the second half of the life cycle. Regardless of your perspective (as a traditional age or nontraditional age student), we hope that you will be able to visualize this time span as a potentially meaningful one.

AGING PHYSICALLY: A PROCESS OF DECLINE

With aging, physical decline will occur. From the fourth decade onward, a gradual decline in vigor and resistance eventually gives way to various types of illnesses. In the opinion of many authorities, people do not die of old age. Rather, old age worsens specific conditions responsible for death. This process of decline can be described on the basis of predictable occurrences.[1]

▼ *Change is gradual.* In aging, there are gradual changes in body structure or function that occur before specific health problems are identified.

▼ *Individual differences occur.* When two people of the same age are compared for the type and extent of change that has occurred with age, major differences can be noted. Even within the same person, different systems decline at differing rates and to varying extents.

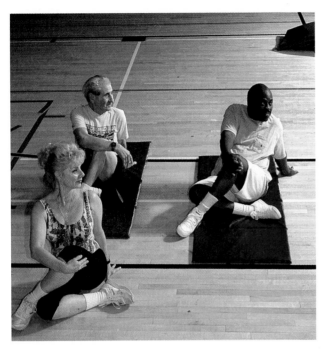

Exercise promotes healthy aging.

▼ *Greatest change is noted in areas of complex function*. In physiological processes involving two or more major body systems, the most profound effects of physiological aging can be noted.

▼ *Homeostatic decline occurs with age*. Becoming older is associated with a growing difficulty in maintaining homeostasis (the dynamic balance among body systems). In the face of stressors, the older adult's system takes longer to respond, does not respond with the same magnitude, and may take longer to return to baseline.

Like growth and development, aging is predictable yet unique for each person. Since the process of aging is extended over the course of time, much living must occur before one is "old." We begin exploring the aging process with middle age.

DEVELOPMENTAL TASKS OF THE MIDLIFE PERIOD

Have you wondered what it would be like to be 20 or 30 years older than you are now? What would you be doing, feeling, and thinking if you were the age of your parents? What are your parents thinking about and trying to accomplish as they move through their midlife years?

One thought that probably recurs all too often is the reality of their own eventual death. Their awareness that they will not live forever is a subtle but profoundly influential force that can cause them to be restless, to renew their religious faith, and to be more highly motivated to master the development tasks of

midlife. This motivation and the awareness of the reality of death combine to produce the dynamic concept of being at the prime of life—a time when there seems to be a great deal to accomplish and less time in which to accomplish it.

Achieving Generativity

In a very real sense, midlife persons are asked to do something they have not been expected to do previously. As a part of their development as unique persons, they are expected to pay back society for the support it has given them, and for the support it will give them during the latter years of their lives. Most persons in midlife begin to realize that the collective society, through its institutions (families, schools, churches), has been generous in its support of their own growth and development and that it is time to replenish these resources. Younger and older persons may have needs that middle-age persons can best meet. By meeting the needs of others, midlife persons can fulfill their own needs to grow and develop. *Generativity* reflects this process of contributing to the collective good.[2] Generativity benefits both midlife persons and society.

The process of repaying society for its support is structured around familiar types of activities. Developmentally speaking, midlife persons are able to select the activities that best use their ability to contribute to the good of society.[3]

The most traditional way in which midlife persons repay society is through parenting. Children, with their potential for becoming valuable members of the next generation, need the support of persons who recognize the contribution they can make. By supporting children, either directly through quality parenting or through institutions that function on behalf of children, middle-age persons repay society for the support they have themselves received. As they extend themselves outward on behalf of the next generation, they ensure their own growth and development. In similar fashion, their support of aging parents and institutions that serve the elderly provides another means to express generativity.

For persons who possess artistic talent, generativity may be accomplished through the pleasure brought to others. Artists, craftsmen, and musicians have unique opportunities to speak directly to others through their talents. Volunteer work serves as another avenue for generativity. Most midlife persons also express generativity through their jobs by providing quality products or services and thus contributing to the well-being of those who desire or need these goods and services.

A sense of intent is important to midlife persons in their quest for generativity. They need to feel that their efforts are important to others. This reinforces their intention to return something of real value to society. Thus generativity exists only when it is recog-

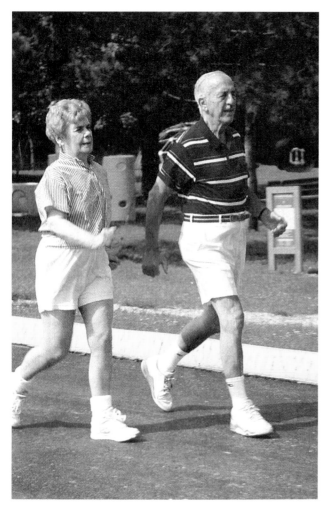

Active midlife adults.

nized in relation to midlife growth and development. The fact that midlife adults work or have children does not ensure that their developmental obligations are being met.

Reassessing the Plans of Young Adulthood

It is also essential for midlife persons to come to terms with the finality of their own deaths. Having done this, they often feel that it is time to think about their goals for adulthood they formulated 25 or more years previously. Their dreams must be revisited.[3] This reassessment constitutes a second developmental task of midlife adults.

By carefully reviewing the aspirations they had as young adults, middle-age persons can more clearly study their short- and long-term goals. Specifically, strengths and limitations that were unrecognizable when they were young adults are now more clearly seen. The inexperience of youth is replaced by the insights gained through experience. A commitment to quality often replaces the desire for quantity during the second half of the life cycle. Time is valued more

highly because it is now seen in a more realistic perspective. The dream for the future is more sharply focused, and the successes and failures of the past are more fully understood as this developmental task of reassessing earlier plans of young adulthood is accomplished.

The Midlife Crisis

As portrayed on television shows, the **midlife crisis** is a drastic and unexplainable "throwing in the towel" on life by a few middle-age men and women. Television viewers ask, "How can they do that? Why would they leave families, jobs, and communities where they have roots to strike out into the world as if they were nothing more than adolescents? Are they crazy?"

We hope that through this discussion of midlife we have helped you better understand why the midlife crisis can occur and why a few men and women make drastic decisions during this period. We are neither condoning nor condemning these kinds of choices. Rather, we are pointing out that midlife can be a precarious time of reflection and reassessment. For many midlife persons this reassessment coincides with a deeply personal sense of time vulnerability—life seems to be slipping by. They sense that personal growth and development should be occurring. If they are not, the alternatives appear to be limited. Dropping out and starting over may seem like an attractive alternative to facing the future. Fortunately, it is far from being a common experience for the middle-aged.

THE JOYS OF MIDLIFE

Contrary to some stereotypical views, the majority of midlife adults do not experience a multitude of problems that fill them with melancholy and despair. The lives of these midlife adults are characterized by positive elements. It is a myth that every midlife adult must have a midlife crisis. Most probably do not experience such an ordeal. Midlife adults may frequently find themselves more reflective than when they were young, but to label these behaviors damaging is to fail to appreciate the value of careful self-examination. Perhaps midlife adults just have more to think about then they did when they were younger.

From our perspective, much of what midlifers think about is positive. Many see themselves as being in the prime of life. Certain potentially difficult aspects of life have been completed. Many have completed a formal education, become established in an occupation, gained financial security, and raised a family. Midlife adults can find great satisfaction with these accomplishments and can begin planning for future challenges.

By being relatively free from financial problems and no longer responsible for young children, midlife adults can pursue some of their own dreams. For example, it is not surprising to see midlife adults travel more than they did earlier in life. Many midlifers rededicate themselves to a fitness program or a hobby, such as reading or gardening. Some seem to love reliving their own college days vicariously through the lives of their college-age children. For many midlifers, joyous moments also come with being grandparents.

Unfortunately, in very recent years the "downsizing" or "rightsizing" of corporate America has cost thousands of midlifers the jobs that they had held for two decades. The impact of midcareer job loss on all dimensions of health will be followed closely for those middle age persons who have been forced to rethink their plans for employment and retirement in the years ahead.

HEALTH CONCERNS OF MIDLIFE ADULTS

The period between 45 and 64 years of age brings with it a variety of subtle changes in the body's structure and function. When life is busy and the mind is active, these changes are generally not evident. Even when they become evident, they are not usually the source of profound concern. Your parents, older students in your class, and persons with whom you will be working are, nevertheless, experiencing these changes[4]:

▼ Decrease in bone mass and density
▼ Increase in vertebral compression
▼ Degenerative changes in joint cartilage
▼ Increase in adipose tissue—loss of lean body mass
▼ Decrease in capacity to engage in physical work
▼ Decrease in visual acuity
▼ Decrease in basal energy requirements
▼ Decrease in fertility
▼ Decrease in sexual function

For some midlife adults these health concerns can be quite threatening, especially those who view aging with apprehension and fear. Some middle-age persons reject these physical changes and convince themselves they are sick. Indeed, *hypochondriasis* is much more common among midlife persons than among young people.

Sexuality and Aging

Students are often curious about how aging affects sexuality. This is understandable because we live in a society that idolizes youth and demands performance. Many younger persons become anxious about growing older because of what they think will happen to their ability to express their sexuality. Interestingly, young adults are willing to accept other physical changes of aging (such as the slowing down of basal

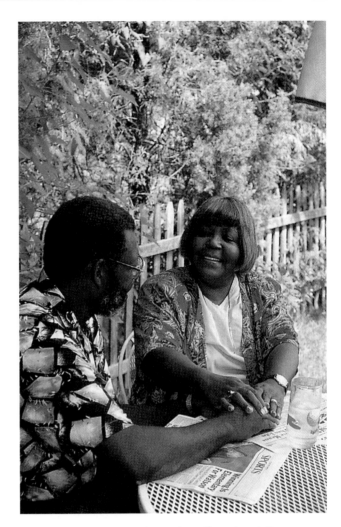

Sexual attraction continues throughout the adult years.

metabolism, reduced lung capacity, and even wrinkles) but not those changes related to sexuality.

Most of the research in this area suggests that older people are quite capable of performing sexually. As with other aspects of aging, certain anatomical and physiological changes will be evident, but these changes do not necessarily reduce the ability to enjoy sexual activity.[5] Most experts in sexuality report that many older persons remain interested in sexual activity. Furthermore, those who are exposed to regular sexual activity throughout a lifetime report being most satisfied with their sex lives as older adults.[5]

> **midlife crisis** period of emotional upheaval noted among some midlife persons as they struggle with the finality of death and the nature of their past and future accomplishments.

As people age, the likelihood of alterations in the male and female sexual response cycles increases. In the postmenopausal woman, vaginal lubrication commonly begins more slowly, and the amount of lubrication usually diminishes. However, clitoral sensitivity and nipple erection remain the same as in earlier years. The female capacity for multiple orgasms remains the same, although the number of contractions that occur at orgasm typically is reduced.

In the older man, physical changes are also evident. This is thought to be caused by the decrease in the production of testosterone between the ages of 20 and 60 years. After age 60 or so, testosterone levels remain relatively steady. Thus many men, despite a decrease in sperm production, remain fertile into their 80s. Older men typically take longer to achieve an erection (however, they are able to maintain the erection longer before ejaculation), have fewer muscular contractions at orgasm, and ejaculate less forcefully. The volume of seminal fluid ejaculated is typically less than in earlier years, and its consistency is somewhat thinner. The resolution phase is usually longer in older men. Despite these gradual changes, some elderly men engage in sexual intercourse with the same frequency as do much younger men.

Menopause

For the vast majority of women in their late 40s through their mid-50s, a gradual decline in reproductive system function, called *menopause*, occurs. Menopause is a normal physiological process, not a disease process.[6] It can, however, become a health concern for some women of middle age who experience unpleasant side effects resulting from this natural stoppage of ovum production and menstruation.

As ovarian function and hormone production diminish, a period of adjustment must be made by the hypothalamus, ovaries, uterus, and other estrogen-sensitive tissues.[6] The extent of menopause as a health problem is determined by the degree to which **hot flashes,** vaginal wall dryness, depression and melancholy, breast changes, and the uncertainty of fertility are seen as problems.

In comparison with past generations, today's midlife women are much less likely to find menopause to be a negative experience. The end of fertility, combined with children leaving the home, makes the middle years a period of personal rediscovery for many women. Many of the nontraditional students in our personal health classes agree on this.

For women who are troubled by the changes brought about by menopause, physicians may prescribe **estrogen replacement therapy** (ERT). This can relieve many symptoms, as well as offer benefits to help reduce the incidence of osteoporosis[7] (see p. 507) and heart disease (see Chapter 10).

Comorbidity

As adults age and move into their middle years (45 to 64), the likelihood of experiencing chronic health problems increases. When two or more diagnosed chronic health problems occur at the same time, a state of **comorbidity** exists. Tables 20-1 and 20-2 identify chronic conditions that can result in comorbidity. In Table 20-1 the 12 most common chronic health problems of midlife men and women are presented in order of prevalence. Table 20-2 depicts a second group of chronic health problems experienced by these men and women. Rather than being ranked by prevalence, however, the conditions in Table 20-2 are those that lead to limitations in primary or secondary activities. Although several health conditions appear on both lists, some of the more prevalent problems do not generate enough limitations to appear in Table 20-2. And, conversely, some chronic problems that cause marked limitations do occur in great prevalence and thus appear in Table 20-1.* For individuals with two, three, or more chronic health problems, several physicians are usually seen, and multiple prescription and OTC drugs may be taken. Consequently, failure to coordinate health care services for comorbidity can lead to drug interactions.[4]

TABLE 20-1   **Prevalent Chronic Health Problems[8]**

Rank	Men (45 to 64 years of age)	Women (45 to 64 years of age)
1	High blood pressure	Arthritis
2	Arthritis	High blood pressure
3	Hearing impairment	Chronic sinusitis
4	Chronic sinusitis	Hearing impairment
5	Coronary artery disease	Hay fever without asthma
6	Orthopedic impairment—lower back	Orthopedic impairment—lower back
7	Hay fever without asthma	Varicose veins
8	Hemorrhoids	Hemorrhoids
9	Orthopedic impairment—lower extremity	Chronic bronchitis
10	Visual impairment	Migraine headache
11	Diabetes	Diabetes
12	Ringing in ear	Bursitis

*Several of the conditions appearing in Tables 20-1 and 20-2 are discussed in other chapters of this textbook. For those conditions not discussed elsewhere, we recommend a basic home health guide, such as The American Medical Association's *Home Medical Encyclopedia.*

TABLE 20-2	Chronic Health Problems Causing Limitation in Activity[8]	
Rank	**Men (45 to 64 years of age)**	**Women (45 to 64 years of age)**
1	Diseases of the heart	Arthritis
2	Arthritis	Diseases of the heart
3	High blood pressure	High blood pressure
4	Orthopedic impairment—lower back	Orthopedic impairment—lower extremity
5	Other musculoskeletal disorders	Other musculoskeletal disorders
6	Orthopedic impairment—lower extremity	Diabetes
7	Diabetes	Orthopedic impairment—lower back
8	Atherosclerosis	Atherosclerosis
9	Emphysema	Cancer
10	Visual impairment	Asthma
11	Other respiratory disease	Depression
12	Paralysis	Digestive disease

Osteoporosis

Osteoporosis is a condition frequently seen in late middle-age women. However, it is not fully understood why white menopausal women are so susceptible to the increase in calcium loss that leads to fracture of the hip, wrist, and vertebral column. Well over 90% of all persons with osteoporosis are white women. The endocrine system plays a large role in the development of osteoporosis. At the time of menopause, a woman's ovaries begin a rapid decrease in the production of *estrogen*, one of the two hormones associated with the menstrual cycle. This lower level of estrogen may decrease the conversion of the precursors of vitamin D into the active form of vitamin D, the form necessary for absorbing calcium from the digestive tract. As a result, calcium may be drawn from the bones for use elsewhere in the body. Recent identification of a gene for the formation of vitamin D receptors may explain why some people are at greater risk for developing osteoporosis than others.[9]

Additional explanations of osteoporosis focus on two other possibilities—*hyperparathyroidism* (another endocrine dysfunction) and the below-average degree of muscle development seen in osteoporotic women. In this latter explanation the reduced muscle mass is associated with decreased activity that in turn deprives the body of the mechanical stimulation needed to facilitate bone growth.

Premenopausal women have the opportunity to build and maintain a healthy skeleton through an appropriate intake of calcium. Current recommendations are for an intake of 1200 mg of calcium per day. Three to four daily servings of low-fat dairy products should provide sufficient calcium. Adequate vitamin D must also be in the diet because it aids in the absorption of calcium.

Many women do not intake an adequate amount of calcium. Calcium supplements, again in combination with vitamin D, can be used to achieve recommended calcium levels. It is now known that calcium carbonate, a highly advertised form of calcium, is no more easily absorbed by the body than are other forms of calcium salts. In fact, calcium citrate may be more completely absorbed by older women. Consumers of calcium supplements should compare brands to determine which, if any, they will buy.

In premenopausal women, calcium deposition in bone is facilitated by exercise, particularly exercise that involves movement of the extremities. Today younger women are encouraged to consume at least the recommended servings from the milk group, engage in regular physical activity that involves the weight-bearing muscles of the legs, such as aerobics, jogging, or walking, and take calcium supplements if dietary sources are less than adequate.[10,11]

Postmenstrual women who are not elderly can markedly slow the resorption of calcium from their bones through the use of estrogen replacement therapy. When combined with a daily intake of 1500 mg of calcium, vitamin D, and regular exercise, estrogen therapy almost eliminates calcium loss. Of course, women will need to work closely with their physicians in monitoring the use of estrogen because of continuing concern over the role of estrogen replacement therapy and the development of endometrial (uterine) cancer.

hot flashes temporary feelings of warmth experienced by women during and following menopause, caused by blood vessel dilation.

estrogen replacement therapy (es tro jen) medically administered estrogen to replace estrogen lost as the result of menopause.

comorbidity (coe more **bid** ah tee) the occurrence of two or more diagnosed chronic health problems at the same time in an individual.

osteoporosis (os te oh po ro sis) loss of calcium from the bone, seen primarily in postmenopausal women.

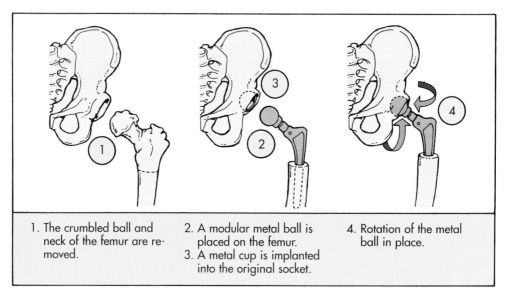

1. The crumbled ball and neck of the femur are removed.

2. A modular metal ball is placed on the femur.
3. A metal cup is implanted into the original socket.

4. Rotation of the metal ball in place.

Figure 20-1 Hip replacement surgery. Surgery usually lasts from 1 to 2 hours followed by hospitialization for several days. Use of crutches and a cane following surgery help reduce pressure on the new joint. Physical therapy with muscle-strenghtening exercises also follows.

Osteoarthritis

Arthritis is an umbrella term for more than 100 forms of joint inflammation. The most common form is **os-teoarthritis.** It is likely that, as we age, all of us will develop osteoarthritis to some degree. Often called wear and tear arthritis, osteoarthritis occurs primarily in the weight-bearing joints of the knee, hip, and spine. In this form of arthritis, joint damage can occur to bone ends, cartilaginous cushions, and related structures as the years of constant friction and stress accumulate. Osteoarthritis is most commonly seen in people over the age of 60.[12]

The object of current management of osteoarthritis (and other forms) is not to cure the disease but rather to reduce discomfort, limit joint destruction, and maximize joint mobility. Aspirin and nonsteroidal antiinflammatory agents are the drugs most frequently used to treat osteoarthritis.

In the last decade joint replacement surgery has become an increasingly popular method to relieve the pain, discomfort, and limited mobility associated with advanced osteoarthritis. As depicted in Figure 20-1, the neck and head of the femur are removed and a new metal or plastic cup is inserted into the acetabulum, or hip socket. Once these are inserted, the metal ball and femoral stem are placed into the shaft of the femur and cemented into place. Following recovery, patients report marked improvement.

It is now believed that osteoarthritis develops most commonly in persons with a genetic predisposition for excessive damage to the weight-bearing joints. Thus the condition seems to run in families. Furthermore, studies comparing the occurrence of osteoarthritis in those persons who exercise and those persons who do not demonstrate the finding that regular activity may decrease the likelihood of a person developing this form of arthritis.

THE ELDERLY YEARS

Most gerontologists, physicians, and other health experts see distinct developmental differences between adults in the midlife years (45 to 64) and those in their elderly years (65 and older). These differences are reflected in the social theories of aging.

Psychosocial Theories of Aging

Several theories have been developed in an attempt to explain how older adults feel and behave. Four of the more familiar of these theories are described. For each, we must anticipate an interplay of expectations and resources on the part of both individuals and society.

DISENGAGEMENT THEORY

Becoming elderly (over 65 years of age) is perceived by many people as a terribly unattractive, undesired, and perhaps even frightening occurrence. These perceptions form a basis for the *disengagement theory* of aging. According to this theory, while society slowly withdraws (disengages) from the elderly, the elderly also withdraw from society.[13] The movement away from cooperation and interaction fosters a sense of isolation. Society no longer wants or needs the elderly, and the elderly comply. Perhaps your generation, initially as younger persons and subsequently as the elderly, will largely reject this interpretation of what it means to grow old.

ACTIVITY THEORY

In contrast to a theory that depicts the elderly as being former members of society, proponents of the *activity theory* of aging see the elderly as being active and contributing for as long as possible. Research clearly shows that the young elderly (ages 65 to 74 years) routinely describe themselves as being middle aged. Most are active at least as long as they can do what they need to do and what they enjoy doing. Particularly for the young elderly living in urban areas and in sunbelt retirement communities, postretirement is a positive and active period of life. These elderly both contribute to the well-being of the society (through volunteer work, as foster grandparents, and as taxpayers) and work to develop or refine interests for themselves. In turn, society encourages their presence, supports their continued involvement, and values their contributions.

In some situations, however, the activity theory of aging may be misused by those working with older adults. When the elderly are forced into planned activities by those who feel that older adults must be active, the opportunity for stress is very real. Not every retired person wants the demanding schedule enjoyed by those elderly who fully subscribe to the activity theory of aging.

CONTINUITY THEORY

Midway between the disengagement and activity theories lies the *continuity theory* of aging.[13] This theory suggests that older adults will follow a familiar level of activity and intensity into their later years. Those who were essentially disengaged as young and middle-age adults will continue to be disengaged as elderly persons. Conversely, those who have been active as younger adults will either continue these activities or replace them with new activities when they reach senior citizen status. According to this theory, the elderly are consistent in their outlook and involvement with life. Furthermore, the continuity of older adults is encouraged by society. Older adults are neither restrained nor pushed, but rather allowed to age comfortably.

ABANDONMENT

Tragically for some elderly, particularly the sick, infirm, and minority elderly, society has little desire to continue contact and support. In turn, these old persons possess few resources and few friends. They allow themselves to become abandoned and are nonplayers in their later years.

Demographic Analysis of the Elderly

Like any segment of the population, today's older adults can be described on the basis of demographic data.[14] The box on p. 512 presents some of these data about *elderly adults* (persons 65 and older). Divisions within this group include the *younger elderly* (those

persons between 65 and 74 years of age) and the *older elderly* (those persons 75 years of age and over). It is interesting to note that the older elderly group represents the most rapidly growing segment of the American population.

Quality of the Elderly Years

For the elderly, as for all adults, the quality of life is often judged on the basis of the status of several traits or conditions. We believe that life will be described as being good by older persons who have not yet shown significant declines in the majority of areas to be described.

▼ *Health.* As long as the person feels well, has sufficient energy, and is not limited in terms of mobility, health is not a distracting factor to a good life.
▼ *Social status.* As long as the elderly person continues to participate in social activities that were enjoyed before retirement or the death of the spouse, social status remains unchanged and is not a negative factor in the quality of life.

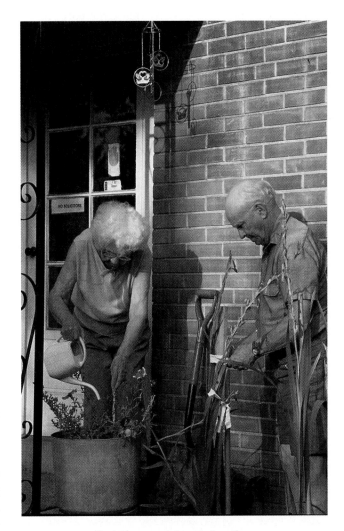

Exploring new interests together.

▼ *Economic status.* As long as income is sufficient to maintain an acceptable lifestyle, provide the basic necessities, and form a cushion against unexpected major expenses, economic status is not a negative factor in a good life.

▼ *Marital status.* For the majority of men, marital status remains unchanged. For women, widowhood can prove to be a significant factor detracting from the quality of life. If a support group can, in a sense, replace the spouse, the impact of a changed marital status can be minimized.

▼ *Living condition.* Only 5% of the elderly are living in nursing homes. As long as residential arrangements are unchanged or, if changed, undertaken with minimal disruption, living conditions are not significant factors in defining the quality of life.

▼ *Educational level.* Educational level in general and an active interest in learning and experimenting in particular seem to foster positive experiences during aging. Limited education may inhibit some elderly persons from learning more about the changing world around them.

▼ *Sexual intimacy.* Assuming the availability of a partner, sexual practices closely follow the patterns established during earlier periods of adulthood. As long as both partners are satisfied, adjustment is not adversely influenced. Divergent expectations can cause difficulty for one or both partners.

▼ For more specific information regarding many of these factors, see the box on p. 512.

WHY DO WE AGE?

Tissue, Cellular, and Subcellular Theories

Among the most intriguing questions in the biological sciences are those associated with an explanation of why humans age. Many diverse theories that focus on changes in organ systems, tissues, and cells have been proposed. Generally, these are grouped into two categories, damage theories and programed theories.[15]

DAMAGE THEORIES OF AGING
Free radical damage
Incomplete cellular oxidative processes result in the formation of highly unstable molecules known as free radicals. In their attempt to regain stability, these free radicals inflict damage to the cell, eventually resulting in diminished function. Some believe that antioxidative agents, such as vitamin E, vitamin A, and vitamin C, should be able to destroy free radicals before they can inflict damage.

> **osteoarthritis** (os te oh arth **rye** tis) arthritis that develops with age; largely caused by weight bearing and deterioration of the joints.

Collagen cross-linking
Collagen, the molecular building material of connective tissue, appears to undergo progressive structural changes with age. Because of the importance of this tissue to the structure of many important organs, collagen changes eventually alter the organs' functions. Free radicals may cause collagen molecules to cross-link.

Accumulation of harmful waste products
Somewhat similar to the free radical theory, this theory suggests that over time, metabolic efficiency within cells decreases. Faulty oxidation of metabolites results in the production of toxic waste products, including *lipofuscin,* a pigment found in the tissue of the elderly. *Amyloid,* a protein-related waste, is also found and probably represents altered oxidative processes.

Accumulation of faulty protein
Whether resulting from defective prescriptions for the composition of protein or faulty synthesis within the cell, the cells of the elderly may produce defective protein. Enzymes, hormones, and cellular structures requiring protein are negatively affected. Then organ systems begin to decline. Some researchers suggest, however, that changes in protein occur, but only after synthesis.

Error accumulation
The growth and repair of tissue require the continuous duplication of cells. The genetic message contained in

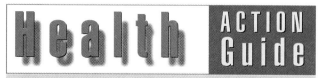

Tips for Talking with Aging Parents

When you are discussing sensitive topics with your aging parents (such as failing health, housing changes, and financial matters), Mark Edinberg, author of *Talking With Your Aging Parents,* suggests the following:

▼ Clearly explain the purpose and objectives of the conversation.
▼ Find out your parents' desires. Let them have a sense of control.
▼ Be assertive when necessary.
▼ Explore options; provide information that can be helpful in making decisions.
▼ Don't be patronizing; learn to accept the impact of potential changes in your parent(s).
▼ Don't make promises you cannot keep.

What Do You Know About Aging?

Erdman Palmore, author of the *The Facts on Aging Quiz: A Handbook,* developed the following quiz to stimulate discussions and identify misconceptions about aging. Test your knowledge about the elderly by answering yes or no to the following items:

	Yes	No
1. A person's height tends to decline in old age.	_____	_____
2. Older people have more acute (short-term) illnesses than people under 65.	_____	_____
3. The aged are more fearful of crime than are people under 65.	_____	_____
4. More of the aged vote than any other age group.	_____	_____
5. There are proportionately more older people in public office than in the total population.	_____	_____
6. Most old people live alone.	_____	_____
7. All five senses tend to decline in old age.	_____	_____
8. When the last child leaves home, the majority of parents have serious problems adjusting to their "empty nest."	_____	_____

	Yes	No
9. Aged people have fewer accidents per driver than drivers under 65.	_____	_____
10. One tenth of the aged live in long-stay institutions like nursing homes.	_____	_____
11. Most old people report they are seldom angry or irritated.	_____	_____
12. Most old people are socially isolated and lonely.	_____	_____
13. Most old people work or would like to have some kind of work (including housework or volunteer work).	_____	_____
14. Medicare pays more than half of the medical expenses for the aged.	_____	_____
15. Social Security benefits automatically increase with inflation.	_____	_____

INTERPRETATION

Answers to the odd-numbered questions are "yes" and to the even-numbered questions are "no."

TO CARRY THIS FURTHER . . .

What were the sources of the information on which you based your responses? How would you describe the quality of the relationships you have had thus far with older adults? What aspects of middle age do you find most and least attractive? Have you identified any misconceptions about older adults that you may have had?

PERSONAL ASSESSMENT

The Elderly: 1993 Data[14]

- ★ In 1992, the elderly population numbered 32.3 million.

- ★ For every 100 elderly men, there were 147 women.

- ★ Those who reach age 65 have an average life expectancy of an additional 17.4 years (19.0 years for females and 15.1 years for males).

- ★ The most rapid increase in the elderly population will be between 2010 and 2030, when the baby boomers reach retirement.

- ★ People age 65 and older will represent 13% of the population by the year 2000 and 20% by the year 2030.

- ★ In 1992, elderly men were nearly twice as likely to be married as elderly women (76% of men and 41% of women).

- ★ The majority of noninstitutionalized elderly (81% of men and 56% of women) lived in families; about 12% lived with children, siblings, or other relatives.

- ★ About 5% of the elderly lived in nursing homes.

- ★ In 1992, about half (52%) of all elderly persons lived in nine states (California, Florida, New York, Pennsylvania, Texas, Illinois, Ohio, Michigan, and New Jersey).

- ★ The median income for elderly persons in 1992 was $14,548 for males and $8,189 for females.

- ★ In 1992, one fifth (20%) of elderly people lived at the poverty or near-poverty level.

- ★ The educational level of the elderly for completion of high school has risen from 28% in 1973 to 60% in 1993.

- ★ Elderly people accounted for 35% of all hospital stays and 47% of all days of care in hospitals.

- ★ Benefits from government programs covered 63% of elderly people's health care expenditures.

the DNA of each cell must be replicated. However, each division exposes the genetic material to insults. At some point the cells' "repair genes" can no longer correct areas of DNA damage, resulting in enough altered cells that function is impaired and organ systems begin to falter.

PROGRAMED THEORIES OF AGING
Hayflict limit
This popular theory suggests that within cells (and thus within the entire organism) there exists a predetermined number of cellular replications (between 30 and 50), after which further activity is turned off. As more and more cells become overly mature (postmitotic), the functional capacity of the tissue declines. In this sense, aging results from the clock ticking down.

Neuroendocrine
A programed hormone appears that results in decreased oxygen consumption, which reduces the effectiveness of cellular oxidation. As oxidation becomes increasingly incomplete, the production of free radicals (damage theory) increases and cellular changes appear, followed by deteriorating function.

Immunological
The body's immune system begins to turn against the body in response to the programed presence of foreign-appearing protein complexes. This autoimmune response eventually weakens the body, resulting in an increase in diseases that eventually lead to death.

Death gene
Largely related to the Hayflict limit theory, this aging theory postulates that there is a gene programed to end life. This would occur by the gene causing gradual change in important biological functions. To date, no death gene has been located within human cells.

The Choices We Make

The choices we make earlier in life are not always the choices we would make again. Many elderly say they would have done some things differently, if they could do it over.*

Saved more money	51%
Traveled more	47%
Different career	31%
Lived elsewhere	18%
Married or married another	11%

*Survey participants could choose more than one response.

At the current time, the extent to which one or more of the many theories of biological aging explains the aging process is far from being resolved. It is apparent, however, that no one escapes the gradual progressive march toward aging and eventual death.

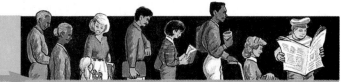

Learning FROM ALL Cultures

Elderly Asian-Americans

The lifestyles of many elderly Asian-Americans clearly reflect the differences between native cultures and traditions and those of their adopted country. The majority of Japanese-American, Filipino-American, and Chinese-American elderly came to the United States as adolescents or young adults.[16] Many of their children and grandchildren have been completely assimilated into American culture and society. Numerous instances can be found in which grandchildren (and even their parents) are unable to speak their grandparents' native language.

Many cultural traditions related to self-restraint and self-respect (including loyalty to family, respect for authority, and the importance of self-sufficiency) have been retained and reinforced by elderly Asian-Americans among family members and friends. Whether they live in the homes of their children and grandchildren or reside in the Chinatowns and Koreatowns of large American cities, in their late years many elderly Asian-Americans retain membership in ethnic support groups and follow religious practices that may no longer appeal to their own children. Although limited familiarity with and use of the American language may sometimes be a factor, a sense of well-being and healthfulness exists among many elderly Asian-Americans.

For those of you who are of Asian-American descent, are these characteristics similar to those that you have observed among your grandparents and older family members? If you were responsible for the de-

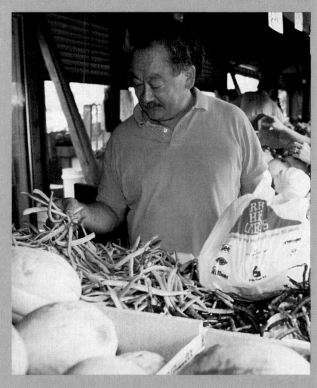

livery of heatlh or social services to older Asian-Americans, how would you work with these unique factors? What can the rest of us learn about our own elderly relatives and other senior citizens? ●

HEALTH CONCERNS OF ELDERLY ADULTS

In elderly persons it is frequently difficult to distinguish between changes caused by aging and those caused by disease. For virtually every body system, biomedical indexes for the old and young can overlap. In the respiratory system, for example, the oxygen uptake capacity of a man 70 years old may be no different from that of a man 55 years old who has a history of heavy cigarette smoking. Is the level in the elderly man to be considered an indicator of a disease, or should it be considered a reflection of normal old age? In dealing with the elderly, physicians frequently must make this kind of distinction.

In elderly persons, as in midlife persons, structural and physiological changes are routinely seen. In some

cases these are closely related to disease processes, but in most cases they reflect the gradual decline that is thought to be a result of the normal aging process. The most frequently seen changes include the following:

▼ Decrease in bone mass
▼ Changes in the structure of bone
▼ Decrease in muscle bulk and strength
▼ Decrease in oxygen uptake
▼ Loss of nonreproducing cells in the nervous system
▼ Decrease in hearing and vision abilities
▼ Decrease in all other sensory modalities, including the sense of body positioning
▼ Slower reaction time
▼ Gait and posture changes resulting from a weakening of the muscles of the trunk and legs

In addition to these changes, the most likely change seen in the elderly is the increased sensitivity of the body's homeostatic mechanism. Because of this sensitivity, a minor infection or superficial injury can be traumatic enough to decrease the body's ability to maintain its internal balance. An illness that would be easily controlled in a younger person could even prove fatal to a seemingly healthy 75-year-old person. Health can be an uncertain commodity for persons beyond the age of 65 years.

Comorbidity in Younger and Older Elderly Adults

As was found with middle-age adults (see Tables 20-1 and 20-2), both younger and older elderly adults can experience multiple chronic health problems.[8] Table 20-3 depicts the 12 most frequently occurring chronic health conditions found among men and women ages 65 to 74, and 75 years of age and older. When compared with comorbidity experienced by midlife adults (see Table 20-1), the elderly experience many of the same health conditions. It is not until men reach age 75 that arthritis and high blood pressure lose their rank as the most frequently experienced conditions. These are then replaced by hearing impairment. Women are even more consistent in terms of their incidence of comorbidity through the middle and elderly years than are men.

In terms of limitations in activity (Table 20-4), similar conditions cause loss of activity in the elderly as were reported for midlife persons (Table 20-2). As expected, the prevalence of limitations in activity is more common in the elderly than in the midlife group.

Alzheimer's Disease (Organic Brain Syndrome)

Although it affects fewer than 2% of elderly persons, organic brain syndrome, in either its acute or chronic form, is an incapacitating, heart-rending, and costly affliction. **Alzheimer's disease** represents the best known of the dementia disorders affecting between 3 and 4 million adults. Today, more than ever before, it is *the* disease associated with those individuals who have lived a long time.

The initial indication of Alzheimer's disease is often subtle and may be confused with mild depression. At this stage of the disease process, however, the person might experience some difficulty answering questions like these:

▼ Where are we now?
▼ What month is it?
▼ What is today's date?
▼ When is your birthday?
▼ Who is the President?

During the ensuing months, victims experience greater memory loss, confusion, and *dementia* (or loss of reasoning). In the most advanced stage, Alzheimer's victims experience incontinence, infantile behavior, and finally total incapacitation resulting from the de-

TABLE 20-3   Chronic Health Problems[8]

Rank	Men (65 to 74 years of age)	Women (65 to 74 years of age)
1	Arthritis	Arthritis
2	High blood pressure	High blood pressure
3	Hearing impairment	Hearing impairment
4	Coronary artery disease	Chronic sinusitis
5	Chronic sinusitis	Cataracts
6	Ringing in ear	Coronary artery disease
7	Diabetes	Diabetes
8	Visual impairment	Varicose veins
9	Other heart diseases	Orthopedic impairment—lower back
10	Atherosclerosis	Ringing in ear
11	Orthopedic impairment—lower back	Hemorrhoids
12	Hemorrhoids	Heart rhythm disorders

Rank	Men (75+ years of age)	Women (75+ years of age)
1	Hearing impairment	Arthritis
2	Arthritis	High blood pressure
3	High blood pressure	Hearing impairment
4	Cataracts	Cataracts
5	Coronary artery disease	Chronic sinusitis
6	Visual impairment	Visual impairment
7	Chronic sinusitis	Coronary artery disease
8	Atherosclerosis	Frequent constipation
9	Other hearing diseases	Atherosclerosis
10	Cerebrovascular disease	Varicose veins
11	Diabetes	Heart rhythm disorders
12	Ringing in ear	Other heart diseases

struction of brain tissue. Institutionalization of persons with advanced Alzheimer's disease is certain.

The precise diagnosis of Alzheimer's disease and other similar disorders remains difficult to make before the death of the victim. At that time, the characteristic *neurofibrillary tangles, neuritic plaques,* and loss of neurons can be identified. Before death, all other conditions capable of leading to dementia are individually ruled out. The initial diagnosis of Alzheimer's disease is made based on a process of elimination.

Several theories exist concerning the cause of Alzheimer's disease. Growing research indicates that

Rank	Men (65+ years of age)	Women (65+ years of age)
1	Diseases of the heart	Arthritis
2	Arthritis	Diseases of the heart
3	High blood pressure	High blood pressure
4	Emphysema	Diabetes
5	Arteriosclerosis	Orthopedic impairment—lower back
6	Visual impairment	Visual impairment
7	Diabetes	Arteriosclerosis
8	Orthopedic impairment—lower extremity	Orthopedic impairment—lower extremity
9	Cerebrovascular disease	Other musculoskeletal disorders
10	Paralysis	Cerebrovascular disease
11	Other musculoskeletal disorders	Paralysis
12	Orthopedic impairment—lower back	Cancer

TABLE 20-4 Chronic Health Problems Causing Limitation in Activity[8]

genetic mutations in chromosomes 14, 19, or 21 may encourage the development of the disease. Three genes on chromosome 19—E_2, E_3, and E_4—control the production of ApoE, a protein associated with amyloid production, and are thought to be related to the development of Alzheimer's disease. Today, people with two E_4 genes are thought to be particularly at risk.[17]

Additional theories suggest possible linkages between Alzheimer's disease and deficiencies in acetylcholine (a neurotransmitter) production, abnormal blood flow, and exposure to infectious agents or toxins.

Drugs to treat Alzheimer's disease effectively have not yet been developed. Although over 10 experimental drugs are currently being tested, none has been shown to have major impact upon reversing the disease. One drug, tacrine (brand name Cognex), has recently been approved for use in treating Alzheimer's disease. Tacrine facilitates the production of acetylcholine and appears to improve function when used early in the course of the disease.[18]

SPECIAL CONCERNS OF AGING ADULTS

Beyond the concerns common to all persons, aging adults have some special concerns, which reflect the many changes associated with aging, including physical change, retirement, and the changing composition of social groups.[19] Because of these concerns, planning for later life should begin in young adulthood. Particularly in regard to employment benefits, life and health insurance (including home care and nursing home care), and investment counseling, it is better to begin sooner rather than later.

Health-Care Services

As people age, the need for health care services increases. This reflects both the greater amount of illness in general, as well as the amount of chronic problems in the elderly. For older adults the frequency and length of hospitalization increase, rehabilitation services are more likely to become necessary, and prescription medication use increases. These services are expensive and likely to occur at the same time that earning potential is lost to retirement and group health insurance is no longer available. Medicare (see Chapter 17) offers some assistance, but many older adults are forced to use their savings to pay their health care bills.

Housing

Housing is an area of concern for many older adults. As children leave home, as income declines, and as physical restrictions become more common, aging adults may need (or want) to consider making some modification in their housing. Today many forms of households are available to older adults. Those listed range from fully independent living to newer and more innovative semiindependent living to familiar nursing home care:

▼ *Fully independent household.* The elderly person does 90% of the household tasks; perhaps a smaller home or a house with a different floor plan has replaced the home in which the individual once lived.
▼ *Semiindependent household.* The household is self-contained, but a greater degree of assistance in food preparation and residential maintenance is required. Various services can be secured to meet those needs that lie outside the ability of the elderly person.
▼ *Congregate housing.* A private household, often in the form of a small apartment, is maintained; food preparation, cleaning, and laundry services are provided. A full-service retirement community is an example.

Alzheimer's disease (alz hy mers) gradual development of memory loss, confusion, and loss of reasoning; can eventually lead to total intellectual incapacitation, brain degeneration, and death.

▼ *Nursing home.* At the skilled-level, this care is available for those who must have all needs met by others. Total care, incuding food, medical care, and personal care, is provided on a continuous basis at a high financial cost.

Transportation

Transportation represents another area of need that influences the elderly more than any other group of adults. The need to shop, visit with family and friends, attend religious services, and see a physician are particularly stressful for those who are unable to drive, no longer own an automobile, or do not have access to public transportation. In some communities the inability of the elderly to get around remains a largely unmet need. Figure 20-2 identifies problems faced by many elderly drivers.

Abuse

Among the nation's 31 million elderly persons, 1.5 million are the victims of neglect and abuse. Particularly vulnerable are elderly men over the age of 75 years. More often than not, the abusers are the spouses or adult children of the victims, who often reside with the abused.[20]

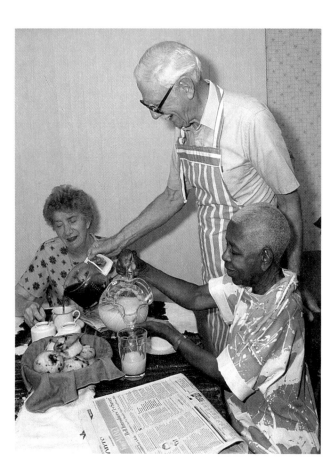

The elderhostel is an example of independent group housing.

Health ACTION Guide

Reducing Accidents

With decline in the accuracy of the senses, reaction time, and balance, the elderly experience a disproportionate number of accidents. More than 20% of all persons 75 years of age or older require medical treatment for injuries sustained during a fall. Most accidents of the elderly occur in the home.

Simple injuries occurring in elderly people who live alone can disrupt routines and force the elderly to care for themselves. Overall health often fails quickly after relatively minor injuries. To reduce accidents the following are suggested:

▼ Choose a single-story residence.
▼ Equip stairs with handrails and nonslip surfaces.
▼ Upgrade lighting.
▼ Equip bathrooms with handrails.

Many elderly persons are hit, kicked, attacked with knives, denied food and medical care, and have their Social Security checks and automobiles stolen. It is likely that this reflects a combination of factors, particularly the stress of caring for failing older persons by middle-age children who are also faced with the additional demands of dependent children and careers. In many cases, when children are the abusers, the children were themselves abused, or there may be a chemical dependence problem. The alternative, institutionalization, is so expensive that is often not an option for either the abused or the abusers.

Although protective services are available in most communities through welfare departments, elder abuse is frequently unseen and unreported. In many cases the elderly persons themselves are afraid to report being abused or neglected because of the fear of embarrassment that they were not good parents to their children or loving spouses. Most recently it has been recognized that much of elder abuse and neglect found by social workers or reported to Adult Protective Service may in fact be self-neglect on the part of elderly.[20] Failure to eat and refusal to take medication are the most common form of this type of abuse or neglect. Regardless of the cause, however, elder abuse must be reported to the appropriate protective service so that intervention can occur.

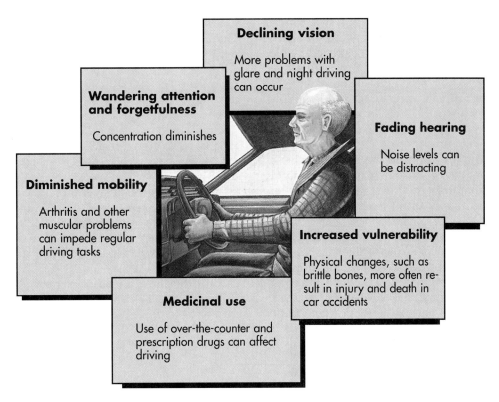

Declining vision

More problems with glare and night driving can occur

Wandering attention and forgetfulness

Concentration diminishes

Fading hearing

Noise levels can be distracting

Diminished mobility

Arthritis and other muscular problems can impede regular driving tasks

Increased vulnerability

Physical changes, such as brittle bones, more often result in injury and death in car accidents

Medicinal use

Use of over-the-counter and prescription drugs can affect driving

Figure 20-2 Although variations among individuals occur, the aging process can introduce problems that affect driving skills.

★ **Who Are the Caregivers?**

For many middle-age persons this period of their lives will include the role of caregiver. For them, becoming a parent to your parent is very real. A survey by the American Association of Retired Persons (AARP) reveals the following:

Average age of caregiver: 46 years old; most are women

Marital status: 66% are married

Living arrangements: 37% live with the care recipient*

Income: 47% have incomes over $25,000

Time: 50% spend approximately 12 hours per week caregiving

Additional expenses: 60% incur additional expenses for travel, telephone calls, special diets, and medicines

*Care recipients are most often the caregivers' mothers, at an average age of 77 years, and 70% have chronic illnesses.

DEVELOPMENTAL TASKS OF THE ELDERLY PERIOD

In this section we focus on the developmental tasks confronted by elderly persons. Accepting the physical decline of aging, maintaining high levels of physical function, and establishing a sense of integrity are tasks of the elderly period.

Accepting the Decline of Aging

The general decline associated with the second half of the life cycle is particularly serious between the seventh and eighth decades. Emotionally, socially, and intellectually, elderly persons must accept at least some decline. Even a spiritual loss may be encountered at those times when life seems less ordered or less humane. Clearly, a developmental task to be accomplished by the elderly is to accept the nature and extent of these losses.

To accept the losses brought about by the aging process, the elderly must first confirm them, usually in one of three ways. The elderly can verify the decline by *testing* for its presence. Depending on the area in question, the elderly can test for losses by trying to take part in activities of which they were previously capable. Failure to perform in an accustomed fashion can confirm the nature and extent of the decline.

Observing others is a second way the elderly can confirm their functional, structural, and emotional losses. When a particular loss can be seen in others, elderly people are able to confirm it in themselves much more easily.

The elderly can also confirm their own decline by *consulting* experts. Physicians and experts in other dimensions of gerontology can assist the elderly in confirming the type and extent of decline that have occurred.

The process of accepting the decline brought about by aging can, we believe, be facilitated by these processes. Actual acceptance of the decline, however, reflects an internalization of that which was confirmed. Of course, whether this will occur in a particular elderly person is a highly individual matter. However, we believe that this acceptance is vital for continued growth and development.

Maintaining High Levels of Physical Function

Because each segment of the life cycle should be approached with the fullest level of involvement possible, the elderly also should strive to maintain the highest level of physical function possible. Two approaches to achieving this level of function are rehabilitation and remediation.

For areas of decline in which some measure of reversal is possible, the elderly are afforded an opportunity to seek **rehabilitation.** Whether through an individually designed program or through the aid of a skilled professional, the elderly can bring back some function to a previously high level.

The second approach, often used in combination with rehabilitation, is **remediation,** whereby an alternative to the area of loss is introduced. Examples of remediation include the use of hearing aids, audio cassettes, and prescription shoes. By using alternative resources, function can often be returned and may actually be improved.

For a growing number of older adults, rehabilitation and remediation are rarely necessary because of the high level of physical fitness that they enjoy. For these older persons, muscular fitness, flexibility, body composition, and cardiorespiratory fitness have been maintained through regular physical conditioning activities (see Chapter 4). For most, only minor modifications are necessary to enjoy injury-free involvement. (see the Health Action Guide on p. 519.)

Should an even greater level of interest in physical fitness develop among adults of all ages, the future holds promise for even higher levels of health, continued independence, and enjoyable participation in day-to-day activities.

Establishing a Sense of Integrity

The third major development task that awaits the elderly is to establish a sense of *integrity,* or a sense of wholeness, concerning the journey that may be nearly complete.[2] The elderly must look back over their lives to see the value in what they were able to accomplish. They must address the simple but critical questions, "Would I do it over again?" "Am I satisfied with what I managed to accomplish?" "Can I accept the fact that others will have experiences to which I can never return?"

If the elderly can answer these questions positively, then they will feel a sense of wholeness, personal value, and self-worth. Having established this sense of integrity, they will believe that their lives have had meaning and fullness and that they have helped society.

Since they have already experienced so much, many elderly people have no fear of death, even though they may fear the process of dying. Their ability to come to terms with death thus reinforces their sense of integrity.

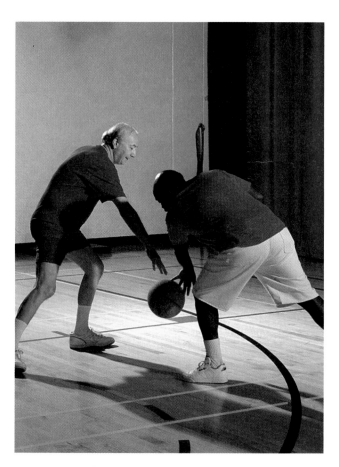

Activity enhances social contact.

Health ACTION Guide

Tips for Exercising Safely

In Chapter 4, physical fitness was described in terms of its components and the benefits to be derived from participation in fitness activities. Cardiovascular fitness was presented as a most beneficial component, and a training program to enhance aerobic capacity was described.

With recent research indicating that life expectancy can be increased through regular physical conditioning, older adults may now be inclined more than ever before to begin or continue an endurance-based conditioning program. This can be done safely and effectively if these steps to safe exercise are considered:

▼ Have a medical checkup and talk with your physician before beginning your program. Continue to consult with your physician during your conditioning program.

▼ If possible, join an exercise class for older adults. Make certain that the instructor is experienced in working with older students. Be certain your instructor is certified in CPR.

▼ Start your participation slowly. Keep records of your progress.

▼ Wear loose, comfortable clothing. Invest in good quality exercise shoes.

▼ Establish a schedule that allows you to exercise three to four times per week. Set aside sufficient time to warm up and cool down.

▼ Exercise 30 to 60 minutes per session, preferably with a friend.

▼ Choose a type of activity that will allow you to have fun when you are exercising. Walking is frequently the most appropriate activity for elderly persons.

▼ Pay attention to your body. Do not exercise if you are ill or injured. Call your doctor if you experience chest pain, breathlessness, joint discomfort, or muscle cramps.

▼ Become involved in your conditioning program—read books and articles. Share your experiences with other participants.

▼ Practice seeing yourself as a healthier, more fit person. Imagery is valuable in obtaining the maximum benefit possible from the fitness program.

When cardiovascular fitness is the focus of the overall fitness program, the formula for intensity presented in Chapter 4 can be used by older adults in calculating a training rate, with a reduction in the percentage of the maximum heart rate used in the calculation. Depending on age and medical status, an intensity rate of 40% to 60% of the maximum heart rate, rather than 75%, will provide a training effect. The frequency and duration of training are consistent with the information presented in Chapter 4. ▼

Like all of the other developmental tasks, this critical area of growth and development is a personal experience. The elderly must assume this last developmental task with the same sense of purpose they used for earlier tasks. When elderly people can feel this sense of integrity, their reasons for having lived will be fully understood.

rehabilitation (re ha bil ih **tay** shun) return of function to a previous level.

remediation (re me dee **ay** shun) development of alternative forms of function to replace those that have been lost or were poorly developed.

*Organizations on Aging

U.S. Commissioner
Administration on Aging
Department of Health and Human Services
Kohen Building
330 Independence Avenue, S.W.
Washington, D.C. 20201
(202) 619-0724

American Association of Retired Persons (AARP)
601 E Street, N.W.
Washington, D.C. 20049
(202) 434-2277

American Health Care Association
1201 L Street, N.W.
Washington, D.C. 20005
(202) 842-4444

American Society on Aging
833 Market Street
Suite 512
San Francisco, CA 94103
(415) 882-2910

Children of Aging Parents
1609 Woodbourne
Suite 302A
Levittown, PA 19057
(215) 345-5104

Foundation for Hospice and Home Care
519 C Street, N.E.
Washington, D.C. 20002
(202) 547-6586

Gray Panthers
2025 Pennsylvania, N.W.
Suite 821
Washington, D.C. 20006
(202) 466-3132

National Association for Home Care
519 C Street, N.E.
Washington, D.C. 20002
(202) 547-7424

National Council of Senior Citizens
1331 F Street, N.W.
Washington, D.C. 20004-1171
(202) 347-8800

National Council on the Aging, Inc.
409 3rd Street, S.W.
2nd Floor
Washington, D.C. 20024
(202) 479-1200

National Hospice Organization
1901 N. Moore Street
Suite 901
Arlington, VA 22209
(703) 243-5900

National Rehabilitation Information Center (NARIC)
8455 Colesville Rd.
Suite 935
Silver Spring, MD 20910
(800) 34-NARIC
(301) 588-9284 (Washington, D.C.)

National Senior Citizens Law Center
1815 H Street, N.W.
Suite 700
Washington, D.C. 20006
(202) 887-5280

The Older Women's League (OWL)
666 11th Street, N.W.
Washington, D.C. 20001
(202) 783-6686

Alzheimer's Association
919 N. Michigan Avenue
Suite 1000
Chicago, IL 60611

Arthritis Consulting Services
(800) 327-3027

Summary

✔ Aging is a positive process of continued growth and development, although physical decline is inevitable.

✔ Midlife adults (ages 45 to 64) have two key developmental tasks: achieving generativity and reassessing the plans of young adulthood.

✔ Although most middle age adults find midlife enjoyable, some experience a midlife crisis.

✔ Health concerns of midlife adults reflect subtle changes in the body's structure and function. Issues surrounding sexuality and menopause are important for midlife adults.

✔ Comorbidity conditions of middle age parallel those of late adulthood.

✔ Osteoporosis and osteoarthritis are conditions experienced for the first time during middle age.

✔ Psychosocial theories of aging look at older people and their environment.

✔ Numerous explanations of physical aging have been developed, but no single theory seems capable of explaining *why* the body ages.

✔ Health concerns of the elderly are, in many cases, a continuation of those same concerns of middle age.

✔ Alzheimer's disease can develop slowly and eventually cause brain degeneration and death.

✔ The elderly have special concerns, including health care, housing, transportation, and abuse and neglect.

✔ Developmental tasks of the elderly years include accepting aging, maintaining physical function, and establishing a sense of integrity.

Review Questions

1. What consistent traits characterize physical aging?
2. What are the principal developmental tasks of middle age?
3. What is a midlife crisis? How can the reality of one's own mortality influence midlife growth and development?
4. What physiological and emotional changes constitute menopause?
5. What comorbidity conditions are prevalent in midlife?
6. Why does osteoporosis develop in women of middle age and older rather than in younger women?
7. What are four principal psychosocial theories of aging and how are they different?
8. What are the principal points within the damage and programed theories of aging?
9. Describe the progression of Alzheimer's disease.
10. What are some of the special concerns of older adults?

Think about This . . .

✔ Based on your contact with middle-age persons, in your opinion, how common is midlife crisis, and what are the precipitating factors?

✔ Projecting forward to your own middle and later adult years, do you think you will be able to accept your own decline? How easy or difficult has that been for older adults you have known?

✔ Would you participate in a high-risk research project if there was some possibility of retarding or reversing the aging process?

✔ If you were now elderly, what would your physical limitations most likely be? Which phychosocial theory of aging would be most reflective of your approach to living? To what extent would you be experiencing a sense of intergrity?

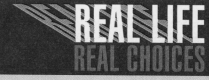

YOUR TURN

▼ What are the psychosocial theories of aging? Which theory seems to apply to both of Josh's grandmothers? Give reasons for your answer.

▼ What are the factors that influence an elderly person's quality of life? Which might apply to either or both of Josh's grandmothers?

▼ What are some steps Josh's Grandmother Washington might take to help herself live a more satisfying life?

AND NOW, YOUR CHOICES . . .

▼ If one or more of your grandparents are living, how would you describe each one's overall attitude and behavior? Do you enjoy being in their company, deliberately avoid them, or feel indifferent toward them? Give reasons for your answer.

▼ Is there an elderly person (relative or not) whom you admire and respect—the kind of person you'd like to be when you yourself are elderly? If so, what qualities do you like in this person and why? ▼

References

1. Cavanaugh J: *Adult development and aging,* Belmont, Calif, 1990, Wadsworth.
2. Erikson E: *Childhood and society,* New York, 1963, WW Norton.
3. Levinson D: *The seasons of a man's life,* New York, 1978, Alfred A Knopf.
4. Ferrini AF, Ferrini RL: *Health in the later years,* ed 2, Madison, Wis, 1992, Brown & Benchmark.
5. Haas K, Haas A: *Understanding sexuality,* ed 3, St Louis, 1993, Mosby.
6. Denney NW, Quadagno D: *Human sexuality,* ed 2, St Louis, 1992, Mosby.
7. Felson D, et al: The effect of postmenopausal estrogen therapy on bone density in elderly women, *N Engl J Med* 329(16):1141-1146, 1993.
8. Verbrugge LM: Recent, present, and future health of American adults, *Ann Rev Pub Health* 10:333, 1989.
9. Mundy GR: Boning up on genes, *Nature* 367:216-217, 1994.
10. Reid I, et al: Effect of calcium supplementation on bone loss in postmenopausal women, *N Engl J Med* 328(7):460-464, 1993.
11. Recker R, et al: Bone gain in young adult women, *JAMA* 268(17):2403-2408, 1992.
12. Hamann B: *Disease: identification, prevention and control,* St Louis, 1994, Mosby.
13. Atchley R: *Social forces and aging,* Belmont Calif, 1991, Wadsworth.
14. A profile of older Americans: 1993, Program Resource Department, Washington, DC, 1993, American Association of Retired Persons.
15. Hampton J: *The biology of human aging,* Dubuque, Iowa, 1991, William C Brown.
16. Hooyman NR, Kiyak HA: *Social gerontology,* ed 3, Needham, Mass, 1993, Allyn & Bacon.
17. Travis J: New piece in Alzheimer's puzzle, *Science,* 261:828-829, 1993.
18. Davis K et al: A double-blind, placebo-controlled multi-center study of tacrine for Alzheimer's disease, *N Engl J Med* 327(18):1253, 1992.
19. *Aging America: trends and projection* (annotated), Washington, DC, 1990, Special Committee On Aging, United States Senate (serial no. 101-j).
20. Deets HB: AARP study sheds new light on elder abuse, *AARP Bulletin* 34(3):3, 1993.

Suggested Readings

Annas GJ: *The rights of patients: the ACLU guide to patient rights,* ed 2, Totowa, NJ, 1992, Humana Press.

This handbook explains patients' rights and how they can be asserted within the medical system. Designed for laypersons, this is written in an easy-to-read question-and-answer format.

Dixon BM, Wilson J: *Good health for African Americans,* New York, 1994, Crown Publishers.

The health gap between black and white Americans of all ages (and income levels) is clearly documented. Introduces a 24-week program for nutritional and lifestyle changes over the course of the life cycle, including the elderly years.

Gordon S, Brecher H: *Life is uncertain . . . eat dessert first,* New York, 1990, Delacorte.

A positive self-help book that shows readers how to enjoy life by approaching day-to-day obstacles with a program of positive thinking and action. A practical, humorous, and beneficial book that older readers will especially enjoy.

Dying and Death

The Last Transitions

The primary goal of this chapter is to help people realize that the reality of death can serve as a focal point for a more enjoyable, productive, and contributive life. Each day in our lives becomes especially meaningful only after we have fully accepted the reality that someday we are going to die. We can then live each day to its fullest, as if it were our last day.

Our mortality provides us with a framework from which to appreciate and conduct our lives. It should help us prioritize our activities so that we can accomplish what we want to accomplish (in our academic work, our relationships with others, our recreation) before we die. Quite simply, death gives us our only absolute reason for living.

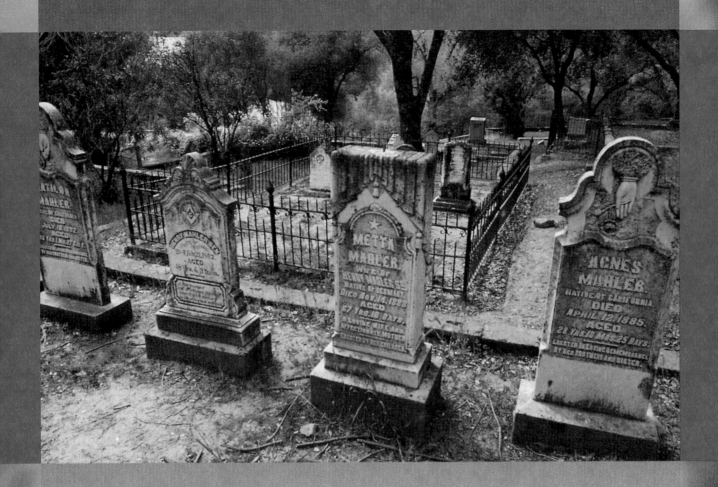

DYING AND DEATH

The following objectives are covered in this chapter:

▼ Increase years of healthy life to at least 65 years. (Baseline: An estimated 62 years in 1980; p. 532.)

▼ Reduce deaths caused by unintentional injuries to no more than 29.3 per 100,000 people. (Age-adjusted baseline: 34.5 per 100,000 in 1987; p. 273.)

▼ Reduce deaths from work-related injuries to no more than 4 per 100,000 full-time workers. (Baseline: Average of 6 per 100,000 in 1983-87; p. 298.)

▼ Reduce infant mortality to no more than 7 per 1000 live births. (Baseline: 10.1 per 1000 live births in 1987; p. 368.)

▼ Reduce coronary heart disease deaths to no more than 100 per 100,000 people. (Age-adjusted baseline: 135 per 100,000 in 1987.)

▼ Reverse the rise in cancer deaths to achieve a rate of no more than 130 per 100,000 people. (Age-adjusted baseline: 133 per 100,000 in 1987; p. 418.)

REAL LIFE
REAL CHOICES
Love and Loss: When a Friend is Dying

▼ **Name:** Wendy DuBois
▼ **Age:** 21
▼ **Occupation:** Physical education student

EXIT 47B-SHORE POINTS reads the green and white sign just ahead on Wendy's right. The cloudless blue sky and brisk offshore breeze promise another perfect beach day, but that's not where Wendy's going. Instead of joining the crawling knot of ocean-bound vehicles in the left lane of the exit ramp, Wendy whisks along the empty right lane, following the sign that says **SOUTH SHORE MEDICAL CENTER.**

No trace of the sparkling summer day follows Wendy through the whispering revolving door at the hospital's entrance. In here, she thinks, the weather is always the same: cool, dim, windless.

The west wing of the fifth floor is quiet this early July afternoon, and patients are sleeping or resting in many of the rooms Wendy passes. At the half-open door to Room 518 she pauses, feeling overwhelmed once again by the surge of conflicting emotions that wash over her every time she sees Jenny in this bed. As always, her impulse is to say, "Come on—let's get out of here," as if those words would magically cause the tubes and needles in Jenny's arms to vanish, the bruises to fade, the glow of health to return to her pale cheeks, the horror of the last several months to seep back into the black hole from which it emerged.

"Hey, Zebra!" As always, Jenny has sensed Wendy's presence without having seen her, and now she turns toward her best friend with the smile that even radiation and chemotherapy haven't dimmed.

"Hey, Wing," Wendy replies, in a ritual that dates back to their days on the junior high field hockey team.

It seems like just last week that they were eager novices at the game they both grew to love. But it was almost 10 years ago, Wendy reflects. How fast the time has gone, how fast it's going now, how suddenly Jenny got sick, how soon she'll…"NO!," screams a voice inside Wendy. No—she isn't dying, she can't, I won't let her. But she's in pain, says another voice. She still laughs, banters with the nurses, is cheerful with me and with her family. But the shadow is over her, it's growing longer every day. I can't stand to let her go, and I can't stand to see how hard she has to work to keep *us* from being afraid.

Fear is just one of the emotions Wendy feels as she helplessly watches her best friend lose ground every day to the ravages of leukemia. Terror, anguish, rage, and hope all do battle within her as she tries to accept the fact Jenny is dying. Sometimes Wendy sees the mute pleading in Jenny's eyes and knows her friend is weary and longing for release from pain, drugs, nausea, from other people's fears and expectations, from the effort it costs her to fight for one more day. For Wendy it seems impossible to choose between encouraging Jenny to hang on and acknowledging her need to let go, between talking about her recovery and dealing with her reality. I love you, Jenny, Wendy says silently. I want to help you do it your way.

As you study this chapter, think about Wendy's feelings as she tries to come to terms with Jenny's dying, and prepare yourself to answer the questions in **Your Turn** at the end of the chapter. ▼

PERSONAL DEATH AWARENESS

Since shortly after the turn of the century, the manner in which people experience death in this society has changed significantly. Formerly most people died in their own homes, surrounded by family and friends. Young children frequently lived in the same home with their aging grandparents and saw them grow older and eventually die. Death was seen as a natural extension of life. Children grew up with a keen sense of what death meant, both to the dying person and the grieving survivors.

Times have indeed changed. Today approximately 70% of people die in hospitals, nursing homes, and extended care facilities, not in their own homes. The extended family is seldom at the bedside of the dying person.[1] Frequently, frantic efforts are made to keep a dying person from death. Although medical technology may have improved our lives, some persons believe that it has reduced our ability to die with dignity. Many are convinced that our way of dying has become more artificial and less civilized than it used to be. (The trend toward hospice care may be a positive response to this high-tech manner of dying; see p. 532.)

Because we have been raised in a society that shields us from death in many ways, it is natural for us to deny the reality of our own deaths.[2] Unfortunately, by doing so we open ourselves to a variety of unpleasant situations. These situations start to present themselves when we begin to fully realize that others around us do die. We may begin to feel uneasy when a friend, grandparent, or parent dies. When we hear about disasters or terrorist bombings, we may start to believe that we, too, may die someday. Most of us persist in ignoring this thought. We continue to deny the inevitability of our own deaths.

Worden and Proctor[3] believe that the confusion or dissonance created with our death denial is unhealthful since it breeds feelings of helplessness and vulnerability, which will eventually lead to one of the following three situations:

▼ *Fear and anxiety.* Unresolved fear and anxiety commonly cause neurotic behavior. Phobias, compulsions, and even hypochondriasis may result.

▼ *Futility and alienation.* The conflicts generated by death denial can lead to an existential type of depression in which a person can have profound doubts about the value of living. Worden and Proctor think such a depression can ultimately lead to suicide or a **willed death.**

▼ *Frustration and anger.* Persons who are unable to cope with the reality of death may react by becoming aggressive. Ultimately, with frustration, rage, and aggression, people can become homicidal. Perhaps they believe that by controlling the fate of another person, they have in some manner mastered their own fate.

Because of the pitfalls associated with the denial of death, many death educators are supporting the concept of *personal death awareness,* or the acceptance of the fact that you are going to die. Personal death awareness allows you to put your life in a clearer, more comfortable, meaningful perspective. The goal is not to make you so cognizant of your own potential death that you live in constant fear of its coming. Rather, the goal is a positive, healthy one. We can best gain personal death awareness by undertaking some of the activities that force us to deal with our own mortality. We discuss many of these activities in the section entitled "Personal Preparation for Death" on p 537.

DEFINITIONS OF DEATH

Upon your death, would you want your estate to spend thousands of dollars a year for your body or head to be frozen in liquid nitrogen to await the development of thawing technology and a medical cure that could bring you back to life? If so, you might be interested in the pseudoscience of **cryonics.** Already a few hundred people have consented to be frozen in hopes of cheating death. Scientists, however, believe that their wait will be very long.

In contrast with cryonics is the science of **cryobiology,** in which the effects of freezing on living tissues are studied. Already cyrobiologists have contributed to our ability to preserve tissue for transplanting, such as fertilized ova. Cryobiologists doubt, however, that science will overcome the enormous problems associated with thawing a frozen human.

Before many of the scientific advancements of the past 30 years, death was relatively easy to define. People were considered dead when a heartbeat could no longer be detected and when breathing ceased. Now, with the technological advancements made in medicine (especially emergency medicine), some patients and accident victims who give every indication of being dead can be resuscitated. Critically ill persons (even those in comas) can now be kept alive for years with many of their body functions maintained by medical devices, including feeding tubes and respirators.

Thus death can be a very difficult concept to define. Numerous professional associations and ad hoc interdisciplinary committees have struggled with this problem and have developed criteria by which to establish death. Some of these criteria have been adopted by state legislatures, although there certainly is no consensus definition of death that all states embrace.

Clinical determinants of death refer to measures of bodily functions. Often judged by a physician (who can then sign a legal document called a medical death certificate), these clinical criteria include the following:

1. Lack of heartbeat and breathing.
2. Lack of central nervous system function, including all reflex activity and environmental responsiveness. Often this can be corroborated by an **electroencephalograph** reading. If there is no brain wave activity following an initial measurement and a second measurement after 24 hours, the person is said to have undergone *brain death.*
3. The presence of **rigor mortis,** indicating that body tissues and organs are no longer functioning at the cellular level. This is sometimes referred to as *cellular death.*

The *legal determinants* used by government officials are established by state law and often adhere closely to the clinical determinants already listed. A person is

willed death a death in which a person gives up the desire to live and merely waits to die.

cryonics (**cry** on icks) an unproven technology in which dead bodies are frozen in hopes of preserving tissues until disease cures are found.

cryobiology (**cry** oh by **ol** ahgee) the science of freezing living tissues.

electroencephalograph (e lek tro en **sef** a low graph) instrument that measures the electrical activity of the brain.

rigor mortis (**rig** er **more** tiz) rigidity of the body that occurs after death.

The Suicide Machine

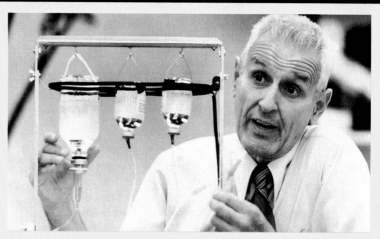

In June 1990 Dr. Jack Kevorkian first used his suicide machine on Janet Adkins, a 54-year-old early-stage Alzheimer's patient. The machine consisted of three bottles: one containing saline solution, another containing a pain killer, and a third containing potassium chloride. After placing an intravenous needle in the patient's arm, Dr. Kevorkian watched his patient push a red button that replaced the saline with the pain killer. Shortly afterward, the deadly potassium chloride replaced the pain killer. Within minutes, the patient's heart stopped beating.

More recently Dr. Kevorkian's technology for "medicide" or "physician-assisted suicide" has involved the use of carbon monoxide. Now after an interview and videotaped request to die, a patient is fitted with a mask that attaches to a cylinder of CO and provided instructions on how to administer the lethal gases.

On March 31, 1993, physician-assisted suicide became illegal in the state of Michigan. Dr. Kevorkian was jailed to await clarification of the Michigan physician-assisted suicide law. On May 3, 1994, a Michigan jury found Dr. Kevorkian innocent of assisting a person to commit suicide. Rather, the jury decided that Dr. Kevorkian had attempted only to help his patient find relief from the pain and discomfort associated with Lou Gehrig's disease. Supporters of physician-assisted suicide hailed the jury's decision, while opponents saw Dr. Kevorkian as being freed by a loophole in the Michigan law against assisted suicide.

Today, polls suggest that nearly 85% of the American public favor some process by which physicians can help people to die with dignity. Police, prosecutors, and medical ethicists are waiting to see whether Congress will adopt a law that provides carefully controlled measures for physicians to assist the dying, or if the Supreme Court will decide that laws preventing physician-assisted suicide are in violation of the Constitution. ★

---

not legally dead until a death certificate is signed (by a physician, **coroner,** or health department officer).

In addition to the constructs for physical and legal death, could it be possible that there are other forms of death? For persons who have lost contact with reality, could psychological death exist? For those who reject all contact with others, could social death exist? For persons who fail to recognize the existence of a supreme being, could spiritual death exist? If so, how many other forms of death can you identify?

EUTHANASIA

There are two types of euthanasia for desperately ill persons: they are either intentionally put to death (direct euthanasia) or allowed to die without being subjected to heroic lifesaving efforts (indirect euthanasia). **Direct (active) euthanasia** usually involves the administration of large amounts of depressant drugs, which eventually causes all central nervous system functions to stop. Although direct euthanasia is commonly practiced on household pets and laboratory animals, it is illegal for humans in the United States, Canada, and other developed countries. However, in February 1992, The Netherlands became the first developed country to enact legislation that permits euthanasia under strict guidelines. Also, see the Star box above, which discusses the suicide machine.

Indirect (passive) euthanasia is increasingly occurring in a number of hospitals, nursing homes, and medical centers. Physicians who withhold heroic lifesaving techniques or drug therapy treatments or who disconnect life support systems from terminally ill patients are practicing indirect euthanasia. Although some people still consider this form of euthanasia a type of murder, indirect euthanasia seems to be gaining legal and public acceptance for victims of certain terminal illnesses—near-death cancer patients, brain-dead accident victims, and hopelessly ill newborn babies. Physicians' orders of "Do Not Resuscitate" and "Comfort Measures Only" (referred to as DNR and CMO) are examples of passive euthanasia that are familiar to hospital personnel.

Because some physicians and families find it difficult to support indirect euthanasia, many people are starting to use legal documents called advance medical directives. One of these medical directives is the living will. This is a document that confirms a dying

★ The Living Will

The living will is a legally binding document in all 50 states and the District of Columbia. This document allows individuals to express their wishes concerning dying with dignity. When such a document has been drawn, families and physicians are better able to deal with the wishes of persons who are near death from conditions from which there is no reasonable expectation of recovery. The following is a generic living will. However, people should use a living will that is specific for the state in which they live. For additional information and materials, contact the Choice in Dying organization by using the toll-free number 1-800-989-WILL. ★

INSTRUCTIONS

Choice In Dying Living Will

PRINT YOUR NAME

I, _____,
being of sound mind, make this statement as a directive to be followed if I become permanently unable to participate in decisions regarding my medical care. These instructions reflect my firm and settled commitment to decline medical treatment under the circumstances indicated below:

I direct my attending physician to withhold or withdraw treatment if I should be in an incurable or irreversible mental or physical condition with no reasonable expectation of recovery.

These instructions apply if I am a) in a terminal condition; b) permanently unconscious; or c) if I am minimally conscious but have irreversible brain damage and will never regain the ability to make decisions and express my wishes.

I direct that treatment be limited to measures to keep me comfortable and to relieve pain, including any pain that might occur by withholding or withdrawing treatment.

While I understand that I am not legally required to be specific about future treatments, if I am in the condition(s) described above I feel especially strongly about the following forms of treatment:

CROSS OUT ANY STATEMENTS THAT DO NOT REFLECT YOUR WISHES

    I do not want cardiac resuscitation (CPR).
    I do not want mechanical respiration.
    I do not want tube feeding.
    I do not want antibiotics.

    However, I do want maximum pain relief, even if it may hasten my death.

ADD PERSONAL INSTRUCTIONS (IF ANY)

Other directions (insert personal instructions):

These directions express my legal right to refuse treatment, under federal and state law. I intend my instructions to be carried out, unless I have rescinded them in a new writing or by clearly indicating that I have changed my mind.

SIGN AND DATE THE DOCUMENT AND PRINT YOUR ADDRESS

Signed: _____ Date: _____

Address: _____

WITNESSING PROCEDURE

I declare that the person who signed this document is personally known to me and appears to be of sound mind and acting of his or her own free will. He or she signed (or asked another to sign for him or her) this document in my presence.

Witness: _____

Address: _____

TWO WITNESSESS MUST SIGN AND PRINT THEIR ADDRESSES

Witness: _____

Address: _____

© 1994 Choice In Dying, Inc. 1/94
200 Varick Street, New York, NY 10014 1-800-989-WILL

PAGE 2

---

person's desire to be allowed to die peacefully and with a measure of dignity if a time should arise when there is little hope for recovery from a terminal illness or major injury. Living will statutes exist in all 50 states and the District of Columbia.[4] The living will requires that physicians or family members carry out a person's wishes to die naturally, without receiving life-sustaining treatments.[5] About 20% of U.S. citizens have signed living wills.[6]

A second important document that can assist terminally ill or incapacitated patients is the **durable power of attorney for health care** document. This legal document authorizes another person to make specific health-care decisions about treatment and care under specified circumstances, most commonly in dire circumstances when patients are in long-term vegetative states and cannot communicate their medical wishes

coroner (core en er) an elected legal official empowered to pronounce death and to determine the official cause of a suspicious or violent death.

direct (active) euthanasia (you than **a** sha) process of inducing death, often through the injection of lethal drugs.

indirect (passive) euthanasia process of allowing a person to die by disconnecting life support systems or withholding lifesaving techniques.

durable power of attorney for health care a legal document that designates who will make health care decisions for persons unable to do so for themselves.

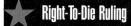

Right-To-Die Ruling

A 1990 Supreme Court ruling should alert all persons to protect themselves in the event that an accident or illness could leave them in a condition called persistent vegetative state (or PVS). There are an estimated 10,000 patients presently living in persistent vegetative states.[7] In this landmark case the U.S. Supreme Court ruled that the State of Missouri could refuse to allow removal of the artificial feeding tube that had helped keep Nancy Cruzan alive.

Nancy had been in a car accident that left her in a vegetative coma for 7 years. Although her parents had wanted to remove her feeding tube to allow her to die, the Supreme Court said the State of Missouri had no clear and convincing evidence that Nancy would have wanted the tube removed. Before her accident at age 25, Nancy had left no instructions about what she would want done if she were left in an incapacitated state. She had not prepared either a living will or a durable power of attorney for health care documents.

Nancy Cruzan's feeding tube was eventually removed after a lower court judge heard testimony from three of Nancy's former co-workers. These co-workers stated that Nancy had told them she would not want to be kept alive in a vegetative state. This testimony was ruled clear and convincing, and the judge allowed Nancy's feeding tube to be removed. She died a peaceful death shortly thereafter.

The Cruzan case points to the need to prepare the appropriate legal documents when you are fully competent.[7] Few people know for certain when (or if) they are going to be in a persistent vegetative state. With increasing medical and technological advances, there will undoubtedly be more and more cases of persons in irreversible comas. By planning ahead, you can ease the burden on your close relatives and, perhaps, have the right to die a more dignified death. ★

(see the box above). This document helps inform hospitals and physicians which person will help make the critical medical decisions. Usually this person is a loving relative. It is recommended that people complete both living will and durable power of attorney for health care documents.

EMOTIONAL STAGES OF DYING

A process of self-adjustment has been observed in persons who have a terminal illness. The stages in this process have helped form the basis for the modern movement of death education. An awareness of these stages may help you understand how people adjust to other major losses in their lives.

Perhaps the most widely recognized name in the area of death education is Dr. Elisabeth Kübler-Ross. As a psychiatrist working closely with terminally ill patients at the University of Chicago's Billings Hospital, Kübler-Ross was able to observe the emotional reactions of dying persons. In her classic book *On Death and Dying,* Kübler-Ross summarized the psychological stages that dying people often experience.[8]

▼ *Denial.* This is the stage of disbelief. Patients refuse to believe that they actually will die. Denial can serve as a temporary defense mechanism and can allow patients the time to accept their prognosis on their own terms.

▼ *Anger.* A common emotional reaction after denial is anger. Patients can feel as if they have been cheated. By expressing anger, patients are able to vent some of their fears, jealousies, anxieties, and frustrations. Patients often direct their anger at relatives, physicians and nurses, religious symbols, and normally healthy people.

▼ *Bargaining.* Terminally ill persons follow the anger stage with a stage characterized by bargaining. Patients who desperately want to avoid their inevitable deaths attempt to strike bargains—often with God or a church leader. Some people undergo religious conversions. The goal is to buy time by promising to repent for past sins, to restructure and rededicate their lives, or to make a large financial contribution to a religious cause.

▼ *Depression.* When patients realize that at best bargaining can only postpone their fate, they may begin an unpredictable period of depression. In a sense, terminally ill people are grieving for their own anticipated death. They may become quite withdrawn and refuse to visit with close relatives and friends. Prolonged periods of silence or crying are normal components of this depression stage and should not be discouraged.

▼ *Acceptance.* During the acceptance stage, patients fully realize that they are going to die. Acceptance ensures a relative sense of peace for most dying persons. Anger, resentment, and depression are usually gone. Kübler-Ross describes this stage as one without much feeling. Patients feel neither happy nor sad. Many are calm and introspective and prefer to be left either alone or with a few close relatives or friends.

One or two additional points should be made about the psychological stages of dying. Just as each person's life is totally unique, so is each person's death. Unfolding deaths vary as much as do unfolding lives. Some people move through Kübler-Ross's stages of dying very predictably. Others do not. It is not uncommon for some dying people to avoid one or more of these stages entirely.

The second important point to be made about Kübler-Ross's stages of dying is that the family members or friends of dying people often pass through similar stages as they observe the dying of their loved ones. When informed that a close friend or relative is dying, many people will also experience varying degrees of denial, anger, bargaining, depression, and acceptance. Because of this, as caring persons we need to recognize that the emotional needs of the living must be fulfilled in ways that do not differ appreciably from those of the dying.

NEAR-DEATH EXPERIENCES

As Bob lay on the gymnasium floor in apparent cardiac arrest, he watched from above as the team trainer and coaches performed CPR. After observing his own attempted resuscitation, he began walking in the direction of his uncle's voice. The last time he had heard his uncle's voice was a few days before his death 4 years earlier. Suddenly, his uncle instructed Bob to stop and turn back because Bob was not yet ready to join him. Over 24 hours later Bob regained consciousness in the cardiac intensive care unit of The Ohio State University Hospital.

Death brings an end to our physical existence. Perhaps this is the ultimate connection between death and our physical dimension of health. Many people believe that, in a positive sense, death brings with it a sense of relief and comfort—two qualities that may be most needed when one is dying. The work of Raymond Moody,[13] who examined reports of people who had near-death experiences, suggests that we may have less to fear about dying than we have generally thought.

In a most recent study of more than 100 persons who had near-death experiences, Kenneth Ring[14] reported these people shared a core experience. This experience was composed of some or all of the following stages:

1. A sense of well-being and peace
2. An out-of-body experience in which the dying person floats above his or her body and is able to witness the activities that are occurring
3. A movement into extreme blackness or darkness
4. A shaft of intense light that generally leads upward or lies in the distance
5. A decision to enter into the light

Central to this experience is the need to make a decision to move toward death or to return to the body that has been temporarily vacated.

Experts are not in agreement as to whether near-death experiences are truly associated with death or more closely associated with the depersonalization that is experienced by some persons during particularly frightening situations. In a scientific sense, near-death experiences are impossible to prove. Science can neither verify nor deny the existence of out-of-body experiences.[1] Some neurologists claim that near-death phenomena result from dreams occurring days or weeks after the person nearly dies that are subsequently deemed the near-death experience itself.[15]

Regardless, for those who had near-death experiences, simply knowing that death might not be such an unpleasant experience appears to be comforting. Most seem to have formed a new orientation toward living.[1]

INTERACTING WITH DYING PERSONS

Facing the impending death of a friend, relative, or loved one is a difficult experience. If you have yet to face this situation, be assured that, as you grow older, your opportunities will increase. This is part of the reality of living.

Most counselors, physicians, nurses, and ministers who spend time with terminally ill people suggest that you display one quality when interacting with dying people. That quality is honesty. Just the thought of talking with a dying person may make you feel uncomfortable. (Most of us have had no training in this sort of thing.) Sometimes, to make ourselves feel less anxious or depressed, we may tend to deny that the person we are with is dying. Our words and nonverbal behavior indicate that we prefer not to face the truth. Our words become stilted as we gloss over the facts and merely attempt to cheer up both our dying friend and ourselves. This behavior is rarely beneficial or supportive—for either party.

As much as possible, we should attempt to be genuine and honest. We should not try to avoid crying if we feel the need to cry. At the same time, we can provide emotional support for dying people by allowing them to express their feelings openly. We should resist the temptation of trying to pull someone out of the denial, anger, or depression. We should not feel obliged to talk constantly and to fill long pauses with idle talk. Sometimes nonverbal communication, including touching, may be much more appreciated than mere talk. Since our interactions with dying persons help fulfill our needs, we too should express our emotions and concerns as openly as possible.

TALKING WITH CHILDREN ABOUT DEATH

Because most children are curious about everything, it is not surprising that they are also fascinated about death. From very young ages, children are exposed to death through mass media (cartoon shows, pictures in newspapers and magazines, and news re-

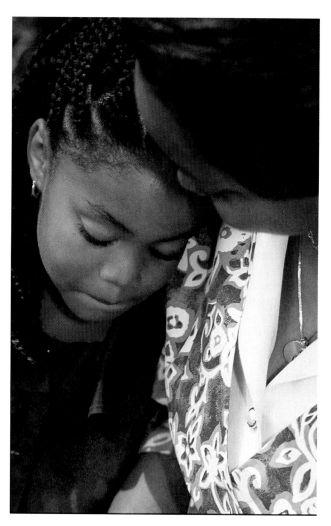

Children need support when dealing with death.

ports), adult conversations ("Aunt Emily died today," "Uncle George is terminally ill"), and their discoveries (a dead bird, a crushed bug, a dead flower). The manner in which children learn about death will have an important impact on their ability to recognize and accept their own mortality and to cope with the deaths of others.

Psychologists encourage parents and older friends to avoid shielding children from or misleading children about the reality of death. Young children need to realize that death is not temporary and it is not like sleeping. Parents are encouraged to make certain they understand children's questions about death before they give an answer. Most children want simple, direct answers to their questions, not long detailed dissertations, which often confuse the issues. For example, when a 4-year old asks her father, "Why is Tommy's dog dead?" an appropriate answer might be, "Because he got very, very sick and his heart stopped beating." Getting involved in a lengthy discussion about "doggy heaven" or the causes of specific canine diseases may not be necessary or appropriate.

Parents should answer questions when they arise and always respond with openness and honesty. In this way young children can learn that death is a real part of life and that sad feelings are a normal part of accepting the death of a loved one.

DEATH OF A CHILD

Adults face not only the death of their parents and friends, but perhaps the death of a child. Whether because of sudden infant death syndrome (SIDS), chronic illness, accident, or suicide, children die and adults are forced to grieve the loss of someone who was "too young to die."

Coping with the death of children presents adults with a difficult period of adjustment, particularly when the death was unexpected. Experts agree the grieving adults, particularly the parents, should express their grief fully and proceed cautiously on their return to normal routines. Many pitfalls can be avoided. Adults who are grieving for dead children should:

▼ *Avoid coping through the use of alcohol or drugs.*
▼ *Make no major life changes.* Moving to a different home, relocating, or changing jobs usually doesn't help parents deal any better with the grief they are experiencing.
▼ *Share their feelings with others.* Grieving adults should share their feelings particularly with other adults who have experienced a similar loss. Group support is available in many communities.
▼ *Avoid trying to erase the death.* Giving away clothing and possessions that belonged to the child cannot erase the memories the adult may have of the child.
▼ *Give themselves the time and space to grieve.* On the anniversary of the child's death or on the child's birthday grievers should give themselves special time just for grieving.
▼ *Don't attempt to replace the child.* Do not quickly have another child or use the deceased child's name for another child.

For some adults, grief over the death of a child will require an extended period of time. Eventually, however, life can return to normal.

HOSPICE CARE FOR THE TERMINALLY ILL

The thought of dying in a hospital ward, with spotless floors, pay television, and strict visiting hours, leaves many people with a cold feeling. Perhaps this thought alone has helped encourage the concept of **hospice care.** Hospice care provides an alternate approach to dying for terminally ill patients and their families. The goal of hospice care is to maximize the quality of life

★ The Grieving Process

The grieving process consists of four phases, each of which is variable in length and unique in form to the individual. These phases are composed of the following:

1 *Internalization of the deceased person's image.* By forming an idealized mental picture of the dead person, the grieving person is freed from dealing too quickly with the reality of the death.

2 *Intellectualization of the death.* Mental processing of the death and the events leading up to its occurrence move the grieving person to a clear understanding that death has occurred.

3 *Emotional reconciliation.* During this third, and often delayed phase, the grieving person allows conflicting feelings and thoughts to be expressed and eventually reconciled with the reality of the death.

4 *Behavioral reconciliation.* Finally, the grieving person is able to comfortably return to a life in which the death has been fully reconciled. Old routines are reestablished and new patterns of living are adopted where necessary. The grieving person has largely recovered.

If a mistake is to be made by the friends of a grieving person, it will be in terms of encouraging a return to normal behavior too quickly. When friends urge the grieving person to return to work right away, make new friends, or become involved in time-consuming projects, they may be preventing necessary grieving from occurring. It is not easy or desirable to forget about the fact that a spouse, friend, or child has recently died. ★

for dying persons and their family members. Popularized in England during the 1960s yet derived from a concept developed during the Middle Ages (where *hospitable lodges* took care of weary travelers), the hospice helps people die comfortably and with dignity by using one or more of the following strategies:

▼ *Pain control.* Dying persons are not usually treated for their terminal disease; they are provided with appropriate drugs to keep them free from pain, alert, and in control of their faculties. Drug dependence is of little concern, and patients can receive pain medication when they feel they need it.

▼ *Family involvement.* Family members and friends are trained and encouraged to interact with the dying person and with each other. Family members often care for the dying person at home. If the hospice arrangement includes a hospice ward in a hospital or a separate building (also called a hospice), the family members have no restrictions on visitation.

▼ *Multidisciplinary approach.* The hospice concept promotes a team approach. Specially trained physicians, nurses, social workers, counselors, and volunteers work with the patient and family to fulfill important needs. The needs of the survivors receive nearly the same priority as those of the patient.

▼ *Patient decisions.* Contrary to most hospital approaches, hospice programs encourage patients to make their own decisions. The patient decides when to eat, sleep, go for a walk, and just be alone. By maintaining a personal schedule, the patient is more apt to feel in control of his or her life, even as that life is slipping away.

Another way in which the hospice approach differs from the hospital approach concerns the care given to the survivors. Even after the death of the patient, the family receives a significant amount of follow-up counseling. Helping families with their grief is an important role for the hospice team.

The number of hospices in the United States has climbed quickly to over 2000.[9] People seem to be convinced that the hospice system does work effectively. Part of this approval may be the cost factor. The cost of caring for a dying person in a hospice is usually less than the cost of full (inpatient) services provided by a hospital. Although insurance companies are delighted to see the lower cost for hospice care, many are still uncertain as to how to define hospice care. Thus not all insurance companies are fully reimbursing patients for their hospice care. Before discussing the possibility of hospice care for members of your family, you should consider the extent of hospice coverage in your health insurance policy.

GRIEF AND THE RESOLUTION OF GRIEF

The emotional feelings that persons experience after the death of a friend or relative are collectively called *grief. Mourning* is the process of experiencing these emotional feelings in a culturally defined manner. See the box above for more information on the grieving process. The expression of grief is seen as a valuable process that gradually permits the people to detach themselves from the deceased. Expressing grief, then, is a sign of good health.

Although people experience grief in remarkable different ways, most people experience some of the following sensations and emotions.

---

hospice care (**hos** pis) approach to caring for terminally ill patients that maximizes the quality of life and allows death with dignity.

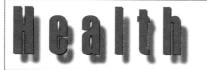

ACTION Guide

Helping the Bereaved

Leming and Dickinson[1] point out that the peak time of grief begins in the week after a loved one's funeral. Realizing that there is no one guaranteed formula for helping the bereaved, friends and caregivers can help by performing some or all of the following:

▼ Make few demands on the bereaved; allow him or her to grieve.
▼ Help with the household tasks.
▼ Recognize that the bereaved person may vent anguish and anger, and that some of it may be directed at you.
▼ Recognize that the bereaved person has painful and difficult tasks to complete; mourning cannot be rushed or avoided.
▼ Do not be afraid to talk about the deceased person; this lets the bereaved know that you care for the deceased.
▼ Express your own genuine feelings of sadness, but avoid pity. Speak from the heart.
▼ Reassure bereaved persons that the intensity of their emotions is very natural.
▼ Advise the bereaved to get additional help if you suspect continuing major emotional or physical distress.
▼ Keep in regular contact with the bereaved; let him or her know you continue to care about them. ▼

▼ *Physical discomfort.* Shortly after the death of a loved one, grieving persons display a rather similar pattern of physical discomfort. This discomfort is characterized by "sensations of somatic distress occurring in waves lasting from twenty minutes to an hour at a time, a feeling of tightness in the throat, choking with shortness of breath, need for sighing, and an empty feeling in the abdomen, lack of muscular power, and an intense subjective distress described as a tension or mental pain. The patient soon learns that these waves of discomfort can be precipitated by visits, by mentioning the deceased, and by receiving sympathy."[16]

▼ *Sense of numbness.* Grieving persons may feel as if they are numb or in a state of shock. They may deny the death of their loved one.

▼ *Feelings of detachment from others.* Grieving persons see other people as being distant from them, perhaps because the others cannot feel the loss. A person in grief can feel very lonely. This is a common response.

▼ *Preoccupation with the image of the deceased.* The grieving person may not be able to complete daily tasks without constantly thinking about the deceased.

▼ *Guilt.* The survivor may be overwhelmed with guilt. Thoughts may center on how the deceased was neglected or ignored. Sensitive survivors feel guilt merely because they still are alive. Indeed, guilt is a common emotion.

▼ *Hostility.* Survivors may express feelings of loss and remorse through hostility, which they direct at other family members, physicians, lawyers, and others.

▼ *Disruption in daily schedule.* Grieving persons often find it difficult to complete daily routines. They can suffer from an anxious type of depression. Seemingly easy tasks take a great deal of effort. Initiation of new activities and relationships can be difficult. Social interaction skills can be lost.

▼ *Delayed grief.* In some people, the typical pattern of grief can be delayed for weeks, months, and even years.

The grief process will continue until the bereaved person can establish new relationships, feel comfortable with others, and look back on the life of the deceased person with positive feelings. Although the duration of the grief resolution process will vary with the emotional attachments one has to a deceased person, grief usually lasts from a few months to a year. Professional help should be sought when grieving is characterized by unresolved guilt, extreme hostility, physical illness, significant depression, and a lack of other meaningful relationships. Trained counselors, physicians, and hospice workers can all play significant roles in helping people through grief.

RITUALS OF DEATH

Our society has established a number of rituals associated with death that help the survivors accept the reality of death, ease the pain associated with the grief process, and provide a safe disposal of the body. Our rituals give us the chance to formalize our goodbyes to a person and to receive emotional support and strength from family members and friends. In recent years more of our rituals seem to be celebrating the life of the deceased. In doing this, our rituals also reaffirm the value of our own lives.

Most of our funeral rituals take place in funeral homes, churches, and cemeteries. *Funeral homes* (or *mortuaries*) are business establishments that provide a variety of services to the families of dead people. The

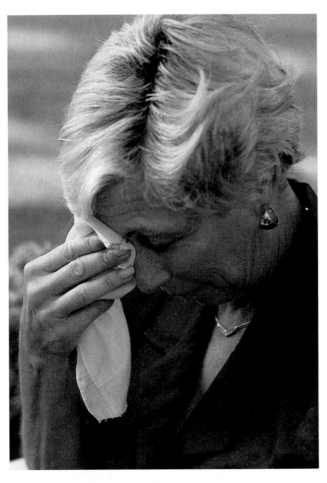

Grief evokes feelings of profound loss.

services are carried out by funeral directors, who are licensed by the state in which they operate. Most funeral directors are responsible for preparing the bodies for viewing, filing death certificates, preparing obituary notices, establishing calling hours, assisting in the preparation and details of the funeral, casket selection, transportation to and from the cemetery, and family counseling. Although licensing procedures vary from state to state, most new funeral directors must complete 1 year of college, 1 year of mortuary school, and 1 year of internship with a funeral home before taking a state licensing examination.[10]

Funeral Services

An ethical funeral director will attempt to follow the wishes of the deceased's family and provide only the services requested by the family. Most families want traditional, **full funeral services.** Three major components of the full funeral services are as follows.

EMBALMING

Embalming is the process of using formaldehyde-based fluids to replace the blood components. Embalming helps preserve the body and return it to a natural look. Embalming permits friends and family members to view the body without being subjected to the odors associated with tissue decomposition. Embalming is often an optional procedure, except when death results from specific communicable diseases or when body *disposition* (disposal) is delayed.

CALLING HOURS

Formerly called a *wake,* this is an established time when friends and family members can gather in a room to share their emotions and common experiences about the dead person. Generally in the same room, the body will be in a casket, with the lid open or closed. Open caskets assist some people to confirm that death truly did occur. Some families prefer not to have any calling hours, sometimes called visiting hours.

FUNERAL SERVICE

Funeral services vary according to religious preference and the emotional needs of the survivors. Although some services are held in a church, most funeral services today take place in a funeral home, where a special room might serve as a chapel. Some services are held at the graveside. Families may also choose to have a simple *memorial service* within a few days after the funeral.

Disposition of the Body

Bodies are disposed of in one of four ways. *Ground burial* is the most common method. About 75% of all bodies are placed in ground burial. The casket is almost always placed in a metal or concrete vault before being buried. The vault serves to further protect the body (a need only of the survivors) and to prevent collapse of ground because of the decaying of caskets. Use of a vault is required by most cemeteries.

A second type of disposition is *entombment.* Entombment refers to nonground burial, most often in structures called **mausoleums.** A mausoleum has a series of shelves where caskets can be sealed in vaultlike areas called *niches.* Entombment can also occur in the basements of buildings, especially in old, large churches. The bodies of famous church leaders are sometimes entombed in vaultlike spaces called **crypts.**

---

full funeral services all of the professional services provided by funeral directors.

mausoleum (moz oh **lee** um) above-ground structure into which caskets can be placed for disposition and which frequently resembles a small stone house.

crypts (krips) burial locations generally underneath churches.

Cremation is a third type of body disposition. In the United States, 19% of all bodies are cremated.[11] This practice is increasing. Generally both the body and casket (or cardboard cremation box) are incinerated so that only the bone ash from the body remains. The body of an average adult produces about 5 to 7 pounds of bone ash. These ashes can then be placed in containers called *urns,* and then buried, entombed, or scattered, if permitted by state law. The cost of cremation (from $200 to $500) is much less than ground burial. Some families choose to cremate after having full funeral services.

A fourth method of body disposition is *anatomical donation.* Separate organs (such as corneal tissue, kidneys, heart) can be donated to a medical school, research facility, or organ donor network. Certain states permit people to indicate on their driver's licenses that they wish to donate their organs. However, family consent (by next of kin) is also required at the time of death for organ or tissue donation to occur. Recently, hospitals have been required by federal law to inform the family of a deceased person about organ donation at the time of his or her death. The need for donor organs is far greater than the current supply. (See the box on p. 537.) For some, the decision to donate body tissue and organs is rewarding and comforting. Organ donors understand that their small sacrifice can help give life or improve the quality of life for another person. In this sense, their death can mean life for others. To become an organ donor, you must fill out a uniform organ donor card like the one in Figure 21-1.

Some people choose to donate their entire body to medical science. Often this is done through prior arrangements with medical schools. Bodies still require embalming. After they are studied, the remains are often cremated and returned to the family, if requested.

Costs

The full funeral services offered by a funeral home average from $2000 to $2500. To this price, one must add other expenses. Casket prices vary significantly, with the average cost between $1500 and $2500. If the family chooses an especially fancy casket, then the costs could spiral up to $10,000 or more. Costs that extend beyond these expenses include (should one choose them) those shown in Table 21-1. When one adds up all of the expenses associated with a typical funeral, the average cost is between $5000 and $6500.

Regardless of the rituals you select for the handling of your body (or the body of someone in your care), most educators are encouraging people to prearrange their plans. Before you die, you can save your survivors a lot of misery by putting your wishes in writing. *Funeral prearrangements* relieve the survivors of many of the details that must be handled at the time of your death. You can gather much of the information

TABLE 21-1 **Estimated Funeral Costs**	
Cemetery lot	$200-700
Opening and closing of grave	$200-700
Vault	$350-1000
Mausoleum space	$1500-5000
Honorarium for minister	$75-100
Organist and vocalists	$50-75 each
Flowers over casket	$100+
Grave marker	$500-1500+
Beautician services	$75+

for your obituary notice and your wishes for the disposition of your body. Prearrangements can be made with a funeral director, family member, or attorney. Many individuals also prepay the costs of their funeral. By making arrangements in advance of need, you can enhance your own peace of mind. Currently about 30% to 40% of funerals are preplanned and prepaid. Interestingly, in the 1960s nearly all funerals were planned by relatives at the time of a person's death.[11]

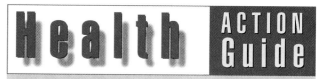

Organ Donations

Making an organ donation is one of the most compassionate, responsible acts a person can do. Only a few simple steps are required:

1. You must complete a uniform donor card. Obtain a card from a physician, a local hospital, or the nearest regional transplant or organ bank.
2. Print or type your name on the card.
3. Indicate which organs you wish to donate. You may also indicate your desire to donate all organs and tissues.
4. Sign your name in the presence of two witnesses, preferably your next of kin.
5. Fill in any additional information (for example, date of birth, city and state in which the card is completed, date the card is signed).
6. Tell others about your decision to donate. Some donor cards have detachable portions to give to your family.
7. Always carry your card with you.
8. If you have any questions, you can call the United Network for Organ Sharing (UNOS) at (800) 24-DONOR, or call (613) 727-1380 in Canada.

Current Organ Donation Issues

At the time of this writing, two key issues face the current organ donation practices in the United States: (a) the continued shortage of organ donors, and (b) the threat of disease transmission in certain donated tissues or organs.

The shortage of organ donors is life threatening to the thousands of patients waiting for a kidney, heart, lung, liver, pancreas, skin, or bone marrow tissue. Although donor cards are widely available and hospitals are now required by law to ask survivors promptly if they will donate the deceased's organs, only a small percentage of organs and tissues are collected.

Why has the donor system not been more effective? Here are some possible reasons. Many people do not prepare living wills; likewise, most people do not prepare a uniform organ donor card. Many survivors also prefer not to consider organ donation during the stressful aftermath of death. Some physicians and hospital staff workers may feel uncomfortable asking survivors about organ donation.

Beyond the psychological obstacles that surround organ donation are some very real difficulties in the administration of organ donation programs. Regulations at different organ banks may vary, as may state and local laws. These regulations may make it difficult for organ banks to prepare and transport tissues or organs from one location to another. Also, a hospital's ability to instantly recognize a patient as a registered donor requires donor registries across the country to be more compatible with each other. Finally, organ donation networks must find better ways to encourage people to understand the urgent need to provide these "gifts of life."

The second problem facing organ donation reached the public's attention in the Spring of 1991. It was discovered that tissues transplanted into multiple persons came from a donor who had died from AIDS. This oversight caused considerable public alarm, but has resulted in more stringent screening of donor candidates, as well as more careful examination and handling of organs and tissues. These tighter procedures are encouraging news for the public. Clearly, everyone waiting for an organ donation deserves the opportunity to receive a healthy organ. ★

UNIFORM DONOR CARD

of _____
(print or type name of donor)

In the hope that I may help others, I hereby make this anatomical gift, if medically acceptable, to take effect upon my death. The words and marks below indicate my wishes:

I give: (a) _____ any needed organs or parts
(b) _____ only the following organs or parts

_____
(specify the organ(s), tissue(s), or part(s))

for the purposes of transplantation, therapy, medical research or education;

(c) _____ my body for anatomical study if needed.

Limitations or special wishes, if any: _____

Signed by the donor and the following two witnesses in the presence of each other:

_____   _____
Signature of Donor   Date of Birth of Donor

_____   _____
Date Signed   City and State

_____   _____
Witness   Witness

This is a legal document under the Anatomical Gift Act or similar laws.
☐ Yes, I have discussed my wishes with my family.
For further information consult your physician or

THE NATIONAL KIDNEY FOUNDATION
30 East 33rd Street   New York, NY 10016

08-21

Figure 21-1 Organ donor card.

PERSONAL PREPARATION FOR DEATH

We hope that this chapter is helping you to discover some new perspectives about death and to develop your own personal death awareness. Remember, the ultimate goal of death education is a positive one—to help you best use and enjoy your life. Becoming aware of the reality of your own mortality is a step in the right direction. Reading about the process of dying, grief resolution, and the rituals surrounding death can also help you imagine that someday you too will die.

There are some additional ways in which you can prepare for the reality of your own death. Preparing a will, purchasing a life insurance policy, making funeral prearrangements, preparing a living will, and considering an anatomical or organ donation are measures that help you prepare for your own death. At the appropriate time, you might also wish to talk with family and friends about your own death. You may discover that an upbeat, positive discussion about death can help relieve some of your apprehensions and those of others around you.

Planning Your Funeral

PERSONAL ASSESSMENT

In line with this chapter's positive theme of the value of personal death awareness, here is a funeral service assessment that we frequently give to our health classes. This inventory can help you assess your reactions and thoughts about the funeral arrangements you would prefer for yourself.

After answering each of the following questions, you might wish to discuss your responses with a friend or close relative.

1. Have you ever considered how you would like your body to be handled after your death?
   _____ Yes _____ No

2. Have you already made funeral prearrangements for yourself?
   _____ Yes _____ No

3. Have you considered a specific funeral home or mortuary to handle your arrangements?
   _____ Yes _____ No

4. If you were to die today, which of the following would you prefer?
   _____ Embalming   _____ Ground burial
   _____ Cremation   _____ Entombment
   _____ Donation to medical science

5. If you prefer to be cremated, what would you want done with your ashes?
   _____ Buried   _____ Entombed
   _____ Scattered
   _____ Other, please specify _____

6. If your funeral plans involve a casket, which of the following ones would you prefer?
   _____ Plywood (cloth covered)
   _____ Hardwood (oak, cherry, mahogany, maple, etc.)
   _____ Steel (sealer or nonsealer type)
   _____ Stainless steel
   _____ Copper or bronze
   _____ Other, please specify _____

7. How important would a funeral service be *for you?*
   _____ Very important
   _____ Somewhat important
   _____ Somewhat unimportant
   _____ Very unimportant
   _____ No opinion

8. What kind of funeral service would you want *for yourself?*
   _____ No service at all
   _____ Visitation (calling hours) the day before the funeral service; funeral held at church or funeral home
   _____ Graveside service only (no visitation)

   _____ Memorial service (after body disposition)
   _____ Other, please specify _____

9. How many people would you want to attend your funeral service or memorial service?
   _____ I do not want a funeral or memorial service
   _____ 1-10 people
   _____ 11-25 people
   _____ 26-50 people
   _____ Over 51 people
   _____ I do not care how many people attend

10. What format would you prefer at your funeral service or memorial service? Select any of the following that you would like.

	Yes	No
Religious music	_____	_____
Nonreligious music	_____	_____
Clergy present	_____	_____
Flower arrangements	_____	_____
Family member eulogy	_____	_____
Eulogy by friend(s)	_____	_____
Open casket	_____	_____
Religious format	_____	_____
Other, please specify		

11. Using today's prices, how much would you expect to pay for your *total* funeral arrangements, including cemetery expenses (if applicable)?
   _____ Less than $4000
   _____ Between $4001 and $5500
   _____ Between $5501 and $7000
   _____ Between $7001 and $8500
   _____ Above $8500

TO CARRY THIS FURTHER . . .

Which items had you not thought about before? Were you surprised at the arrangements you selected? Will you share your responses with anyone else? If so, whom?

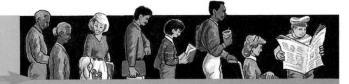

Learning FROM ALL Cultures

Funeral and Burial Rituals

Funeral rituals typically reflect people's religious beliefs and practices. In North America, most people are buried according to Protestant traditions. People pay their respects to the deceased, a minister conducts a service, and in 75% of the cases, the body is buried after a graveside ceremony.

The rest of the human population, however, bury their dead in a variety of ways. The Parsis, a group of people in India, follow an ancient religion called *Zoroastrianism*. They perform their burial rituals at the seven Towers of Silence, outside of Bombay. The corpse is brought to one of the towers by six individuals dressed in white. The body is left on a tower for vultures to devour, leaving only the skeleton. A few days later the bones are put into a pit. The Parsis believe this method keeps the air, soil, and water from becoming contaminated.[12]

Hindus believe that the physical body must be gone for the soul to continue on to reincarnation. Their ritual consists of washing the dead body and dressing it in a shroud adorned with flowers. The body is carried to a funeral pyre, and the closest male relative lights the fire, walks around the burning body three times, and recites Hindu verses.[12]

Buddhists, who live mostly in China, Japan, Sri Lanka, Myanmar, Vietnam, and Cambodia, also cremate their dead. They believe cremation was favored by Buddha.

Unlike Hindus and Buddhists, Muslims do not believe in cremation. Their ritual is to wash the dead body, dress it in three pieces of white cloth, and put it in a wooden coffin. Burial is within 24 hours of death, since there is no embalming unless dictated by law. The body is taken out of the coffin and buried with the head turned toward Mecca.[12]

Most people do not like to think about their own death or plan for it, but there are some individuals who plan their funerals to the last detail. What would be your wishes concerning your own funeral and burial? ●

Another suggestion to help you emotionally prepare for your own death is to prepare an *obituary notice* or **eulogy** for yourself. Include all the things you would like to have said about you and your life. Now compare your obituary notice and eulogy with the current direction your life seems to be taking. Are you doing the kinds of activities for which you want to be known? If so, great! If not, perhaps you will want to consider why your current direction does not reflect how you would like to be remembered. Should you make some changes to restructure your life's agenda in a more personally meaningful fashion?

Another suggestion to help make you aware of your own eventual death is to write your own **epitaph.** Before doing this, you might want to visit a cemetery. (Unfortunately, most of us visit cemeteries only when we are forced to.) Reading the epitaphs of others may help you to develop your own epitaph.

Further awareness of your own death might come from attempting to answer these questions in writing (since this pushes you beyond mere thinking): (1) If I had only one day to live, how would I spend it? (2) What one accomplishment would I like to make before I die? (3) Once I am dead, what two or three things will people miss most about me? By answering these questions and accomplishing a few of the tasks suggested in this section, you will have a good start on accepting your own death and the value of life itself.

> **eulogy** (you **la** gee) composition or speech that praises someone; often delivered at a funeral or memorial service.
>
> **epitaph** (**ep** ah taff) inscription on a grave marker or monument.

Summary

✔ Personal death awareness encourages one to live a meaningful life.

✔ Death denial tends to breed feelings of helplessness and vulnerability.

✔ Death is determined primarily by clinical and legal factors.

✔ Euthanasia can be undertaken with either direct or indirect measures.

✔ The most current advance medical directives are the living will and the durable power of attorney for health care. Both documents permit critically ill persons (especially those who cannot communicate) to die with dignity.

✔ Denial, anger, bargaining, depression, and acceptance are the five classic psychological stages that dying people commonly experience, according to Dr. Kübler-Ross.

✔ Hospice care provides an alternate approach to dying for terminally ill persons and their families.

✔ The expression of grief is a common experience that can be expected when a friend or relative dies. The grief process can vary in intensity and duration.

✔ Death in our society is associated with a number of rituals to help survivors cope with the loss of a loved one and to ensure proper disposal of the body.

Review Questions

1. Define "personal death awareness." What is meant by "death denial"?

2. According to Worden and Proctor, death denial can lead to one of three situations. Identify and explain each of these situations.

3. Identify and explain the clinical and legal determinants of death and indicate who establishes each of them.

4. Explain the difference between direct and indirect euthanasia.

5. How does a "living will" differ from a "durable power of attorney for health care" document? Why are these advance medical directives becoming increasingly popular?

6. Identify the five psychological stages that dying people tend to experience. Explain each stage.

7. Identify and explain the four strategies that form the basis of hospice care. What are the advantages of hospice care for the patient and the family?

8. Explain what is meant by the term *grief*. Identify and explain the sensations and emotions most people have when they experience grief. When does the grieving process end? How can adults cope with the death of a child? How can we assist grieving people?

9. What purposes do the rituals of death serve? What are the major components of the full funeral service? What are the four ways in which bodies are disposed?

10. What activities can we undertake to become better aware of our own mortality?

Think about This . . .

✔ How were issues related to death handled in your family when you were growing up?

✔ Will hospice care be an option you might choose someday?

✔ Have you or any of your relatives prepared a living will or a durable power of attorney for health care document?

✔ At your death, would you want your organs or body tissue donated to help another person? Are there any organs you would prefer not to donate?

✔ If you found out you were going to die tomorrow, what would you do today?

✔ If it were determined that you were in a persistent vegetative state, would you want your life support disconnected?

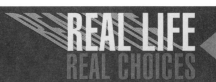

YOUR TURN

▼ According to Elisabeth Kübler-Ross, what are the five psychological stages often experienced by both a dying person and his or her family and friends?

▼ Which of those stages do you think Jenny has gone through with respect to her own death? What about Wendy?

▼ Have you ever experienced the dying and death of a family member or close friend? If so, which of the five stages did the dying person go through? Which stages did you experience?

AND NOW, YOUR CHOICES...

▼ If your best friend had a terminal illness, how would you try to reconcile your feelings with your friend's needs?

▼ If you were terminally ill, how could your best friend be most helpful to you? ▼

References

1. Leming MR, Dickinson GE: *Understanding dying, death, and bereavement*, ed 2, Ft Worth, 1990, Holt, Rinehart, & Winston.
2. Spiegel D: *Living beyond limits: new hope and help for facing life-threatening illness*, New York, 1993, Times Books.
3. Worden J, Proctor W: *PDA: personal death awareness*, Englewood Cliffs, NJ, 1976, Prentice Hall.
4. Smith DA: Ruling undercuts pregnancy restrictions, *Choice in Dying Newsletter* 1(3):4, 1992.
5. Burnell GM: *Final choices: to live or die in an age of medical technology*, New York, 1993, Plenum Press.
6. Choice in Dying: personal correspondence, May 25, 1994.
7. Beck J: Right-to-die ruling unhelpful, *Muncie Star*, July 16, 1990, p 4.
8. Kübler-Ross E: *On death and dying*, New York, 1969, Macmillan Publishing.
9. Baer K: Dying with dignity: a guide to hospice care, *Harvard Health Letter* (special supplement), April 1993, p 9.
10. Bowman J (licensed funeral director), personal correspondence, May 26, 1994.
11. Weaver G, Caleca, LG: Fading grandeur: the traditional funeral is slowly losing ground, *Indianapolis Star*, July 29, 1993, p 1A.
12 Whalen WJ: How different religions pay their funeral respects. In Dickinson G, Leming M, Mermann M, editors: *Dying, death, and bereavement*, Guilford, Conn, 1993, Dushkin Publishing.
13. Moody RA: *Life after life*, New York, 1975, Bantam Books.
14. Ring K: *Life at death: a scientific investigation of the near-death experience*, New York, 1980, Coward, McCann & Geoghegan.
15. Benedetto W: Near-death experiences are likely to be dreams, *USA Today*, Jan 2, 1991, p 9A.
16. Lindemann E: Symptomatology and management of acute grief. In Fulton et al, editors: *Death and dying: challenge and change*, Reading, Mass, 1978, Addison-Wesley.

Suggested Readings

Spiegel D: *Living beyond limits: new hope and help for facing life-threatening illness*, New York, 1993, Times Books.

A psychiatrist writes about the importance of mind-body interactions for people diagnosed with serious illnesses. Using examples from his many years of clinical practice, Spiegel encourages people to face their situations squarely, engage themselves with others, and learn to live "beyond the limits."

Quill T: *Death and dignity: making choices and taking charge*, New York, 1993, WW Norton.

Quill is a physician who gained notoriety after helping a terminally ill patient commit suicide by taking a lethal dose of a prescribed medication. In this book, Quill supports the concept of comfort care, in which the main goal is to relieve pain and suffering. Assisted suicide must be reserved for only a few patients under strict guidelines.

Burnell GM: *Final choices: to live or to die in an age of medical technology*, New York, 1993, Plenum Press.

In the past 20 years technological advancements have dramatically changed the way people die in the United States. This author is a physician who writes about death and dying choices, including viable options, considerations, and responsibilities for young adults and elderly.

Studying about aging and death should help you master the developmental tasks that are meaningful for your emotional growth.

☷ Forming an Initial Adult Identity

It may be obvious that discovering your identity (that which makes you unique) involves first coming to grips with who you are right now—this minute or this day. However, is it also possible that your identity could be related to both past experiences and those awaiting you in the future?

We think so. It would be hard to deny that past experiences play a major role in providing a foundation for developing identity. Clearly, we are products of our past experiences.

But we may also be products of future experiences. How we feel about the impact of our own aging and eventual death is reflected in our self-identities *now*. To fear these inevitable processes may make us tentative, frightened persons during our entire lives. To ignore our aging and eventual death may cause us to live unfocused, less meaningful lives. To acknowledge and accept the reality of aging and dying may be the healthiest approach of all.

☷ Establishing Independence

Being independent is a fragile quality. Most of us will never be completely independent from other people. What comes as a surprise to many independent young and midlife adults is the probability of someday becoming the "parent" to your own parents. By under-standing the needs of older adults, you will be better prepared for this reversal of dependence.

Are you prepared to alter your own independence to help aging parents make decisions? For example, will you be able to tell your parents that they should no longer drive an automobile? Can you be truly sensitive to the loss that parents might feel if you must finally encourage them to move into a retirement community or apartment? Can you envision comforting your parents in death as they once held and comforted you in sickness and disappointment?

☷ Assuming Responsibility

With increasing age and maturity, you will be expected (by the collective society) to assume more and more responsibility. Although you may not consciously think about it, most young adults are probably glad to shoulder more responsibility. Indeed, by successfully assuming increasing levels of responsibility, you can improve mental health and your overall perspective on life.

Concerning dying and death, responsibility can gradually develop in many ways. For example, you can prepare a will, make funeral prearrangements, or plan organ donation. You can also learn to become more responsible to other people by helping survivors cope with the deaths of family or friends. Finally, you can help younger family members or your own children develop healthy attitudes toward death by remaining open and honest when they come to you with questions and concerns about death.

☷ Developing Social Skills

The everyday references you see to the loneliness that comes with aging, death experiences, and the grieving process might lead you to believe that these experiences are solitary ones. In fact, most of the time they are not. Many persons come in contact with older people, including family members, friends, neighbors, nurses, doctors, ministers, and social service employees. Growing older and dying should not be equated with isolation from other persons.

For this reason, it is important to maintain and sharpen communication skills over your entire lifetime. Your continued social involvement as an active, interested older person will make life more enjoyable to you and more meaningful to others.

☷ Developing Intimacy

What better gift could there be to take into the later years of life than the life-long intimacy provided by a spouse, friend, or important teacher from your youth? As we age, our ability to pursue new relationships diminishes. Trusted friends made in earlier life can provide comfort and support through the end of life. The support and understanding derived from close relationships help in dealing with the death of a spouse, child, friend, or associate, and extend the gift of intimacy during some of life's most difficult transitions.

1

Commonly Used Over-the-Counter Products

Pain Relievers

Product	Physiological function	Potential side effect	Product	Physiological function	Potential side effect
Aspirin (only)	Analgesic (pain relief)	Hypersensitivity	Acetaminophen (with caffeine)		
Aspirin (with caffeine)	Antipyretic (fever reduction)	Gastrointestinal disturbance	Acetaminophen (with aspirin and caffeine)		
	Antirheumatic (inflammation reduction)	Internal bleeding	Ibuprofen		
	Anticoagulant (slowed clotting time)	Ototoxicity (toxic action on the ear)		Analgesic (pain relief)	Gastrointestinal disturbance
		Prothrombin depression		Antirheumatic (inflammation reduction)	Headache Nervousness
		Overdose potential			Vision distortion
		Reye's syndrome			Fluid retention
					Rash
Acetaminophen (only)	Analgesic (pain relief)	Liver damage			
Acetaminophen (with aspirin)	Antipyretic (fever reduction)	Gastric erosion Kidney failure Irregular heartbeat			

Cold and Cough Products

Active ingredient*†	Physiological function	Potential side effect	Active ingredient *†	Physiological function	Potential side effect
Decongestant (sympathomimetic amine)			Cough suppressant		
Phenylephrine hydrochloride	Vasoconstriction, which decreases blood flow into nasal tissues, thus decreasing fluid loss	Nervousness, sweating	Dextromethorphan hydrobromide	Suppression of sensitivity of the brain's cough control center and reduced CNS activity, thus reducing coughing and facilitating sleep	Mild sedation
Antihistamine			Codeine		
			Alcohol		
Chlorpheniramine maleate	Blockage of histamine's vasodilating effect on capillaries within nasal tissue, thus reducing fluid loss (runny nose)	Drowsiness, drying of the mouth			
Analgesic			20% to 25% per unit volume	CNS depression	Reduction in inhibitions when taken in quantity
Acetaminophen	Pain relief and fever reduction	Generally few side effects with the amounts found in cold and cough preparations—see p. A1 for additional information on side effects			

*Popular cold and cough medications generally contain an ingredient from each of the five categories listed.
†Expectorants, *which stimulate respiratory tract secretions, and* bronchodilators, *which increase the diameter of air passages, have also been used in the formulations of cold and cough medications. Their roles are to some degree controversial and are currently under study.*

Deodorant and Antiperspirant Products

Two avenues exist for controlling odor resulting from the action of microbes on the organic matter in the perspiration of the apocrine sweat glands.

Function/Product	Active agents	Adverse side effects	Function/Product	Active agents	Adverse side effects
Control or mask odor			**Reduce release of perspiration**		
Mild deodorant soaps	Hexachlorophene (0.75% or less)	Swelling; blistering on exposure to sun	Antiperspirants	Aluminum chloride	Allergic reactions
Deodorant (toilet water, colognes, perfumes, deodorants)	Triclocarban (TCC)	Allergic reactions		Aluminum chlorohydrate	Should not be used for excessive, offensive, or colored perspiration
	Tribromosalicylanilide (TBS)			Aluminum sulfate	
	Alcohol				
	Essential oils				
	Vitamin E				

Sun Tanning Products

Sun Protection Factors and Classifications

2   Dark tan for skin that tans easily; minimal protection from sunburn
4   Dark tan for normal skin; minimal to moderate protection from sunburn
6   Golden tan for normal skin; moderate protection from sunburn
8   Gradual tan for normal skin; extra protection from sunburn
15 Gradual tan for sun-sensitive skin; maximal protection from sunburn
25 Protection for sun-sensitive skin; ultraprotection from sunburn
30 Protection for sun-sensitive skin for prolonged exposure

Safe and Effective Sunscreens

Aminobenzoic acid
Cinoxate
Diethanolamine *p*-methoxycinnamate
Digalloyl trioleate
Dioxybenzone
Ethyl 4-bis (hydroxypropyl) aminobenzoate

2-Ethylhexyl 2-cyano-3,3 diphylacrylate
Ethylhexyl *p*-methoxycinnamate
2-Ethylhexyl salicylate
Glyceryl aminobenzoate
Homosalate
Lawsone with dihydroxyacetone
Menthyl anthranilate
Oxybenzone

Padimate A
Padimate O
2-Phenylbenzimidazole-5-sulfonic acid
Red petrolatum
Sulisobenzone
Titanium dioxide
Triethanolamine salicylate

Adverse Reactions to Excessive Sun Tanning

Skin cancer   Photosensitivity
Skin aging   Allergies

Personal Dental Hygiene Products

Product	Recommendations for selection or use	Product	Recommendations for selection or use
Toothbrush	Round, soft bristles in four rows; use 3 to 4 minutes with a proven technique; replace brush every 2 to 3 months, weekly when ill	Dental irrigator	Device using a pressurized stream of water to "pick" food debris lodged between teeth; model with a self-contained pump is considered more effective than one using household water pressure
Disclosing solution	Use periodically to familiarize yourself with the locations in which plaque accumulates and to assess the effectiveness of your brushing and flossing technique; sequence: disclose-brush-inspect-brush-re-disclose	Mouthwash	Freshens the breath; capable of effecting some plaque reduction only when used in combination with regular brushing and flossing; fluoridated dental rinses can contribute to the prevention of dental caries when used in combination with brushing and flossing.
Dental floss	Waxed or unwaxed cotton fiber thread for use in removing food debris from areas not generally reached by brushing alone; pull thread through adjoining tooth surfaces, gently elevating gingival tissues	Anti-plaque dental rinse	Solution whose effervescent action dislodges plaque from dental surfaces. Vigorous swishing of the solution should be followed by regular brushing. Then a second application of the anti-plaque rinse should follow
Toothpaste	Tartar-control toothpaste is recommended. Select a fluoridated product in the midrange of abrasiveness; products designed to "brighten" or "whiten" teeth are generally too abrasive for general use; dentifrice intended for use with the false teeth should not be used on natural teeth		

Acne Products

Active ingredient	Representative brands	Effectiveness
Benzoyl peroxide medications	PanOxyl bar Oxy-5 and Oxy-10 Clearasil cream Noxzema Acne 12	The most effective OTC active ingredient, benzoyl peroxide aids in the prevention of new lesion formation
Salicylic acid cleaners	Clearasil Medicated Cleanser Stri-Dex Maximum Strength Pads PROPA pH Cleaning Pads and Lotion	Salicylic acid aids in unseating blackheads; alcohol base helps remove surface oils; no suppression of lesion formation is associated with these products
Sulfur-based medications	Acnomel Cream Fostril Lotion	Does not prevent lesion formation; active ingredient does help dry areas associated with lesions
Alcohol-based cleansers	Sea Breeze Antiseptic for the Skin Noxema Antiseptic Skin Cleanser	Noneffective
Scrubs	Epi-Clear Scrub Cleanser Komix Cleanser	Too abrasive
Medicated soaps	Clearasil Antibacterial Soap Fostex Medicated Cleansing Bar	No more effective than ordinary soap and water

APPENDIX

2

First Aid

Accidents are the leading cause of death for people ages 1 to 37. Injuries sustained in accidents can often be tragic. They are grim reminders of our need to learn first aid skills and to practice preventive safety habits.

First aid knowledge and skills allow you to help people who are in need of immediate emergency care. They also can help you save yourself if you should become injured. We recommend that our students enroll in Red Cross first aid and safety courses, which are available in local communities or through colleges or universities. In this appendix we will briefly present some information about common first aid emergen-

cies. (Please note that our information is *not* a substitute for comprehensive Red Cross first aid instruction.)

FIRST AID

▼ Keep a list of important phone numbers near your phone (your doctor, ambulance service, hospital, poison control center, police and fire departments).

▼ In case of serious injury or illness, call the appropriate emergency service immediately for help (if uncertain, call "911" or "0").

Specific problem	What to do
Asphyxiation	
Victim stops breathing and skin, lips, tongue, and fingernail beds turn bluish or gray.	Adult: Tip head back with one hand on forehead and other lifting the lower jaw near the chin.
	Look, listen, and feel for breathing.
	If not breathing, place your mouth over victim's mouth, pinch the nose, get a tight seal, and give 2 slow breaths.
	Recheck the breathing; if still not breathing, give breaths once every 5 seconds for an adult, once every 3 seconds for a child, once every 3 seconds for infants (do not exaggerate head tilt for babies).
Bleeding	
Victim bleeding severely can quickly go into shock and die within 1 or 2 minutes.	With the palm of your hand, apply firm, direct pressure to the wound with a clean dressing or pad.
	Elevate the body part if possible.
	Do not remove blood-soaked dressings; use additional layers, continue to apply pressure, and elevate the site.

Specific problem

Choking

Accidental ingestion or inhalation of food or other objects causes suffocation that can quickly lead to death. There are over 3,000 deaths annually, mostly of infants, small children, and the elderly.

Hyperventilation

A situation in which a person breathes too rapidly; often the result of fear or anxiety; may cause confusion, shortness of breath, dizziness, or fainting. Intentional hyperventilation before an underwater swim is especially dangerous, since it may cause a swimmer to "pass out" in the water and drown.

Bee stings

Not especially dangerous except for persons who have developed an allergic hypersensitivity to a particular venom. Those who are not hypersensitive will experience swelling, redness, and pain.
Hypersensitive persons may develop extreme swelling, chest constriction, breathing difficulties, hives, and shock signs.

Poisoning

Often poisoning can be prevented with adequate safety awareness. Children are frequent victims.

Shock

A life-threatening depression of circulation, respiration, and temperature control, recognized by a victim's cool, clammy, pale skin; weak and rapid pulse; shallow breathing; weakness; nausea; or unconsciousness.

Burns

Burns can cause major tissue damage and lead to serious infection and shock.

What to do

The procedure is easy to learn; however, the Heimlich maneuver must be learned from a qualified instructor. The procedure varies somewhat for infants, children, adults, pregnant women, and obese persons.

Have the person relax and rest for a few minutes. Provide reassurance and a calming influence. Having the victim take a few breaths in a paper bag (not plastic) may be helpful. Do not permit swimmers to practice hyperventilation before attempting to swim.

For nonsensitive persons: Scrape stinger from skin and apply cold compresses or over-the-counter topical preparation for insect bites.
For sensitive persons: Get professional help immediately. Scrape the stinger from skin; position the person so that the bitten body part is below the level of the heart; help administer prescribed medication (if available); apply cold compresses.

Call the poison control center immediately; follow the instructions provided.
Keep syrup of ipecac on hand.

Provide psychological reassurance.
Keep victim calm and in a comfortable, reclining position; loosen tight clothing.
Prevent loss of body heat; cover if necessary.
Elevate legs 8 to 12 inches (if there are no head, neck, or back injuries, or possible broken bones involving the hips or legs).
Do not give food or fluids.
Seek further emergency assistance.

Minor burns: immerse in cold water and then cover with sterile dressings; do not apply butter or grease to burns.
Major burns: seek help immediately; cover affected area with large quantities of clean dressings or bandages; do not try to clean the burn area or break blisters.
Chemical burns: flood the area with running water.

Specific problem	What to do
Broken bones	
Fractures are a common result of car accidents, falls, and recreational accidents.	Do not move the victim unless absolutely necessary to prevent further injury. Immobilize the affected area. Give care for shock while waiting for further emergency assistance.

Epilepsy: Recognition and First Aid

Seizure type	What it looks like	Often mistaken for	What to do	What not to do
Convulsive				
Generalized tonic-clonic (also called grand mal)	Sudden cry, fall, rigidity, followed by muscle jerks, frothy saliva on lips, shallow breathing or temporarily suspended breathing, bluish skin, possible loss of bladder or bowel control, usually lasts 2-5 minutes; normal breathing then starts again; there may be some confusion and/or fatigue, followed by return to full consciousness	Heart attack Stroke Unknown but life-threatening emergency	Look for medical identification Protect from nearby hazards Loosen ties or shirt collars Place folded jacket under head Turn on side to keep airway clear; reassure when consciousness returns If single seizure lasted less than 10 minutes, ask if hospital evaluation wanted If multiple seizures, or if one seizure lasts longer than 10 minutes, take to emergency room	Don't put any hard implement in the mouth Don't try to hold tongue. It can't be swallowed Don't try to give liquids during or just after seizure Don't use oxygen unless there are symptoms of heart attack Don't use artificial respiration unless breathing is absent after muscle jerks subside, or unless water has been inhaled Don't restrain
Nonconvulsive				
	This category includes many different forms of seizures, ranging from temporary unawareness (petit mal) to brief, sudden, massive muscle jerks (myoclonic seizures)	Daydreaming, acting out, clumsiness, poor coordination, intoxication, random activity, mental illness, and many others	Usually no first aid necessary other than to provide reassurance and emotional support. Any nonconvulsive seizure that becomes convulsive should be managed as a convulsive seizure. Medical evaluation is recommended.	Do not shout at, restrain, expect verbal instructions to be obeyed, or grab a person having a nonconvulsive seizure (unless danger threatens)

APPENDIX

3

A Look at Canadian Health

Canada's Population[1] (Thousands)

	Nfld.	PEI	NS	NB	Que.	Ont.	Man.
1921		88.6	523.8	387.9	2,360.5	2,933.7	610.1
1931		88.0	512.8	408.2	2,874.7	3,431.7	700.1
1941		95.0	578.0	457.4	3,331.9	3,787.7	729.7
1951	361.4	98.4	642.6	515.7	4,055.7	4,597.6	776.5
1961	457.9	104.6	737.0	597.9	5,259.2	6,236.1	921.7
1971	522.1	111.6	789.0	634.6	6,027.8	7,703.1	988.2
1981	567.7	122.5	847.4	696.4	6,438.2	8,624.7	1,026.2
1991[2]	575.7	131.2	901.0	727.6	6,847.4	9,917.3	1,094.4
1992[3]	577.5	130.5	906.3	729.3	6,925.2	10,098.6	1,096.8

	Sask.	Alta.	BC	YT	NWT	Canada
1921	757.5	588.5	524.6	4.1	8.1	8,787.4
1931	921.8	731.6	694.3	4.2	9.3	10,376.7
1941	896.0	796.2	817.8	5.0	12.0	11,506.7
1951	831.7	939.5	1,165.2	9.1	16.0	14,009.4
1961	952.2	1,332.0	1,629.1	14.6	23.0	18,265.3
1971	926.2	1,627.9	2,184.6	18.4	34.8	21,568.3
1981	968.3	2,237.3	2,744.2	23.2	45.7	24,341.7
1991[2]	994.2	2,521.6	3,212.1	26.7	55.2	27,004.4
1992[3]	993.2	2,562.7	3,297.6	27.9	56.5	27,402.1

[1]*As of June 1.*
[2]*Final postcensal estimates.*
[3]*Updated postcensal estimates.*

*Source: Statistics Canada. Appendix 3 is adapted from Canada Year Book 1994, Catalogue No. 11-402E/1994, pp. 112, 120-124, 148-151, 211, 215, 216. Reproduced by authority of the Minister of Industry, 1994. *Readers wishing further information on data provided through the cooperation of Statistics Canada may order copies of related publications by mail from: Publications Sales, Statistics Canada, Ottawa, Ontario, Canada K1A 0T6, by calling 1-613-951-7277 or toll-free 1-800-267-6677. Readers may also facsimile their order by dialing 1-613-951-1584.*

Number of Employed, by Occupation Group[1,2] (Thousands)

Occupation	1984	1989	1991	Percentage change 1989-1991
Managerial and administrative	1,169	1,545	1,660	7.4
Natural sciences, engineering and mathematics	388	457	488	6.8
Social sciences	181	218	263	20.6
Religion	32	32	29	− 9.4
Teaching	473	528	561	6.3
Medicine and health	540	628	674	7.3
Art, literature and recreation	182	233	231	− 0.9
Clerical	1,876	2,090	2,029	− 2.9
Sales	1,043	1,171	1,192	1.8
Service	1,491	1,655	1,642	− 0.8
Farming, horticultural and animal-husbandry	497	435	459	5.5
Fishing, hunting and trapping	32	37	40	8.1
Forestry and logging	64	55	46	− 16.4
Mining and quarrying	63	61	56	− 8.2
Processing	366	410	341	− 16.8
Machining	220	228	183	− 19.7
Product fabricating, assembling and repairing	942	1,050	930	− 11.4
Construction trades	568	744	660	− 11.3
Transport equipment operating	398	469	450	− 4.1
Material handling	261	281	254	− 9.6
Other crafts and equipment operating	144	155	151	− 2.6
All occupations	10,932	12,486	12,339	− 1.2

[1]Annual averages.
[2]Standard Occupational Classification 1980.

Religious Composition, 1991 (Percent)

	Canada	Nfld	PEI	NS	NB	Quebec	Ontario	Man.	Sask.	Alta.	BC	Yukon	NWT
Catholic	45.7	37.0	47.3	37.2	54.0	86.1	35.5	30.4	32.5	26.5	18.6	20.2	38.2
Roman Catholic	45.2	37.0	47.3	37.2	53.9	86.0	35.1	27.2	30.4	25.4	18.3	20.0	38.0
Ukrainian Catholic	0.5	0.0	0.0	0.0	0.0	0.1	0.4	3.1	2.1	1.0	0.2	0.2	0.1
Protestant	36.2	61.0	48.4	54.1	40.1	5.9	44.4	51.0	53.4	48.4	44.5	43.1	50.0
United Church	11.5	17.3	20.3	17.2	10.5	0.9	14.1	18.6	22.8	16.7	13.0	8.7	5.7
Anglican	8.1	26.2	5.2	14.4	8.5	1.4	10.6	8.7	7.2	6.9	10.1	14.8	32.0
Presbyterian	2.4	0.4	8.6	3.5	1.4	0.3	4.2	1.5	1.2	1.9	2.0	1.3	0.7
Lutheran	2.4	0.1	0.1	1.3	0.2	0.2	2.3	5.1	8.4	5.4	3.3	2.4	1.2
Baptist	2.5	0.2	4.1	11.1	11.3	0.4	2.7	1.9	1.6	2.5	2.6	3.6	1.2
Pentecostal	1.6	7.1	1.0	1.2	3.2	0.4	1.7	2.0	1.8	2.1	2.2	2.2	3.9
Other Protestant	7.9	9.8	9.0	5.5	4.9	2.3	8.8	13.2	10.5	12.9	11.4	10.2	5.2
Eastern Orthodox	1.5	0.1	0.1	0.3	0.1	1.3	1.9	1.9	2.0	1.7	0.7	0.3	0.3
Jewish	1.2	0.0	0.1	0.2	0.1	1.4	1.8	1.3	0.1	0.4	0.5	0.2	0.1
Eastern Non-Christian	2.8	0.3	0.4	0.6	0.3	1.5	3.9	1.6	0.8	3.2	5.1	1.3	0.9
Islam	0.9	0.1	0.0	0.2	0.0	0.7	1.5	0.3	0.1	1.2	0.8	0.1	0.1
Hindu	0.6	0.1	0.0	0.1	0.1	0.2	1.1	0.3	0.2	0.4	0.6	0.1	0.1
Buddhist	0.6	0.0	0.0	0.2	0.1	0.5	0.7	0.5	0.2	0.8	1.1	0.1	0.1
Sikh	0.5	0.0	0.1	0.0	0.0	0.1	0.5	0.3	0.1	0.5	2.3	0.1	0.1
Other Non-Christian	0.1	0.0	0.1	0.1	0.1	0.0	0.1	0.1	0.1	0.1	0.2	0.7	0.4
No Religion[1]	12.7	1.7	3.8	7.7	5.5	3.9	12.7	14.0	11.3	19.9	30.7	35.2	10.7

[1]Includes Para-religious groups and others not elsewhere classified.

Marriages, First Marriages and Remarriages

	Number of marriages	Number of first marriages		Number and proportion of marriages in which at least one spouse had been previously married		Number and proportion of remarriages in which the two spouses had been previously married	
		Males	Females	Number	%	Number	%
1971	191,324	168,944	169,072	31,698	16.6	12,934	40.8
1981	190,082	151,978	154,506	52,340	27.5	21,340	40.8
1990	187,738	143,637	145,350	60,393	32.2	26,094	43.2
1991	172,251	131,996	133,584	55,578	32.3	23,644	42.5

Number of Divorces

	1985	1986	1987	1988	1989	1990
Newfoundland	561	610	1,002	884	981	973
Prince Edward Island	213	191	246	260	243	268
Nova Scotia	2,337	2,550	2,640	2,478	2,524	2,347
New Brunswick	1,360	1,700	1,952	1,665	1,647	1,643
Quebec	15,814	18,399	19,315	19,825	19,790	19,405
Ontario[1]	20,854	28,653	38,223	29,873	31,202	28,183
Manitoba	2,314	2,917	3,771	2,998	2,847	2,677
Saskatchewan	1,927	2,395	2,751	2,463	2,451	2,227
Alberta	8,102	9,386	9,170	8,644	8,227	9,314
British Columbia	8,330	11,176	11,697	10,591	10,630	9,649
Yukon and Northwest Territories	168	183	218	191	174	173
Canada	61,980	78,160	90,985	79,872	80,716	76,859
Total Divorce Rate	3,121	3,799	4,314	3,748	3,928	3,827

[1]Data have been adjusted to take account of approximately 2,000 cases granted in Ontario in 1986 and 4,000 in Ontario in each of 1987 and 1988 that are not on the data base due to incomplete information.

Prevalence Rates[1] of Common-Law Unions in Canada

	1981	1986	1991
Newfoundland	2.19	3.50	9.34
Prince Edward Island	3.18	5.20	8.51
Nova Scotia	4.92	7.40	10.67
New Brunswick	4.02	6.48	11.04
Quebec	8.13	13.65	21.66
Ontario	5.63	7.20	7.42
Manitoba	5.26	7.03	10.32
Saskatchewan	4.25	6.35	9.57
Alberta	6.61	8.15	11.30
British Columbia	8.12	9.90	13.49
Yukon	15.41	18.30	23.13
Northwest Territories	9.63	14.22	14.76
Canada	6.40	9.18	13.50

[1]Rate per 100 persons living in couples.

Families Headed by a Single Parent (Percent)

Percent of families with children	1981	1986	1991
Newfoundland	12.7	14.2	15.9
Prince Edward Island	16.7	17.5	18.5
Nova Scotia	17.3	19.0	20.4
New Brunswick	16.8	18.5	19.7
Quebec	17.6	20.8	21.7
Ontario	16.3	17.8	19.3
Manitoba	16.9	18.7	20.4
Saskatchewan	14.6	17.0	18.5
Alberta	15.0	17.6	19.0
British Columbia	17.3	20.1	20.3
Yukon	18.1	21.3	21.7
Northwest Territories	16.4	20.0	20.2
Canada	16.6	18.8	20.0

Average Family Income

	Current dollars				
	1981	1986	1989	1990	1991
Newfoundland	25,870	30,383	39,648	40,770	41,654
Prince Edward Island	23,455	32,029	38,726	39,701	42,779
Nova Scotia	24,862	35,352	43,123	44,385	45,130
New Brunswick	24,608	33,313	40,670	42,356	44,323
Quebec	28,568	38,110	44,860	47,158	48,634
Ontario	32,322	45,778	57,330	57,027	58,634
Manitoba	28,606	37,875	46,551	47,178	46,621
Saskatchewan	30,575	37,025	42,978	44,234	45,930
Alberta	36,279	43,729	49,734	51,985	55,552
British Columbia	33,687	40,590	49,442	54,448	54,895
Canada	30,973	41,240	50,083	51,633	53,131

Average Family Income (concluded)

	Constant (1991) dollars				
	1981	1986	1989	1990	1991
Newfoundland	43,229	38,346	43,875	43,064	41,654
Prince Edward Island	39,193	40,423	42,855	41,934	42,779
Nova Scotia	41,544	44,617	47,721	46,882	45,130
New Brunswick	41,120	42,044	45,006	44,739	44,323
Quebec	47,737	48,098	49,643	49,811	48,634
Ontario	54,010	57,776	63,443	60,235	58,634
Manitoba	47,801	47,801	51,514	49,832	46,621
Saskatchewan	51,091	46,729	47,560	46,723	45,930
Alberta	60,622	55,190	55,037	54,910	55,552
British Columbia	56,291	51,228	54,714	57,511	54,895
Canada	51,756	52,048	54,423	54,538	53,131

Life Expectancy (years)

	Males				Females			
	At birth	20 years	40 years	60 years	At birth	20 years	40 years	60 years
1931	60.00	49.05	31.98	16.29	62.10	49.76	33.02	17.15
1941	62.96	49.57	31.87	16.06	66.30	51.76	33.99	17.62
1951	66.33	50.76	32.45	16.49	70.83	54.41	35.63	18.64
1961	68.35	51.51	32.96	16.73	74.17	56.65	37.45	19.90
1971	69.34	51.71	33.22	16.95	76.36	58.18	38.99	21.39
1976	70.19	52.09	33.59	17.23	77.48	58.95	39.67	21.96
1981	71.88	53.39	34.72	17.96	78.98	60.08	40.73	22.85
1986	73.04	54.27	35.52	18.41	79.73	60.65	41.20	23.17
Gains								
1931-76	10.19	3.04	1.61	0.94	15.38	9.19	6.65	4.81
1931-86	13.04	5.22	3.45	2.12	17.63	10.89	8.18	6.02

Canada's Infant Mortality Rate per 1,000 Live Births

Year	Male	Female	Year	Male	Female
1921	98.2	77.4	1981	10.8	8.4
1931	95.7	76.0	1986	8.7	7.0
1941	68.3	53.0	1987	8.4	6.2
1951	42.7	34.0	1988	8.2	6.4
1961	30.5	23.7	1989	8.0	6.2
1971	19.9	15.1	1990	7.5	6.1

Therapeutic Abortions

Residence	Number of therapeutic abortions		
	1986	1989	1990
Newfoundland	367	467	462
Prince Edward Island	13	8	51
Nova Scotia	1,704	2,030	1,871
New Brunswick	358	509	542
Quebec	12,410	13,854	14,438
Ontario	26,928	31,644	31,224
Manitoba	2,568	2,766	2,529
Saskatchewan	1,048	1,339	1,336
Alberta	6,313	6,585	6,621
British Columbia	11,386	11,098	11,518
Yukon	119	136	142
Northwest Territories	248	261	335
Residence not reported	-	8	23
Canada	63,462	70,705	71,092

Leading Causes of Death, 1990

	Male		Female	
	No.	Rate[1]	No.	Rate[1]
Diseases of the circulatory system	38,823	296.3	36,266	269.0
Cancer	28,865	220.3	23,560	174.8
Respiratory diseases	9,351	71.4	6,921	51.3
Accidents and adverse effects	9,064	69.2	3,993	29.6
Diseases of the digestive system	3,691	28.2	3,303	24.5
Endocrine diseases, etc.	2,533	19.3	2,939	21.8
Diseases of the nervous system	2,275	17.4	2,580	19.1
All other causes	9,358	71.2	8,434	62.7
Total, causes	103,960	793.3	87,996	652.8

[1]Per 100,000 population.

Cancer Deaths, 1990

Cause	ICD-9[1]	Rank	Number	Percentage	Rate[2]
Males					
Lung	162	1	9,536	33.0	72.8
Prostate	185	2	3,212	11.1	24.5
Colon	153	3	2,216	7.7	16.9
Pancreas	157	4	1,329	4.6	10.1
Site unspecified	199	5	1,313	4.5	10.0
Stomach	151	6	1,305	4.5	10.0
Other of lymphoid and histiocytic tissue	202	7	846	2.9	6.4
Bladder	188	8	821	2.8	6.3
Rectum	154	9	777	2.7	5.9
Brain	191	10	742	2.6	5.7
Total, all cancers	140-208		28,865	100.0	220.3
Females					
Breast	174	1	4,712	20.0	34.9
Lung	162	2	4,168	17.7	30.9
Colon	153	3	2,215	9.4	16.4
Pancreas	157	4	1,282	5.4	9.5
Ovary	183	5	1,222	5.2	9.1
Site unspecified	199	6	1,160	4.9	8.6
Stomach	151	7	795	3.4	5.9
Other of lymphoid and histiocytic tissue	202	8	763	3.2	5.7
Other and ill-defined sites	159	9	672	2.8	5.0
Rectum	154	10	577	2.5	4.3
Total, all cancers	140-208		23,560	100.0	174.8

[1]International Classification of Diseases, 9th Revision.
[2]Per 100,000 population.

Number of Reported Cases of Selected Notifiable Diseases, 1990

	Canada	Nfld	PEI	NS	NB	Que.	Ont.	Man.	Sask.	Alta.	BC	Yukon	NWT
AIDS	1,183	6	—	17	10	436	437	4	14	83	176	—	—
Amoebiasis	1,965	5	—	13	2	135	1,007	50	69	138	545	1	—
Campylobacteriosis	11,817	130	90	223	382	2,151	5,768	—	298	842	1,916	10	7
Chickenpox	20,254	1,338	—	852	170	—	—	—	1,370	14,314	1,702	147	361
Giardiasis	8,786	46	18	119	134	688	3,462	—	649	354	2,235	39	42
Gonococcal infections[1]	13,822	49	10	310	62	1,966	6,148	1,079	903	1,255	1,500	85	455
Hepatitis A	1,939	4	1	4	5	315	412	91	275	274	556	1	1
Hepatitis B	3,001	7	1	115	85	1,039	656	35	34	102	914	10	3
Measles	1,033	3	3	51	12	85	741	—	7	23	107	—	1
Pertussis	8,030	11	31	191	27	1,626	850	117	73	4,851	197	28	28
Salmonellosis[2]	8,947	127	72	336	401	1,962	3,605	310	313	791	991	11	28
Shigellosis	1,652	3	3	12	62	418	530	42	233	117	229	3	—
Syphilis	1,444	2	—	3	26	200	979	13	—	100	120	—	1
Tuberculosis	1,964	8	1	18	32	405	704	95	223	156	270	10	22

[1]Includes all 098 categories except 098.4.
[2]Excludes typhoid 002.0 and paratyphoid 002.1 to 02.09.

A P P E N D I X

4

Mental Disorders

CATEGORIES OF MENTAL DISORDERS

Anxiety Disorders

Anxiety disorders are characterized by a fear that leads to overarousal of heartbeat, muscle tension, and shakiness.

- ▼ *Phobic disorder.* Excessive irrational fears. Examples are agoraphobia (fear of open places), claustrophobia (fear of enclosed places), and acrophobia (fear of heights).
- ▼ *Pain disorder.* Overwhelming fear of losing control or going crazy. Panic attacks can last from a minute to an hour or more. No clear reason exists as to why panic attacks occur.
- ▼ *Generalized anxiety disorder.* Continued, free-floating anxiety that lasts for at least 1 month.
- ▼ *Obsessive-compulsive disorder.* Obsessive behavior is characterized by recurring, irrational thoughts that remain out of control. Compulsive behavior reflects an irresistible urge to act repeatedly.

Dissociative Disorders

Dissociative disorders in which there is a sudden, temporary change in consciousness or self-identity.

- ▼ *Psychogenic amnesia.* Inability to recall a stressful event.
- ▼ *Psychogenic fugue.* Disorder in which a person loses memory of his or her past, moves to another locale, and takes on a new identity.
- ▼ *Multiple personality.* Disorder characterized by several distinct personalities occupying the same person.

Somatoform Disorders

Persons with somatoform disorders complain of a physical ailment, yet no physical abnormality can be found.

- ▼ *Conversion disorder.* Major, unexplained loss of some physical ability (such as eyesight or use of the legs).
- ▼ *Hypochondriasis.* The belief that one is sick, although no medical evidence can be found.

Affective Disorders

In affective disorders a disturbance exists in a person's ability to express emotions.

- ▼ *Dysthymic disorder.* Persistent feelings (lasting for at least 2 years) characterized by lack of energy, loss of self-esteem, pessimistic outlook, inability to enjoy other people or pleasurable activities, and thoughts about suicide. The disorder is likely the most common psychological problem in humans.
- ▼ *Major depressive disorder.* Depression more severe than dysthymic disorder. Evidenced by poor appetite and major weight loss, psychomotor symptoms, impaired reality testing, and recurrent thoughts of suicide.
- ▼ *Bipolar disorder.* Mood swings from elation to depression (formerly known as manic-depression).

Schizophrenic Disorders

Schizophrenic disorders are largely recognized by a person's verbal behavior. These disorders are characterized by disturbances in thought, perception, and attention. Schizophrenics may speak in a meaningless fashion, switch from topic to topic, and convey little important information. They may have delusions of grandeur or persecution, hallucinations, or excited or slowed motor activity. Usually schizophrenics do not think that their thoughts and actions are abnormal.

▼ *Disorganized type*. Characterized by disorganized delusions and frequent hallucinations that may be sexual or religious in nature. Exaggerated social impairment is common.

▼ *Catatonic type*. Characterized by a marked impairment in motor activity. May hold one body position for hours and not respond to the speech of others.

▼ *Paranoid type*. Characterized by delusions of persecution, often ones that are complex and systemized. Paranoid schizophrenics may experience vivid hallucinations that support their delusions.

THERAPEUTIC APPROACHES TO MENTAL DISORDERS

A variety of approaches can be used to help persons who have mental disorders. These approaches involve psychotherapy or the use of biological therapies. A brief outline of the more widely known strategies follows, as a comprehensive presentation on this topic is beyond the scope of this appendix.

Insight-Oriented Therapies

Underlying this category of therapeutic approaches is the belief that the client must gain insight into the experiences that led up to his or her problem or maladaptive behavior. By being able to recognize the underlying motives for one's behavior, a client will be better able to objectively view his or her beliefs, feelings, and thinking patterns. These underlying motives often are beneath the person's level of consciousness. Insight-oriented forms of psychotherapy include cognitive therapy, psychoanalysis, person-centered therapy, transactional analysis, and gestalt therapy.

Behavior Therapy

Discussed briefly in Chapter 6, behavior therapy (also called behavior modification) attempts to produce behavior change in a client by using scientifically tested principles of classical and operant conditioning and observational learning. Techniques of behavior therapy include operant conditioning (behavior reinforcement), aversive conditioning, systematic desensitization, assertiveness training, and self-control techniques.

Group Therapy

This form of therapy involves a therapist and several clients who have similar problems. Examples might be group therapy for persons with eating disorders, smoking concerns, sexual problems, family problems, or relationship concerns. By meeting together and working to resolve their similar concerns, clients often receive support from other group members. With multiple members, a larger volume of pertinent information exists for clients to share. In a practical sense, group therapy is usually less expensive than individual therapy and the therapist can reach more clients at once.

Biological Therapies

Psychiatrists and other physicians are qualified to approach mental disorders from a medical framework. They are able to use chemotherapy (tranquilizers, antidepresants, lithium), electroconvulsive therapy (ECT or shock therapy), and even psychosurgery (brain surgery). Often these approaches are used with clients who have especially serious psychiatric disorders or who do not respond well to psychotherapy.

APPENDIX

5

Body Systems

THE CIRCULATORY SYSTEM

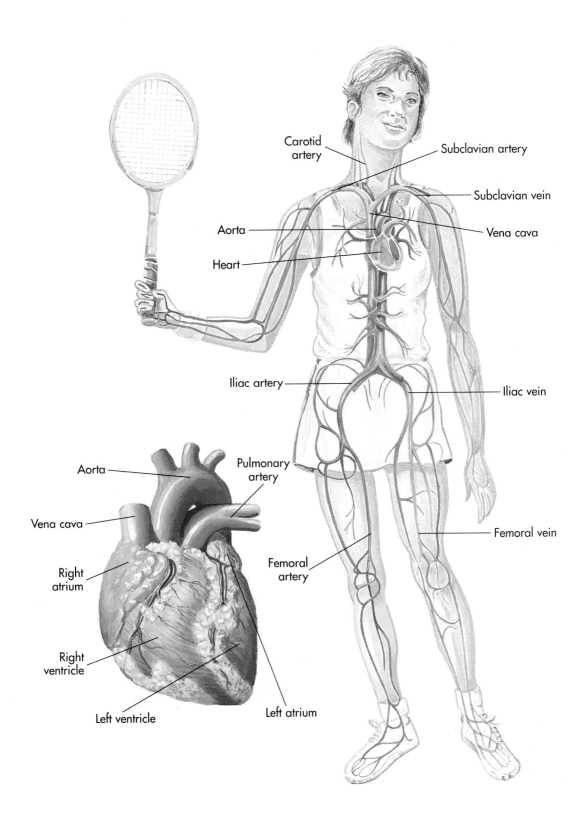

Carotid artery

Subclavian artery

Subclavian vein

Aorta

Vena cava

Heart

Iliac artery

Iliac vein

Aorta

Pulmonary artery

Vena cava

Right atrium

Femoral artery

Femoral vein

Right ventricle

Left ventricle

Left atrium

THE RESPIRATORY SYSTEM

Terminal end of bronchiole

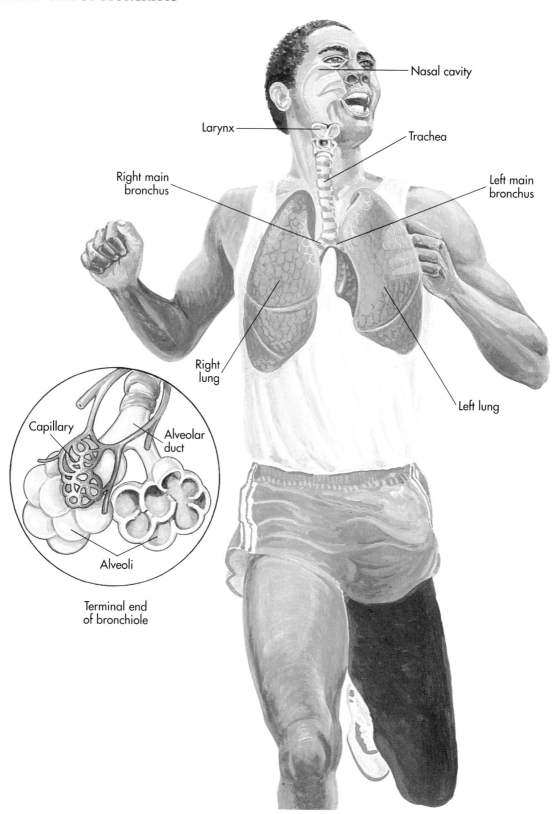

Nasal cavity

Larynx

Trachea

Right main bronchus

Left main bronchus

Right lung

Left lung

Capillary

Alveolar duct

Alveoli

Terminal end of bronchiole

THE MUSCULAR SYSTEM
Ligaments

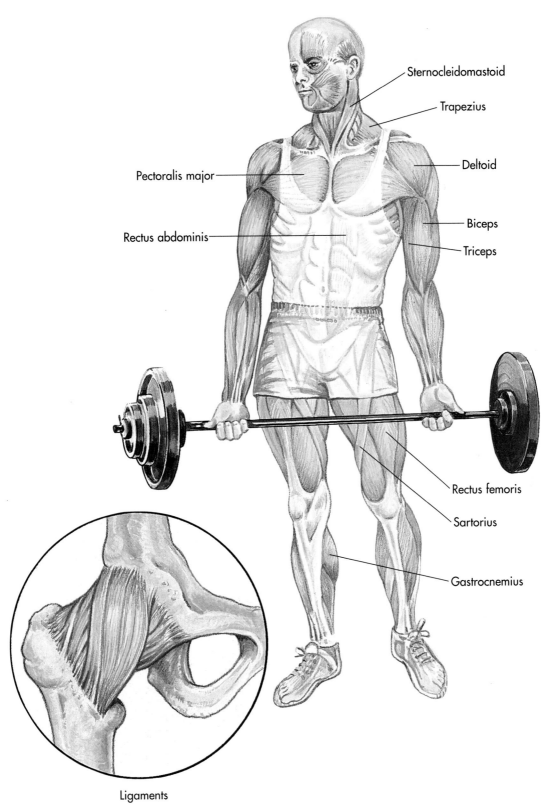

Sternocleidomastoid

Trapezius

Deltoid

Pectoralis major

Biceps

Rectus abdominis

Triceps

Rectus femoris

Sartorius

Gastrocnemius

Ligaments

THE SKELETAL SYSTEM

Cross section of bone

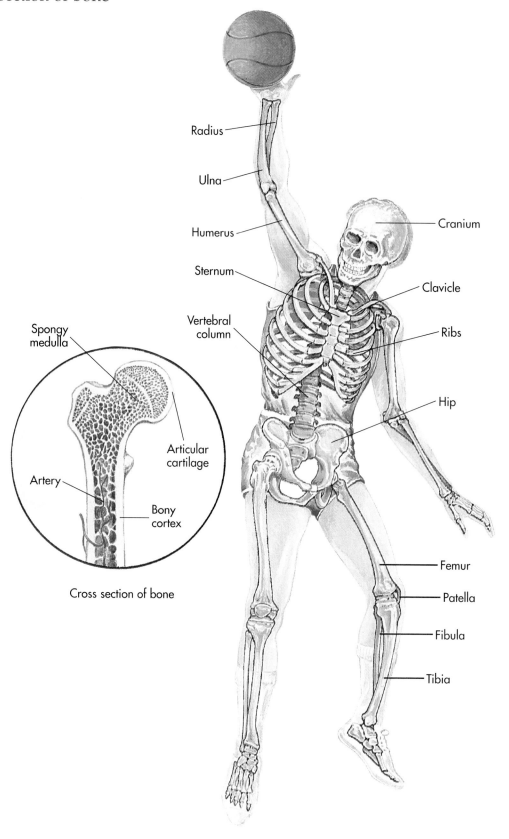

Cross section of bone

THE NERVOUS SYSTEM

Spinal cord detail

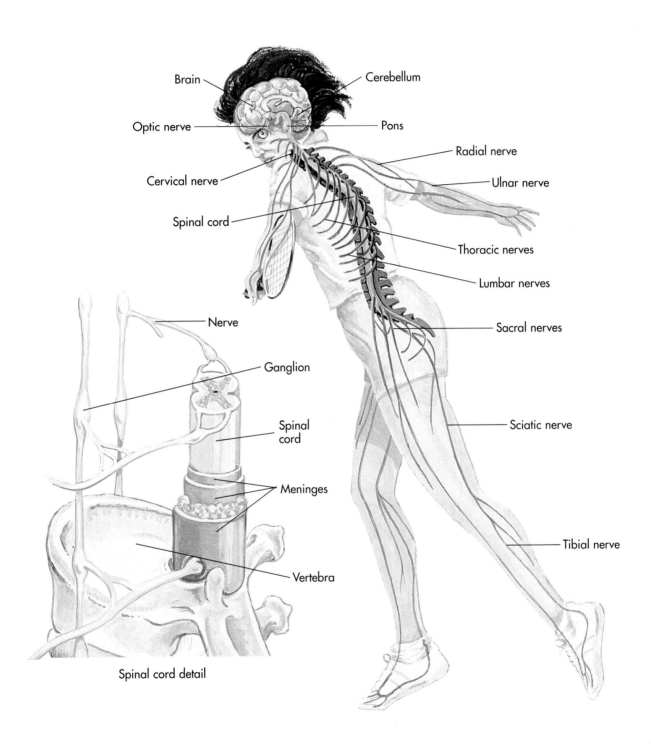

Brain
Cerebellum
Optic nerve
Pons
Cervical nerve
Radial nerve
Spinal cord
Ulnar nerve
Thoracic nerves
Lumbar nerves
Sacral nerves
Nerve
Ganglion
Spinal cord
Sciatic nerve
Meninges
Vertebra
Tibial nerve

Spinal cord detail

THE DIGESTIVE SYSTEM

Cross section of intestine wall

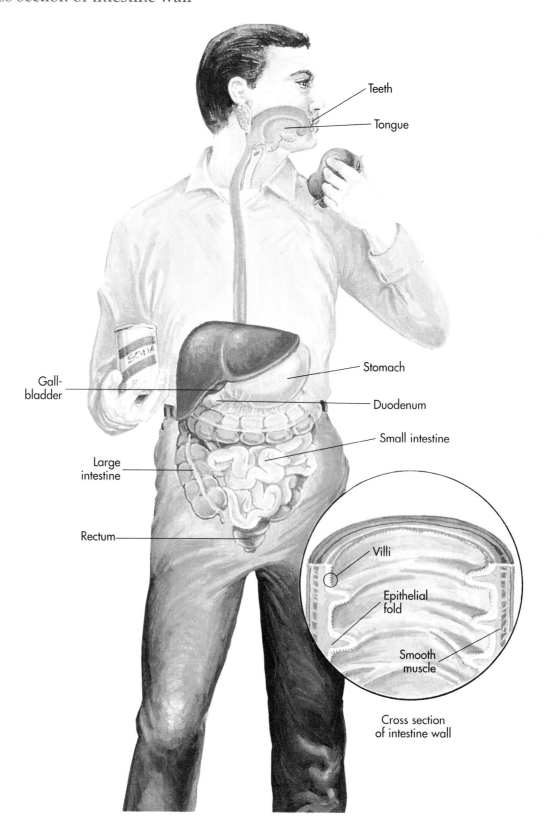

Teeth

Tongue

Stomach

Duodenum

Small intestine

Gall-bladder

Large intestine

Rectum

Villi

Epithelial fold

Smooth muscle

Cross section of intestine wall

THE URINARY SYSTEM

Cross section of kidney

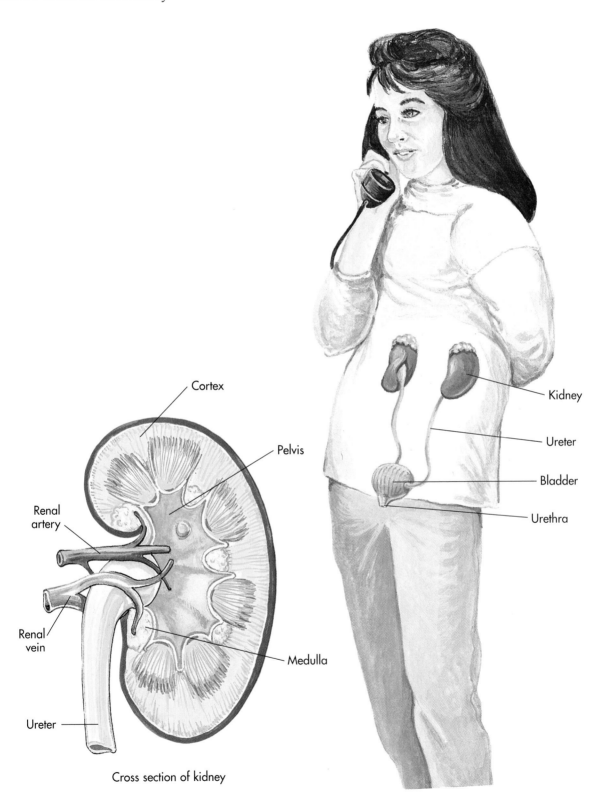

Cortex

Pelvis

Renal artery

Renal vein

Ureter

Medulla

Cross section of kidney

Kidney

Ureter

Bladder

Urethra

THE ENDOCRINE SYSTEM

NOTE: Refer to Figures 13-2 and 13-3 for detailed anatomical illustrations of the reproductive systems.

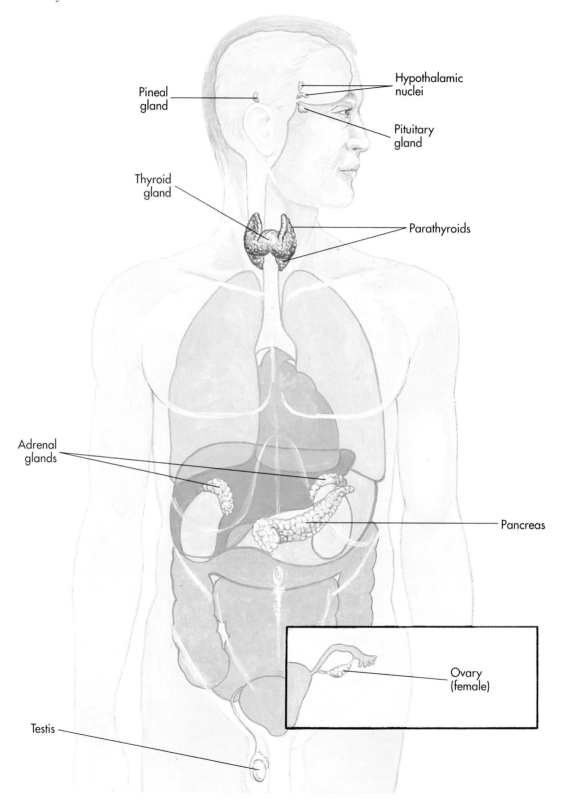

Pineal gland

Hypothalamic nuclei

Pituitary gland

Thyroid gland

Parathyroids

Adrenal glands

Pancreas

Ovary (female)

Testis

Glossary

A

abortion induced premature termination of a pregnancy.

absorption passage of nutrients or alcohol through the walls of the stomach or intestinal tract into the bloodstream.

abuse any use of a legal or illicit drug that is detrimental to health.

acid-base balance acidity-alkalinity of body fluids.

acid rain rain that has a lower pH (more acidic) than that normally associated with rain.

ACOAs (Adult Children of Alcoholics) grown children who were raised in a family with one or more alcoholic parents.

acquaintance rape forced sexual intercourse between individuals who know each other.

acquired immunity (AI) major component of the immune system associated with the formation of antibodies and specialized blood cells that are capable of destroying pathogens.

ACTH adrenocorticotropic hormone.

activity requirement Calories required for daily physical work.

activity theory theory of aging that suggests that the elderly must (and desire to) remain in familiar and/or new areas of involvement.

acupuncture insertion of fine needles into the body to alter electroenergy fields and cure disease.

acute begins abruptly and subsides after a short period.

acute alcohol intoxication potentially fatal elevation of blood alcohol concentration, often resulting from heavy, rapid consumption of large amounts of alcohol.

acute rhinitis the common cold; the sudden onset of nasal inflammation.

adaptive thermogenesis physiological response of the body to adjust its metabolic rate to the presence or absence of Calories.

addiction term used interchangeably with physical dependence.

additive effect combined (but not exaggerated) effect produced by the concurrent use of two or more drugs.

adipose tissue tissue comprised of fibrous strands around which specialized cells designed to store liquified fat are ordered.

adrenal cortex outer cell layers of the adrenal glands; cells of the cortex on stimulation by ACTH, produce corticoids.

adrenal glands paired triangular endocrine glands located at the top of each kidney; site of epinephrine and corticoid production.

adrenaline common name for epinephrine.

adrenocorticotropic hormone (ACTH) hormone produced in the pituitary gland and transmitted to the cortex of the adrenal glands; stimulates production and release of corticoids.

aerobic energy production body's production of energy when the respiratory and circulatory systems are able to process and transport sufficient amounts of oxygen to muscle cells.

affective pertaining to beliefs, values, and predispositions.

agent causal pathogen of a particular disease.

AIDS Acquired Immunodeficiency Syndrome; viral-based destruction of the immune system leading to illness and death from a variety of factors, including opportunistic infections.

alcoholism a primary, chronic disease with genetic, psychosocial, and environmental factors influencing its development and manifestations.

allergens environmental substances to which persons may be hypersensitive; allergens function as antigens.

allopathy system of medical practice in which specific remedies are used to produce effects different from those produced by a disease or injury.

alveoli thin, saclike terminal ends of the airways; the site at which gases are exchanged between the blood and inhaled air.

Alzheimer's disease gradual development of memory loss, confusion, and loss of reasoning; can eventually lead to total intellectual incapacitation, brain degeneration, and death.

amino acids "building blocks" of protein; manufactured by the body or obtained from dietary sources.

amotivational syndrome behavioral pattern characterized by widespread apathy toward productive activities.

anabolic steroids drugs that function like testosterone to produce increases in weight, strength, endurance, and aggressiveness.

anaerobic energy production body's production of energy when needed amounts of oxygen are not readily available.

analgesic drugs drugs that reduce the sensation of pain.

anaphylactic shock life-threatening congestion of the airways resulting from hypersensitivity to a foreign protein.

androgens male sex hormones.

androgyny the blending of both masculine and feminine qualities.

anemia condition reflecting abnormally low levels of hemoglobin.

anesthetics drugs capable of blocking pain sensations.

aneurysm a ballooning or outpouching on a weakened area of an artery.

angina pectoris chest pain that results from impaired blood supply to the heart muscle.

angiogenesis factor chemical messenger that stimulates the development of additional capillaries into the tumor.

angioplasty surgical insertion of a balloon-tipped catheter into the coronary artery to open areas of narrowing.

anorexia nervosa disorder of emotional origin in which appetite and hunger are suppressed, and marked weight loss occurs.

anovulatory not ovulating; refers to a time period when the ovaries fail to release an ovum.

antagonistic effect effect produced when one drug reduces or offsets the effects of a second drug.

antibodies chemical compounds produced by the immune system to destroy antigens and their toxins.

antigens disease-producing microorganisms or foreign substances that on entering the body trigger an immune response.

aortic valve valve that controls the blood flow into the aorta from the left ventricle of the heart.

arrhythmias irregularities of the heart's normal rhythm or beating pattern.

arteriosclerosis calcification within the artery's wall that makes the vessel less elastic, more brittle, and more susceptible to bursting; hardening of the arteries.

artificial insemination depositing of sperm in the female reproductive tract in an attempt to impregnate; sperm may be those of the partner or of a donor.

artificially acquired immunity (AAI) type of acquired immunity resulting from the body's response to pathogens introduced into the body through immunizations.

asbestos fibrous material found in insulation and many other building materials; asbestosis.

asphyxiation death resulting from lack of oxygen to the brain.

atherosclerosis buildup of plaque on the inner wall of arteries.

attention deficit disorder (ADD) above-normal physical movement; often accompanied by an inability to concentrate on a specified task; also called hyperactivity.

audiologists health care professionals trained to assess auditory function.

auditory acuity clarity or sharpness at which a particular sound can be heard.

authentic self positive self-identity that underlies the individual's more temporary mood identities; the most basic self-concept.

autoimmune immune response against the cells of a person's own body.

axon portion of a neuron that conducts electrical impulses to the dendrites of adjacent neurons; neurons typically have one axon.

ayurveda traditional Indian medicine based on herbal remedies.

AZT (azidothymidine) the first drug approved for use in the treatment of AIDS, capable of reducing symptoms and possibly extending life expectancy of the HIV-infected person.

B

balanced diet diet featuring food selections from each food group.

ballistic stretching a "bouncing" form of stretching in which a muscle group is lengthened repetitively to produce multiple quick, forceful stretches.

bariatrician physician who specializes in the study and treatment of obesity.

basal cells foundation cells that underlie the epithelial cells.

basal metabolic rate (BMR) the amount of energy (in Calories) your body requires to maintain basic functions.

behavior modification behavioral therapy designed to change the learned behavior of an individual.

being needs needs associated with actualization and spiritual growth.

benign noncancerous; tumors that do not spread.

bestiality alternate term for zoophilia.

beta blockers drugs that prevent overactivity of the heart, which results in angina pectoris.

bias and hate crimes criminal acts directed at a person or group solely because of a specific characteristic such as race, religion, ethnic background, or political belief.

binge drinking consuming five or more alcoholic drinks during one drinking occasion.

biochemical oxygen demand index of water pollution based on the rate and extent that organic matter uses dissolved oxygen from a sample of water.

biofeedback self-monitoring of physiological processes as they occur within the body.

biological sexuality male and female aspects of sexuality.

biological toxins poisons produced by microorganisms during the course of an infectious disease.

biologically available term used to describe the ability of a particular material to be used by the body.

birth control all of the procedures that can prevent the birth of a child.

birthing rooms hospital facilities that serve as both a labor and a delivery room.

bisexual a sexual orientation in which there is an attraction to same-sex and opposite-sex partners.

blackout temporary state of amnesia experienced by an alcoholic; an inability to remember events that occur during a period of alcohol use.

blood alcohol concentration (BAC) percentage of alcohol in a measured quantity of blood.

blood analysis chemical analysis of various substances in the blood; helps determine changes and possible disturbances in the body.

body fat analysis determination of the percentage of body tissue composed of fat.

body image subjective perception of how one's body appears.

bodybuilding sports activity in which the participants train their bodies to reach desired goals of muscular size, symmetry, and proportion.

body mass index (BMI) numerical expression of body weight based on height and weight.

bonding important, initial recognition established between the newborn and those adults on whom the newborn will depend.

brain death the absence of brain wave activity after an initial measurement followed by a second measurement 24 hours later.

brand name specific name assigned to a drug by its manufacturer.

Braxton Hicks contractions false labor contractions; mild and of irregular spacing.

breakthrough bleeding midcycle uterine bleeding; spotting.

breast augmentation enlarging breasts for cosmetic purposes.

breech position birth position in which the baby's feet or buttocks are presented first.

bulimarexia binge eating followed by purging the body of the food.

bulimia disorder of emotional origin in which binge eating patterns are established; usually accompanied by purging.

C

caffeinism chronic, heavy consumption of caffeine.

calcium channel blockers drugs that prevent arterial spasms; used in the long-term management of angina pectoris.

calendar method form of periodic abstinence in which the variable lengths of a woman's menstrual cycle are used to calculate her fertile period.

calipers device to measure the thickness of a skinfold from which percent body fat can be calculated.

caloric balance caloric input equals caloric output; weight remains constant.

Calories units of heat (energy); specifically, 1 Calorie equals the heat required to raise 1 kilogram of water 1° C.

cannula hollow metal or plastic tube through which materials can be aspirated.

carbohydrates chemical compounds comprising sugar or saccharide units; the body's primary source of energy.

carbon monoxide (CO) gaseous compound that can inactivate red blood cells.

carcinogens a tracing that stimulate the development of cancer.

carcinoma in situ cancer at its site of origin.

cardiac pertaining to the heart.

cardiac muscle specialized, smooth muscle tissue that forms the middle (muscular) layer of the heart wall.

cardiogram a tracing of heart and lung function from a cardiograph machine.

cardiovascular pertaining to the heart (cardio) and blood vessels (vascular).

cardiorespiratory endurance ability of the heart, lungs, and blood vessels to process and transport oxygen required by muscle cells so that they can sustain aerobic energy production.

carjacking a crime that involves a thief's attempt to steal a car while the owner is behind the wheel; carjackings are usually random, unpredictable, and frequently involve handguns.

CAT scan computerized axial tomography; x-ray procedure designed to visualize structures within the body that would not normally be seen through conventional x-ray procedures.

catabolism metabolic process of breaking down tissue for the purpose of converting it into energy.

cauterize to apply a small electrical current and permanently close a tube or vessel; to burn.

celibacy the practice of being sexually abstinent.

cell-mediated immunity form of acquired immunity that uses specialized white blood cells to destroy specific antigens that enter the body.

cellular cohesiveness tendency of normal cells to "stick together" rather than to move independently throughout the body.

central nervous system the brain and spinal cord.

cereal germ highly nutritious portions of the cereal grain, often removed during milling.

cerebral cortex outer covering of the brain; site of intellect, memory, thought processes, and rationalization.

cerebral hemorrhage bleeding from the cerebral arteries within the brain.

cerebrovascular accident stroke; brain tissue damage resulting from impaired circulation within blood vessels in the brain.

cerebrovascular occlusions blockages to arteries supplying blood to the cerebral cortex of the brain; strokes.

cervical cap small, thimble-shaped contraceptive device designed to fit over the cervix.

cesarean delivery surgical removal of a fetus through the abdominal wall.

chemical name name used to describe the molecular structure of a drug.

chemoprevention cancer prevention based on the selection of foods whose nutrient composition is thought to protect the body from certain forms of cancer.

child abuse harm that is committed against a child; usually referring to physical abuse, sexual abuse, or child neglect.

chippers a small percentage of smokers who can smoke a few cigarettes on a daily basis without becoming dependent.

chiropractic manipulation of the vertebral column to relieve pressure and cure illness.

chlamydia the most prevalent sexually transmitted disease; caused by a nongonococcal bacterium.

chlorofluorocarbons (CFCs) gaseous compounds that contain chlorine and fluorine.

cholesterol a primary form of fat found in the blood; lipid material manufactured with the body, as well as derived through dietary sources.

chorionic villi fingerlike extensions of the fetal portion of the placenta; these extensions carry fetal blood vessels close to the maternal blood vessels.

chorionic villi sampling (CVS) microscopic examination of the cells of the chorionic villi; process for identifying genetic defects earlier than can be done with amniocentesis.

chronic develops slowly and persists for a long period.

chronic bronchitis persistent inflammation and infection of the smaller airways within the lungs.

chronic fatigue syndrome (CFS) illness that causes severe exhaustion, fatigue, aches, and depression; mostly affects women in their thirties and forties.

cilia small, hairlike structures that extend from cells that line the air passages.

cirrhosis pathological changes to the liver resulting from chronic, heavy alcohol consumption; a frequent cause of death among heavy alcohol users.

clinical stage stage of an infectious disease at which symptoms are most fully expressed; acute stage.

clitoris small shaft of erectile tissue located in front of the vaginal opening; the female homolog of the male penis.

cochlea small, snail-shaped organ of the inner ear in which the energy of sound is converted into electrical energy for transmission to the brain.

codependence a strong, unconscious attraction to a chemically dependent person; codependent persons may exhibit behaviors that include both denial and enabling.

coenzyme vitamin-based organic compound that assists a particular enzyme in performing its role in regulating biochemical reactions.

cohabitation sharing of a residence by two unrelated, unmarried people; living together.

coitus penile-vaginal intercourse.

coitus interruptus (withdrawal) a contraceptive practice in which the erect penis is removed from the vagina before ejaculation.

cold turkey immediate, total discontinuation of use of a drug; associated withdrawal discomfort.

coliform bacteria intestinal tract bacteria; presence in a water supply suggests contamination by human or animal waste.

colostomy surgically created opening on the abdominal wall for the elimination of body wastes.

comorbidity two or more diagnosed chronic health problems that occur at the same time in an individual.

companionate love friendly affection and deep attachment, based on extensive familiarity with another person.

complex carbohydrates carbohydrates composed of long molecular chains containing many saccharide units; starches.

compliance willingness to follow the directions provided by another person.

compulsion compelling emotional desire to engage in a particular behavior.

condom latex shield designed to cover the erect penis and retain semen upon ejaculation; "rubber".

conflict-habituated marriage marriage characterized by unending conflict and disagreement.

confrontation an approach to convince drug-dependent people to enter treatment.

congestive heart failure inability of the heart to pump out all the blood that returns to it; can lead to dangerous fluid accumulations in veins, lungs, and kidneys.

consumer fraud marketing of unrealiable and ineffective services, products, or information under the guise of curing disease or improving health; quackery.

contact inhibition ability of a tissue, on reaching its mature size, to suppress additional growth.

contraception any procedure that prevents fertilization.

contraceptive sponge soft, spongy disk that is moistened and inserted over the cervical area.

contraindications factors that make the use of a drug inappropriate or dangerous for a particular person.

cool down stretching and walking after exercise.

coronary arteries vessels that supply oxygenated blood to heart muscle tissue.

coronary artery bypass surgery surgical procedure designed to improve blood flow to the heart by providing alternate routes for blood to take around points of blockage.

coroner an elected official empowered to pronounce death and to determine the official cause of a suspicious or violent death.

corpus luteum cellular remnant of the graafian follicle after the release of an ovum.

corticoids hormones generated by the adrenal cortex; corticoids influence the body's control of glucose, protein, and fat metabolism.

CPR cardiopulmonary resuscitation; first aid procedure designed to restore breathing and heart function.

crack a crystalline form of cocaine that is smoked; has an instantaneous effect and is highly dependence producing.

creativity innovative ability; insightful capacity to solve problems; ability to move beyond analytical or logical approaches to experiences.

cross-tolerance transfer of tolerance from one drug to another within the same general category.

crosstraining use of more than one aerobic activity to achieve cardiovascular fitness.

crowning first appearance of the fetal head at the vaginal opening.

cruciferous vegetables vegetables that have flowers with four leaves in the pattern of a cross.

cryobiology the science of freezing living tissue.

cryonics an unproven technology in which dead bodies are frozen in hopes of preserving tissues until disease cures are found.

crypts burial locations generally underneath churches.

cunnilingus oral stimulation of the vulva or clitoris.

cystitis infection of the urinary bladder.

D

date rape a form of acquaintance rape that involves forced sexual intercourse by a dating partner.

deficiency needs survival requirements; needs associated with normal function as a physical being.

dehydration abnormal depletion of fluids from the body; severe dehydration can lead to death.

delirium tremens (DTs) uncontrollable shaking associated with withdrawal from heavy chronic alcohol use.

dendrite portion of a neuron that receives electrical stimuli from adjacent neurons; neurons typically have several such branches or extensions.

denial in this case, the failure to acknowledge that alcohol or drug use seriously affects one's life.

dependence general term that reflects the need to keep consuming a drug for psychological or physical reasons, or both.

depressants the psychoactive drugs that reduce the function of the central nervous system.

depression an emotional state characterized by exaggerated feelings of sadness, melancholy, dejection, worthlessness, emptiness, and hopelessness that are inappropriate and out of proportion to reality.

designated driver a person who abstains or carefully limits alcohol consumption to be able to safely transport other people who have been drinking.

designer drugs drugs that chemically resemble drugs on the FDA Schedule 1.

desirable weight weight range deemed appropriate for persons of a specific sex, age, and frame size.

devitalized marriage marriage that lacks the vitality or dynamic nature it once possessed.

diagnosis-related groups (DRGs) prospective billing categories established by the federal government for Medicare reimbursements to hospitals for patients' illnesses, injuries, and surgical procedures.

diaphragm soft, rubber vaginal cup designed to cover the cervix.

diastolic pressure blood pressure against blood vessel walls when the heart relaxes.

dietary cholesterol cholesterol obtained from food sources.

diffusion movement of a substance across a membrane from an area of greater concentration to an area of lesser concentration.

dilation gradual expansion of an opening or passageway.

dilation and curettage (D & C) surgical procedure in which the cervical canal is dilated to allow the uterine wall to be scraped.

dilation and evacuation (D & E) surgical procedure using cervical dilation and vacuum aspiration to remove uterine wall material and fetal parts.

direct (active) euthanasia process of inducing death, often through the injection of a lethal drug.

disaccharides sugars composed of two monosaccharide units; sucrose, lactose, and maltose.

disengagement theory theory of aging that suggests that society slowly withdraws from the elderly and they in turn slowly withdraw from society.

dissonance feeling of uncertainty that occurs when a person believes two equally attractive but opposite ideas.

distillation production of alcohol by the vaporization and condensation of plant material; the process that produces liquor.

distress stress that diminishes the quality of life; commonly associated with disease, illness, and maladaptation.

diuresis increased discharge of fluid from the body; frequent urination.

doubling mitotic reproductive division undertaken by cells of a particular tissue.

diuretic drugs drugs that aid the body in removing excess fluid.

dose related drug-related response pattern that changes according to the amount of a drug within the body.

drug synergism enhancement of a drug's effect as a result of the presence of additional drugs within the system.

durable power of attorney for health care a legal document that designates who will make health care decisions for persons unable to do so for themselves.

duration length of time one needs to exercise at the target heart rate to produce the training effect.

dynamic in a state of change; health is dynamic because it can change from day-to-day.

E

ECG pattern electrocardiograph; an instrument to measure and record the electrical activity within the heart.

echocardiography procedure that uses high-frequency sound waves to visualize the structure and function of the heart.

ecosystem an ecological unit made up of both animal and plant life that interact to produce a stable system.

ectopic pregnancy a pregnancy wherein the fertilized ovum implants at a site other than the uterus, typically in the fallopian tube.

EEG patterns patterns reflecting the type and extent of electrical activity occurring in the cerebral cortex of the brain.

effacement a thinning and pulling back of the cervical opening to allow movement of the fetus from the uterus.

electrical impedence method to test for the percentage of body fat using an electrical current.

electroencephalogram instrument that measures the electrical activity of the brain.

electrolyte balance proper concentration of various minerals within the blood and body fluids.

embolism potentially fatal condition in which a circulating blood clot lodges itself in a smaller vessel.

embryonic stage stage of human development from the second through the eighth weeks of pregnancy.

emotional health subjective value-oriented responses to changing situations reflected in feelings of joy, anger, compassion, sympathy, and frustration.

empowerment process in which people gain increasing measures of control over their health.

empty Calories Calories obtained from foods that lack most other important nutrients.

enabling in this case, the inadvertent support that some people provide to alcohol or drug abusers.

endocrine system ductless glands that secrete one or more chemical messengers (hormones) into the bloodstream.

endometriosis growth of endometrial tissue into pelvic areas outside the uterus.

endometrium innermost lining of the uterus, broken down and discharged during menstruation.

enriched process of returning to foods some of the nutritional elements (B vitamins and iron) removed during processing.

Environmental Protection Agency (EPA) federal agency charged with the protection of natural resources and the quality of the environment.

environmental tobacco smoke tobacco smoke that is diluted and stays within a common source of air.

enzymes organic substances that control the rate of physiological reactions but are not altered in the process.

epidemic rapid spread of a disease among individuals within a given area or population.

epinephrine powerful adrenal hormone whose presence in the bloodstream prepares the body for maximal energy production and skeletal muscle response.

episiotomy a surgical procedure to enlarge the vaginal opening before giving birth.

epitaph inscription on a grave marker or monument.

erection the engorgement of erectile tissue with blood; characteristic of the penis, clitoris, nipples, labia minora, and scrotum.

erotic dreams dreams whose content elicits a sexual response.

essential amino acids nine amino acids that can be obtained only from dietary sources.

essential hypertension hypertension (high blood pressure) resulting from chronic widespread constriction of arterioles.

estrogen ovarian hormone that initiates the development of the uterine lining.

estrogen replacement therapy medically administered estrogen to replace estrogen lost as the result of menopause.

eulogy composition or speech that praises someone; often delivered at a funeral or memorial service.

eustress stress that adds a positive, enhancing dimension to the quality of life.

eutrophication enrichment of a body of water with nutrients, which causes overabundant growth of plants.

excitement stage initial arousal stage of the sexual response pattern.

exhibitionism exposure of one's genitals for the purpose of shocking other persons.

expectorants drugs that help bring mucus and phlegm up from the respiratory system.

expressionistic sexuality complete expression of one's personally defined concept of sexuality.

F

faith the purposes and meaning that underlie an individual's hopes and dreams.

fallopian tubes paired tubes that allow passage of ova from the ovaries to the uterus: the oviducts.

false labor conditions that tend to resemble the start of true labor; may include irregular uterine contractions, pressure, and discomfort in the lower abdomen.

false negative in this case, a test result that indicates "no pregnancy" when, in fact, there is a pregnancy.

false positive in this case, a test result that indicates "pregnancy" when, in fact, there is no pregnancy.

fast foods convenience foods; foods featured in a variety of restaurants, including hamburgers, pizza, and tacos.

fast-twitch (FT) fibers type of muscle cells especially suited for anaerobic activities.

fat density percentage of a food's total Calories that are derived from fat; above 30% reflects higher fat density.

fat soluble capable of being dissolved in fats or lipids.

fatty acid acid component that in combination with glycerol forms the dietary fat molecule.

FDA Schedule 1 list comprising drugs that hold a high potential for abuse but have no medical use.

fecundity the ability to produce offspring.

fellatio oral stimulation of the penis.

femininity behavioral expressions traditionally observed in females.

fermentation chemical process whereby plant products are converted into alcohol by the action of yeast on carbohydrates.

fertility ability to reproduce.

fertilization the union of ovum and sperm resulting in a fertilized egg; conception.

fetal alcohol syndrome characteristic birth defects noted in the children of some women who consume alcohol during their pregnancies.

fetal stage stage of human development from the end of the eighth week of

gestation until the time of birth.

fetishism choice of a body part or inanimate object as a source of sexual excitement.

fiber cellulose-based plant material that cannot be digested; found in cereal, fruits, and vegetables.

fight-or-flight response the reaction to a stressor by confrontation or avoidance.

five dimensions of health major areas of health in which specific strengths or limitations will be found: physical, emotional, social, intellectual, and spiritual.

flaccid nonerect; the state of erectile tissue when vasocongestion is not occurring.

flashback unpredictable return of a psychedelic trip.

flexibility ability of joints to function through an intended range of motion.

folacin folic acid; a vitamin of the B-complex group; used in the treatment of nutritional anemia.

follicle-stimulating hormone (FSH) gonadotrophic hormone required for initial development of ova (in the female) and sperm (in the male).

food additives chemical compounds that are intentionally or unintentionally added to our food supply.

food supplements nutrients taken in addition to those obtained through the diet: includes powdered protein, vitamins, and mineral extracts.

foreplay activities, often involving touching and caressing, that prepare individuals for sexual intercourse.

formaldehyde chemical found in many common buildup materials and home furnishings.

fraternal twins twins resulting when two separate ova are fertilized by different sperm.

freebase altered form of cocaine that can be smoked.

frequency (1) number of times per week one should exercise to achieve a training effect. (2) rate at which a sound source vibrates, measured in cycles per second.

fructose monosaccharide that provides a source of simple sugar; fruits and berries.

full funeral services all of the professional services provided by funeral directors.

G

gait pattern of walking.

gamete intrafallopian transfer (GIFT) retrieved ovum and partner's sperm are positioned in the fallopian tube for fertilization and subsequent movement into the uterus for implantation.

gaseous phase portion of tobacco smoke containing carbon monoxide and many other physiologically active gaseous compounds.

gateway drugs easily obtained legal or illegal drugs (alcohol, tobacco, marijuana) whose use may precede the use of less common illegal drugs.

gender general term reflecting a biological basis of sexuality; the male gender or the female gender.

gender adoption lengthy process of learning the behaviors that are traditional for one's gender.

gender identification achievement of a personally satisfying interpretation of one's masculinity or femininity.

gender identity recognition of one's gender.

gender preference emotional and intellectual acceptance for the gender that one is.

gender schema mental image of the cognitive, affective, and performance characteristics appropriate to a particular gender; a mental picture of being a man or a woman.

general adaptation syndrome sequenced physiological response to the presence of a stressor; the alarm, resistance, and exhaustion stages of the stress response.

generativity midlife developmental task; repaying society for its support through contributions associated with parenting, creativity, and occupation.

generic name common or nonproprietary name of a drug.

genetic counseling medical counseling regarding the transmission and management of inherited conditions.

genetic predisposition inherited tendency to develop a disease if necessary environmental factors exist.

genital sexuality sexuality that is centered in the recreational use of reproductive structures; the sexuality that encompasses sexual performance and eroticism.

glucose blood sugar; the body's primary source of energy.

goblet cells cells within the epithelial lining of the airways that produce the mucus required for cleaning the airways.

gonads male or female sex glands; testes produce sperm and ovaries produce ova (eggs).

greenhouse effect warming of the Earth's surface that is produced when solar heat becomes trapped by layers of carbon dioxide and other gases.

grief the emotional feelings associated with death.

H

habituation term used interchangeably with psychological dependence.

hallucinogens psychoactive drugs capable of producing hallucinations (distortions of reality).

hardiness the capacity to respond to change quickly and effectively.

hashish resins collected from the flowering tops of marijuana plants.

hate crimes see bias crimes.

health maintenance organizations (HMOs) groups that supply prepaid comprehensive health care with an emphasis on prevention.

health promotion movement in which knowledge, practices, and values are transmitted to people for use in lengthening their lives, reducing the incidence of illness, and feeling better.

healthy body weight weight range based on waist and hip measurements and reflecting an acceptable, healthy amount of fat within the central body cavity.

heart catheterization procedure wherein a thin catheter is introduced through an arm or leg artery into the coronary circulation to visualize areas of blockage.

heart-lung machine device that oxygenates and circulates blood during bypass surgery.

hemorrhaging bleeding; often implies profuse bleeding.

herbicides chemical agents used to destroy unwanted plants and weeds.

heterosexual a sexual orientation in which there is an attraction to opposite-sex partners.

HIV human immunodeficiency virus.

holistic health a view of health in terms of its physical, emotional, social, intellectual, and spiritual makeup.

homicide the intentional killing of one person by another.

homosexual a sexual orientation in which there is an attraction to same-sex partners.

hospice care approach to caring for terminally ill patients that maximizes the quality of life and allows death with dignity.

host negligence a legal term that reflects the failure of a host to provide reasonable care and safety for persons visiting the host's residence or business.

hot flashes temporary feelings of warmth experienced by women during and following menopause; caused by blood vessel dilation.

human chorionic gonadotropin (HCG) gonadotropic hormone that maintains the ovaries' production of progesterone.

Human Genome Project an international project in which geneticists are attempting to identify all genes on each chromosome.

human papilloma virus (HPV) sexually transmitted virus capable of causing precancerous changes in the cervix; causative agent for genital warts.

humoral immunity form of acquired immunity that uses antibodies to counter specific antigens that enter the body.

hurry sickness excessive time dependence; seen in persons whose lives are geared to rigid schedules and high achievement aspirations.

hydrostatic weighing weighing the body while it is submerged in water.

hypercellular obesity form of obesity seen in individuals who possess an abnormally large number of fat cells.

hyperglycemia elevated blood glucose levels; an important indicator of diabetes mellitus.

hyperparathyroidism condition reflecting the overactive production of parathyroid hormone by the parathyroid glands.

hypertonic saline solution salt solution with a concentration higher than that found in human fluids.

hypertrophic obesity form of obesity in which fat cells are enlarged, but not excessive in number.

hypervitaminosis excessive accumulation of vitamins within the body; associated with the fat-soluble vitamins.

hypochondriasis neurotic conviction that one is ill or afflicted with a particular disease.

hypothalamus portion of the midbrain that provides a connection between the cerebral cortex and the pituitary gland.

hypothyroidism condition in which the thyroid gland produces an insufficient amount of its hormone, thyroxin.

hysterectomy surgical removal of the uterus.

I

identical twins twins resulting when only one ovum is fertilized but divides into two zygotes early in its development.

immune system system of cellular elements that protect the body from invading pathogens and foreign materials.

immunizations laboratory-prepared pathogens that are introduced into the body for the purpose of stimulating the body's immune system.

in vivo fertilization and embryo transfer (IVF-ET) fertilization in the laboratory of an ovum taken from the woman with subsequent return of the developing embryo into the woman's uterus.

incest marriage or coitus (sexual intercourse) between closely related individuals.

incubation stage time required for a pathogen to multiply significantly enough for signs and symptoms to appear.

independent practice association (IPA) a modified HMO in which a group of physicians provide prepaid health care, but not from a central location within an HMO.

indirect (passive) euthanasia process of allowing a person to die by disconnecting life support systems or withholding lifesaving techniques.

indulgence strong emotional desire to engage in a particular behavior solely for one's own enjoyment or benefit.

infatuation an often shallow, intense attraction to another person.

inferior vena cava large vein that returns blood from lower body regions to the right atrium of the heart.

infertility inability of a male to impregnate, or of a female to become pregnant.

inhalants psychoactive drugs that enter the body through inhalation.

inhibitions inner controls that prevent a person's engaging in certain types of behavior.

insoluble fibers that can absorb water from the intestinal tract.

insulin pancreatic hormone required by the body for the effective metabolism of glucose.

insulin-dependent diabetes mellitus (type 1) form of diabetes generally seen for the first time in childhood or adolescence; juvenile onset diabetes.

intensity (1) level of effort put into an activity. (2) strength or loudness of a particular sound, measured in decibels.

intentional injuries injuries that are purposefully committed by a person.

interstitial cell stimulating hormone (ICSH) a gonadotropic hormone of the male required for the production of testosterone.

interstitial cells specialized cells within the testicles that on stimulation by ICSH produce the male sex hormone testosterone.

intimacy any close, mutual verbal or nonverbal behavior within a relationship.

intrauterine device (IUD) small, plastic, medicated or unmedicated device that when inserted in the uterus prevents continued pregnancy.

introspective looking inward to examine one's feelings and beliefs.

ionizing radiation form of radiation capable of releasing electrons from atoms.

isokinetic exercises muscular strength training exercises that use machines to provide variable resistances throughout the full range of motion.

isometric exercises muscular strength training exercises that use a resistance so great that the resistance object cannot be moved.

J

junk foods foods that contribute little healthful nutrition other than providing additional Calories; includes foods that fit the "fats, oils, and sweets" food group.

K

kwashiorkor protein deficiency disease, associated with early weaning of children and a diet lacking complete protein.

L

labia majora the larger, more external skin folds that surround the vaginal opening.

labia minora the smaller skin folds immediately adjacent to the vaginal opening.

lactating breastfeeding; nursing.

lactator female who is producing breast milk.

lactovegetarian diet vegetarian diet that includes the consumption of milk and dairy products.

laminaria plugs made of seaweed that on exposure to moisture expand and dilate the canal into which they have been placed.

lead toxicity blood lead level above 25 micrograms/deciliter. (If adopted, the new standard will be 10 micrograms/deciliter.)

legumes peas and beans; plant sources high in the essential amino acids.

lesbianism female homosexuality.

life cycle artificial segmenting of the life span; each segment represents a developmental period.

lightening movement of fetus deeper into the pelvic cavity before the onset of the birth process.

lipogenesis process whereby the body develops (and fills) adipose cells.

lipoprotein protein-like structure in the bloodstream to which circulating fatty materials attach; various lipoprotein profiles are associated with cardiovascular disease.

liposuction vacuum aspiration used to remove fat cells.

living will document confirming a person's desire to be allowed to die peacefully and with a measure of dignity in case of terminal illness or major injury.

low tar and nicotine brands cigarettes containing 15 mg of tar or less.

luteinizing hormone (LH) a gonadotropic hormone of the female required for fullest development and release of ova; ovulating hormone.

Lyme disease bacterial infection transmitted by deer ticks.

M

macrobiotic diet vegetarian diet composed almost entirely of brown rice.

macrocytic anemia form of anemia in which large red blood cells predominate, but in which total red blood cell count is depressed.

macronutrients minerals needed in relatively high amounts.

mainstream smoke the smoke inhaled and then exhaled by a smoker.

maltose disaccharide derived from germinating cereals and lactose (the carbohydrate found in human and animal milk).

mammogram x-ray examination of the breast.

masculinity behavioral expressions traditionally observed in males.

masochism sexual excitement while being injured or humiliated.

mastectomy removal of breast tissue.

mastery when applied to growth within the young adult segment of the life cycle, mastery implies becoming more self-aware, independent, responsible, and socially interactive.

masturbation self-stimulation of the genitals.

maternal supportive tissues general term referring to the development of the placenta and other tissues specifically associated with pregnancy.

mausoleum above-ground structure into which caskets can be placed for disposition; frequently resembles a small stone house.

maximum heart rate maximum number of times the heart can beat per minute.

Medicaid noncontributory governmental health insurance for persons receiving other types of public assistance.

Medicare contributory governmental health insurance, primarily for persons 65 years of age or older.

meltdown the overheating and eventual melting of the uranium fuel rods in the core of a nuclear reactor.

memorial service form of funeral service in which the body or casket often is not present.

menarche time of a female's first menstrual period (cycle).

menopause decline and eventual cessation of hormone production by the female reproductive system.

menstrual extraction procedure using vacuum aspiration to remove uterine wall material within 2 weeks following a missed menstrual period.

menstrual phase phase of the menstrual cycle during which the broken-down lining of the uterus (endometrium) is discharged from the body.

menstruate to undergo cyclic buildup and destruction of the uterine wall.

metabolic rate rate or intensity at which the body produces energy.

metastasis spread of cancerous cells from their site of origin to other areas of the body.

micronutrients minerals needed in relatively small amounts.

midlife period between 45 and 65 years of age.

midlife crisis period of emotional upheaval noted among some midlife persons as they struggle with the finality of death and the nature of their past and future accomplishments.

minerals chemical elements that serve as structural elements within body tissue or participate in physiological processes.

minipills low-dose progesterone oral contraceptives.

misuse inappropriate use of legal drugs intended to be medications.

mitral (bicuspid) valve two-cusp valve that regulates blood flow between the left atrium and the left ventricle of the heart.

monogamous paired relationship with one partner.

mononuclear leukocytes large white blood cells that have only one nucleus.

mononucleosis ("mono") viral infection characterized by weakness, fatigue, swollen glands, and low-grade fever.

monosaccharides simple sugars; carbohydrate compounds of one saccharide unit.

monounsaturated fats fats made of compounds in which one hydrogen-bonding position remains to be filled; semisolid at room temperature; derived primarily from peanut and olive oils.

morning-after pill high-dose combination oral contraceptive sometimes prescribed to terminate a possible pregnancy.

motorized scraper a motor-driven cutter that shaves off plaque deposits from inside artery walls.

mourning culturally defined manner of expressing grief.

mucus clear, sticky material produced by specialized cells within the mucous membranes of the body; mucus traps much of the suspended particulate matter within tobacco smoke.

MRI scan magnetic resonance imaging; an imaging procedure that uses a powerful magnet to generate an image of body tissue.

Mullerian inhibiting substance a hormone produced by the developing testes that helps prevent the development of female reproductive structures.

multiorgasmic capacity potential to have several orgasms within a single period of sexual arousal.

murmur atypical heart sound that suggests a backwashing of blood into a chamber of the heart from which it has just left.

muscular endurance ability of a muscle or muscle group to function over time; supported by the respiratory and circulatory systems.

muscular strength ability to contract skeletal muscles to engage in work; the force that a muscle can exert.

mutagenic capable of promoting genetic alterations in cells.

myelin white, fatty, insulating material that surrounds the axons of many nerve cells.

myocardial infarction heart attack; the death of heart muscle as a result of a blockage in one of the coronary arteries.

myotonia buildup of a neuromuscular tonus.

N

narcolepsy sleep-related disorder in which a person has a recurrent, overwhelming, and uncontrollable desire to sleep.

narcotics opiates; psychoactive drugs derived from the oriental poppy plant; narcotics relieve pain and induce sleep.

naturally acquired immunity (NAI) type of acquired immunity resulting from the body's response to naturally occurring pathogens.

necrosis cell death.

needle biopsy procedure minor surgical procedure in which a needle is inserted into an anesthetized portion of a muscle tissue and a sample of that tissue is removed for microscopic examination.

negative dependence behavior behavior that can not only create psychological dependence but can also harm structure and function.

nerve blockers drugs that can stop the flow of electrical impulses through the nerves into which they have been injected.

neuritic plaques characteristic changes to brain tissue found in association with Alzheimer's disease.

neurofibrillary tangles characteristic changes to brain tissue found in association with Alzheimer's disease.

neuromuscular tonus level of nervous tension within the muscle.

neuron nerve cell; the structural unit of the nervous system.

neurotransmitters chemical messengers released by neurons that permit electrical impulses to be transferred from one nerve cell to another.

nicotine physiologically active, dependence-producing drug found in tobacco.

nitroglycerin a blood vessel dilator used by some cardiac patients to relieve angina.

nocturnal emission ejaculation that occurs during sleep; "wet dream."

nodes in this case, the electrical centers found in cardiac muscle.

nomogram graphic means for finding an unknown value.

nonessential amino acids the eleven amino acids the body can make itself.

noninsulin-dependent diabetes mellitus (type 2) form of diabetes generally seen for the first time in adulthood; adult onset diabetes.

nonoxynol-9 a spermicide commonly used with contraceptive devices.

nontraditional students administrative term used by colleges and universities for students who, for whatever reason, are pursuing undergraduate work at an age other than that associated with traditional college years (18-22).

norepinephrine adrenalin-like neurotransmitter produced within the nervous system.

nurse practitioners registered nurses who have taken specialized training in one or more clinical areas and are able to engage in limited diagnosis and treatment of illnesses.

nutrient density quantity of selected nutrients in 1000 Calories of food.

nutrients elements in food that are required for energy, growth, repair, and the regulation of body processes.

O

obesity condition in which a person's excess fat accumulation results in a body weight that exceeds desirable weight by 20% or more.

obituary notice biographical sketch that appears in a newspaper shortly after a person's death.

oncogenes genes that are believed to activate the development of cancer.

oogenesis production of ova in a biologically mature female.

oral contraceptive pill pill taken orally, composed of synthetic female hormones that prevent ovulation or implantation; "the pill."

orgasmic platform expanded outer third of the vagina that during the plateau phase of the sexual response grips the penis.

orgasmic stage third stage of the sexual response pattern; the stage during which neuromuscular tension is released.

orthodontics dental specialty that focuses on the proper alignment of the teeth.

osteoarthritis arthritis that develops with age.

osteopathy system of medical practice which combines allopathic principles with specific attention to postural mechanics of the body.

osteoporosis loss of calcium from the bone seen primarily in postmenopausal women.

outercourse sexual behaviors that do not involve intercourse.

ovary female reproductive structure that produces ova and the female gonadal sex hormones estrogen and progesterone.

overload principle principle whereby a person gradually increases the resistance load that must be moved or lifted; also applies to other types of fitness training.

overweight condition in which a person's excess fat accumulation results in a body weight that exceeds desirable weight by 1% to 19%.

ovolactovegetarian diet diet that excludes the use of all meat but does allow the consumption of eggs and dairy products.

ovulation the release of a mature egg from the ovary.

oxidation process that removes alcohol from the bloodstream.

oxygen debt physical state that occurs when the body can no longer process and transport sufficient amounts of oxygen for continued muscle contraction.

ozone layer layer of triatomic oxygen that surrounds the Earth and filters much of the sun's radiation before it can reach the Earth's surface.

P

pacemaker sinoatrial or SA node; an area of cells within the heart that controls its electrical activity.

palliative measure taken to reduce pain and discomfort but not to cure a disease.

pandemic spread of a disease process over a wide geographic area.

Pap smear cancer screening procedure in which cells removed from the cervix are examined.

paracervical anesthetic anesthetic injected into tissues surrounding the cervical opening.

particulate phase portion of tobacco smoke composed of small suspended particles.

particulate pollutants class of air pollutants composed of small solid particles and liquid droplets.

partner abuse violence committed against a domestic partner.

parturition childbirth.

passionate love state of extreme absorption in another; tenderness, elation, anxiety, sexual desire, and ecstacy.

passive smoking inhalation of air that is heavily contaminated with tobacco smoke.

passive-congenial marriage marriage that primarily supports the outside interests of the partners.

passively acquired immunity (PAI) temporary immunity achieved by providing antibodies to a person exposed to a particular pathogen.

pathogen disease-causing agent.

patient education health education delivered in a hospital or health care setting.

pedophilia sexual contact with children

as a source of sexual excitement.

pelvic inflammatory disease (PID) acute or chronic infections of the peritoneum or lining of the abdominopelvic cavity; associated with a variety of symptoms and a potential cause of sterility; generalized infection of the pelvic cavity that results from the spread of an infection through a woman's reproductive structures.

periodic abstinence birth control methods that rely on a couple's avoidance of intercourse during the ovulatory phase of a woman's menstrual cycle; also called fertility awareness or natural family planning.

periodontal disease destruction to soft tissue and bone that surround the teeth.

peripheral artery disease (PAD) damage resulting from restricted blood flow to the extremities, especially the legs and feet.

peritonitis inflammation of the peritoneum or lining of the abdominopelvic cavity.

personality the distinctive and unique emotional characteristics of a person.

pesticide agent used to destroy pests.

phenol chemical found in tobacco smoke thought to inactivate the cilia lining air passages.

phenylpropanolamine (PPA) active chemical compound found in most over-the-counter diet products.

physical dependence need to continue using a drug to maintain normal body function and to avoid withdrawal illness; also called addiction.

pituitary gland "master gland" of the endocrine system; the wide variety of hormones produced by the pituitary are sent to structures throughout the body.

placebo pills pills that contain no active ingredients.

placenta structure through which nutrients, metabolic wastes, and drugs (including alcohol) pass from the bloodstream of the mother into the bloodstream of the developing fetus.

plateau stage second stage of the sexual response pattern; a leveling off of arousal immediately before orgasm.

platelet adhesiveness tendency of platelets to clump together, thus enhancing speed at which the blood clots.

platonic close association between two

people that does not include a sexual relationship.

podiatrists specialists who treat a variety of ailments of the feet.

polychlorinated biphenyls (PCBs) class of chlorinated organic compounds similar to the herbicide DDT.

polyneuropathy gradual destruction of nervous system functioning resulting from influence of alcohol on nerve cells.

polysaccharide complex carbohydrate; a compound of a long chain of glucose units; found primarily in vegetables, fruits, and grains.

polyunsaturated fats fats composed of compounds in which multiple hydrogen-bonding positions remain open; these fats are liquids at room temperature; derived from a variety of vegetable sources.

positive caloric balance caloric intake greater than caloric expenditure.

postpartum period of time after the birth of a baby during which the uterus returns to its prepregnancy size.

potentiated effect phenomenon whereby the use of one drug intensifies the effect of a second drug.

preferred provider organization (PPO) a group of physicians who market their professional services to an insurance company at predetermined fees.

premenstrual syndrome (PMS) a collection of physical and psychological signs and symptoms that recur in the same phase of the menstrual cycle, typically in the week before menstruation begins.

primary care physician (PCP) the physician who sees a patient on a regular basis, rather than a specialist who sees the patient only for a specific condition or procedure.

private hospitals profit-making hospitals; proprietary hospitals.

problem drinking alcohol use pattern in which a drinker's behavior creates personal difficulties or difficulties for other persons.

procreation reproduction.

prodromal stage stage of an infectious disease process in which only general symptoms appear.

progesterone ovarian hormone that continues the development of the uterine wall that was initiated by estro-

gen.

progressive resistance exercises muscular strength training exercises that use traditional barbells and dumbbells with fixed resistances.

proliferative phase first half of the menstrual cycle.

proof twice the percentage of alcohol by volume in a beverage; 100 proof alcohol is 50% alcohol.

prospective pricing system system of establishing in advance the reimbursement rates for health services.

prostaglandin inhibitors drugs that block the production of prostaglandins, thus eliminating the hormonal stimulation of smooth muscles.

prostaglandin intrauterine injection an injection of hormone-like chemicals into the uterine wall that causes uterine muscles to contract and expel fetal contents.

prostaglandins chemical substances that stimulate smooth muscle contractions.

prosthodontics dental specialty that focuses on the construction and fitting of artificial appliances to replace missing teeth.

proteins compounds composed of chains of amino acids; primary components of muscle and connective tissue.

protooncogenes normal genes that hold the potential of becoming cancer-causing oncogenes.

psychoactive drug any substance capable of altering one's feelings, moods, or perceptions.

psychological dependence need to consume a drug for emotional reasons; also called habituation.

psychological health functional application of psychic traits, such as language, memory, perceptual processes, awareness states, and mind-body interaction.

psychosocial sexuality masculine and feminine aspects of sexuality.

psychosomatic disorders physical illnesses of the body generated by the effects of stress.

puberty achievement of reproductive ability.

public hospitals hospitals operated by governmental agencies and supported by tax dollars.

pulmonary pertaining to the lungs and breathing.

pulmonary emphysema irreversible disease process in which the alveoli are destroyed.

pulmonary valve valve that controls the flow of blood into the pulmonary arteries from the right ventricle of the heart.

purging use of vomiting or laxatives to remove undigested food from the body.

putrefaction decomposition of organic matter.

Q

quackery marketing of unreliable and ineffective services, products, or information under the guise of curing disease or improving health.

R

radiation sickness illness characterized by fatigue, nausea, weight loss, fever, bleeding from mouth and gums, hair loss, and immune deficiencies, resulting from overexposure to ionizing radiation.

radionuclide imaging a diagnostic test which injects small amounts of radioactive substances (radionuclides) into the bloodstream; computer-generated pictures are than able to see how well the heart muscle is functioning.

radon gas a naturally occurring radioactive gas produced by the decay of uranium.

range of motion distance through which a joint can be moved; measured in degrees.

rape an act of violence against another person wherein that person is forced to engage in sexual activities.

rapid eye movement (REM) sleep dream stage of sleep characterized by twitching movements of the eyes beneath the eyelids.

raves all-night dancing parties where electronically mixed music is often combined with video and laser light shows.

rebound effect excessive congestion that results from the overuse of nose-drops and sprays.

recovery stage stage of an infectious disease at which the body's immune system has overcome the infectious agent and recovery is underway; convalescence stage.

recycling ability to convert disposable items into reusable materials.

reflexology massage applied to specific areas of the feet in order to treat illness and disease in other areas of the body.

refractory phase that portion of the male's resolution stage during which sexual arousal cannot occur.

refractory errors incorrect patterns of light wave transmission through the structures of the eye.

regulatory genes genes within the cell that control cellular replication or doubling.

rehabilitation return of function to a previous level.

relaxation training the use of various techniques to produce a state of relaxation.

remediation development of alternative forms of function to replace those which had been lost or were poorly developed.

repair gene gene intended to repair DNA, the cells' genetic blueprint, following mutational change.

reproductive sexuality sexuality that is centered in the structural, functional, and behavioral aspects of reproduction.

resolution stage fourth stage of the sexual response pattern; the return of the body to a preexcitement state.

retinal hemorrhage uncontrolled bleeding from arteries within the eye's retina.

rheumatic heart disease chronic damage to the heart (especially heart valves) resulting from a streptococcal infection within the heart; a complication associated with rheumatic fever.

rheumatoid arthritis the result of autoimmune deterioration of the joints.

rigor mortis rigidity of the body that occurs after death.

role of health mission of health within a person's life cycle.

rubella German (or 3-day) measles.

rubeola red or common measles

S

sadism sexual excitement achieved while inflicting injury or humiliation on another person.

sadomasochism combination of sadism and masochism into one sexual activity.

salt sensitive description of people who overreact to the presence of sodium by retaining fluid, and thus experience an increase in blood pressure.

satiety a feeling of no longer being hungry; a diminished desire to eat.

saturated fats fats that are difficult for the body to use; these are fats in solid form at room temperature; primarily animal fats.

sclerotic changes thickening or hardening of tissues.

screenings relatively superficial evaluations designed to identify deviations from normal.

secondary bacterial infection bacterial infection that develops as a consequence of a primary infection.

secretory cells specialized cells within the breast that will, on stimulation, produce milk.

secular recovery programs recovery programs based on a person's self-reliance and self-determination, and not upon the recognition of a higher power.

sediments fine particles of soil that are washed into a body of water, become suspended, and eventually settle to the bottom.

self-actualization highest level of personality development; self-actualized persons recognize their roles in life and use personal strengths to reach their fullest potential.

self-care movement trend toward individuals taking increased responsibility for prevention or management of certain health conditions.

self-concept perception or mental picture of oneself.

self-esteem the quality of feeling good about yourself and your abilities; self-acceptance.

semen secretion containing sperm and other nutrients discharged from the male urethra at ejaculation.

sensory modalities vision, hearing, taste, touch, and smell; pathways for stimuli to register within the body.

serum lipid analysis analysis of fat substances in the bloodstream; includes cholesterol and triglyceride measurements.

set point genetically programmed range of body weight.

sex flush reddish skin response that results from increasing sexual arousal.

sex reassignment operation surgical procedure designed to remove the external genitalia and replace them with genitalia appropriate to the opposite sex.

sexual fantasies fantasies with sexual themes; sexual daydreams or imaginary events.

sexual harassment unwanted attention of a sexual nature that creates embarrassment or stress.

sexual orientation the sex to which one is attracted.

sexual victimization sexual abuse of children, family members, or subordinates by a person in a position of power.

sexuality the quality of being sexual; can be viewed from many biological and psychosocial perspectives.

sexually transmitted diseases (STDs) infectious diseases that are spread primarily through intimate sexual contact.

shaft body of the penis.

shingles viral infection affecting the nerve endings of the skin.

shock profound collapse of many vital body functions; evident during acute alcohol intoxication and other serious health emergencies.

sidestream smoke the smoke that comes from the burning end of a cigarette, pipe, or cigar.

singlehood the state of not being married.

skinfold measurement measurement to determine the thickness of the fat layer that lies immediately beneath the skin.

sliding scale method of payment by which patient fees are scaled according to income levels.

slow wave (SW) sleep stage of sleep characterized by minimal dream activity.

slow-twitch (ST) fibers type of muscle cell specialty suited for aerobic activities.

smegma cellular discharge that can accumulate beneath the clitoral hood and the foreskin of an uncircumcised penis.

smog air pollution composed of a combination of smoke, photochemical compounds, and fog.

smokeless tobacco tobacco products (chewing tobacco and snuff) that are chewed or sucked rather than smoked.

snuff finely shredded smokeless tobacco; used for dipping.

sodomy penile-anal intercourse.

soluble fiber that turns to a gel within the intestinal tract and then binds to liver bile which has cholesterol at-

tached; may be valuable in lowering blood cholesterol levels.

sonogram images of internal structures produced by high-frequency sound waves; also called ultrasound and ultrasonography.

specificity training concept that fitness components can be increased for very specific tasks or functions.

spermatogenesis process of sperm production.

spermicides chemicals capable of killing sperm.

stalking a crime involving an assailant's planned efforts to pursue an intended victim.

starch complex carbohydrate; a polysaccharide; a compound of long-chain glucose units.

static stretching the slow lengthening of a muscle group to an extended level of stretch; followed by holding the extended position for a recommended time period.

sterilization generally permanent birth control techniques that surgically disrupt the normal passage of ova or sperm.

stewardship acceptance of responsibility for the wise use and protection of the Earth's natural resources.

stillborn baby that is dead at the time of birth.

stimulants psychoactive drugs that stimulate the function of the central nervous system.

stress physiological and psychological state of disruption caused by the presence of an unanticipated, disruptive, or stimulating event.

stress test examination and analysis of heart-lung function while the body is undergoing physical exercise; generally accomplished when the client walks or runs on a treadmill device while being monitored by a cardiograph.

stressors factors or events, real or imagined, that elicit a state of stress.

subcutaneous fat fat layer immediately beneath the skin.

subdermal implants contraceptive devices that consist of surgically implanted rods containing synthetic progesterone.

sucrose a disaccharide; table sugar.

sudden cardiac death immediate death resulting from a sudden change in the rhythm of the heart.

superfund $12 billion fund to be used in cleaning-up selected toxic waste sites; EPA controlled.

superior vena cava body's largest vein; the vessel that brings blood from the upper body regions back to the right atrium of the heart.

suppressor gene gene intended to monitor cell regulatory activity and stop faulty regulatory activity.

surrogate parenting one of several arrangements in which a woman becomes pregnant and gives birth for an infertile couple.

sustainable environment an environment capable of supporting habitation; made possible by the efforts of individuals, organizations, and all levels of government.

sympto-thermal method method of periodic abstinence that combines the basal body temperature method and the cervical mucus method.

synapse location at which an electrical impulse from one neuron is transmitted to an adjacent neuron; synaptic junction.

synergistic drug effect heightened, exaggerated effect produced by the concurrent use of two or more drugs.

synesthesia perceptual process in which a stimulus produces a response from a different sensory modality.

systemic throughout the body.

systolic pressure blood pressure against blood vessel walls when the heart contracts.

T

tar particulate phase of tobacco smoke with nicotine and water removed.

target heart rate (THR) number of times per minute that the heart must contract to produce a training effect.

teaching hospital hospital in which pre-professional students and graduates receive clinical experience.

temperment personality traits which may be genetically conditioned such as shyness and aggressiveness.

teratogenic capable of producing birth defects.

testes male reproductive structures that produce sperm and the gonadal hormone testosterone.

testosterone male sex hormone that stimulates tissue development.

thermic effect the energy the body requires for the digestion, absorption, and transportation of food.

thorax the chest; portion of the torso above the diaphragm and within the rib cage.

thrombi stationary blood clots.

titration a particular level of a drug within the body.

tolerance an acquired reaction to a drug; continued intake of the same dose has diminishing effects.

total marriage marriage in which the needs and goals of each partner are assigned a lower priority for the good of the partnership.

total person holistic view of the person, incorporating the dynamic interplay of physical, emotional, social, intellectual, and spiritual factors.

toxic shock syndrome potentially fatal condition resulting from the proliferation of certain bacteria in the vagina, that enter the general blood circulation.

trace elements minerals whose presence in the body occurs in very small amounts; micronutrient elements.

training effect significant positive effect that exercise has on the heart, lungs, and blood vessels.

transcenders self-actualized people who have achieved a quality of being ordinarily associated with higher levels of spiritual growth.

transcervical balloon tuboplasty the use of inflatable balloon catheters to open blocked fallopian tubes; a procedure used for some women with fertility problems.

transient ischemic attack (TIA) strokelike symptoms caused by temporary spasm of cerebral blood vessels.

transition the third and last phase of the first stage of labor; full dilation of the cervix.

transsexualism the profound rejection of the gender to which the individual has been born.

transvestism recurrent, persistent cross-dressing as a source of sexual excitement.

tricuspid valve three-cusp (leaf) valve that regulates blood flow between the right atrium and the right ventricle of the heart.

triglycerides fats made up of glycerol units, each having three fatty acid molecules; high blood levels are associated with increased risk of car-

diovascular disease.

triphasic pills oral contraceptives in which the progesterone levels vary every seven days during the cycle while the estrogen levels remain constant.

trimester three-month period of time; human pregnancies encompass three trimesters.

tropical oils oils extracted from coconut, palm, and palm kernel that contain much higher levels of saturated fat than other vegetable oils.

tubal ligation sterilization procedure in which the fallopian tubes are cut and the ends tied back or cauterized.

tumescence state of being swollen or enlarged.

tumor mass of cells; may be cancerous (malignant) or noncancerous (benign).

twelve step programs recovery programs based on the twelve steps to recovery used by Alcoholics Anonymous.

type 1 alcoholism inherited predisposition supported by environmental factors favoring alcoholism.

type II alcoholism male-limited alcoholism; an inherited form of alcoholism passed from father to son.

U

ultralow tar and nicotine brands cigarettes containing less than 4 mg of tar.

ultrasound high-frequency sound waves used to create an image of internal body structures; or to elevate the internal temperature of cancer cells, thus killing the cells.

unbalanced diet diet lacking adequate representation from each of the food groups.

underweight condition in which body weight is below desirable weight.

unintentional injuries injuries that occur without anyone intending that any harm be done.

urethra passageway through which urine leaves the urinary bladder.

urethritis infection of the urethra.

uterine perforation penetration of a foreign object through the uterine wall.

V

vacuum aspiration abortion procedure in which the cervix is dilated and vacuum pressure is used to remove the uterine contents.

vaginal contraceptive film (VCF) spermicide-impregnated film that clings to the cervical opening.

variant different from the statistical average.

vas deferens (pl. vasa deferentia) passageway through which sperm move from the epididymis to the ejaculatory duct.

vascular system body's blood vessels; arteries, arterioles, capillaries, venules, and veins.

vasectomy surgical procedure in which the vasa deferens are cut to prevent the passage of sperm from the testicles; the most common form of male sterilization.

vasocongestion retention of blood within a particular tissue.

vasodilators drugs that relax muscles in the walls of blood vessels (especially the arterioles); these drugs allow blood vessels to dilate (widen).

vegan vegetarian diet vegetarian diet that excludes the use of all animal products, including eggs and dairy products.

vegetarian diet relies on plant sources for nutrients needed by the body.

vicariously formed stimuli erotic stimuli that originate in one's imagination.

virulent capable of causing disease.

vital marriage marriage in which the needs and goals of the individual, as well as the needs of the marital union, are given top priority.

vitamins organic compounds that facilitate the action of enzymes.

voluntary hospitals nonprofit hospitals operated by a variety of organizations, including religious orders and fraternal groups.

voyeurism watching others undressing or engaging in sexual activities.

vulval tissues tissues surrounding the vaginal opening.

W

waist to hip ratio (WHR) see healthy body weight.

wake an established time for people to view the body of a dead person; the calling hours.

warm-up physical and mental preparation for exercise.

water soluble capable of being dissolved in water.

wellness a broadly based term used to

describe a highly developed level of health.

wellness centers units within hospitals or clinics that provide a wide range of rehabilitation, disease prevention, and health enhancement programs.

whole-grain flour flour made from grain that has received only minimal processing (milling); flour containing many nutrients lost in more highly processed flour.

will legal document that describes how a person wishes his or her estate to be disposed of after death.

willed death a death in which a person gives up the desire to live and merely waits to die.

withdrawal illness uncomfortable, perhaps toxic response of the body as it attempts to maintain homeostasis in the absence of a drug; also called abstinence syndrome.

work movement of mass over distance.

Y

yeast single-cell plant responsible for the fermentation of plant products.

young adult years segment of the life cycle from ages 18 to 22; a transitional period between adolescence and adulthood.

yo-yo syndrome the repeated weight loss, followed by weight gain, experienced by many dieters.

Z

zero tolerance laws laws that severely restrict the right to drive for underage drinkers who have been convicted of driving under *any* influence of alcohol.

zoophilia sexual contact with animals as a preferred source of sexual excitement; bestiality.

Index

A

AA; *see* Alcoholics Anonymous
AAI; *see* Artificially acquired immunity
AARP; *see* American Association of Retired Persons
Abandonment, aging and, 513
Abortion, 386–391
   dilation and curettage in, 389
   dilation and evacuation in, 390–391
   hypertonic saline procedure in, 391
   menstrual extraction in, 389
   prostaglandin procedure in, 391
   RU-486 in, 389–390
   vacuum aspiration in, 389
Absorption of alcohol, 196–197, 198
Abstinence
   as contraceptive, 373–377
   drug use and, 164
   sexual, 350
Abuse, 165
   of child, 480–481, 486
   of drugs; *see* Drug use
   of elderly, 516
   emotional, 480
   of partner, 479–480
Accident, 488–491, 492
   alcohol and, 202
   elderly and, 516
   firearm safety and, 490

Accident—cont'd
   home accident prevention and, 491, 492
   motor vehicle safety and, 490–491
   nuclear reactor, 464–467
   personal safety and, 488–489
   recreational safety and, 489
   residential safety and, 489
Accutane, 401
Acetaminophen, 439
Acid rain, 451
Acid-base balance, 97
Acme, term, 299
Acne, 401
ACOAs; *see* Adult Children of Alcoholics
Acquaintance rape, 485–486
Acquired immunity, 300
Acquired immunodeficiency syndrome, 310–314
   cause of, 311
   diagnosis and treatment of, 313
   in health-care setting, 313–314
   Pneumocystis carinii pneumonia in, 306
   prevention of, 314
   signs and symptoms of, 312
   transmission of, 311–312
   in workplace, 296
ACSM; *see* American College of Sports Medicine
ACTH; *see* Adrenocorticotropic hormone
Activity; *see* Physical activity
Activity theory of aging, 513

Acupuncture, 147, 427
Acute alcohol intoxication, 198–200
Acute community-acquired pneumonia, 306
Acute rhinitis, 303–304
Acute stage of infection, 299
Acyclovir, 318
ADA; *see* Americans with Disabilities Act
Adaptive thermogenesis, 136, 137
ADD; *see* Attention deficit disorder
Addictive behavior
    drug use and, 163–164
    dynamics of, 165–169
Addictive effect of drugs, 181
Adenocarcinoma, 272
Adipose tissue, 128, 129, 136
Adoptive Families of America, Inc., 410
Adrenal glands, 45
Adrenaline, 45–47
Adrenocorticotropic hormone, 45, 220
Adult Children of Alcoholics, 207–208
Advance medical directive, 528–529
Advertising
    addictive personality and, 169
    alcohol and, 211
    health consumerism and, 421
    sexually oriented, 364, 488
    tobacco use and, 217–218, 224–225
Advil, 439
Aerobic energy production, 67
Aerobic exercise, 79–82
    low-impact, 82
    shoe for, 80–81
Affective, term, 341
Afterbirth, 406
Age
    basal metabolism rate and, 140
    body mass index and, 132
    nutrition and, 121
    oral contraceptives and, 384
    recommended dietary allowances and, 105
Aged; *see* Older adult
Agent, pathogenic, 297
Aging, 502–503
    acceptance of, 517–518
    organizations on, 520
    personal assessment of, 511
    process of, 509–513
        damage theories of, 509–510
        programmed theories of, 510–512
        psychosocial theories of, 512–513
    sexuality and, 505–506
AI; *see* Acquired immunity
AIDS; *see* Acquired immunodeficiency syndrome
AIDS hot line, 314
Air pollution, 449–455
    health implications of, 455
    indoor, 454–455

Air pollution—cont'd
    sources of, 450–454
    temperature inversions and, 454
Airborne transmission of infection, 298
Al-Anon, 210
Al-Anon Adult Family Groups, 208
Alateen, 210
Alcohol, 188–213
    accidents and, 202
    advertising and, 211
    cancer and, 275, 288
    choosing to drink, 190
    combination drug effects with, 181
    coronary heart disease and, 256
    crime and violence and, 202
    cross-tolerance and, 164
    date rape and, 485
    dietary guidelines for, 114, 116, 121
    driving and, 204–205
    fetal alcohol syndrome and, 200–202
    hosting responsible party and, 203
    hypertension and, 258
    nature of, 194–200
        absorption in, 196–197, 198
        acute intoxication and, 198–200
        blood alcohol concentration and, 197–198
        sobering up and, 198
    organizations supporting responsible drinking, 203–204
    personal assessment of, 15–16, 199, 265
    problem drinking and alcoholism, 204–208
    suicide and, 202
    usage patterns of, 190–194
    women and, 211
Alcohol dehydrogenase, 197
Alcohol Hot Line, 182
Alcoholics Anonymous, 210
Alcoholism, 204–208
    adult children of alcoholics and, 207–208
    codependence and, 207
    defined, 206
    denial and enabling in, 206–207
    family and, 190, 208
    rehabilitation and recovery in, 208–210
Allergen, 303
Allergic disorders, 303
Allied health care professional, 430
Allopathy, 426–427
Alveolus, tobacco use and, 229
Alzheimer's Association, 520
Alzheimer's disease, 514–515
Amenorrhea, 384
American Association of Retired Persons, 520
American Board of Medical Specialists, 429
American Cancer Society National Hot Line, 286
American College of Radiology, 286
American College of Sports Medicine, 72–73

American Dietetic Association, 109
American Fertility Society, 410
American Health Care Association, 520
American Hospital Association, 422
American Medical Association, 422
American Pharmaceutical Association, 422
American Society on Aging, 520
Americans with Disabilities Act, 8
Amino acids, 96
Aminophylline, 145
Amniocentesis, 408
Amniotic fluid level assessment, 408
Amniotic sac, 403
Amotivational state, 30–31, 179
Amphetamines, 172
Amyloid, 510
Anabolic steroids, 83–84
ANAD; *see* National Association of Anorexia Nervosa
  and Associated Disorders
Anaerobic energy production, 67
Analgesics, 406
Anatomical donation, 536
Androgens, 328
Androgyny, 331–332
Anesthetics, 406
Aneurysm, 259
Angel dust, 178–179
Anger
  in dying, 530
  personal death awareness and, 527
  stress and, 57
Angina pectoris, 226, 252–253
Angiogenesis factor, 272
Angioplasty, 255
Angry heart, term, 57
Animals in research, 438
Anorexia nervosa, 150–151, 152, 153
Anorgasmic, term, 347
Anovulatory, term, 329
Antabuse, 208
Antagonistic effect of drugs, 181
Antibody, 300, 302, 303
Antidepressant drugs, 31
Antigen, 302, 303
Antihypertensives, 258
Anxiety
  personal death awareness and, 527
  in test taking, 51
Aorta, 248, 249
Aortic valve, 248, 249
Appetite center, 134–135
Appetite suppressants, 144–145, 172
Arm, steroids and, 84
Arm hang exercise, 74
Arrhythmias, 253
Arteries, 247–248
  atherosclerosis and, 251

Arteries—cont'd
  hypertension and, 258
Arteriole, 247
Arteriosclerosis, 258
Arthritis, 508
Arthritis Consulting Services, 520
Artificial heart, 256
Artificial insemination, 409
Artificially acquired immunity, 300
Asbestosis, 453–454
Ascorbic acid, 99
Asphyxiation, acute alcohol intoxication and, 200
Aspirin, 256, 439
Assertiveness, 38
Asthma, 290–291
Atherosclerosis, 251–252, 258
Athlete
  drug abuse and, 168
  shoe guidelines for, 80–81
Atrium, 248, 249
Attention deficit disorder, 172
Attitude, addictive personality and, 166–167
Audiologist, 467
Auditory acuity, 467
Autocrine motility factor, 273
Autoimmune, term, 290
Axon, 169, 170
Ayurveda, 427
Azidothymidine, 313
AZT; *see* Azidothymidine

B

B cell, 300, 303
BAC; *see* Blood alcohol concentration
BACCHUS; *see* Boost Alcohol Consciousness
  Concerning the Health of University Students
Bacteria
  in infectious disease, 297
  in Lyme disease, 308
  in syphilis, 318
  in urethritis, 314–315
  in water, 456
Balanced diet, 104–105
  for infant, 136
  portion control and, 143
Ballistic stretching, 71
Band-aid surgery, term, 386
Barbiturates, 177
Bariatrician, 136
Bartholin's glands, 335
Basal body temperature method of contraception, 376
Basal cell carcinoma, 281
Basal ganglia, 166
Basal metabolism
  body energy needs and, 139–141
  weight management and, 135–136, 137

Bayer aspirin, 439
Beer, 195, 196
Behavior
    alcoholism recovery and, 209
    in dating and mate selection, 354
    variant sexual, 364
    weight reduction and, 147–149
Beliefs, addictive personality and, 166–167
Benign tumor, 272
Bereavement, 533–534
Bestiality, 364
Beta blockers, 253
Betaseron, 290
Beverages, 110, 172
Bias and hate crimes, 483–484
Bicuspid valve, 248, 249
Billings cervical mucus method of contraception,
    376–377
Binge drinking, 192
Biochemical oxygen demand, 456
Biofeedback, stress management and, 56
Biofeedback Society of America, 56
Biological magnification, 456
Biological sexuality, 328
Biological toxin, 109
Biopsy, 275
Biotin, 99, 104
Bipolar depression, 30
Birth; see Childbirth
Birth control
    choice of, 371
    contraception versus, 370–371
    methods of, 373–391
        abortion in, 386–391
        cervical cap in, 381
        condom in, 378–379
        contraceptive sponge in, 381–382
        diaphragm in, 380–381
        intrauterine device in, 382
        periodic abstinence in, 373–377
        sterilization in, 385–386
        subdermal implants in, 384
        vaginal spermicide in, 377
        withdrawal in, 373, 374–375
    personal assessment of, 388
Birth defects, 401
Birth technology, 408–411
Birthing room, 408
Bisexuality, 362, 363
Blackout, alcohol and, 204
Bladder, 319–320
Blastocyst, 400
Blood, 249–250
Blood alcohol concentration, 197, 205
Blood clot
    in myocardial infarction, 251
    nicotine and, 226

Blood clot—cont'd
    stress and, 47
Blood pressure
    hypertension and, 257
    personal assessment of, 264
Blood vessels, 247–248
    hypertension and, 258
    metastasis and, 273
Bloody show, 403
Blue baby, 260
BMI; see Body mass index
Body
    alcohol absorption and, 197
    anatomical donation of, 536
    infectious disease and, 299–303
        immune response in, 302–303
        immune system in, 300
        immunizations in, 300–302
    physical fitness and, 71
Body fat
    health problems and, 129
    liposuction and, 147
    measurement of, 131–132, 133
    stress and, 47
Body image, 128, 129, 132–133
Body mass index, 131–132, 133
Body weight management; see Weight management
Bodybuilding, 82
Bonding, childbirth and, 406
Bone disorders
    excess body fat and, 129
    osteoarthritis and, 508
    osteoporosis and, 507
Boost Alcohol Consciousness Concerning the
    Health of University Students, 203–204
Brady Bill, 480
Brain
    cocaine and, 173
    nicotine and, 219–220
    psychoactive drugs and, 166
    steroids and, 84
Brain death, 527
Brainstem, 166
Brand name drug, 438
Braxton Hicks contraction, 402
Bread, 108
    additional intake of, 121
    daily servings of, 106
    personal intake assessment of, 118
Breast
    cancer of, 274–276, 284
    exercise support for, 79
    implants in, 279
    self-examination of, 278
    sexual response and, 349
    steroids and, 84
Breast-feeding, 231, 406–407

Breech position, 405
Bronchitis, chronic, 229
Bufferin, 439
Bulbourethral glands, 333, 334
Bulimia Anorexia Nervosa Association, 152
Bulimia nervosa, 151, 152, 153
Burial, 535
Burns, alcohol and, 202
Buttermilk, 108
Byssinosis, 453

C

Caffeine, 172, 230
Caffeinism, 230
Calcium, 101
    in dairy products, 108
    dietary recommendations for, 105, 116
    milk consumption and, 117
    osteoporosis and, 507
Calcium channel blockers, 253
Calendar method of contraception, 374–376
Caliper, 132, 133, 134
Caloric balance, 137–138
Calories, 92
    in alcohol, 195, 196
    calculation of, 97
    in candy, 95
    in dairy products, 108
    empty, 121
    in fast foods, 109, 110
    obesity and, 129–130
    weight management and, 137–138
Campus safety, 494
Cancer, 270–288
    breast, 274–276
    cell regulation in, 270–271
    colorectal, 280–281
    diagnosis of, 282–283
    dietary guidelines in, 115
    environmental factors in, 287–288
    excess body fat and, 129
    incidence and mortality in, 274
    lung, 274
    marijuana and, 179
    ovarian, 279
    pancreatic, 281
    personal risk assessment of, 284–285
    prostate, 279–280
    radiation exposure and, 464
    skin, 270, 281–282, 284
    smoking and, 220
    testicular, 280
    tissue types of, 272–273
    treatment of, 283–287
    uterine, 276–278
    vaginal, 278–279

Candida albicans, 318
Candidiasis, 318–319
Candlelighters Childhood Cancer Foundation, 286
Candy, 95
Caning, 482
Cannabis, 179–180
Cannula in menstrual extraction, 389
Capillary, 247–248
Carbohydrates, 92–93
    calories in, 97
    in dairy products, 108
    dietary guidelines for, 114, 116
    in fast foods, 110
Carbon dioxide, 451
Carbon monoxide
    cardiovascular disease and, 226–227
    placenta and, 230
    as pollutant, 451
    tobacco use and, 225–226
Carbonation, 197
Carboxyhemoglobin, 226, 227
Carcinogen, 271, 464
Carcinogenic effects, 457
Carcinoma, 272
Cardiac muscle, 249
Cardiopulmonary resuscitation, 253
Cardiorespiratory endurance, 67–68
Cardiorespiratory fitness program, 72–85
    aerobic exercise in, 79–82
    athletic shoe and, 80–81
    bodybuilding in, 82
    breast support in, 79
    commercial clubs and, 82–83
    cross training and, 83
    danger signs in, 87
    duration of training in, 76
    fluid replacement in, 82
    frequency of training in, 73
    intensity of training in, 73–76
    jumping rope in, 78–79
    low-impact aerobic exercise in, 82
    mode of activity in, 72–73
    muscle fiber and, 85
    older adult and, 77–78
    physical examination before, 78
    proper equipment in, 82
    resistance training in, 76–77
    safety precautions in, 77
    steroids and, 83–84
    warm-up, workout, and cool-down in, 77
Cardiovascular disease, 244–267
    congenital, 260
    coronary, 251–256
    dietary guidelines in, 115
    excess body fat and, 129
    exercise and, 250
    hypertension and, 257–258

Cardiovascular disease—cont'd
  normal heart function and, 247–250
  peripheral artery disease and, 261
  personal assessment of, 264–265
  pervasiveness of, 246–247
  rheumatic, 260–261
  risk factors in, 261–263
  saturated fats and, 94
  smoking and, 226–227
  stroke and, 258–260
Caregiver, 517
Carjacking, 483
Carotenoids, 98
Carotid artery, 76
CAT scan; *see* Computerized axial tomography
Catabolism, 143
Celibacy, 350
Cell
  aging of, 510
  body defenses and, 300
  cohesiveness of, 272
  death of, 527
  malignant, 272
  regulation of, 270–271
Cell-mediated immunity, 300
Central nervous system
  alcohol and, 196
  appetite center and, 134
  depressants and, 177
  drug impact on, 169, 170
  nicotine and, 219–220
  psychoactive drugs and, 166
  stressors and, 45
Cereal germ, 108
Cereals, 108
  additional intake of, 121
  daily servings of, 106
  personal intake assessment of, 118
Cerebral aneurysm, 259
Cerebral cortex
  psychoactive drugs and, 166
  stressors and, 45
Cerebral hemorrhage, 259
Cerebrovascular accident, 258–260
Cerebrovascular occlusion, 259
Cervical cap, 374, 381
Cervical mucous plug, 403
Cervical mucus
  contraception and, 376–377
  fertilization and, 397
Cervical os, 336
Cervix, 336
  cancer of, 285
  labor and, 403–405
Cesarean delivery, 318, 406
CFCs; *see* Chlorofluorocarbons
CFS; *see* Chronic fatigue syndrome

Chain of infection, 297–299
Cheese, 106, 107, 108
Chemical name drug, 438
Chemical waste, 460–461
Chemotherapy
  in cancer, 286
  monitoring of, 272
Chernobyl, 464–467
Chest, steroids and, 84
Chest pain, 252–253
Chewing gum, nicotine-impregnated, 234
Chewing tobacco, 224, 231–232
Chicken, fast food, 110
Chickenpox, 302
Child
  abuse of, 480–481, 486
  biological sexuality and, 328–329
  death and, 531–532
  early years of, 411–412
  home accident prevention and, 491, 492
  neglect of, 481
  obesity and, 136
  parental smoking and, 234
  physical fitness and, 85
Childbirth, 402–408
  breast-feeding and, 406–407
  cervical effacement and dilation in, 403–405
  cesarean delivery in, 406
  delivery of fetus in, 405–406
  medications and, 406
  placenta delivery in, 406
  preparation for, 407–408
Children of Aging Parents, 520
Children of Alcoholics Foundation, Inc., 208
Chippers, 219
Chiropractic medicine, 427
Chlamydial infection, 314–315
Chlordane, 457
Chlordecone, 457
Chlordiazepoxide, 177
Chloride, 101, 105
Chlorinated hydrocarbons, 457
Chlorine, 458
Chlorofluorocarbons, 452
Choice in Dying, 529
Cholecalciferol, 98
Cholesterol, 95
  atherosclerosis and, 251–252, 253
  in dairy products, 108
  dietary fat and, 94
  dietary recommendations for, 116
  in fast foods, 110
  measurement of, 253
  oat bran and, 104
  personal assessment of, 264
Chorionic villi sampling, 408
Chromium, 103, 104

Chronic bronchitis, 229
Chronic fatigue syndrome, 307
Chronic illness, 268–293
    aging and, 506, 507, 514
    asthma as, 290–291
    cancer as, 270–288; *see also* Cancer
    diabetes mellitus as, 288–290
    multiple sclerosis as, 290
    physical activity and, 506, 507, 515
    tobacco use and, 229
Chronic obstructive pulmonary disease, 229
Cider, 196
Cigarette smoking; *see* Smoking
Cilia
    tobacco use and, 228
    of vas deferens, 334
Circulatory system, alcohol and, 201
Cirrhosis, 209
Civil rights, 235
Clear cell cancer, 279
Clear Water Act, 458
Clinical depression, 30–31
Clinical stage of infection, 299
Clitoris, 334–335, 348–349
Clomiphene citrate, 410
Clotting time, stress and, 47
Cluster headache, 54
CMO; *see* Comfort Measures Only
Cobalamin, 99
Cocaine, 173–177
    crack, 174–175
    freebasing of, 174
    society and, 175–177
Cocaine Abuse Hot Line, 182
Cocaine Anonymous, 182
Cocarcinogen, 271
Cocktail, 196
Cocoa, 172
Coconut oil, 95
Codependence, alcoholism and, 207
Coenzymes, 97
Coffee
    caffeine in, 172
    tobacco use and, 230
Cohabitation, 362
Coinsurance, 433
Coitus, 347, 353
Coitus interruptus, 373, 374–375
Cold, common, 303–304, 305
Cold remedies, 172
Cold turkey
    in drug use, 180
    in tobacco use, 234
Coliform bacteria, 456
Collagen cross-linking theory of aging, 509
College student
    alcohol and, 190–192

College student—cont'd
    campus safety and, 494
    with disabilities, 6–7
    insurance coverage for, 434
    minority, 6
    nontraditional, 6, 7
    traditional, 5–6
Colon cancer, 280–281
Color Additive Amendments, 111
Colostomy, 281
Colostrum, 406
Coma, diabetic, 289
Comfort Measures Only, 528
Commercials
    addictive personality and, 169
    alcohol and, 211
    health consumerism and, 421
    sexually oriented, 364, 488
    tobacco use and, 217–218, 224–225
Common cold, 303–304, 305
Communication
    with aging parent, 510
    developing skills of, 33–34
Community
    addictive personality and, 168
    drug use support services of, 184
Comorbidity
    in elderly, 514
    in midlife period, 506, 507
Companionate love, 354–356
Compensation as defense mechanism, 33
Complete fast, 143
Complete protein foods, 96
Compliance, 424
Compulsion
    addiction and, 163
    tobacco use and, 219
Computed tomography, 132
Computer, stress reduction and, 55
Computerized axial tomography, 260
Condom, 378–379
    effectiveness of, 374
    in oral-genital contact, 351
Condyloma acuminata, 315
Conflict-habituated marriage, 357
Confrontation therapy, 184
Congenital heart disease, 260, 262–263
Congenital rubella syndrome, 260
Congestive heart failure, 261
Congregate housing, 515
Consultation, 425
Consumer advocacy groups, 424
Consumer fraud, 421, 439–441
Consumer Information Center, 422
Consumerism; *see* Health consumerism
Consumers Union of the United States, Inc., 422
Contact inhibition, 272

Continuity theory of aging, 513
Contraception; *see also* Fertility control
    birth control *versus*, 370–371
    breast-feeding and, 407
    selecting method of, 373
    theoretical *versus* use effectiveness in, 373
Contraceptive sponge, 374, 381–382
Contraction
    Braxton Hicks, 402
    in labor, 403–405
    of muscle, 68
Contraindication, defined, 385
Convalescence stage of infection, 299
Cooking oil, 95
Cool-down, 77
COPD; *see* Chronic obstructive pulmonary disease
Coping
    with divorce, 360
    with stressors, 55–56
    with test anxiety, 51
Copper, 102, 104
Copper T380A, 382
Corona of penis, 334
Coronary artery, 248, 249
Coronary artery bypass surgery, 254–255
Coronary heart disease, 251–256
    alcohol and, 256
    angina pectoris in, 252–253
    aspirin and, 256
    atherosclerosis in, 251–252
    diagnosis and treatment of, 254–255
    dietary guidelines in, 115
    emergency response to, 253, 254
    heart transplantation in, 256
    risk factors for, 262
Coroner, 528
Corpus luteum, 338
Corpus of uterus, 336
Corticoids, 45
Cosmetics, 439
Cost of living, 54
Cough, smoker's, 228
Council of Environmental Quality, 469
Counseling
    in divorce, 360
    in eating disorders, 152
    emotional growth and, 38
Court shoe, 80–81
Cousteau Society, 469
Cowper's glands, 333, 334
CPR; *see* Cardiopulmonary resuscitation
Crabs, 318
Crack, 174–175
Cream, 108
Creative expression, 36
Creativity, 36, 37
Cremation, 536

Crime, 478–484
    alcohol and, 202
    bias and hate, 483–484
    on campus, 494
    domestic violence, 479–481
    gangs and, 481–483
    guns and, 483
    homicide and, 478–479
    personal assessment of, 493
    sexual victimization and, 484–488
        commercialization of sex in, 488
        rape and sexual assault in, 484–486
        sexual abuse of child in, 486
        sexual harassment in, 486–488
    stalking and, 484
Cross training, 83
Cross-tolerance to drugs, 164
Crowning, 405
CRS; *see* Congenital rubella syndrome
Cruciferous vegetables, 107
Cryobiology, 527
Cryonics, 527
Crypt, 535
Crystal meth, 173
Cultural diversity, 4, 7
    in aging, 512
    in alcohol use, 195
    in breast cancer, 277
    in diet, 123
    in eating habits, 152
    in fertility control, 390
    in funeral and burial rituals, 539
    in hallucinogens and religious ceremonies, 178
    in health consumerism, 436
    in heart disease, 248
    in hepatitis B, 310
    in humor, 28
    in land pollution, 462
    in marriage customs, 358
    in physical fitness, 79
    in pregnancy and childbirth, 403
    in reducing stress, 53
    in tobacco use, 217
    in violence, 482
Cunnilingus, 351
Curette, 389
Curl-up exercise, 75
CVA; *see* Cerebrovascular accident
CVS; *see* Chorionic villi sampling
Cynicism, stress and, 57
Cystitis, 319–320
Cytomegalovirus retinitis, 311

D

Darvon; *see* Propoxyphene
Date rape, 478, 485–486, 487

Dating, 353–354
D&C; *see* Dilation and curettage
DDT; *see* Dichlorodiphenyltrichloroethane
D&E; *see* Dilation and evacuation
Death, 524–542
    cancer and, 274
    cardiovascular disease and, 247
    of child, 532
    definitions of, 527–528
    emotional stages of, 530–531
    euthanasia and, 528–530
    excess body fat and, 129
    grief and, 533–534
    hospice care and, 532–533
    interacting with dying person, 531
    leading causes of, 3
    near-death experiences and, 531
    personal awareness of, 526–527
    personal preparation for, 537–539
    rituals of, 534–535
    smoking and, 220
    talking with child about, 531–532
    tobacco use and, 226
Death gene, 512
Decibel, 467, 468
Decline stage of infection, 299
Deductible amount, 433
Deer tick, 308
Defense mechanisms, 33
Dehydration, 100
Delirium tremens, 206
Delivery room, 408
Dementia, 514
Demerol; *see* Meperidine
Dendrite, 169, 170
Denial
    alcoholism and, 206–207
    as defense mechanism, 33
    of dying, 530
Dental care, 428
Dentist, 427–428
Deoxyribonucleic acid, 510
Department of Energy, 469
Department of Health and Human Services, 520
Department of Interior, 469
Dependence
    on alcohol, 206
    on caffeine, 230
    drug use and, 164–165
    on tobacco, 219–225
    treatment costs of, 184
Depo-Provera, 375, 384
Depressants, 177, 196
Depression, 30–31
    in dying, 530
    loneliness and, 32
DES; *see* Diethylstilbestrol

Desensitization, 303
Designated driver, 203
Designer drugs, 178
Desirable weight, defined, 129
Detoxification, 208–210
Developmental tasks
    addictive personality and, 167
    of elderly, 517–519
    of midlife period, 503–504
    of young adult period, 8–10
Devitalized marriage, 357–358
Dextrose, 92
Diabetes mellitus, 288–290
    dietary guidelines in, 115
    excess body fat and, 129
    personal assessment of, 265
Diagnosis-related groups, 435
Diaphragm, contraceptive, 374, 380–381
Diastolic pressure, 257
Diazepam, 177
Dichlorodiphenyltrichloroethane, 457
Didanosine, 313
Didoxycytidine, 313
Diet, 117–121
    alcohol consumption and, 121
    balanced, 104–105
        for infant, 136
        portion control and, 143
    cancer and, 287
    cardiovascular disease and, 263
    choice of, 146
    cultural diversity in, 123
    fad, 117, 143, 144–145
    grain products in, 120
    guidelines for, 113, 114, 115
    lifestyle and, 92
    macrobiotic, 117
    milk consumption in, 117
    nutrient density and, 121
    personal assessment of, 118–119
    protein in, 117
    recommendations for, 116
    types of, 144–145
    unbalanced, 117
    on vacation, 93
    vegetarian, 114–117
        lactovegetarian, 115
        ovolactovegetarian, 114–115
        vegan, 116–117
    vitamin C and A in, 120
    weight management and, 141, 143–144
    yo-yo, 128
Dietary aids, 99, 100
Dietary fat, 93–94
Dietary fiber, 93, 103–104
    intake of, 120
    recommendations for, 116

Dietary Guidelines for Americans, 131
Dietary thermogenesis, 141
Diethylstilbestrol, 278–279
Differentiation of cell, 271
Diffusion, alcohol absorption and, 196–197
Digestive system
    alcohol and, 201
    stress and, 47
Dilation, labor and, 403, 405
Dilation and curettage, 389
Dilation and evacuation, 390–391
Diphtheria, 301
Direct euthanasia, 528
Direct transmission of infection, 298
Disability insurance, 434
Disabled student, 6–7
Disaccharides, 92
Disengagement theory of aging, 513
Displacement as defense mechanism, 33
Distillation, 194
Distilled spirits, 196
Distress, 49
Diuresis, 289
Diuretics
    caffeine in, 172
    in hypertension, 258
Divorce, 359–360
Do Not Resuscitate, 528
Doctor; see Physician
DOM, designer drug, 178
Domestic violence, 479–481
Doubling of cell, 271
Dream, erotic, 350
DRGs; see Diagnosis-related groups
Drinking; see Alcohol
Drinking water, 456
Driving, alcohol and, 204–205
Drowning, 202
Drug testing, 182–183
Drug treatment programs, 184, 207
Drug use, 160–187
    addictive behavior and, 163–164
    addictive personality and, 165–169
    alcohol in, 188–213; see also Alcohol
    amphetamines in, 172
    caffeine in, 172
    central nervous system and, 169
    cocaine in, 173–177
    college and community support services for, 184
    combination drug effects in, 181
    depressants in, 177
    hallucinogens in, 177–179
    homicide and, 478–479
    inhalants in, 181
    marijuana in, 179–180
    narcotics in, 180–181
    personal assessment of, 15–16, 176, 185

Drug use—cont'd
    reduction of, 184
    society's response to, 181–183
    stimulants in, 169–172
    terminology in, 164–165
Drugs
    abuse of; see Drug use
    childbirth and, 406
    defined, 164
    generic versus brand name, 438
    health consumerism and, 423
    over-the-counter, 438–439
    personal supply of, 442
    prescription, 437
    research and development of, 437–438
    synergism of, 203
Dry beans, 106
DTs; see Delirium tremens
Due date in pregnancy, 402
Durable power of attorney for health care, 529
Duration of training, 76
Dying, 524–542
    child and, 532
    death definitions in, 527–528
    emotional stages of, 530–531
    euthanasia and, 528–530
    grief and, 533–534
    hospice care in, 532–533
    near-death experiences and, 531
    personal death awareness and, 526–527
    personal preparation for, 537–539
    rituals in, 534–535
    talking with child about, 531–532
Dyspareunia, 352

E

Eating disorders, 150–152
    anorexia nervosa in, 150–151, 152
    bulimia nervosa in, 151
    treatment for, 152
Economic factors
    in aging, 509
    in cardiovascular disease, 247
    in contraception selection, 373
    in death, 536
    in drug use, 184
    in health-care, 432–437
        government insurance plans and, 435–436
        health insurance and, 433–434
        health maintenance organizations and, 434
        national health care and, 436–437
    in hospitalization, 432
    in stress, 51, 54
Ecosystem, 462
Ecstasy, designer drug, 180
Ectopic pregnancy, 384

EEG; *see* Electroencephalogram
Effacement, 402–406
Eggs, 106, 107–108
Ego, 33
Ejaculation, 334, 349
    rapid, 352
    sperm number in, 397
Ejaculatory duct, 333, 334
Elderhostel, 516
Elderly; *see also* Older adult
    abuse of, 516
    aging process and, 509–513
        damage theories of, 509–510
        programmed theories of, 510–512
        psychosocial theories of, 512–513
    demographic analysis of, 508, 510
    developmental tasks of, 517–519
    health concerns of, 513–514
    health-care services for, 515
    housing for, 515–516
    quality of life, 508–509
    transportation for, 516, 517
Electrical impedance, 132
Electroencephalogram, 527
    nicotine and, 225
    sleep patterns and, 86
Electrolyte balance, 208
Electromagnetic radiation, 463–464
ELISA; *see* Enzyme-linked immunosorbent assay
Embalming, 535
Embolism
    in myocardial infarction, 251
    oral contraceptives and smoking and, 231
    in stroke, 259
Embryo transfer, 410
Embryonic stage, 400
Emission of semen, 334
Emotional abuse, 480
Emotional health, 24–41
    characteristics of, 26
    communication skills and, 33–34
    creative expression and, 36
    defined, 11
    dying and, 530–531
    enhancement of, 37–38
    Maslow's hierarchy of needs in, 34–35
    personality and, 27
    psychological health *versus*, 26–27
    range of emotions in, 27–33
        depression in, 30–31
        happiness and sense of humor in, 28
        loneliness in, 32–33
        seasonal affective disorder in, 31, 32
        self-esteem in, 28–30
        shyness in, 33
        suicide in, 31–32
    spiritual development and, 36

Emphysema, 229
Employment
    drug testing and, 183
    as stressor, 49
Empowerment, 4–5
Empty calories, 121
Enabling, alcoholism and, 206–207
Endocarditis, 261
Endocrine system
    aging and, 512
    obesity and, 136
    stressors and, 45–47
Endometriosis, 338
Endometrium, 336
Endurance, muscular, 70
Energy
    aerobic, 67
    anaerobic, 67
    body needs of, 138–141
        activity requirements in, 138–139
        basal metabolism and, 139–141
        dietary thermogenesis and, 141
        life-time weight control and, 141
    dietary recommendations for, 116
    fats and, 93
    glucose and, 92
    stressors and, 47–48
Enriched, term, 108
Entombment, 535
Environment, 446–475
    addictive personality and, 167–168
    air pollution and, 449–455
        health implications of, 455
        indoor, 454–455
        sources of, 450–454
        temperature inversions and, 454
    balance of, 472
    cancer and, 287–288
    chain of infection and, 298
    land pollution and, 459–462
        chemical waste in, 460–461
        pesticides in, 461–462
        solid waste in, 459–460
    noise pollution and, 467–468
     organizations concerned with, 469
    personal assessment of, 470–471
    personality and, 27
    postindustrial society transition and, 448–449
    radiation and, 462–467
        electromagnetic, 463–464
        health effects of, 463
        nuclear reactor accidents and, 464–467
        personal assessment of, 465
        radon gas and, 466, 467
        sunglasses and, 463
    water pollution and, 455–459
        health effects of, 459

Environment—cont'd
  water pollution and—cotn'd
    sources of, 456–458
      wetlands and, 458–459
  world population growth and, 449
Environment Canada, 469
Environmental Protection Agency, 469
  on chemical waste, 460–461
  on water pollution, 457
Environmental tobacco smoke, 232
Enzyme-linked immunosorbent assay, 313
Enzymes, 97
EPA; *see* Environmental Protection Agency
Epidemic, 296
Epididymis, 333, 334
Epinephrine, 45–47, 225
Episiotomy, 406
Epitaph, 539
Epstein-Barr virus, 306
Erection, 347, 352
Ergo-calciferol, 98
Erotic dream, 350
Erythroplakia, 232
Esophagus, alcohol and, 201
Essential amino acids, 96
Essential hypertension, 257
Estrogen, 337, 338
  in oral contraceptives, 382–383
  osteoporosis and, 507
  replacement therapy for, 506
Ethanol; *see* Alcohol
Ethyl alcohol, 194, 195–196
Eulogy, 539
Eustress, 48–49
Euthanasia, 528–530
Eutrophication, 456
Excitement stage of sexual response, 347, 348
Exclusion policy, 433–434
Exercise
  aerobic, 79–82
  cardiorespiratory fitness program and, 72–85
    aerobic exercise in, 79–82
    athletic shoe and, 80–81
    bodybuilding in, 82
    breast support in, 79
    commercial clubs and, 82–83
    cross training and, 83
    danger signs in, 87
    duration of training in, 76
    fluid replacement in, 82
    frequency of training in, 73
    intensity of training in, 73–76
    jumping rope in, 78–79
    low-impact aerobic exercise in, 82
    mode of activity in, 72–73
    muscle fiber and, 85
    older adult and, 77–78

Exercise—cont'd
  cardiorespiratory fitness program and—cont'd
    physical examination before, 78
    proper equipment in, 82
    resistance training in, 76–77
    safety precautions in, 77
    steroids and, 83–84
    warm-up, workout, and cool-down in, 77
  cardiovascular health and, 250
  elderly and, 519
  hypertension and, 258
  isokinetic, 69
  isometric, 68
  isotonic, 68–69
  personal assessment of, 264
  progressive resistance, 68–69
  stress management and, 56, 57
  weight control and, 141, 148–149
Exhaustion, stress and, 48, 49
Exhibitionism, 364
Expectorants, 304
Expressionistic sexuality, 341
Extended care insurance, 436
Externality, 136

F

Fad diet, 117, 143, 144–145
FAE; *see* Fetal alcohol effect
Faith, 36, 37, 53–54
Fallopian tube, 336
  fertilization and, 397
  ligation of, 386
False labor, 402–403
False negative, 399
False positive, 399
Family
  addictive personality and, 167
  alcoholism and, 190, 208
  death and, 533
  health consumerism and, 421
  obesity and, 137
  as stressor, 51–53
Fantasy
  as defense mechanism, 33
  sexual behavior and, 350
FAS; *see* Fetal alcohol syndrome
Fast foods, 109, 110
Fasting, controlled, 143
Fasting starvation diet, 145
Fast-twitch fiber, 85
Fat density, 109
Fat soluble vitamins, 97, 98, 104
Fats, 108–109
  calories in, 97
  in candy, 95
  daily servings of, 106

Fats—cont'd
    in dairy products, 108
    dietary recommendations for, 116
    in fast foods, 110
    intake of, 120
    low-calorie substitutes for, 96
    as nutrients, 93–94
    reducing intake of, 96
Fatty acids, 93–94
Federal Trade Commission, 422
Fellatio, 351
Female condom, 378
Female reproductive system, 335–336
    ovum fertilization and, 400
    sexual response and, 348–349
Females; see Women
Fermentation, 194
Fertility
    defined, 371
    tobacco use and, 230
Fertility control, 368–393
    birth control methods in, 373–391
        abortion and, 386–391
        cervical cap and, 381
        condom and, 378–379
        contraceptive sponge and, 381–382
        diaphragm and, 380–381
        intrauterine device and, 382
        periodic abstinence and, 373–377
        sterilization and, 385–386
        subdermal implants and, 384
        vaginal spermicide and, 377
        withdrawal and, 373, 374–375
    birth control versus contraception in, 370–371
    choice of, 371
    contraception selection in, 373
    cultural diversity in, 390
    personal assessment of, 372
    theoretical versus use effectiveness in, 373
Fertilization, 397–399
Fetal alcohol effect, 200–202
Fetal alcohol syndrome, 200–202
Fetishism, 364
Fetus, 400–401
    cesarean delivery of, 406
    damaging agents to, 401–402
    delivery of, 405–406
    maternal smoking and, 226, 230
Fiber, dietary, 93
    intake of, 120
    recommendations for, 116
Fibrocystic breast condition, 339
Fight-or-flight response, 48
Filter cigarette, 220
Fimbriae, 338
Fire
    alcohol and, 202

Fire—cont'd
    smoking and, 220
Firearm
    safety precautions for, 490
    violence and, 483
First aid, 198–200
Fish, 107–108
    daily servings of, 106
    fast food, 110
    tips for cooking, 457
Fitness club, 82–83
Fitness program, 72–85
    aerobic exercise in, 79–82
    athletic shoe and, 80–81
    bodybuilding in, 82
    breast support in, 79
    commercial clubs and, 82–83
    cross training and, 83
    danger signs in, 87
    duration of training in, 76
    fluid replacement in, 82
    frequency of training in, 73
    intensity of training in, 73–76
    jumping rope in, 78–79
    low-impact aerobic exercise in, 82
    mode of activity in, 72–73
    muscle fiber and, 85
    older adult and, 77–78
    physical examination before, 78
    proper equipment in, 82
    resistance training in, 76–77
    safety precautions in, 77
    steroids and, 83–84
    warm-up, workout, and cool-down in, 77
Fixed indemnity benefit, 433
Flaccid, term, 334, 335
Flashback, 177
Flexibility, physical fitness and, 70–71
Flood, 459
Fluids
    daily intake of, 103
    in fitness program, 82
Fluoride, 103, 104, 116
Folacin, 120, 121
Folate, 99, 105
Folic acid, 99
Folklore, health consumerism and, 422
Follicle, 338
Follicle-stimulating hormone, 333, 337, 338
Food, Drug and Cosmetic Act, 111
Food additives, 109–111
Food Additives Amendment, 111
Food and Drug Administration
    on cosmetics, 439
    on designer drugs, 178
    on food labels, 111
    on food supplements, 99

Food and Drug Administration—cont'd
  Office of Consumer Affairs, 422
  on over-the-counter drugs, 438–439
  on prescription drugs, 437, 438
Food groups, 104–108, 111
  breads, cereals, rice, and pasta in, 108
  fats, oils, and sweets in, 108–209
  fruits in, 105
  meat, poultry, fish, and eggs in, 107–108
  milk, cheese, and yogurt in, 107, 108
  vegetables in, 105–107
Food intake
  alcohol and, 197
  caloric balance and, 138
  changing pattern of, 148
  controlled fasting and, 143
  dietary thermogenesis and, 141
  low-calorie, 143
Food labels, 111–113
Food supplements
  Food and Drug Administration and, 99
  ovolactovegetarian diet and, 115
Foreplay, 350
Foundation for Hospice and Home Care, 520
Fraternal twins, 401, 402
Fraud Division of U.S. Postal Service, 422
Free radical damage theory of aging, 509
Freebasing, 174
French fries, 110
Frenulum, 334
Frequency of training, 73
Friendship, 356
Fructose, 92
Fruits, 105
  daily servings of, 106
  personal intake assessment of, 118
FSH; see Follicle-stimulating hormone
FT fiber, 85
Full funeral services, 535
Fully independent household, 515
Funeral services, 535–536, 538
Fungus, 297

G

Gait, multiple sclerosis and, 290
Gallstones, 129
Gamete intrafallopian transfer, 410
Gang violence, 481–483
Gaseous pollutants, 450–453
Gastric resection, 147
Gastrointestinal disease, 115
Gastroplasty, 147
Gateway drugs, 168
Gender
  alcohol absorption and, 197
  defined, 330

Gender—cont'd
  sex reassignment operation and, 364
Gender adoption, 330–331
Gender identification, 331
Gender identity, 330
Gender preference, 330
Gene alteration, food technology and, 122
General adaptation syndrome, 48–49
General anesthetics, 406
Generativity, 503–504
Generic name drug, 438
Genetic predisposition, 288
Genetics
  in addictive personality, 165
  in alcoholism, 206
  in Alzheimer's disease, 515
  in biological sexuality, 328
  in obesity, 134
  in oncogene formation, 271
  personality and, 27
Genital herpes, 317
Genital sexuality, 339–341, 346
  genital contact in, 350–351
  oral-genital stimulation in, 351
  shared touching in, 350
Genital warts, 315
Genitalia
  female, 335–336
  male, 332–334
  steroids and, 84
German measles, 302, 307
GIFT; see Gamete intrafallopian transfer
Glans, 334
Glucose, 92
  diabetes mellitus and, 288–289
  stress and, 47
Glycogen, 47
Goals
  self-esteem and, 30
  in weight reduction, 150
Goblet cell, 228
Gonads, 328, 332, 333
Government agencies
  health consumerism and, 424
  insurance plans and, 435
Graafian follicle, 338
Grade point average, drinks per week by, 193
Grain alcohol, 194
Gray Panthers, 520
Great Flood of 1993, 459
Green Plan, 462
Greenhouse effect, 450–451
Greenpeace USA, 469
Grief
  death and, 533–534
  divorce and, 360
Ground burial, 535

Group plan insurance, 434
Gulf War syndrome, 451
Gum disease, 232
Gun
    safety precautions for, 490
    violence and, 483
GWS; *see* Gulf War syndrome

H

Habitrol, 234
Habituation, tobacco use and, 219
Haemophilus influenzae, 301
Hallucinogens, 177
Hamburger, 110
Hantavirus pulmonary syndrome, 308–309
Happiness, emotional health and, 28
Hard cider, 196
Hardiness, 56
Hash, 179–180
Hashish, 179–180
Hate crime, 483–484
Hayflick limit theory, 510
Hazardous waste, 460–461
HDLs; *see* High-density lipoproteins
Headache, 54
Health, 1–21
    college student and
        developmental tasks of, 8–9
        with disabilities, 6–7
        minority, 6
        nontraditional, 6
        traditional, 5–6
    composition of, 10–12
    current concerns in, 2, 3
    definitions of, 2–5
        empowerment in, 4–5
        health promotion in, 3–4
        Healthy People 2000 in, 5
        holistic, 3
        traditional, 2–3
        wellness in, 4, 5
    environmental factors in, 446–475
        air pollution and, 449–455
        balance of, 472
        land pollution and, 459–462
        noise pollution and, 467
        organizations related to, 469
        personal assessment of, 470–471
        postindustrial society transition and, 448–449
        radiation and, 462–467
        water pollution and, 455–459
        world population growth and, 449
    personal evaluation of, 13–19
    role of, 10
Health care provider, 425–430
    allied professional as, 430

Health care provider—cont'd
    consultation of, 425–426
    nonallopathic practitioner as, 427
    nurse as, 429–430
    physician as, 426–427
    restricted practice, 427–429
Health clinic, 431
Health club, 82–83
Health consumerism, 418–445
    costs and reimbursement in, 432–437
        government insurance plans and, 435–436
        health insurance and, 433–434
        health maintenance organizations and, 434
        national health care and, 436–437
    drugs and, 437–439
    health care providers and, 425–430
        allied professional in, 430
        consultation of, 425–426
        nonallopathic practitioner in, 427
        nurse in, 429–430
        physician in, 426–427
        restricted practice, 427–429
    information sources in, 420–425
    personal assessment of, 18–19, 440
    quackery and consumer fraud and, 439–441
    self-care and, 430
    skills in, 442–443
Health educator, 424
Health insurance, 433–434, 435
Health maintenance organization, 434
Health promotion, 3–4, 430
Health reference publications, 424
Health-care
    aging and, 515
    costs and reimbursement in, 432–437
        government insurance plans and, 435–436
        health insurance and, 433–434
        health maintenance organizations and, 434
        national health care and, 436–437
    quackery and, 439–441
Health-care worker
    acquired immunodeficiency syndrome and, 313–314
    health consumerism and, 424
Healthy People 2000, 5
Hearing loss, noise-induced, 467
Heart
    bodybuilding and, 82
    catheterization of, 254
    cocaine and, 173
    disease of; *see* Cardiovascular disease
    exercise and, 250
    hypertension and, 258
    normal function of, 247–250
    rheumatic fever and, 260
    steroids and, 84
    stress and, 47, 57

Heart—cont'd
  target rate of, 73
  tobacco use and, 226–227
  transplantation of, 256
Heart attack; *see* Myocardial infarction
Heart murmur, 260
Heart-lung machine, 255
Heavy drinker, 192
Height-weight tables, 130
Helper T-cell, 302, 303
Hemoglobin, smoking and, 226
Hemorrhage
  in delivery of placenta, 406
  retinal, 258
  in stroke, 259
Hepatitis, 310
Hepatitis B, 301
Hepatoma, 273
Herbal medicine, 427
Herbicides, 462
Heredity, personal evaluation of, 17–18
Heroin, 180
Herpes simplex infection, 315–318
HFCs; *see* Hydrofluorocarbons
High-carbohydrate diet, 145
 High-density lipoproteins, 252
High-fiber, low-calorie diet, 144
High-protein, low carbohydrate diet, 144
Hip replacement surgery, 508
HIV; *see* Human immunodeficiency virus
HMO; *see* Health maintenance organization
Holistic health, 3
Home health test, 430
Home pregnancy test, 399
Homicide, 478–479
Homosexuality, 362–363
Hormones
  in biological sexuality, 328
  menstrual cycle and, 337
  in oral contraceptives, 382
  premenstrual syndrome and, 338–339
Hospice care, 532–533
Hospital, 431–432
Hospital insurance, 434
Host negligence, 203
Hot flash, 506
Housing, older adult and, 515–516
HPV; *see* Human papillomavirus
HSV; *see* Herpes simplex infection
Human chorionic gonadotropin, 399
Human immunodeficiency virus, 310–314
Human papillomavirus, 315
Humor, 28
Humoral immunity, 300
Hydration, alcoholism and, 208
Hydrocarbons, chlorinated, 457
Hydrofluorocarbons, 452

Hydrostatic weighing, 132, 133
Hymen, 335–336
Hyperbaric therapy, 286
Hypercellular obesity, 136
Hyperglycemia, 288
Hyperparathyroidism, 507
Hypertension, 257–258
  excess body fat and, 129
  risk factors for, 262
Hyperthermia, 286
Hypertonic saline procedure, 391
Hypertrophic obesity, 136
Hypervitaminosis, 97
Hypnosis for weight reduction, 148
Hypochondriasis, 505
Hypothalamus, 45
  appetite center and, 134
  psychoactive drugs and, 166
Hypothyroidism, 136
Hysterectomy, 386, 391
Hysterotomy, 391

I

Ibuprofen, 439
Ice, 173
Ice beer, 195
Ice cream, 108
ICSH; *see* Interstitial cell stimulating hormone
IDDM; *see* Insulin-dependent diabetes mellitus
Ideal weight, defined, 129
Identical twins, 401, 402
Identity formation, 8
Illness
  as stressor, 55
  tobacco use and, 226
  uncontrolled stress and, 49
Immune response, 302–303
Immune system, 300
  aging and, 512
  human immunodeficiency virus and, 311
  stress and, 47
Immunizations, 300–302
Immunotherapy, 303
  in asthma, 290
  in cancer, 286
Implant, breast, 279
In vitro fertilization and embryo transfer, 410
Inactivity, obesity and, 137
Incest, 364
Incineration of waste, 459–460
Income protection insurance, 434
Incomplete protein foods, 96
Incubation stage, 299
Independence, establishment of, 8
Independent practice association, 434
Indirect euthanasia, 528

Indirect transmission of infection, 298
Individual insurance policy, 434
Indoor air pollution, 454–455
Infant
    breast-feeding and, 406–407
    maternal tobacco use and, 231
    obesity and, 136
Infatuation, 353–354
Infection
    chain of, 297–299
    defined, 297
    immune response and, 302–303
    opportunistic, 311
    stages of, 299
    vaginal, 318–319
Infectious diseases, 294–323
    acquired immunodeficiency syndrome in, 310–314
    body defenses and, 299–303
        immune response in, 302–303
        immune system in, 300
        immunizations in, 300–302
    chronic fatigue syndrome in, 307
    common cold in, 303–304
    hantavirus pulmonary syndrome in, 308–309
    hepatitis in, 310
    influenza in, 304–305
    Lyme disease in, 308
    measles in, 307
    mononucleosis in, 306–307
    mumps in, 307
    pneumonia in, 306
    in the 1990s, 296
    sexually transmitted, 314–320
        chlamydia in, 314–315
        cystitis and urethritis in, 319–320
        herpes simplex infection in, 315–318
        human papillomavirus in, 315
        pubic lice in, 318
        syphilis in, 318
        vaginal infection in, 318–319
    toxic shock syndrome in, 309
    transmission of, 296–299
        chain of infection in, 297–299
        pathogens in, 296–297
    tuberculosis in, 305–306
Inferior vena cava, 248, 249
Infertility, 396
    birth technology in, 408–411
    tobacco use and, 230
Influenza, 304–305
Infrared light transmission, 132
Inhalants, 181
Inhibitions, alcohol and, 190
Insoluble fiber, 103
Insulin, 288
Insulin-dependent diabetes mellitus, 289–290
Insurance, health, 433–434, 435

Intellectual health, 12
Intellectualization, 33
Intensity of training, 73–76
Intentional injuries, 478–484
    bias and hate crimes in, 483–484
    domestic violence in, 479–481
    gang and youth violence in, 481–483
    gun violence in, 483
    homicide in, 478–479
    stalking in, 484
Intercourse, 353
Interferon, 286
Interleukin-2, 286
Interpersonal skills, 167
Interstitial cell stimulating hormone, 333
Intestinal bypass operation, 147
Intimacy, 10, 356–357
Intoxication, 198–200
Intrauterine device, 375
Inversion, temperature, 454
Iodide, 102
Iodine, 105
Ionizing radiation, 462
IPA; *see* Independent practice association
Iron, 102
    dietary recommendations for, 105, 116
    supplements of, 117
Isokinetic exercise, 69
Isolation as defense mechanism, 33
Isometric exercise, 68
Isotonic exercise, 68–69
IVF-ET; *see* In vitro fertilization and embryo transfer

J

Jet skiing, 490
Joint disorders, 129
Journal keeping, 38
Juice, term, 83
Jumping rope, 78–79
Junk food, 109, 118

K

Kaposi's sarcoma, 311
Killer T-cell, 302, 303
Kissing disease, 306
Kübler-Ross stages of dying, 530–531
Kwashiorkor, 97

L

Labeling
    of food, 111–113
    health consumerism and, 421–422, 423
Labia majora, 334, 335
Labia minora, 334, 335

Labial herpes, 315
Labor, 402–406
    cervical effacement and dilation in, 403–405
    delivery of fetus in, 405–406
    placenta delivery in, 406
Labor room, 408
Lactation, 406
    body fat and, 132
    recommended dietary allowances in, 104–105
    vegan vegetarian diet and, 116
Lactose, 92
Lactovegetarian diet, 115
Laminaria, 391
Land pollution, 459–462
    chemical waste and, 460–461
    pesticides and, 461–462
    solid waste and, 459–460
Laparoscopy, 386
Larynx, tobacco use and, 228
LDLs; see Low-density lipoproteins
Lead toxicity, 454
Leg, steroids and, 84
Lesbianism, 362
Leukemia, 273
Leukoplakia, 232
Levulose, 92
Librium; see Chlordiazepoxide
Lice, pubic, 318
Licensed practical nurse, 430
Lifestyle
    cardiovascular disease and, 262
    diet and, 92
    weight control and, 141
Lightening, 402
Limbic system, 166
Lipectomy, 147
Lipids, 93–94
Lipofusion, 510
Lipogenesis, 136
Lipoplasty, 147
Lipoproteins
    atherosclerosis and, 251–252, 253
    nicotine and, 226
Liposuction, 147
Liqueur, 196
Liver
    alcohol and, 201, 209
    steroids and, 84
Living will, 529
Local anesthetics, 406
Loneliness, 32–33
Loss of control, addiction and, 163
Loss of property, 54
Love, 354–356
Low-calorie, high-protein supplement diet, 144
Low-density lipoproteins, 252
Lower body obesity, 131

Low-impact aerobic exercise, 82
LSD; see Lysergic acid diethylamide
Ludes, term, 177
Lung
    cancer of, 274
    stress and, 47
    tobacco use and, 228–230
Luteinizing hormone, 337, 338
Lyme disease, 308
Lymphoma, 273, 311
Lysergic acid diethylamide, 177–178

M

Macrobiotic diet, 117
Macrocytic anemia, 120, 121
Macronutrients, 100, 101
Macrophage, 303
MADD; see Mothers Against Drunk Drivers
Magnesium, 101, 105
Magnetic resonance imaging
    in body composition measurement, 132
    in breast cancer, 275
    in coronary heart disease, 254
    in stroke, 260
Mainstream smoke, 232
Major depression, 30–31
Major medical coverage, 434
Male reproductive system, 332–334
Males; see Men
Malignancy, 272, 283–287; see also Cancer
Malnutrition
    alcohol and, 201
    fad diet and, 117
    obesity and, 128–129
    vegan vegetarian diet and, 116–117
    Zen macrobiotic diet and, 117
Maltose, 92
Mammary glands, 406
Mammography, 275
Manganese, 103, 104
Mania, 30
Manic-Depressive Illness Foundation, 31
Marijuana, 179–180
Marriage, 357–360
    alternatives to, 359–362
        cohabitation in, 362
        divorce in, 360
        single parenthood in, 362
        singlehood in, 360–361
    forms of, 357–359
    improvement of, 358
    older adult and, 509
Maslow's hierarchy of needs, 34–35
Masochism, 364
Mass media exposure, 422–423
Mastectomy, 279

Mastery, 10, 11
Masturbation, 350–351
Mate selection, 353–354
Maternal supportive tissues, 136
Mature adult; *see* Older adult
Mausoleum, 535
MDMA, designer drug, 178, 180
MDR; *see* Multiple drug-resistant
Measles, 307
Meat, 107–108
    daily servings of, 106
    USDA safety guide for, 113
Mechanical body defenses, 300
Medicaid, 435–436
Medicare, 435
Medicare supplement policies, 436
Medicine, term, 164
Medicine cabinet, 442
MEDIGAP; *see* Medicare supplement policies
Melanoma, 272, 281–282
Meltdown, 464–467
Memory T-cell, 302, 303
Men
    alcohol absorption and, 197
    cardiovascular disease and, 246
    infertility in, 408–409
    recommended dietary allowances for, 104–105
    sexual response pattern of, 347
Menaquinone, 98
Menarche, 329, 336
Menopause, 329, 506
Menses, 336
Menstrual cycle, 336–339
    alcohol and, 197
    determination of, 377
Menstrual extraction, 389
Menstruation, 336
Mental health, 24–41
    characteristics of, 26
    communication skills and, 33–34
    creative expression and, 36
    enhancement of, 37–38
    Maslow's hierarchy of needs in, 34–35
    personality and, 27
    psychological health *versus*, 26–27
    range of emotions in, 27–33
        depression in, 30–31
        happiness and sense of humor in, 28
        loneliness in, 32–33
        seasonal affective disorder in, 31, 32
        self-esteem in, 28–30
        shyness in, 33
        suicide in, 31–32
    spiritual development and, 36
Mental picture
    self-esteem and, 37, 38
    stress management and, 58

Mentor, 30
Meperidine, 181
Mercury, 456–457
Mescaline, 177, 178
Metabolic rate, 47
Metastasis, 272, 273
Methamphetamine, 173
Methaqualone, 177
Methyl mercury, 456–457
Micronutrients, 100, 102
Midlife crisis, 504
Midlife period
    developmental tasks of, 503–504
    health concerns of, 505–508
        comorbidity in, 506, 507
        menopause in, 506
        osteoarthritis in, 508
        osteoporosis in, 507
        sexuality in, 505–506
    joys of, 504–505
Mifepristone, 389–390
Migraine, 54, 420
Military, gays in, 363
Milk, 107, 108
    additional consumption of, 117
    daily servings of, 106
    personal intake assessment of, 118
Minerals, 100, 101–103, 105
Minilaparotomy, 386
Minipill, 384
Minor depression, 30
Minority student, 6
MIS; *see* M;auullerian-inhibiting substance
Miscarriage, 231
Misuse, term, 165
Mitral valve, 248, 249
Mixed drink, 196
Mode of transmission, 298
Modeling
    addictive personality and, 169
    tobacco use and, 224
Molybdenum, 103, 104
Monilial infection, 318–319
Mono, term, 306–307
Monoclonal antibody, 286
Monogamous, term, 360
Mononuclear leukocytes, 306
Mononucleosis, 306–307
Monosaccharides, 92
Monospot blood smear, 306
Monounsaturated fats, 94
Mons pubis, 334, 335
Morning-after pill, 383
Morphine, 180
Mortality; *see* Death
Mortuary, 534–535
Mothers Against Drunk Drivers, 203

Motor vehicle accident, 202, 204–205
Motor vehicle safety, 490–491
Mourning, 533–534
Mouth, smokeless tobacco and, 232
MPPP, designer drug, 178
MRI; *see* Magnetic resonance imaging
MS; *see* Multiple sclerosis
MSW; *see* Municipal solid wastes
Mucus
    cervical, 336
    tobacco use and, 228
M;auullerian-inhibiting substance, 328
Multiorgasmic capacity, 347
Multiple birth, 401, 402
Multiple drug-resistant, 306
Multiple sclerosis, 290
Mumps, 302, 307
Municipal solid wastes, 459
Murder, 478–479
Murmur, 260
Muscle, 68–70
    exercise and, 85
    stress and, 47
Mutagenic effects, 457
Myelin, 290
Myocardial infarction
    atherosclerosis and, 251
    death and, 247
    emergency response to, 253, 254
    reducing risk of, 263
    tobacco use and, 226
    warning signals of, 254
Myotonia, 350

N

NAI; *see* Naturally acquired immunity
Napping, 86
Narcolepsy, 172
Narcotics, 180–181
Narcotics Anonymous, 182
NARIC; *see* National Rehabilitation
    Information Center
National Adoption Center, 410
National Association for Home Care, 520
National Association of Anorexia Nervosa and
    Associated Disorders, 152
National Cancer Institute Cancer Information
    Service, 286
National Clearinghouse for Alcohol and Drug
    Information, 182
National Coalition for Cancer Survivorship,
    286
National Cocaine Hot Line, 182
National Committee for Adoption, 410
National Consumers' League, 422
National Council of Senior Citizens, 520

National Council on Alcoholism and Drug
    Dependence, 208
National Council on the Aging, Inc., 520
National Federation of State High School
    Associations Target Programs, 182
National Foundation for Depressive Illness, 31
National health care, 436–437
National Health Information Clearinghouse, 182
National Hospice Organization, 520
National Institute of Mental Health, 31
National Institute on Alcohol and Drug Abuse Hot
    Line, 182
National Institutes of Health, 286–287
National Kidney Foundation, 537
National Mental Health Association, 31
National Oceanic and Atmospheric Administration,
    469
National Rehabilitation Information Center, 520
National Senior Citizens Law Center; *see* National
    Rehabilitation Information Center
National Wildlife Federation, 469
Naturally acquired immunity, 300
Nature Conservancy, 461
NCADA; *see* National Council on Alcoholism and
    Drug Dependence
Near-death experience, 531
Necrosis, 272
Needle sharing, 312
Neglect, child, 481
Neonatal herpes, 318
Neonate; *see* Newborn
Nerve blockers, 290
Neuritic plaque, 514
Neuroanatomy, 166
Neuroblastoma, 272
Neuroendocrine system, 512
Neurofibrillary tangles, 514
Neuromuscular tonus, 350
Neuron, 169
Neurotransmitters
    nicotine and, 219
    psychoactive drugs and, 169, 170
Neutron activation, 132
Newborn
    herpes simplex virus and, 318
    maternal tobacco use and, 231
Niacin, 99, 105
Nicoderm, 234
Nicorette, 234
Nicotine, 225
    cardiovascular disease and, 226
    dependence and, 219–224
    placenta and, 230–231
Nicotine patch, 234
Nicotinic receptors, 225
NIDDM; *see* Noninsulin-dependent diabetes mellitus
Nitrogen, 451

Nitroglycerin, 252–253
Nitrous oxide, 452
Nocturnal emission, 329
Nodes in cardiac muscle, 249
Noise pollution, 467–468
Noise-induced hearing loss, 467
Nomogram, 131, 133
 Nonappetite suppressant pharmaceutical agents, 145–147
Nonessential amino acids, 96
Noninsulin-dependent diabetes mellitus, 288–289
Nonspecific urethritis, 314–315
Nontraditional student, 6, 7
Nonverbal communication, 34
Norepinephrine, 225
Norplant, 384
North American Council on Adoptable Children, 410
Novocain, 406
NSU; *see* Nonspecific urethritis
Nuclear energy, 462
Nuclear reactor accident, 464–467
Nuprin, 439
Nurse practitioner, 430
Nursing home, 431, 516
Nutrients, 92–104
    carbohydrates in, 92–93
    density of, 121
    fats in, 93–94
    fiber in, 103–104
    minerals in, 100, 101–103
    proteins in, 96–97
    tropical oils in, 95
    vitamins in, 97–100
    water in, 100–103
Nutrition, 90–125
    alcohol consumption and, 121
    diet and
        fad, 117
        guidelines for, 113, 114, 115
        macrobiotic, 117
        vegetarian, 114–117
    fast foods and, 109, 110
    food additives and, 109–111
    food exchange system and, 109
    food groups and, 104–108
        breads, cereals, rice, and pasta in, 108
        fats, oils, and sweets in, 108–209
        fruits in, 105
        meat, poultry, fish, and eggs in, 107–108
        milk, cheese, and yogurt in, 107, 108
        vegetables in, 105–107
    food labels and, 111–113
    food technology and, 122
    grain products and, 120
    international concerns in, 121–122
    milk consumption and, 117
    nutrients and, 92–104

Nutrition—cont'd
    nutrients and—cont'd
        carbohydrates in, 92–93
        density of, 121
        fats in, 93–94
        fiber in, 103–104
         minerals in, 100, 101–103
        proteins in, 96–97
        tropical oils in, 95
        vitamins in, 97–100
        water in, 100–103
    older adult and, 121
    personal assessment of, 15, 118–119
    protein and, 117
    vitamin C and A and, 120
Nuts, 106

O

Oat bran, 104
Obesity
    appetite center in, 134–135
    controlled fasting and, 143
    decreasing basal metabolism rate in, 137
    endocrine influence in, 136
    externality in, 136
    family dietary practices in, 137
    genetics in, 134
    inactivity in, 137
    infant and adult feeding patterns in, 136
    older adult and, 129
    pregnancy and, 136–137
    set point theory and, 135–136
Obituary notice, 539
Obstetrics, 408
Occlusion, cerebrovascular, 259
Occupation, cancer and, 287
Ocean dumping, 460
Office of Consumer Affairs, 422
Office of Minority Health, 7
Oil spill, 457–458
Oils, 106, 108–109
Older adult, 500–523
    aging and, 502–503, 509–513
        damage theories of, 509–510
        programmed theories of, 510–512
        psychosocial theories of, 512–513
    air pollution and, 452
    demographic analysis of, 508, 510
    developmental tasks of, 503–504, 517–519
    exercise for, 77–78
    health concerns of, 505–508
        Alzheimer's disease in, 514–515
        comorbidity in, 506, 507
        menopause in, 506
        osteoarthritis in, 508
        osteoporosis in, 507

Older adult—cont'd
　health concerns of—cont'd
　　sexuality in, 505–506
　　health-care service and, 515
　　home accident prevention and, 491, 492
　　housing and, 515–516
　　joys of midlife and, 504–505
　　nutrition and, 121
　　obesity and, 129
　　organizations for, 520
　　quality of life, 508–509
　　transportation and, 516, 517
Older Women's League, 520
OMH; see Office of Minority Health
Oncogene, 271
Oogenesis, 336
Open dumping, 459
Opium, 180
Opportunistic infection, 311
Optician, 428–429
Optometrist, 428
Oral cavity
　alcohol and, 201
　smokeless tobacco and, 232
Oral contraceptives, 382–384
　breast cancer and, 275
　effectiveness of, 375
　tobacco use and, 231
Oral herpes, 317
Oral-genital stimulation, 351
Organ donation, 536–537
Organic brain syndrome, 514–515
Orgasm, 334, 347, 349
　difficulties in, 352
　genital contact and, 350–351
Orgasmic platform, 336
Orlistat, 145
Orthodontics, 427
Osteoarthritis, 508
Osteopathic medicine, 426–427
Osteoporosis, 117, 507
OTC drugs; see Over-the-counter drugs
Outercourse, 370–371
Ovariectomy, 386
Ovary, 336
　aging of, 506
　cancer of, 279
Overload principle, 68
Over-the-counter drugs, 438–439, 441
Overweight, defined, 128–130
Oviduct, 336
Ovolactovegetarian diet, 114–115
Ovral, 383
Ovulation, 338
Ovum, 336, 338, 397, 400
OWL; see Older Women's League
Oxidation of alcohol, 198

Oxygen, hyperbaric, 286
Oxygen debt, 67
Oxytocin
　breast-feeding and, 406
　in labor, 403
Ozone layer, 452–453

P

Pacemaker, cardiac, 249
PAD; see Peripheral artery disease
PAI; see Passively acquired immunity
Pain
　cardiorespiratory fitness program and, 87
　death and, 533
　in labor, 403–405
Pain relievers, 172, 439
Palliative measure, 283–286
Palm oil, 95
Pancreas
　alcohol and, 201
　cancer of, 281
　insulin and, 288
Pandemic, 296
Pantothenic acid, 99, 104
Pap test, 276–278
Paracervical anesthetic, 389
Parasitic worm, 297
Parenthood, 396–397
　drug use and, 162
　early years of, 411–412
　midlife period and, 503
　personal assessment of, 398
　single, 362
Parent's Resource Institute for Drug Education, 182
Particulate pollutants, 453–454
Partner abuse, 479–480
Parturition, 402
Passionate love, 354–356
Passive smoking, 232–234
Passive-congenial marriage, 358
Passively acquired immunity, 300
Pasta, 106, 108
Pathogens, 296–297, 456
Patients' institutional rights, 432
PCBs; see Polychlorinated biphenyls
PCP; see Phencyclidine hydrochloride
Pedophilia, 364
Peers, addictive personality and, 168
Pelvic inflammatory disease, 315, 377
Penis
　anatomy and physiology of, 332, 333, 334
　sexual response and, 348–349
Pergonal, 410
Pericarditis, 261
Periodic abstinence, 373–377
Periodontal disease, 232

Peripheral artery disease, 261
Peripheral nervous system, 225
Peripheral vascular system, 225
Peritonitis, 315
Personal death awareness, 526–527
Personal safety, 488–489, 493
Personality, 27
    addictive, 166–167
    alcoholism and, 206
    stress and, 57
Pesticides, 457, 461–462
Peyote, 177, 178
Phantasticants, 177
Phencyclidine hydrochloride, 178–179
Phenylpropanolamine, 145
Phosphorus, 101, 105
Phototherapy, 31
Phylloquinone, 98
Physical activity
    calories expended during, 140
    chronic illness and, 506, 507, 515
    elderly and, 518
    energy needs of body and, 138–139
    hypertension and, 258
    during pregnancy, 407
    for weight reduction, 148–149
Physical dependence, 164, 219
Physical examination, 78
Physical fitness, 11, 64–89
    body composition and, 71
    cardiorespiratory endurance and, 67–68
    cardiorespiratory fitness program in, 72–85
        aerobic exercise in, 79–82
        athletic shoe and, 80–81
        bodybuilding in, 82
        breast support in, 79
        commercial clubs and, 82–83
        cross training and, 83
        danger signs in, 87
        duration of training in, 76
        fluid replacement in, 82
        frequency of training in, 73
        intensity of training in, 73–76
        jumping rope in, 78–79
        low-impact aerobic exercise and, 82
        mode of activity in, 72–73
        muscle fiber and, 85
        older adult and, 77–78
        physical examination before, 78
        proper equipment in, 82
        resistance training in, 76–77
        safety precautions in, 77
        steroids and, 83–84
        warm-up, workout, and cool-down in, 77
    child and, 85
    common attitudes toward, 66–67
    flexibility and, 70–71

Physical fitness—cont'd
    muscular endurance and, 70
    muscular strength and, 68–70
    personal assessment of, 13–14, 74–75
    sleep and, 85–86
    weight management and, 148–149
Physician, 426–427
Physicians' Desk Reference, 437
PID; *see* Pelvic inflammatory disease
Pipe smoking, 218–219
Pituitary gland, 45
Placebo pill, 383
Placenta, 400–401
    alcohol and, 200
    delivery of, 404, 406
    tobacco use and, 230–231
Planned Parenthood Federation of America, 410
Plateau stage of sexual response, 347, 348
Platelet adhesiveness, 226
Platonic, term, 360
PMS; *see* Premenstrual syndrome
Pneumocystis carinii pneumonia, 306, 311
Pneumonia, 306
Podiatrist, 428
Polio, 302
Pollutants
    gaseous, 450–453
    particulate, 453–454
    in water, 456
Pollution
    air, 449–455
        health implications of, 455
        indoor, 454–455
        sources of, 450–454
        temperature inversions and, 454
    land, 459–462
        chemical waste and, 460–461
        pesticides and, 461–462
        solid waste and, 459–460
    noise, 467–468
    postindustrial society transition and, 448–449
    water, 455–459
        effects on health, 459
        sources of, 456–458
        wetlands and, 458–459
Polychlorinated biphenyls, 457
Polyneuropathy, 209
Polysaccharides, 93
Polyunsaturated fats, 94
Polyvalent vaccine, 305
Population growth, 449
Portal of entry, 298
Portal of exit, 298
Positive caloric balance, 130
Postpartum, 406
Posttraumatic stress syndrome, 486
Pot, 179–180

Potassium, 101, 105
Potentiated effect of drugs, 181
Poultry, 106, 107–108
Poverty, 448
Power nap, 86
PPA; *see* Phenylpropanolamine
PPO; *see* Preferred provider organization
Preferred provider organization, 434
Pregnancy, 338, 339, 394–402
    birth technology and, 408–411
    cultural diversity in, 403
    determination of, 399
    due date in, 402
    excess body fat and, 129
    fertilization and, 397–399
    fetal life and, 400–401
    multiple births and, 401, 402
    obesity and, 136–137
    parenting issues and, 396–397
    physical activity during, 407
    recommended dietary allowances in, 104–105
    rubella and, 307
    signs of, 400
    tobacco use and, 230–231
Premature death, tobacco use and, 226
Premeasured food plan, 144
Premenstrual syndrome, 338–339
Prepuce, 334, 335
Prescription drugs, 437
PRIDE; *see* Parent's Resource Institute for Drug
    Education
Primary care physician, 427
Primary depression, 30
Private hospital, 431
Problem drinking, 204
Problem solving, weight control and, 92
Procreation, 339, 353
Prodromal stage of infection, 299
Progestasert, 382
Progesterone, 337, 338, 382–383
Progressive resistance exercise, 68–69, 76–77
Projection as defense mechanism, 33
Proof, term, 194
Propoxyphene, 181
Prospective pricing system, 435
Prostaglandins
    in abortion procedure, 391
    in labor, 403
Prostate, 333, 334
    cancer of, 279–280
    steroids and, 84
Prostatic specific antigen, 280
Prostep, 234
Prosthodontics, 427
Protein
    additional consumption of, 117
    aging and, 510

Protein—cont'd
    calories in, 97
    in dairy products, 108
    dietary guidelines for, 104, 114
    in fast foods, 110
    as nutrient, 96–97
    personal intake assessment of, 118
Protein-sparing, modified fat diet, 144
Protooncogene, 271
Protozoa
    in infectious disease, 297
    in water, 456
Prozac, 31
PSA; *see* Prostatic specific antigen
Psilocybin, 177
Psychedelic drugs, 177
Psychiatric disorders, 209
Psychiatrist, 428
Psychoactive drugs, 164
Psychological dependence, 164, 219
Psychological health; *see* Emotional health
Psychologist, 428
Psychosocial sexuality, 329–331
Psychosocial theories of aging, 512–513
Psychosomatic disorders, 48
Psyllium, 104
Puberty, 329
Pubic lice, 318
Public hospital, 431
Pulmonary disease
    air pollution and, 452
    excess body fat and, 129
    tobacco use and, 229
Pulmonary valve, 248, 249
Purging, 151
Push-ups, 75
Putrefaction, 456
Pyridoxine, 99

Q

QI; *see* Queteletindex
Quaalude, 177
Quackery, 439–441
Quasi-synthetic narcotics, 180
Queteletindex, 131
Quieting, stress management and, 56

R

Radial artery, 76
Radiation, 462–467
    electromagnetic, 463–464
    exposure to
        fetus and, 401–402
        health effects of, 463
        personal assessment of, 465

Radiation—cont'd
   nuclear reactor accidents and, 464–467
   radon gas and, 466, 467
   sunglasses and, 463
Radiation inversion, 454
Radiation sickness, 463
Radiation therapy, 283–286
Radionuclide imaging, 254
Radon gas, 466, 467
Rain forest, 450
Range of motion, 69
Rape, 484–486
   alcohol and, 202
   date, 478, 485–486
   help procedures in, 487
   prevention of, 486
Rapid eye movement sleep, 86
Rational Recovery Systems, 211
Rationalization as defense mechanism, 33
Rave, 180
Reaction formation, 33
Reactive depression, 30
Rebound effect, 304
Recommended dietary allowances, 104–105
Recovery
   in alcoholism, 208–210
   in infection, 299
Recreational safety, 489
Rectal cancer, 280–281
Recycling, 460, 461
Red measles, 302
Reflexology, 427
Refractory error, 428
Refractory phase of sexual response, 347
Regional anesthetics, 406
Regression, 33
Regulatory gene, 271
Rehabilitation, 208–210, 518
Rehabilitation center, 431
Relaxation
   personal evaluation of, 18
   stress management and, 56
   as stressor, 55
Religious ceremonies, 178
REM sleep, 86
Remediation, 518
Repair gene, 271
Repression, 33
Reproductive sexuality, 339
Reproductive system, 332–339
   alcohol and, 201
   male, 332–334
   menstrual cycle and, 336–339
   tobacco use and, 230–231
Reservoir in chain of infection, 298
Residential safety, 489
Resistance training, 76–77

Resolution stage of sexual response, 347, 349
Resource Center, 286
Responsibility, 8
Rest, personal evaluation of, 18
Restricted calorie, balanced food plan, 145
Reticular activating system, 166
Retinal hemorrhage, 258
Retinoids, 98
Rheumatic fever, 260
Rheumatic heart disease, 260–263
Rheumatoid arthritis, 301
Rhinitis, 303–304
Rhythmic pelvic thrusting, 347
Riboflavin, 99, 105
Rice, 108
   daily servings of, 106
   Zen macrobiotic diet and, 117
Rice bran, 104
Rickettsia, 297
Right-to-die, 530
Rigor mortis, 527
Roe v. Wade, 386
Roid rage, term, 83
Roids, term, 83
Rollerblading, 82
Rooming in, 408
RRS; *see* Rational Recovery Systems
RU-486, 389–390
Rubella, 260, 302, 307
Rubeola, 307
Runner's nipple, 79
Running shoe, 80–81

S

SA node, 249
SAD syndrome; *see* Seasonal affective disorder
SADD; *see* Students Against Driving Drunk
Sadism, 364
Sadomasochism, 364
Safety, 476–496
   campus, 494
   in cardiorespiratory fitness program, 77
   in contraception selection, 373
   intentional injuries and, 478–484
      bias and hate crimes and, 483–484
      domestic violence in, 479–481
      gangs and, 481–483
      guns and, 483
      homicide in, 478–479
      stalking and, 484
   personal assessment of, 16, 493
   sexual victimization and, 484–488
      commercialization of sex in, 488
      rape and sexual assault in, 484–486
      sexual abuse of child in, 486
      sexual harassment in, 486–488

Safety—cont'd
  unintentional injuries and, 488–491, 492
    firearm safety and, 490
    home accident prevention and, 491, 492
    motor vehicle safety and, 490–491
    personal safety and, 488–489
    recreational safety and, 489
    residential safety and, 489
Salivation, 47
Salmonella, 311
Salt
  hypertension and, 258
  intake of, 120
Sanitary landfill, 459
Sarcoma, 272
Satiety, 93
Saturated fats, 94
  in dairy products, 108
  dietary guidelines for, 114
Scarlet fever, 260
Sclerotic changes, 273
Screening for cancer, 276–277, 283, 425
Scrotum, 332–333
Seasonal affective disorder, 31, 32
Seat belt, 491
Secondary bacterial infection, 305
Secondary depression, 30
Secondary hypertension, 257–258
Secular Organizations for Sobriety, 211
Secular recovery programs, 210–211
Sedatives, 177
Sediment, 458
Selenium, 102, 105
Self-acceptance, 27, 37
Self-actualization, 35
Self-care
  personal evaluation of, 16–17
  weight reduction programs and, 143–144
Self-concept, self-ideal *versus*, 29
Self-esteem
  emotional health and, 28–30
  Maslow's hierarchy of needs and, 35
Self-examination
  of breast, 278
  of testicle, 280
Self-hypnosis, 56
Self-protection, 488–489
Semen, 334
Semi-independent household, 515
Seminal vesicle, 333, 334
Seminiferous tubule, 333
Sense of humor, 28
Serotonin-reuptake inhibitors, 31
Set point theory, 135–136
Sewage treatment, 456
Sex; *see* Gender
Sex flush, 347

Sex reassignment operation, 364
Sex role, 328
Sexual abuse, 481, 486
Sexual assault, 484–486
Sexual behavior patterns, 350–353
  celibacy in, 350
  dysfunctional, 352
  fantasy and erotic dreams in, 350
  genital contact in, 350–351
  intercourse in, 353
  masturbation in, 350
  oral-genital stimulation in, 351
  shared touching in, 350
  variant, 364
Sexual harassment, 486–488
Sexual orientation, 362–364
  bisexuality in, 363
  homosexuality in, 362–363
  transsexualism in, 363–364
  variant sexual behaviors in, 364
Sexual victimization, 484–488
  of child, 486
  commercialization of sex in, 488
  rape and sexual assault in, 484–486
  sexual harassment in, 486–488
Sexuality, 326–367
  aging and, 505–506, 509
  androgyny and, 331–332
  biological bases of, 328–329
  commercialization of, 364
  dating-mate selection and, 353–354
  expressionistic, 341
  friendship and, 356
  genital, 339–341
  human sexual response pattern in, 346–350
  intimacy and, 356–357
  love and, 354–356
  marriage and, 357–360
  personal assessment of, 340
  psychosocial bases of, 329–331
  reproductive, 339
  reproductive systems and, 332–339
    female, 335–336
    male, 332–334
    menstrual cycle and, 336–339
  sexual behavior patterns in, 350–353
    celibacy in, 350
    fantasy and erotic dreams in, 350
    genital contact in, 350–351
    intercourse in, 353
    masturbation in, 350
    oral-genital stimulation in, 351
    shared touching in, 350
  sexual orientation and, 362–364
    bisexuality in, 363
    homosexuality in, 362–363
    transsexualism in, 363–364

Sexuality—cont'd
  sexual orientation and—cont'd
    variant sexual behaviors in, 364
  therapy for dysfunctional, 352
Sexually transmitted diseases, 314–320
  chlamydia in, 314–315
  cystitis and urethritis in, 319–320
  herpes simplex infection in, 315–318
  human papillomavirus in, 315
  oral-genital contact and, 351
  personal assessment of, 316
  pubic lice in, 318
  syphilis in, 318
  vaginal infection in, 318–319
  vaginal spermicide and, 377
Shaft of penis, 334
Shake, fast food, 110
Sherbet, 108
Shingles, 315
Shoe, athletic, 80–81
Short stature, 129
Shyness, 33
Sick building syndrome, 455
Sickle cell disease, 409
Sidestream smoke, 232
Sierra Club, 469
Silicosis, 453
Singlehood, 360–361
Sinoatrial node, 249
Sinsemilla, 179
Sit and reach exercise, 74
Skin
  cancer of, 281–282
    personal risk assessment of, 284
    tanning and, 270
  excess body fat and, 129
Skinfold measurement, 132, 133, 134, 135
Sleep
  personal evaluation of, 18
  physical fitness and, 85–86
Slow wave sleep, 86
Slow-twitch fiber, 85
Smart drinks, 180
Smegma, 335
Smog, 451–452
Smoke detector, 489
Smokeless tobacco, 231–232
Smoker's cough, 228
Smoking
  caffeine and, 230
  cancer and, 227–229, 274, 287
  carbon monoxide and, 225–226
  cardiovascular disease and, 226–227, 262
  cessation of, 234–235, 236
  chronic obstructive pulmonary disease and, 229–230
  dependence on, 219–225

Smoking—cont'd
  health concerns in, 230
  illness and premature death in, 226
  indoor air pollution and, 454–455
  nicotine and, 225–226
  nonsmokers versus smokers, 236
  oral contraceptives and, 231, 384
  passive, 232–234
  personal assessment of, 222–223, 264
  pipe, 218–219
  reproduction and, 230–231
  restrictions on, 233
  rights in, 235
  society and, 216–218
Snuff, 224, 231–232
Sobering up, 198
Social health, 11
Social relationships
  older adult and, 509
  personal evaluation of, 14
  self-esteem and, 30
Social skills, 9–10
Society
  addictive personality and, 168
  cocaine and, 175–177
  drug use and, 181–183
  tobacco use and, 216–218
Sodium, 100
  dietary allowances of, 105, 116
  in fast foods, 110
  hypertension and, 258
  intake of, 120
Soft drinks, 110, 172
Solid waste, 459–460
Soluble fiber, 103–104
Sonogram, 408
Sopor, 177
Sore throat, 260
SOS; see Secular Organizations for Sobriety
Sound, 467
Sour cream, 108
Soybeans, 115
Specificity in physical fitness, 69–70
Sperm, 329, 333, 334
  fertilization and, 397–399
  vasectomy and, 386
Spermicide, 377
  with cervical cap, 381
  with contraceptive diaphragm, 380
  effectiveness of, 374
Sphygmomanometer, 257
Spiritual health, 12
  development of, 36
  personal evaluation of, 14
Sports bra, 79
Squamous cell carcinoma, 281
ST fiber, 85

Stacking, term, 83
Stalking, 484
Staphylococcus aureus, 309
Starches, 92, 93
Starvation response, 135–136
Static stretching, 71
STDs; *see* Sexually transmitted diseases
Stenosis, rheumatic heart disease and, 260
Sterilization, 385–386
Steroids, 83–84
Stillborn birth, 231
Stimulants, 169–172
Stomach
   alcohol and, 201
   stapling of, 147
STP, designer drug, 178
Strep throat, 260, 262
Stress, 42–61
   coping and, 55–56
   disease states and, 49
   general adaptation syndrome and, 48–49
   hypertension and, 257
   inevitability of, 49
   personal assessment of, 52, 264
   stress management techniques and,   56–58
   stressors and, 44–48
      college-centered, 49–54
      life-centered, 54–55
Stress management
   personal evaluation of, 13
   techniques of, 56–58
Stressors, 44–48
   cerebral cortex and, 45
   college-centered, 49–54
      cultural conflicts and, 53
      employment and, 49
      faculty and, 54
      family and, 51–53
      financial, 51
      institutional, 49
      personal expectations as, 51
      religious faith and, 53–54
      time management and, 53
   endocrine system and, 45–47
   energy release and, 47–48
   epinephrine and, 47
   generalized physiological response to,   45, 46
   intensity of, 48
   life-centered, 54–55
   noise, 467
   personal assessment of, 50
   positive or negative, 48–49
   reaction to, 55–56
   response variation to, 44
   sensory modalities and, 45
Stretching, 71
Stroke, 258–260
   dietary guidelines in, 115

Stroke—cont'd
   risk factors for, 262
Student; *see* College student
Students Against Driving Drunk, 203
Subclinical depression, 30
Subscapular skinfold measurement, 134, 135
Subsidence inversion, 454
Sucrose, 92–93
Sudden cardiac death, 226
Sugars, 92–93
   dietary recommendations for, 116
   intake of, 120
Suicide, 31–32
   alcohol and, 202
   assisted, 528
Sulfur, 101
Sulfur dioxide, 452
Sulfur oxide, 451
Sunburn, 282
Sunglasses, 463
Sunlight
   cancer and, 287–288
   seasonal affective disorder and, 31
Sunscreen, 282
Superfund, 461
Superior vena cava, 248, 249
Support group
   for cancer victim, 286
   emotional growth and, 38
Suppressor gene, 271
Suppressor T-cell, 302, 303
Surgeon General, 219
Surgery
   for cancer, 283
   insurance coverage for, 434
   for weight reduction, 147
Surrogate parenting, 410, 411
Surviving: Support group, 286
Susceptible host, 298–299
SW sleep, 86
Sweating, 47
Sweets, 106, 108–109
Symptothermal method of periodic abstinence,
  376–377
Synapse, 169, 170
Synergistic drug effect, 181
Synesthesia, 177
Synthetic narcotics, 181
Syphilis, 318, 319
Syrup of ipecac, 151
Systemic circulation, 225
Systolic pressure, 257

T

T cell
   human immunodeficiency virus and, 311
   immune response and, 302

T cell-mediated immunity, 300
Tacrine, 515
Tampon, 309, 338
Tanning, 270
Target heart rate, 73–76
TB; *see* Tuberculosis
Tea, 172
Teaching hospital, 431
Teeth, 232
Temperament, 27
Temperature inversion, 454
Tennis shoe, 80–81
Tension headache, 54
Teratogenic effects, 457
Terminal illness, 532–533
Test anxiety, 51
Testicle, 332–333
    cancer of, 280
    self-examination of, 280
Testimonials, health consumerism and, 422
Testosterone, 131, 333
Tetanus, 302
Tetrahydrocannabinol, 179
Textured vegetable protein, 115
Thalamus, 166
THC; *see* Tetrahydrocannabinol
Thebaine, 180
Thermal pollution, 458
Thermic effect of food, 141
Thiamin, 99, 105
Thorax, 248
THR; *see* Target heart rate
Three-minute step test, 74
Throat
    steroids and, 84
    tobacco use and, 228
Thrombus
    in myocardial infarction, 251
    in stroke, 259
Thrush, 318–319
TIA; *see* Transient ischemic attack
Time management, 53
Titration, 219
Tobacco use, 214–241
    caffeine and, 230
    cancer and, 227–229, 287
    carbon monoxide and, 225–226
    cardiovascular disease and, 226–227, 262
    cessation of, 234–235, 236
    chronic obstructive pulmonary disease and, 229–230
    dependence on, 219–225
    health concerns in, 230
    illness and premature death in, 226
    indoor air pollution and, 454–455
    involuntary, 232–234
    nicotine and, 225
    nonsmokers *versus* smokers, 236

Tobacco use—cont'd
    oral contraceptives and, 231
    personal assessment of, 15–16, 222–223
    reproduction and, 230–231
    rights in, 235
    smokeless, 231–232
    society and, 216–218
Tocopherol, 98
Tocotrienol, 98
Tolerance to drugs, 164
Total marriage, 359
Touch, sexual behavior and, 350
Toughlove, 182
Toxic shock syndrome, 309
Toxic waste, 460–461
Toxicity
    of alcohol, 196
    of minerals, 100–103
    of vitamins, 97, 98, 99
Toxins
    biological, 109
    in water, 456–457
Toxoplasmosis, 311
Trace elements, 100, 102–103, 454
Training effect, 73
Tranquilizers, 177
Transcendental meditation, 56
Transcender, 35
Transcervical balloon tuboplasty, 410
Transient ischemic attack, 259
Transition in labor, 405
Transportation, older adult and, 516, 517
Transsexualism, 363–364
Transvestism, 364
Treponema pallidum, 318, 319
Trial separation, 360
Triceps skinfold measurement, 134, 135
Trichomonas vaginalis, 319
Tricuspid valve, 248, 249
Triglycerides, 95
Trimester, 402
Triphasic pill, 382–383
Tropical oil, 95
TSS; *see* Toxic shock syndrome
Tubal ligation, 375, 385, 386
Tuberculosis, 305–306
Tuboplasty, transcervical balloon, 410
Tumescence, 347
Tumor, 272
Tumor necrosis factor, 286
Twelve-step program, 210
Twins, 401, 402
Tylenol, 439

U

Unbalanced diet, 117
Undernutrition, 152–153

Underwater weighing, 132
Underweight, defined, 128, 129
Unintentional injuries, 488–491, 492
   firearm safety and, 490
   home accident prevention and, 491, 492
   motor vehicle safety and, 490–491
   personal safety and, 488–489
   residential safety and, 489
Union Carbide, 462
Unipolar depression, 30
Uniqueness, self-esteem and, 30
United Network for Organ Sharing, 536
United States Consumer Product Safety
  Commission Hotline, 422
United States Department of Agriculture
   food guide of, 107
   on meat handling, 113
United States Fish and Wildlife Service, 469
United States Postal Service Fraud Division, 422
Unsaturated fats, 114
Upper body obesity, 131
Urethra, 333, 334
Urethritis
   chlamydia in, 314–315
   sexually transmitted, 319–320
USDA; see United States Department of
  Agriculture
Uterus, 335, 336
   aging of, 506
   cancer of, 276–278
   labor and, 404–405

V

Vacuum aspiration, 389
Vagina, 335, 336
   cancer of, 278–279
   childbirth and, 405
   fertilization and, 397
   infection of, 318–319
   spermicide and, 377
Vaginal contraceptive film, 378
Vaginismus, 352
Valium; see Diazepam
Variant sexual behavior, 364
VariVax, 302
Vas deferens, 333, 334
Vascular system, 247–248
Vasectomy, 334, 375, 385–386
Vasocongestion, 334, 350
Vasodilators, 258
VCF; see Vaginal contraceptive film
Vector, 298
Vegan vegetarian diet, 116–117
Vegetable oil, 94
Vegetables, 105–107
   daily servings of, 106

Vegetables—cont'd
   personal intake assessment of, 118
   water-soluble vitamins in, 98
Vegetarian diet, 114–117
   additional protein-rich sources for, 117
   ovolactovegetarian, 114–115
   vegan, 116–117
Veins, 247–248
Vena cava, 248, 249
Venereal disease; see Sexually transmitted
  diseases
Ventricle, 248, 249
Ventricular fibrillation, 253
Venule, 247–248
Verbal communication, 34
Vernix, 406
Very low-density lipoproteins, 252
Vestibule of labia minora, 335
Violence, 476–496
  alcohol and, 202
  on campus, 494
  intentional injuries and, 478–484
    bias and hate crimes and, 483–484
    domestic violence in, 479–481
    gangs and, 481–483
    guns and, 483
    homicide in, 478–479
    stalking and, 484
  personal assessment of, 493
  sexual victimization and, 484–488
    commercialization of sex in, 488
    rape and sexual assault in, 484–486
    sexual abuse of child in, 486
    sexual harassment in, 486–488
  unintentional injuries and, 488–491, 492
    firearm safety and, 490
    home accident prevention and, 491, 492
    motor vehicle safety and, 490–491
    personal safety and, 488–489
    recreational safety and, 489
    residential safety and, 489
Virulent, term, 297
Virus, 297
  in hantavirus pulmonary syndrome,
   308–309
  herpes simplex, 315–318
  immune response and, 303
  in influenza, 304–305
  in mononucleosis, 306
  in mumps, 307
  in oncogene formation, 271
  in water, 456
Vital marriage, 359
Vital Options: Support group for young
  adults, 286
Vitamin, 97–100
  fats and, 93

Vitamin—cont'd
  vegan vegetarian diet and, 116
Vitamin A, 98
  additional intake of, 120
  recommended dietary allowances of,
    104
Vitamin B$_6$, 99, 105
Vitamin B$_{12}$, 99, 105
Vitamin C, 99
  additional intake of, 120
  recommended dietary allowances of,
    104
Vitamin D, 98
  osteoporosis and, 507
  recommended dietary allowances of,
    104
Vitamin E, 98, 104
Vitamin K, 98, 104
VLDLs; see Very low-density lipoproteins
Voluntary health agency, 424
Voluntary hospital, 431
Vomiting, 200
Voyeurism, 364
Vulva, 334, 335

W

Waist-to-hip ratio, 131
Wake, 535
Walking pneumonia, 306
Warm-up, 77
Waste disposal, 459–460, 464–467
Wasting syndrome, 311
Water
  for fluid replacement, 82
  as nutrient, 100–103
  pollution of, 455–459
    effects on health, 459
    sources of, 456–458
    wetlands and, 458–459
Water soluble vitamins, 97–98, 99, 105
Weight loss industry, 150
Weight management, 126–157
  body energy needs in, 138–141
    activity requirements and, 138–139
    basal metabolism and, 139–141
    dietary thermogenesis and, 141
    life-time weight control and, 141
  body image and, 128, 129, 132–133
  caloric balance in, 137–138
  cancer and, 287
  in diabetes mellitus, 289
  dietary recommendations for, 116
  eating disorders and, 150–152
  healthy body weight and, 130–132
  height-weight tables and, 130
  hypertension and, 258

Weight management—cont'd
  obesity and, 134–137
  personal assessment of, 142, 264
  techniques of, 141–150
    acupuncture in, 147
    appetite suppressants in, 144–145
    behavior modification in, 147–148
    combination approach in, 149–150
    dietary alterations in, 143–144
    hypnosis in, 148
    liposuction in, 147
    nonappetite suppressant pharmaceutical
      agents in, 145–147
    physical activity in, 148–149
    surgical, 147
  undernutrition and, 152–153
  weight loss industry and, 150
Wellness, 4, 5
Wellness center, 431
Western blot, 313
Wet dream, 350
Wetlands, 458–459
Wheezing, 290
Whiskey, 196
WHO; see World Health Organization
Whole-grain flour, 108
Whooping cough, 301
WHR; see Waist-to-hip ratio
Wilderness Society, 469
Willed death, 527
Wine, 196
Withdrawal
  as birth control method, 373, 374–375
  from drugs, 164
Womb, 335, 336
Women
  abuse of, 480
  alcohol and, 197, 211
  cardiovascular disease and, 246–247
  infertility in, 409
  osteoporosis in, 507
  recommended dietary allowances for,
    104–105
  sexual response pattern of, 347
Workout, 77
World Health Organization, 2–3
World population growth, 449

X

X-ray, 402, 463

Y

Year 2000 National Health Objectives, 5
Yeast
  in alcohol fermentation, 194

Credits

Chapter 1

p. 3 (Table 1-1), National Center for Health Statistics: Births, marriages, divorces, and deaths for May, 1993. *Monthly Vital Statistics Report:* 42:5, Hyattsville, Md, Public Health Service, October 21, 1993, pp. 18-19; **p. 3,** Source: Guyton R, et al: College students and national health objectives for the year 2000: a summary report, *Journal of American College Health* July 1989, 38:9-14; **p. 5 (Figure 1-1),** *Healthy People 2000: National Health Promotion and Disease Prevention Objectives,* Department of Health and Human Services, Washington, DC, 1991.

Chapter 2

p. 29, From Study Guide and Personal Explorations for *Psychology applied to modern life: adjustment in the 80s,* by Wayne Weiten. Copyright © 1983 by Wadsworth, Inc. Reprinted by permission of Brooks/Cole Publishing, Pacific Grove, CA 93950; **p. 30 (Figure 2-1),** Depression is a sign of illness, not a sign of weakness, *Ball State University Campus Update* December 12, 1988, p. 1; **p. 32 (Figure 2-2),** From Carbohydrates and Depression, by Richard J Wurtman and Judith J Wurtman. Copyright © January, 1989, by SCIENTIFIC AMERI-

Illustration by Andrew Christie; **p. 32 (Star Box),** From Blumenthal SJ: Suicide: a guide to risk factors: assessment and treatment of suicidal patients. *Medical Clinics of North America* 72:937-971, 1988; **p. 35, (Figure 2-3),** "HIERARCHY OF NEEDS" from MOTIVATION AND PERSONALITY, 3rd ed. by ABRAHAM H. MASLOW. Revised by Robert Frager, James Fadiman, Cynthia McReynolds, and Ruth Cox. Copyright 1954, © 1987 by Harper & Row, Publishers, Inc. Copyright © 1970 by Abraham H. Maslow. Reprinted by permission of Harper Collins Publishers, Inc.

Chapter 3

p. 50, Modified from Holmes TH and Rahe RH: The social adjustment rating scale, *Journal of Psychosomatic Research,* 11:213-218, 1967; **p. 52,** Modified from an inventory developed by Rosellen Bohlen, University of Scranton; **p. 56,** Adapted from Hafen BQ, Thygerson AL, and Frandsen KJ: *Behavioral guidelines for health and wellness,* Denver, 1988, Morton Publishers.

Chapter 4

p. 70, (Health Action Guide), Source: Dr. Steven Blair, Director of Epidemiology

at the Aerobics Institute, Dallas, and author of *Living with exercise,* American Health Publishing Co., 1991; **pp. 71 (Star Box) and 77 (Health Action Guide),** From Prentice WE: *Fitness for college and life,* ed 4, St Louis, 1994, Mosby; **pp. 74-75,** Data from the National Fitness Foundation; **pp. 80-81 (Star Box),** Copyright 1986, *USA Today,* excerpted with permission, art by Donald O'Connor; **p. 84 (Figure 4-2),** Copyright 1987, *USA Today,* excerpted with permission, art by Donald O'Connor.

Chapter 5

p. 94 (Figure 5-1), Adapted from Procter & Gamble, 1989; **p. 95 (Star Box),** Source: Top-10 listing from DEBSICC Snacs Report; fat content from Center for Science in the Public Interest; **pp. 98-103, 106 (Tables 5-1, 5-2, 5-4, 5-5, 5-7),** From Wardlaw G, Insel P, and Seyler M: *Contemporary nutrition: issues and insights,* ed. 2, St. Louis: Mosby, 1994; **p. 100 (Table 5-3),** Source: Council for Responsible Nutrition; **pp. 104-105 (Table 5-6),** Modified from Food and Nutrition Board, National Research Council: *Recommended dietary allowances,* ed 10, Washington, DC, 1989, National Academy of Sciences; **p. 107 (Figure 5-**

2), US Department of Agriculture/US Department of Health and Human Services, August, 1992; **p. 108 (Table 5-8),** Data from USDA Handbook #8; **p. 110 (Star Box),** Modified from Hegarty V: *Decisions in nutrition,* St Louis, 1988, Mosby-Year Book; **p. 112, (Figure 5-3),** Source: Food and Drug Administration, and Wardlaw G, Insel P, and Seyler M: *Contemporary nutrition: issues and insights,* ed. 2, St. Louis: Mosby, 1994; **p. 113 (Health Action Guide),** Source: USDA; **pp. 115 (Table 5-9) and 116 (Health Action Guide),** US Department of Health and Human Services, Public Health Service: *The Surgeon General's report on nutrition and health,* Washington, DC, 1988, US Government Printing Office; **p. 118,** data on four food groups from Guthrie H: *Introductory nutrition,* ed 7, St. Louis, 1989, Mosby-Year Book; **p. 120 (Health Action Guide),** © 1986, American Diabetic Association, Inc., and The American Dietetic Association. HEALTH FOOD CHOICES, Used with permission. Art by Donald O'Connor.

Chapter 6
p. 129 (Table 6-1), From Wardlaw G, Insel P, and Seyler M: *Contemporary nutrition: issues and insights,* ed. 2, St. Louis: Mosby, 1994; **p. 130 (Table 6-2),** Reprinted with permission of the Metropolitan Life Insurance Company; **p. 131 (Table 6-3),** US Department of Agriculture, **p. 132, (Figure 6-1),** Adapted from Guthrie H: *Introductory nutrition,* ed 7, St Louis, 1989, Mosby-Year Book, pp. 205-206; **p. 133 (Figure 6-2),** Modified from George A. Bray; **p. 135 (Figure 6-4),** From Prentice WE: *Fitness for college and life,* ed 4, St Louis, 1994, Mosby; **p. 140 (Table 6-5),** Based on data from Bannister EW and Brown SR: The relative energy requirements of physical activity. In HB Falls, editor: *Exercise physiology,* New York, 1968, Academic Press Inc; Howley ET and Glover ME: The caloric costs of running and walking one mile for men and women, *Medicine and Science in Sports* 6:235, 1974; and Passmore R and Durnin JVGA: Human energy expenditure, *Physiological Reviews* 35:801, 1955; **p. 142,** Modified from Foreyt J, and Goodrick GK: Living without dieting, Houston: Harrison Publishing; **pp. 144-145 (Table 6-6),** Adapted from Guthrie H: *Introductory nutrition,* ed 7, St Louis, 1989, Mosby-Year Book, pp. 226-227; **p. 146 (Health Action Guide),** © 1987,

USA Today, excerpted with permission, art by Donald O'Connor; **p. 147 (Figure 6-7),** From Hegarty V: *Decisions in nutrition,* St Louis, 1988, Mosby-Year Book.

Chapter 7
p. 162 (Figure 7-1), Source: Johnston LD, O'Malley PM, Bachman JG: National survey results on drug use from the Monitoring the Future Study, 1975-1992, Vol II: College students and young adults, National Institute on Drug Abuse, NIH Pub No 93-3598, 1993, p. 157; **p. 163 (Star Box),** Source: Intragency Drug Alcohol Council: Why people use drugs, Ft. Wayne, IN, The Council; **p. 168 (Star Box),** Source: Caryn Oftedahl of Hazelden Services, Inc., Center City, Minnesota; **pp. 170-171, (Table 7-1),** Modified from the Muncie Star © 1987. Reprinted with permission; **p. 172 (Table 7-2),** Caffeine data obtained from Consumers Union, Food and Drug Administration, National Coffee Association, National Soft Drink Association, and Physicians' Desk Reference for Non-Prescription Drugs. Reprinted from *Caffeine and endurance performance* by permission of the Gatorade Sports Science Institute, Chicago, IL; **p. 174 (Star Box),** Sources: Congressional Research Service, State Department, Drug Enforcement Administration; **p. 175 (Star Box),** Source: US Department of Health and Human Services: 1992 estimates of drug-related emergency room episodes; advance report number 4, Substance Abuse and Mental Health Services Administration, September 1993.

Chapter 8
p. 191 (Figure 8-1), From US Bureau of the Census: *Statistical abstracts of the United States, 1993,* ed 113, Washington, DC, 1993, US Government Printing Office; **p. 192 (Table 8-1),** US Department of Health and Human Services: Alcohol and health: fourth special report to the US Congress, Washington DC 1981 DHHS Pub No ADM 81-1080; **p. 193 (Figures 8-2 and 8-3),** Source: Presley, CA, Meilman, PW: *Alcohol and drugs on American college campuses: a report to college presidents,* June 1992, US Department of Education, Drug Prevention in Higher Education Program, (FIPSE Grant), Southern Illinois University Student Health Program Wellness Center; **p. 194 (Figure 8-4),** Reproduced from Kinney J

and Leaton G: *Loosening the grip: a handbook of alcohol information,* ed. 5, St. Louis, 1995, Mosby, artwork by Stuart Copans, MD, Dartmouth Medical School; **p. 196 (Table 8-2),** US Department of Transportation, National Highway Safety Administration: Adapted from Alcohol and the impaired driver, (AMA); **p. 204 (Health Action Guide),** Modified from brochure of the Indiana Alcohol Countermeasure Program; **p. 207 (Star Box),** Modified from Woititz JG: *Adult children of alcoholics,* Pompano Beach, Florida, 1983, Health Communications, Inc. In Pinger R, Payne W, Hahn D, Hahn E: *Drugs: issues for today,* St Louis, 1995, Mosby; **p. 210 (Star Box),** The Twelve Steps are reprinted with permission of Alcoholics Anonymous World Services, Inc. Permission to reprint this material does not mean that AA has reviewed or approved the contents of this publication, nor that AA agrees with the views expressed herein. AA is a program of recovery from alcoholism only. Use of the Twelve Steps in connection with programs and activities which are patterned after AA, but which address other problems, does not imply otherwise.

Chapter 9
pp. 220 (Star Box) and 235 (Health Action Guide), Reproduced with permission of the American Cancer Society; **p. 221 (Figure 9-1),** Centers for Disease Control and Prevention; **pp. 221 (Star Box) and 233 (Star Box),** From Pinger R, Payne W, Hahn D, Hahn E: *Drugs; issues for today,* St. Louis, 1995, Mosby.

Chapter 10
pp. 247 (Figure 10-1) and 250 (Table 10-1), Source: 1993 Heart and Stroke Facts, American Heart Association; **p. 253 (Table 10-2),** Report of the Expert Panel on Detection, Evaluation, and Treatment of High Blood Cholesterol in Adults, US Department of Health and Human Services (PHS: NIH Pub No 89-2925), 1989, Washington, DC, US Government Printing Office; **p. 254 (Star Box),** Reproduced with permission, © 1988, American Heart Association: Heart Facts; **p. 255 (Figure 10-4),** 1990 Heart Facts, art by Donald O'Connor; **p. 256 (Figure 10-5),** Source: Registry for the International Society for Heart Transplantation; **pp. 260 (Star Box), and**

263 (bottom Star Box), Source: American Heart Association; pp. 264-265, From Howard E: *Health risks,* Tucson, 1986, Body Press.

Chapter 11

p. 273 (Figure 11-1), National Cancer Institute: *Horizons of cancer research,* NIH Pub No 89-3011, © 1989; pp. 274 (Figure 11-2), 276-277 (Star Box), 278 (Health Action Guide), 280 (Health Action Guide), 283 (Star Box), and 287 (Health Action Guide), Reprinted with permission of the American Cancer Society, Inc.; p. 274 (bottom), Source: National Cancer Institute; pp. 284-285, Modified from American Cancer Society, Inc.

Chapter 12

p. 302, Sources, Centers for Disease Control and Prevention and American Academy of Pediatrics;
p. 303 (Figure 12-3), Artwork by Allen Carroll and Dale Glasgow, © National Geographic Society; p. 316, Centers for Disease Control and Prevention, Atlanta.

Chapter 14

p. 355, Modified from *USA Today;*
p. 360, (Health Action Guide), Adapted from Haas K and Haas A: *Understanding sexuality,* ed 3, St Louis, 1993, Mosby; p. 361, Quiz from *The joy of being single,* by Janice Harayda, copyright © 1986 by Janice Harayda, used by permission of Doubleday, a division of Bantam Doubleday, Dell Publishing Group, Inc.

Chapter 15

p. 372, Modified from Hatcher RA, et al: *Contraceptive technology: 1986-1987,* ed 13, New York, 1986, Irvington Publishers, Inc.: pp. 374-375 (Table 15-1), Source: Hatcher RA, et al: *Contraceptive technology:* ed 16, New York, 1994, Irvington Publishers; p. 388, From Haas K and Haas A: *Understanding sexuality,* ed 3, St. Louis, 1993, Mosby.

Chapter 16

p. 407 (Health Action Guide), Source: Prentice WE: *Fitness for college and life,* ed. 4, St. Louis, 1994, Mosby.

Chapter 17

p. 423 (Figure 17-1), From Marion Laboratories, Inc., Pharmaceutical Division, Kansas City, Mo; p. 426 (Health Action Guide), Source: Pell AR: *Making the most of Medicare,* DCI Publishing, 1990, in *in-sync,* Erie, Pa, Spring, 1994, Erie Insurance Group; p. 428 (Star Box), Modified from *Keeping your dental health: an adult thing to do,* American Dental Association (1987); p. 430 (Health Action Guide), Modified from Farley D: Do-it-yourself medical testing, *FDA Consumer,* 20:22-28, February, 1986; p. 432 (Table 17-1), Source: American Hospital Association; p. 433 (Figure 17-3), Source: SAMHSA News, Vol I, #4, p. 3; p. 442 (Star Box), From Subak-Sharpe GJ, editor: *The physician's manual for patients,* by the Biomedical Information Corporation, © 1984, reprinted by permission of Random House, Inc.

Chapter 18

p. 449 (Figure 18-1), Source: U.N. Population Fund; pp. 450 and 451 (Figure 18-2 and Table 18-1), World Resources, 1988-1989; p. 452 (Figure 18-3), Source: Environment Canada; p. 453 (Figure 18-4), © 1987 Time Inc, all rights reserved, reprinted by permission from TIME; p. 455 (Table 18-2), Source: Water Pollution Control Federation; p. 460 (Figure 18-5), and p. 466 (Figure 18-7), Source: Environmental Protection Agency; p. 465, Modified from LIVING IN THE ENVIRONMENT: AN INTRODUCTION TO ENVIRONMENTAL SCIENCE, fourth edition, by G. Tyler Miller, Jr. © 1985 by Wadsworth, Inc., reprinted by permission of the publisher; p. 466 (Figure 18-6), Adapted by permission of Practical Home-owner magazine, formerly New Shelter, © Rodale Press, Inc., all rights reserved; p. 468 (Star Box), Modified from American Academy of Otolaryngology, *Head and neck surgery: noise, ears, and hearing,* 1985, Washington, DC: p. 469, logos courtesy of The Wilderness Society, USDA, Forest Service, and Sierra Club; Greenpeace logo courtesy of Greenpeace USA, a nonprofit, environmental organization, 1436 U Street, NW, Washington, DC 20009; Cousteau Society logo used with permission of the Cousteau Society, © 1990, a non-profit, membership-supported organization, dedicated to the protection and improvement of the quality of life for present and future generations; pp. 470-471, Modified from *Being green: some tips on how to help the earth,* Scripps Howard News Service.

Chapter 19

p. 481 (Figure 19-1), Courtesy of the National Committee to Prevent Child Abuse, Chicago, Ill; p. 487 (bottom Health Action Guide), From the American College Health Association.

Chapter 20

p. 508 (Figure 20-1), Source: USA Today research, Dr. David Fisher, Orthopedics Indianapolis; p. 511 From the Facts on Aging Quiz, by Erdman Palmore © 1988, Springer Publishing Company, New York, used by permission; p. 513 (Star Box), Source: Marriott Seniors' Attitudes Survey of Adults 65 and over; p. 517 (Figure 20-2), Source: *The Detroit News* and USA Today.

Chapter 21

p.529 (Star Box), Reprinted by permission of Choice In Dying, formerly Concern for Dying/Society for the Right to Die, 200 Varick Street, New York, NY 10014, (212) 366-5540; p. 537 (Figure 21-1), The National Kidney Foundation Uniform Donor Card is reprinted with permission from the National Kidney Foundation, Inc. Copyright 1970, 1991, New York, NY; p. 538, Courtesy Bowman, Meeks Mortuary, Muncie, IN.

Appendix 1 From Cornacchia H and Barrett S: *Consumer health: a guide to intelligent decisions,* St Louis, 1993, Mosby-Year Book.
Appendix 2 Source: Bever DL: *Safety: a personal focus,* ed 3, St Louis, 1992, Mosby-Year Book.
Appendix 4 Source: Rathus SA: *Psychology,* New York, 1987, Holt, Rinehart, & Winston.

PHOTO CREDITS

Chapter 1

pp. 1,2, Courtesy Hanover College, Hanover, IN; pp. 6, 11 (right), CLG Photographics; pp. 7, 10, 11 (left), 12, Ed Self/Photographic Services, Ball State University.

Chapter 2

pp. 25, 27, 39, Courtesy Hanover College, Hanover, IN; pp. 26, 37, CLG Photographics.

Chapter 3

pp. 43, 44, CLG Photographics; pp. 48, 51, 55, Ed Self/Photographic Services,

Ball State University; **p. 58,** Courtesy Hanover College, Hanover, IN.

Chapter 4
p. 65, Courtesy Hanover College, Hanover, IN; **p. 66,** CLG Photographics; **p. 68,** Krebs/Zefa, H. Armstrong Roberts, Inc.; **pp. 69, 72, 76, 78, 83, 86,** Ed Self/ Photographic Services, Ball State University; **p. 71,** Bill Horsman, Stock, Boston; **pp. 74, 75,** Linsley Photographics.

Chapter 5
p. 91, CLG Photographics; **pp. 95, 115,** Ed Self/Photographic Services, Ball State University; **p. 96,** Nutrasweet, Monsanto Corp.; **p. 122,** © Neil Rabinowitz 1992.

Chapter 6
p. 127, Ed Self/Photographic Services, Ball State University; **pp. 130, 148,** CLG Photographics; **p. 134,** Linsley Photographics; **p. 139,** Bob Daemmrich, Stock, Boston; **p. 146,** Kathy Sedovic; **p. 149,** Courtesy Hanover College, Hanover, IN.

Chapter 7
p. 161, CLG Photographics; **p. 179,** S. Ekstrand, H. Armstrong Roberts; **p. 180,** From Drug Enforcement Administration: Drugs of abuse, US Department of Justice; **p. 183,** Charles Gupton, The Stock Market.

Chapter 8
p. 189, Kristin Hardgrove/CLG Photographics; **p. 190,** CLG Photographics; **p. 191,** V. Keith McManus, Archive Pictures, Inc.; **p. 194,** From G. Heileman Brewing Company, Inc., LaCrosse, Wisconsin; **p. 201 (Figure 8-6),** From Streissguth, A: Teratogenic effects of alcohol in humans and laboratory animals, *Science,* 209:353, July 18, 1980, © 1980 by the

AAAS; **p. 205,** U.S. Department of Transportation; **p. 209,** Bob Daemmrich, Stock, Boston.

Chapter 9
p. 215, Ed Self/Photographic Services, Ball State University; **pp. 216, 219, 224, 231, 233, 234,** CLG Photographics; **p. 229,** Courtesy, American Cancer Society; **p. 237,** Wolff Communications.

Chapter 10
pp. 245, 255, 257, Ed Self/Photographic Services, Ball State University; **p. 246,** CLG Photographics.

Chapter 11
p. 269, Ed Self/Photographic Services, Ball State University; **pp. 270, 272,** CLG Photographics; **pp. 275, 288,** Courtesy, American Cancer Society; **pp. 281, 282,** Courtesy, American Academy of Dermatology.

Chapter 12
p. 295, CLG Photographics; **pp. 299, 301,** Ed Self/Photographic Services, Ball State University; **p. 304,** Ellis Herwig, Taurus Photos; **p. 311,** Courtesy, Beth and William Keyt; **pp. 313, 317, 318,** Centers for Disease Control and Prevention, Atlanta.

Chapter 13
pp. 327, 341, CLG Photographics; **p. 330,** Ed Self/Photographic Services, Ball State University; **p. 332,** AP/Wide World Photos.

Chapter 14
pp. 345, 346, 353, 356, 359, CLG Photographics; **p. 351,** Ed Self/Photographic Services, Ball State University; **p. 365,** Courtesy, Loren and Kevin Wilson.

Chapter 15
p. 369, CLG Photographics; **pp. 371, 378 (right),** Linsley Photographics; **pp. 377,**

383, Courtesy, Ortho Pharmaceutical Corp.; **p. 378 (left),** Courtesy, Apothecus, Inc.; **pp. 379, 381, 382 (top & bottom),** Laura J. Edwards; **p. 382 (middle),** Courtesy, Alza Corporation; **p. 384,** Courtesy, Wyeth-Ayerst Laboratories; **p. 387 (top),** A. Tannenbaum, SYGMA; **p. 387 (bottom),** J.L. Atlan, SYGMA.

Chapter 16
p. 395, Courtesy, the Schwent Family; **pp. 396, 407, 411,** CLG Photographics; **p. 397,** Francis Long, Photo Researchers, Inc.; **p. 401,** Petit Format/Science Source, Photo Researchers; **p. 408,** Washington University School of Medicine; **p. 409,** Bill Longacre, Photo Researchers, Inc.

Chapter 17
pp. 419, 420, 421, 425, 426, 428, 437, CLG Photographics; **p. 441,** The Image Works.

Chapter 18
pp. 447, 448, 451, 454, 458, 459, 472, CLG Photographics; **p. 461,** Ed Self/Photographic Services, Ball State University; **p. 464,** © Looney/ Greenpeace.

Chapter 19
pp. 477, 480, 485, 491, CLG Photographics; **p. 490,** © Neil Rabinowitz 1992.

Chapter 20
pp. 501, 502, 503, 504, 505, 509, 512, 516, 518, CLG Photographics.

Chapter 21
p. 525, David W. Hamilton, The Image Bank; **p. 528,** *Detroit News,* Gamma-Liason; **pp. 532, 535,** CLG Photographics.